Promoting Continence

A Clinical and Research Resource

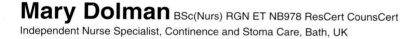

Edited by

Kathryn Getliffe BSc(Hons) MSc PhD RGN DN PGCEA
Professor of Nursing, School of Nursing & Midwifery, University of Southampton, Southampton, UK

Mary Dolman BSc(Nurs) RGN ET NB978 ResCert CounsCert
Independent Nurse Specialist, Continence and Stoma Care, Bath, UK

Foreword by

Sue Thomas BA(Hons) RGN RM DN CPT
Nursing Policy and Practice Adviser, Royal College of Nursing, London, UK

SECOND EDITION

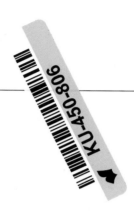

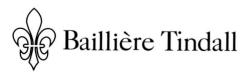

Baillière Tindall

BAILLIÈRE TINDALL
An imprint of Elsevier Science Limited

First Edition 1997
Second Edition 2003
Reprinted 2003

ISBN 0 7020 2637 9

British Library Cataloguing in Publication Data
A catalogue record for this book is available from the British Library

Library of Congress Cataloging in Publication Data
A catalog record for this book is available from the Library of Congress

Note
Medical knowledge is constantly changing. As new information
becomes available, changes in treatment, procedures, equipment and
the use of drugs become necessary. The editors, contributors and
publishers have taken care to ensure that the information given in this
text is accurate and up to date. However, readers are strongly advised
to confirm that the information, especially with regard to drug usage,
complies with the latest legislation and standards of practice.

 your source for books,
journals and multimedia
in the health sciences

www.elsevierhealth.com

The
publisher's
policy is to use
**paper manufactured
from sustainable forests**

Printed in China

Contents

Contributors

Michael Craggs BSc(Hons) PhD CBiol MIBiol MIPEM
Professor in Applied Neurophysiology,
University College London, London, UK;
Director, Spinal Research Centre, Royal
National Orthopaedic Hospital NHS Trust,
Stanmore, Middlesex, UK; Honorary Consultant
Clinical Scientist, University College London
Hospitals NHS Trust, London, UK; Director of
Clinical Research, Institute of Urology and
Nephrology, University College London,
London, UK

Mary Dolman BSc(Nurs) RGN ET NB978 ResCert CounsCert
Independent Nurse Specialist, Continence and
Stoma Care, Bath, UK

Claire Edwards RGN NDN FETC
Clinical Nurse Specialist/Continence, South
Buckinghamshire NHS Trust, Marlow
Community Health Clinic, Glade Road, Marlow,
Buckinghamshire, UK

Mandy Fader BSc (Hons) PhD RN
Lecturer/Research Fellow, Continence Group,
Department of Medicine, University College
London, London, UK; Nursing Director,
Continence Product Evaluation Network,
University College London, London, UK

Kathryn Getliffe BSc(Hons) MSc PhD RGN DN PGCEA
Professor of Nursing, School of Nursing &
Midwifery, University of Southampton,
Southampton, UK

Tracey Heath BSc(Hons) MSc RGN
Lecturer in Nursing/Senior Nurse Evidence
Based Practice, School of Nursing, Social Work
and Applied Health Studies, The University
of Hull, Hull, UK

Nicky Horton RGN
Biofeedback Nurse Specialist, Physiology Unit,
St Mark's Hospital, Harrow, UK

Diane Lukeman MA Dip Psych C Psychol
Head of Child Clinical Psychology Services,
Thelma Golding Centre, Hounslow,
Middlesex, UK

Linda Smith MA MSc
Consultant Clinical Psychologist, Northgate and
Prudhoe NHS Trust, Sanderson Centre,
Newcastle upon Tyne, UK

Mel Smith BPharm MRPharms ACPP MI PharmM
Global Professional Relations Manager, Reckitt
Benckiser Healthcare, Hull, UK

Paul Smith MA MSc PhD
Consultant Clinical Psychologist, County
Durham and Darlington Priority Services NHS
Trust, Earls House Hospital, Durham, and
University of Newcastle upon Tyne, UK

Roger Watson BSc PhD RGN CBiol MIBiol
Professor of Nursing, School of Nursing,
Social Work and Applied Health Studies,
The University of Hull, Hull, UK

Helen White RGN RHV
Formerly Director Promocon, Promocon,
Redbank House, Manchester, UK

Lesley Wilson BSc(Hons) RGN CertEd FETC
Continence Services Manager, Continence
Advisory Service, Hythe Medical Centre, Hythe,
Southampton, UK

Foreword

It is estimated that worldwide more than 200 million people of all ages are incontinent; around 4 million of these people reside in the UK. Although there have been several national reports drawing attention to inequitable continence services in the NHS, in comparison to many diseases there had been little 'real action' in commissioning services until recently. For individuals with the problem, services have fallen short of what might be expected for modern continence management. One of the main reasons for this was, without doubt, the fact that continence care was not seen as a priority and there has been a lack of investment in good continence services.

Perhaps nothing has been more significant in raising awareness and improving services nationally than the Continence Campaign of the late 1990s which resulted in publication of the Department of Health guidance *Good Practice in Continence Services* (DoH 2000). This policy now sets out a vision for integrated continence services and presents a golden opportunity to move continence care forward into a fertile service model for the future.

Good Practice in Continence Services is the starting point for continence service commissioning in this third millennium, but the key to effective management of individuals is undoubtedly the individual client assessment and direction to appropriate management. This new edition of *Promoting Continence: A Clinical and Research Resource* could not have come at a better time as the Government increases its emphasis on continence, with further policy giving this once taboo subject a much more prominent role.

Good Practice in Continence Services states that continence services should extend to faecal as well as urinary incontinence, to children as well as adults, and to people living at home, in hospital or in long-term care. It states that services should also cover prevention as well as treatment and management of incontinence, with the heaviest responsibility for delivering appropriate continence services placed on primary care teams.

With great clarity this text, accompanied by very useful illustrations, diagrams and charts, will give readers helpful evidence-based guidance to help meet the current Government's aims for continence management. The research studies, case studies and key points for practice are an additional resource giving both novice and skilled practitioners sound information for action and reflection. Particularly welcome in this revised publication is the inclusion of Chapter 6 (Focus on older people), not because incontinence is an inevitability of older age but because older people are one of the priority groups targeted by the continence guidance. A greater national awareness of the continence needs in this client group is being achieved through the inclusion of targets for the delivery of integrated continence services in the National Service Framework for Older People (DoH 2000) and the focus of the National Institute of Clinical Excellence to develop audit tools for urinary and faecal continence care in older people (NICE 2002). This policy will generate greater interest towards continence in older people and up-to-date publications like *Promoting Continence: A Clinical and Research Resource* will be in great demand. Chapter 11 (Continence problems in neurological disability) will prove to be a further asset and resource for the proposed National Service Framework for neurology and chronic disease expected in 2004, where continence as a major quality of life issue will, without doubt, be addressed.

This book and its evidence-based approach will be of interest and worth to practitioners who are already involved or wish to be involved with continence care. It will also be a valuable addition to nursing and medical libraries.

Current policy is presenting real opportunities for improving continence management, and coupled with clinical governance, this focus must truly mean that at last continence care is moving out of the shadows. Continence promotion, early recognition assessment and management of incontinence will be a central theme for all patient care in the future. It will be ably assisted by valuable resources like *Promoting Continence: A Clinical and Research Resource*; I thus commend this book with much pleasure.

Sue Thomas

Preface

This book aims to provide practical and theoretical knowledge about incontinence to practitioners caring for all age groups in community and hospital environments. Incontinence is not only a distressing physical problem which can have a major psychological and social impact on the lives of those who live with it, but it also places huge demands on health service resources. However, incontinence is no longer the taboo subject it has been for generations. Not only is the extensive prevalence of the problem being revealed, but research-based knowledge is increasingly being applied to the understanding and management of the condition. For many people incontinence can be cured, and even where this is not possible it can almost always be improved.

Early recognition of the problem and its underlying cause, together with planning and provision of appropriate treatment, are fundamental to promoting continence. Equally important is the need for professional knowledge to be linked with an understanding of the impact of incontinence on the individual's life, and for decisions on care to be made together wherever possible.

This book addresses the practicalities of both promoting continence and/or managing incontinence, by providing information that is underpinned by clearly presented research evidence. It aims to be of direct use to practitioners by providing clinical guidance and highlighting useful practical points, together with examples of appropriate charts and information handouts for use in practice.

Summaries of some key research studies are printed in boxes to allow the reader to either stop and read them or skip over them and continue with the main text, as appropriate. An additional feature is the inclusion of case studies to illustrate problems frequently encountered by practitioners. These may provide added insight into care planning, or may be useful as a focus for teaching sessions. To assist with easy identification of case studies, research studies and summaries of key points, these are presented in tinted boxes throughout the book.

Chapter 1 (Incontinence in perspective) begins with a comprehensive overview of incontinence from a range of perspectives, including attitudes, prevalence, impact and service development. In this new edition, there is increased emphasis on governmental policy initiatives that have taken place in recent years. Continence is gaining a more prominent role in policy agendas at national and local levels as the costs in personal and economic terms are recognized. Clinical governance demands that care is based on the best evidence available and structures are in place to monitor quality of provision. Quality of life issues are increasingly acknowledged as important outcome measures in evaluations of treatments and management strategies and are examined in more detail in this edition.

In *Chapter 2* (Normal and abnormal bladder function) a consideration of the anatomy of the lower urinary tract and of normal and abnormal physiological control of micturition provides a basis for the assessment of incontinence.

The subject of promotion of continence and management of incontinence in adults has been divided into two chapters, entitled 'Mostly female' (*Chapter 3*) and 'Mostly male' (*Chapter 4*). Whilst it is recognized that many causes of incontinence and approaches to treatment are common to both males and females, some conditions are far more common in one sex than the other. For example, genuine stress incontinence is considerably more common in females than in males, but urinary retention is more frequently experienced by males. This strategy allows in-depth discussion of theory and research underpinning practice, particularly where anatomical differences are important or where other sexual differences such as childbirth or enlargement of the prostate gland exert an influence. Issues or problems that could overlap into both chapters, such as problems of urge incontinence, are discussed principally in *Chapter 3* since the overall prevalence of incontinence is relatively higher in females than in males. In *Chapter 5* (Mainly children: childhood enuresis and encopresis) problems of enuresis and encopresis, which occur most commonly in childhood, are addressed.

Throughout the book the term 'incontinence' refers to urinary incontinence unless otherwise stated, but extensive consideration of faecal problems takes place in *Chapters 5* and *7*, and the topic is also discussed in other places. A new inclusion in this edition is *Chapter 6* – 'Focus on older people'. This chapter has been written in recognition of the increasing prevalence of incontinence with advancing age and the need to provide a source of information which is easily accessed by nurses and other health and social carers who work with this client group. Although many of the causes and treatments of incontinence are similar to those in younger people, there are some additional factors which can increase the risks of incontinence for some older individuals. However, the most important message is that incontinence is not an inevitable part of growing older and that age alone should not prevent people receiving appropriate assessment and treatment.

In the second half of the book *Chapter 7* (Down, down and away) examines the causes and treatment of faecal incontinence. The appropriateness and cost-effectiveness of laxative use has been questioned in recent years and has been the focus of several government-funded studies. Biofeedback techniques, frequently used for urinary incontinence, have now been extended to faecal incontinence and are also discussed in this chapter. *Chapter 8* (Medication and continence), which provides information on pharmaceutical resources, has been updated to include consideration of changes in nurse prescribing, and has also changed its title from the first edition. This chapter includes not only medications that may be used as part of planned care to treat either urinary or faecal incontinence, but also medications that can contribute to these problems.

In *Chapter 9* (Catheters and catheterization) the use of catheters and management of catheter-associated problems are addressed in some detail, including suprapubic and clean intermittent self-catheterization as well as urethral catheterization. This chapter includes information on careful selection of equipment and on patient monitoring, together with practical advice in the form of a 'troubleshooting' guide. However, non-invasive approaches to dealing with incontinence are preferable to techniques of catheterization or surgery in most cases, and *Chapter 10* (Continence training in intellectual disability) – written by new contributors – provides an account of the principles of behavioural modification.

Since the causes of incontinence are common to many different underlying medical conditions, the book is not structured on specific disease states. However, problems of incontinence are extremely common in certain conditions involving neurological impairment such as multiple sclerosis (MS), stroke and spinal injury. With this in mind, and the fact that many of these patients will be living at home in the community where expert advice may be less readily available, *Chapter 11* (Continence problems and neurological disability) is devoted to the promotion of continence in this client group.

Two interrelated themes run throughout the book: the importance of evidence-based assessment and treatment interventions, and the importance of clinical governance strategies to evaluate the accessibility and quality of care provided. As a result there is no longer a specific chapter dedicated to the auditing of services. The final section of the book – *Chapter 12* (Resource information) – provides contact numbers, websites and addresses for a range of useful sources of information, suppliers and support groups related to continence issues. Since such information is constantly changing and being added to, the purpose of this section is to act as a guide or starting point rather than to be fully comprehensive.

This book is written for all health professionals and other carers with an interest in continence. It is hoped that it will be of value to clinical specialists, community and hospital-based nurses and those working in nursing homes. It may also be a resource for students at all levels undertaking general or specialist courses. In addition, it may be useful to other members of the multidisciplinary team, including general practitioners, physiotherapists and occupational therapists, health promotion departments and social services.

Whatever your role or interest in incontinence, we hope this book contributes to your knowledge, enhances your practice and stimulates you to discover more.

Southampton and Bath 2002   Kathy Getliffe
                                  Mary Dolman

CHAPTER CONTENTS

1

Incontinence in perspective

Helen White
Kathryn Getliffe

'Few things are impossible to diligence and skill… Great works are performed not by strength but by perseverance.'

Samuel Johnson (1709–1784)

INTRODUCTION

Continence care enters the third millennium as a key issue for policy makers, purchasers and providers of health care. Worldwide there are over 200 million people who have significant incontinence and many more with mild bladder problems (Abrams et al 2002). In the UK there are between 2.5 and 4 million people with incontinence (Royal College of Physicians 1995) and in the average primary care organization (population of around 102 700) there are likely to be around 5600 people with urinary incontinence and 900 with faecal incontinence. The associated costs to primary care organizations are in the order of £750 000 per year. This is indicative of a total expenditure for the UK of more than £420 million (approximately 1/120th of the total cost of the NHS) as at the year 2000. NHS purchases of absorbent products alone is in the order of £80 million a year (Euromonitor 1997, 1999). Clearly the costs of incontinence are high both to individuals and health services. 'The lesson of this high cost is not that large savings can be made but that it is essential to derive the maximum return in better health on the investment' (Continence Foundation 2000a).

In recognition of the extent of need and increasing costs to the NHS, and as a result of an extensive lobbying campaign, the Department of

1

Health published its guidance on *Good Practice in Continence Services* in 2000 (DoH 2000a) (subsequently referred to as the Guidance). The Guidance (discussed further below) sets out a model of good practice to help achieve more responsive, equitable and effective continence services. The emphasis is on primary care to be the first contact point for people with incontinence and a number of targets are suggested, together with effective interventions which can be implemented at minimum cost but maximum gain for primary care. The Guidance also calls for proactive identification of people with continence problems and stresses the need to help carers understand incontinence and possible treatments. Continence problems can often be the final straw that influences whether a patient can be managed at home or is admitted to institutional care (Thom 1997). Promoting independence is a fundamental theme throughout this book and is a national priority for the government as well as for individuals and for health and social care services.

The aim of this book is to give providers and purchasers of health and social care a deeper understanding of the promotion of continence and to enable them to be comfortable and confident with a subject that is not easy to talk about. Throughout the book the term 'incontinence' will refer to urinary incontinence unless otherwise stated, but Chapter 7 addresses faecal incontinence, and some consideration of this problem also occurs in other chapters. The current chapter examines the raising of public awareness of continence issues and addresses continence from historical, epidemiological and service policy perspectives as well as recognizing the psychological and social impact on those living with incontinence.

Urinary incontinence is a common condition, affecting people of all ages from all social and cultural backgrounds. It is a *symptom* with many causes. Whilst the physical effects may not be clinically life threatening, the symptoms can have a devastating effect on the quality of life of these people, their families and friends. Feelings of anger, guilt and frustration are frequently expressed both by those with the problem and by their carers. Embarrassment and ignorance about the subject prevent many people seeking help. It is these social consequences that make incontinence the concern of every health and social care worker. With the correct diagnosis and appropriate treatment, it is a condition that can often be cured and mostly improved, often by simple non-invasive methods. For health and social care staff, the promotion of continence can be one of the most challenging and rewarding aspects of their work.

The recent shift in government policy from institutional to community care and the emphasis on self-care has seen more and more people coming forward for incontinence help. People with congenital and acquired disabilities surviving into old age, together with the very large numbers of elderly people in the population, have the greatest need for these resources. This unprecedented demand has placed incontinence higher on the political and public agenda and tackling incontinence is acknowledged to contribute to a range of Department of Health priorities, including: 'promoting independence'; 'reducing accidents'; National Service Frameworks (NSF) (e.g. NSF for stroke and NSF for older people); the 'expert patients programme' and more.

The emphasis of care is moving from containment (Audit Commission 1999) to promotion of continence through conservative or more complex treatments to reduce the prevalence of treatable incontinence and improve the quality of life in those with intractable incontinence. Collaboration and commitment by policy makers and professionals are essential and the Guidance argues for investment in integrated continence services to bring together professionals from many different disciplines. The evidence base for effective care is growing, with recent increases in the number of well-designed, multicentred studies to validate assessment and treatment standards and procedures. However, there is no room for complacency and much more remains to be done.

HISTORICAL PERSPECTIVES

The importance attached to bladder and bowel control is as old as the human race. Latrine-like receptacles thought to date back 10 000 years have been excavated in the Orkney Isles. The Romans at Pompeii had sophisticated flush toilet facilities and the flush toilet we know today was invented by Sir James Harrington in 1596 (Smith & Smith 1987).

Incontinence is one of the oldest medically recorded complaints in the history of mankind (Smith 1979). The first known cure for incontinence was recorded in 1550 BC. The Papyrus Ebers states that a 'mixture of juniper berries, cyprus and beer' is a remedy for incontinence of urine. Throughout the world various methods for treating people to control this basic bodily function have been recommended. Many of these took the form of beverages made from a variety of infusions – such as shaving down the testicles of the hare into a fragrant wine; infusing the flowers of the white chrysanthemum; adding tepid water to the powdered burnt crop of the cock; and drinking a mixture of catmint and myrrh as an aperitif before supper. One remedy used in the Middle Ages included tying a frog around the waist, but the success of this treatment is not recorded!

The 19th century saw attention to food playing a major role in maintaining continence. It was recommended that salt, sharp and sour foods, malt liquor, tea and coffee should be avoided. Some of these remedies, including limiting tea and coffee, remain today. This was also a period during which pilgrimage and prayer were employed to achieve a cure. St Catherine of Alexandria is considered to be the patron saint of urinary incontinence, and St Vitus from western Germany that for constipation.

It is also interesting to mention some of positive uses of urine. Robert Record, in his *Urinal of the Physik* (1651), suggests that 'if a man lets his own urine drop upon his feet in the morning, it is good against all evil'. The same author recommends human urine as a cure for spots on the face; canine urine as a cure for corns and warts; and male ass's urine to reduce baldness and stimulate new hair growth. The urea in urine has been used for centuries as a fixing agent in dyeing cloth and until recently urine was stored for the treatment of wool in the tweed industry. Even today, in some

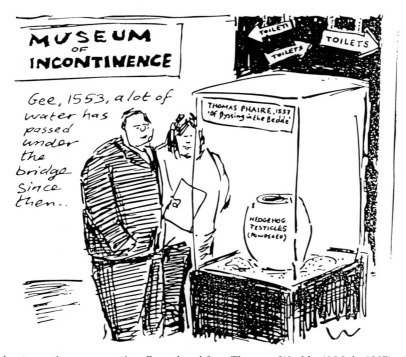

Early approaches to continence promotion. Reproduced from Therapy Weekly *(16 July 1987) with permission.*

countries, human excreta are preciously collected and used to manure the crops.

DEVELOPMENT OF CONTINENCE SERVICES

The 1970s saw the beginning of a concerted approach to promoting continence. Attitudes were gradually changing, with greater awareness of treatments and potential cure. Health professionals, scientists and bioengineers were working together pioneering assessment tools and interventions, and at the same time nurses were being appointed to specialist posts, mainly in urodynamics units.

The Chief Nursing Officer at the Department of Health and Social Security, Dame Phyllis Friend, led the way to encouraging local continence service development. In the first of a series of letters concerned with nursing practice, she recommended to senior nurse managers that district health authorities appoint a nursing officer to take responsibility for meeting the needs of people with incontinence problems and to act as a point of reference to nursing staff (*Standards of Nursing Care: Promotion of Continence and Management of Incontinence* – CNO (SNC) (77)).

The first national incontinence advisory service was established in 1974 as the Disabled Living Foundation Incontinence Advisory Service (this has now been integrated with the Continence Foundation). This service was at the forefront in raising professional and public awareness on the extent of the problem and the needs of the client. Information and fact sheets were produced for the professionals and public, study days were open to all disciplines and an innovative fashion show with students modelling incontinence garments was hosted. A brief interview on radio or TV, an article in the press or a women's magazine would produce a deluge of letters to the service from people eager for information. Following one TV programme there were 12 000 requests for information.

The momentum continued during the 1980s with the setting up of continence services and appointment of continence advisors. The Incontinence Action Group, comprising representatives from the health and social care professions and from industry, was charged with reviewing the provision of continence services and the training of professionals. Their report, *Action on Incontinence* (King's Fund 1983), highlighted the absence of continence as a topic in the pre- and postregistration training of doctors and nurses and the need to educate professionals and the public. It also recommended that an incontinence clinic with some form of urodynamics assessment and a continence nurse advisor should be available in each district. This was followed by a report of the Royal College of Physicians (1986), entitled *Physical Disability in 1986 and Beyond*, which set out the general principles for the operation of a urinary continence service and advocated a written district policy.

Within a decade there were over 300 nurses and two physiotherapists in these specialist posts (Mandelstam 1990). The development of the posts and the services provided varied around the country, depending on the way in which the posts were initially created and funded (Roe 1990). In many instances the services were based on economic grounds rather than the needs of the local population, and the role of the advisor depended on the source of funding for the post. At the time there were no recognized qualifications to prepare health professionals for these new clinical posts. The English National Board subsequently validated a short course primarily aimed at nurses (ENB course 978: An introduction to the promotion of continence and management of incontinence) but, recognizing the multidisciplinary nature of the subject, professionals from other disciplines were encouraged to participate. Several universities now offer a range of postregistration diploma and degree courses for nurses and physiotherapists and courses for occupational therapists are in preparation (Cowley 2001).

As continence services developed, professionals and the public saw a greater need for information, education and support. In 1981 over 100 healthcare professionals from across the UK met in response to a questionnaire asking health authorities to identify professionals concerned with continence. From this meeting the Association of

Continence Advisors (now the Association for Continence Advice) was founded. A few years later the Royal College of Nursing set up a special interest group for continence (now the Continence Care Forum). In 1988 the Enuresis Resource and Information Centre (ERIC) emerged as a support group for children with nocturnal enuresis and their parents and carers. This service has extended to include daytime wetting, encopresis, physical and learning needs (see Chapter 5).

In the following year a group of patients established a self-help group called the National Action on Incontinence (now known as *In*contact – National Action on Incontinence). This consumer-led group continues to play a major role in developing government policy and public awareness. The Continence Foundation was formed in 1994 as an umbrella group bringing together all the continence organizations and now focuses on advice, awareness and advocacy, campaigning for improvements in policy and services. Two years later PromoCon was established as a joint initiative of the Continence Foundation and the Disabled Living Centres Council, Manchester, providing a national resource of continence products, coordinating resources within disabled living centres and piloting public awareness campaigns. This network of continence organizations meets twice a year as the UK Continence Alliance – 'a forum to aid clarification, communication, collaboration and support between continence organisations'.

Public awareness campaigns

Writing in the British Medical Journal in 1999, the President of the Patients' Association acknowledged, 'A public education campaign is the only way to break through social stigma associated with bladder problems and encourage people to seek help for conditions they may never have discussed before'. Opportunities for raising public awareness have increased over the last 20 years or so. For example, in the 1980s the word 'incontinence' could not be used in television advertisements and the advertisement could not be screened 3 hours before or after children's programmes or religious broadcasts. The Advertising Standards Authority have now revised some of

their stringent rules on content and screening times of advertisements and incontinence pads are advertised on television at peak times. Other advertisements, previously tucked away on the back pages of weekly papers, offering plastic pants and male appliances and guaranteeing discreet mailing, are now replaced by high-profile glossy pictures in women's magazines and national papers.

Continence-related commercial companies continue to invest substantially in raising public awareness through products and non-product initiatives such as self-help leaflets, videos and helplines. Articles and interviews with professionals and incontinent people regularly appear in local and national press and on radio. Boots the Chemist, in collaboration with *In*contact held the first Continence Awareness Month in 1993. There were displays of continence products in prominent positions in many major stores, supported by *In*contact's information leaflets. A few stores held advisory sessions, giving customers an opportunity to meet with their local continence advisors.

It was in 1994 that incontinence went public with major government support. 'Don't suffer in silence' was the slogan for the first government-funded national public awareness campaign. The aim was to increase public knowledge about incontinence and to encourage people to seek help. This Department of Health initiative was led by the Continence Foundation in collaboration with all the national continence organizations. The Department of Health distributed in excess of one and a half million leaflets, posters and toilet stickers to healthcare professionals, relevant voluntary organizations, libraries, national rail and coach companies, fast-food chains and a host of other organizations. In addition, press packs which included case histories of people willing to be interviewed were sent to journalists in the professional and public media and a booth at London's Waterloo Station proffered information to mystified commuters. (A similar event held in Manchester's Piccadilly Station in 2001 saw travellers actively requesting information.) The national Incontinence Information Helpline was given government funding to extend its opening times and remained open for 12 hours a day throughout the campaign.

A second national awareness campaign, Dry Day–Dry Night, with the slogan 'It's time to talk about it', was held in 1995. Funded by the Department of Health and led by the Continence Foundation and their affiliated organizations, the campaign focused on enuresis in children and adults and information for people from the ethnic minority groups. The Department of Health distributed stickers in English and ten ethnic minority languages to pharmacists for their window displays, and issued bookmarks in the ethnic minority languages. The bookmarks provided a freephone number, which people could ring to listen to a recorded message in their own language about the causes and treatments of incontinence and how to seek help. The Enuresis Resource Information Centre (ERIC) and Continence Foundation helplines remained open for the 24 hours. Early morning callers appreciated the opportunity to speak when no-one was about.

The Department of Health funded a third public awareness campaign in 1996 – 'Your baby, your bladder and your bowels' with the theme of prevention and early diagnosis. Midwives, health visitors, school nurses and practice nurses were groups who were specifically targeted as well as the public. The 1997 campaign focused on the pelvic floor with Olympic swimmer Sharon Davies launching a highly successful National Pelvic Floorathon. Over 300 events were held throughout the country involving soap opera stars, aerobics classes and continence advisors. The annual campaign has continued with themes on dispelling myths about bladder problems (1998); 'the well-behaved bladder' (1999); women and childbirth (2000) and 'helping you to help yourself' (2001). The 2001 theme was particularly concerned with raising awareness of the psychological impact of incontinence.

A comprehensive service

A multidisciplinary approach to continence care has long been advocated (King's Fund 1983) but the most radical changes have taken place in continence services in the past decade. An extensive review of continence services carried out in 1991 by the Department of Health found that current government policies for these services were sound but for a variety of reasons their implementation was patchy. The report, *Agenda for Action for Continence Services* (Sanderson 1991), was the result of wide consultation with professionals and leading incontinence support groups. It acknowledged that good practice existed, and could provide a framework for continence services, but that central action was needed to stimulate progress. The report also concluded that thorough assessment of need was ten times more cost-effective than the currently predominant practice of containment and supply of disposable continence products. However, responsibility for continence services remained unclear with Rooker (1992) (Shadow Minister for community care at that time) describing 'a continence lottery' based on location and Rhodes (1993) describing incontinence as a 'football kicked between the nursing and medical professions in their attempt to define professional boundaries'.

The NHS Executive made implementing the Agenda for Action guidelines a priority for purchasers in 1994–5. This was supported by additional guidance to purchasers of services distributed by the Continence Foundation (Norton 1995) and based on a report of the Royal College of Physicians Multidisciplinary Working Party (1995) which stated:

A comprehensive continence service should include professional and public education, prevention strategies, comprehensive assessment and investigation, a range of treatment options and a support and management service for people with intractable incontinence. It should not primarily focus on supply of continence products.

The report was important in raising the profile of continence services to managers, planners, professionals and carers, in moving the focus on from containment to assessment and treatment, and in helping to negate entrenched perceptions of continence services as 'pad services'.

As part of the NHS Executive strategy (1993) for development of national clinical guidelines, Button et al (1998) undertook a systematic review of the continence literature. This was used to inform the production of consensus clinical guidelines on promoting continence in primary care and to provide a rationale for treatment interventions based on current evidence. The guidelines provided a framework which could be adapted locally and emphasized that individuals have a right to be involved in the decision-making process about their care and to have an awareness of the options available. They also articulated the need for greater multidisciplinary continence education of all health professionals at pre- and postregistration levels.

Also in 1998, an interprofessional consensus meeting of nurses and physiotherapists was held at the King's Fund Centre to examine current research on prevalence, treatment and services for incontinence (ICCC 1998). At the same time the PACE programme (Promoting Action on Clinical Effectiveness), supported by the King's Fund, looked at current information on services from a range of sources and reported on pressures such as waiting lists for treatment, continence care in residential homes and issues of continence product supplies.

Guidance on good practice in continence services (DoH 2000a)

A review of continence services was instituted by the government in 1998 and the Working Group was charged with updating the guidance previously issued in the 1991 Agenda for Action. Key organizations active in the continence field were invited to nominate representatives for the Working Group and included both professional and voluntary organizations. The Group's aim was to ensure nation-wide availability of high-quality services for people with incontinence by:

- highlighting the extent of the problem
- setting out clear and achievable targets for service
- giving advice about clinical and managerial approaches that ensure the targets are met
- setting out an approach for implementation with systematic processes for monitoring progress.

Due account was taken of new guidance issued to the NHS in recent years and a summary of key documents which informed the consultation is provided at the end of this chapter. The review of continence services identified a number of problems across the country including:

- lack of involvement of users at all levels of service planning and delivery
- geographical variations in the range and quantities of treatment provided and the time spent waiting
- geographical variations in the number of staff trained and the quality of the education and the training given
- gross differences in the NHS Trust policies for the provision of continence supplies. For example, the most common maximum pad allowance/24 h was five, with the lowest two and the highest seven (Anthony 1998).

The Guidance calls for integrated continence services 'based upon and evolved from existing local continence services'. These services are expected to be 'cohesive and comprehensive', covering urinary and faecal incontinence in all age groups – children to older people – in hospital, at home or in care. Services should be provided at different levels and through different bodies, not necessarily the NHS, and based on agreed evidence-based policies, procedures and guidelines with group audit and review (Fig. 1.1). Within this integrated service, primary care is viewed as responsible for: identifying the local population with incontinence; ensuring appropriate resources; providing first-line assessment and treatment, using agreed care pathways; auditing the service, and making the results available for research. In order to fulfil this role primary care and community professionals need to be trained appropriately to implement the prevention, assessment and treatment of incontinence.

The Guidance sets out clear targets, interventions and indicators for clinical audit for the following:

- primary healthcare and community teams
- health authorities and primary care trusts

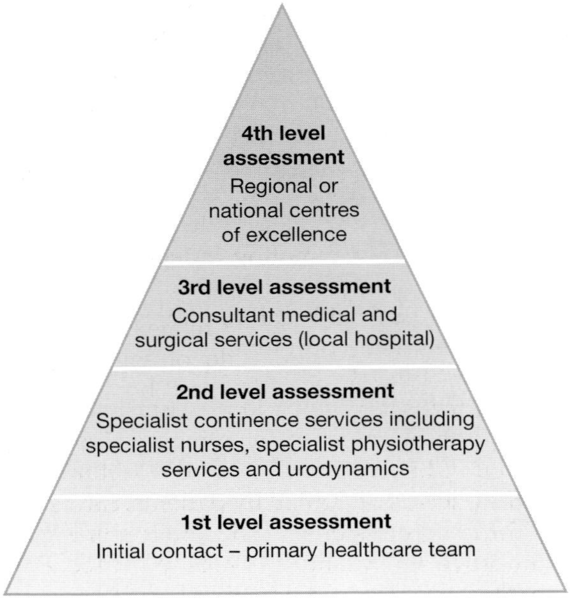

Figure 1.1 Continence service pathways. Local integrated services, led by a Director of Continence Services, will include levels 1–3. Local services should have specific referral arrangements with level 4 provision.

- joint targets for health and local authorities with respect to children, and to residential care and nursing homes
- inpatient care.

An annexe to the Guidance recognizes the need for continence products and recommends that supplies should be governed by clinical need and not cost alone. However, it is also noted that a better knowledge and understanding by health professionals is needed about products such as hand-held urinals (especially female urinals) and lifestyle aids and adaptations which can often prevent the need for continence products such as pads.

Leading continence services

The Guidance recommends that a Director, usually a specialist nurse or physiotherapist, leads the service, coordinating continence specialist nurses, physiotherapists and hospital-based specialists and services. The Director is expected to take a lead in developing shared policies, protocols and pathways that will make for a cohesive and comprehensive service and to coordinate all staff in primary, secondary and tertiary care with outside agencies, including social services, education authorities, care home providers, users and carers.

Informed and effective commissioning are crucial in developing continence services but the agenda for primary care trusts (Pacts) is so broad that continence services may not receive high priority since the Guidance is not mandatory. The Continence Foundation (2000a) have published a source book on *Making the Case for Investment in an Integrated Continence Service* which offers comprehensive advice on getting incontinence on the agenda, including compilation and analysis of population profiles, and estimating costs to the service.

Clinical governance and performance monitoring

There is now a substantial evidence base on proactive identification, assessment, treatment and management of urinary incontinence and to a lesser extent on faecal incontinence. The introduction of clinical governance (DoH 1996) has provided further impetus to the drive for evidence-based health care and plays a key role in ensuring that services have in place systems to monitor and improve treatment and clinical care standards, by placing responsibility at Trust board level. Audit and performance monitoring are important in demonstrating progress in service development and providing feedback at a range of levels within the organization. A range of outcome indicators is provided within the Guidance and others are discussed by Brocklehurst et al (1999), Button et al (1998) and Roe et al (1996). There are two audit tools available for use by all members of primary healthcare teams, both of which have been extensively piloted and peer reviewed: 'Audit protocol: assessment of patients with urinary incontinence' (Cheater et al 1998) and 'Promoting continence: clinical audit scheme for the management of urinary and faecal incontinence' (RCP 1998). Care pathways can also provide an effective strategy to support evidence-based assessment, treatment and management and are becoming more common in continence care (Bayliss et al 2001). Published tools can provide a strong, and often well-tested framework for audit and monitoring, but different strategies may be appropriate in different settings and in order to achieve local ownership and commitment some local adaptation of published tools can be helpful.

The role of nurse consultant was introduced in 1999 (DoH 1999b) as part of the modernization of career frameworks. The nurse consultant, while retaining clinical expertise, has a central role in initiating and leading significant development in practice, education and research. There are relatively few nurse consultants in continence to date, but these posts have the potential to offer great opportunities and also present great challenges.

Linking incontinence with other NHS priorities

Good continence services can contribute directly and indirectly to the public health agenda in a number of areas, even when continence is not explicitly identified. Although there is no immediate reference to incontinence in the NHS Plan (DoH 2000b), the implications for planning and delivering continence services are clear. The plan refers to new extensions to nursing roles including the nurse prescribing agenda. It also refers to nurse-led clinics, management of caseloads, receiving referrals and ordering diagnostic investigations, all of which may be components of integrated care pathways. Of the four priority areas identified in *Saving Lives: Our Healthier Nation* (DoH 1999a), continence care contributes directly to stroke care and to reducing accidents. There is evidence that 42% of stroke survivors are incontinent and 18% are still incontinent on leaving hospital (Rudd et al 1999), but good continence care can reduce the effects of the stroke and enhance self-esteem and rehabilitation. Incontinence can lead to falls and with urge incontinence the risk of falls has been shown to increase by 30% and the risk of fractures by 3% (Brown 2000). The White Paper also sets out requirements for health authorities to make local health improvement plans (HImPs). Continence care has relevance to

a number of the potential target areas within such plans, such as diabetes, learning disabilities, etc. (Continence Foundation 2000a; DoH 2001a).

Incontinence has close links with the National Service Frameworks for Older People (DoH 2001b) (see also Chapter 6), and the NSFs for Children and for Neurological disorders (to be published). It also has clear connections with the national priority 'promoting independence'; the expert patient programme, which is designed to help people deal with chronic illness; and with the benchmarking programme initiated in the *Essence of Care* (DoH 2001c). The latter programme focuses on the 'fundamental and essential aspects of care', and continence (including bladder and bowel care) is one of eight areas of health concerns identified by patients, carers and healthcare professionals. The programme aims to improve the quality of care by a process of benchmarking, which identifies good practice and continuous development through comparison and sharing.

Ethnic and other minority groups

Promoting healthcare in a multicultural society is challenging on a number of accounts, particularly on cultural issues and language barriers (DoH 1998, O'Neale 2000). The taboos and inhibitions connected with continence demand understanding, respect and provision for religious and cultural needs. For example, douching facilities are required for Muslims who cleanse with water after toileting, and women from certain cultures require a female doctor. Describing incontinence symptoms and treatments in any language is problematic: clinical terminology may not be easy to translate, advice easy to understand or treatments culturally acceptable.

An award-winning project initiated by the Tower Hamlets Strategy group in London included raising continence awareness through health promotion sessions. A continence-care trained, bilingual advocate worked with a continence advisor to enable Bangladeshi women to access local continence services (Haggar 1995). At the end of the project a booklet was made available to care workers interested in cultural aspects of incontinence. A similar project was successfully piloted in a mother and baby clinic in the West Midlands. Initiatives focusing on ethnic groups are continuing at local levels and the Continence Foundation acts as a clearing-house for information on minority group issues. It provides leaflets in Asian, African and European languages.

There is a real need for similar work to address the needs of other minority/special groups. The Guidance draws attention to the following groups as likely to encounter problems with continence or have access difficulties:

- People with long-term physical difficulties, neurological conditions and learning disabilities
- Prisoners, asylum seekers and refugees
- Homeless people and those living in hostels
- Older people in residential care and nursing homes.

The Guidance recommends that to ensure fair access to services health commissioners and providers should take particular note of difficulty in accessing services for:

- ethnic minority communities
- children in foster care and at boarding schools
- travelling people.

Ethical issues

The ability to have bladder and bowel control is a basic right for each one of us. However, an ethical conflict can sometimes arise when there are differences between consumer and professional choices. People are encouraged to make choices, but the resources are not always available to cope with demand or the services offered are not acceptable to the potential users.

Differing perceptions of treatments from professionals' and carers' perspectives can also be a source of concern. Some procedures are simply intended to relieve symptoms. The outcome may be satisfactory to the professional but a bitter disappointment to the person who had expected to be cured. For example, a clam-augmentation cystoplasty (see Chapter 3) may resolve the symptoms of an overactive detrusor muscle, but having to self-catheterize several times a day for the remainder of one's life may not be an acceptable price to pay. Procedures such as cystodistension (stretching of the bladder) are often performed with little explanation of the technique involved and the need to do bladder training afterwards. Intermittent catheterization (see Chapter 9) has become very popular with clinicians as a highly effective way of controlling some forms of incontinence. It is generally seen as a simple procedure by nursing staff, but frequently may be frightening to the client or carer. Carers may sometimes be expected to perform this procedure on a partner or relative when one or both find this unacceptable.

Diagnostic tools used for urinary and faecal investigations are not always understood by or acceptable to clients. Urodynamics (see Chapter 2) is frequently cited as an example. This investigation is used for the accurate diagnosis of dysfunction and has an important role to play in research but it is a highly invasive procedure, which many people find embarrassing and undignified. Although the broad concerns highlighted by these issues are not exclusive to continence care this does not make them any less important.

PREVALENCE OF INCONTINENCE
Defining incontinence

People from differing cultures and disciplines may sometimes find the meaning of the word incontinence problematic and it is worth considering the meaning of continence as well as incontinence. Continence has been described as having the ability to store urine in the bladder or faeces in the bowel and to excrete voluntarily where and when it is socially appropriate. In children continence is about being able to alternate voluntarily and comfortably between the storing and emptying phases of the bladder and bowel. The age of achieving continence varies according to the individual's physical and social development, the natural maturation of the central nervous system and the cultural background (see Chapters 2 and 5).

Studies on the prevalence of incontinence frequently use differing definitions of incontinence (or sometimes do not state their definition at all). It is important to have a clear understanding of the definition used by the author when comparing results of research studies or prevalence data. The International Continence Society (ICS) promotes use of common definitions and common data collection criteria where possible to facilitate such comparisons. The *Good Practice in Continence Services* guidance (DoH 2000a) defines incontinence as 'the involuntary or inappropriate passing of urine and/or faeces that has an impact on social functioning or hygiene. It also includes nocturnal enuresis (bedwetting)'.

Faecal incontinence is far less common than urinary incontinence but the social consequences can be more severe. The definition of faecal incontinence adopted by the WHO 2nd International Consultation on Incontinence (Norton et al 2001) is more detailed than that of the Guidance: 'anal incontinence is the involuntary loss of flatus, liquid or solid stool that is a social or hygiene problem'. However, both definitions make allowances for the fact that the impact of similar symptoms on social functioning may be very different for different people. For example, loss of flatus is hardly noticed by some but is perceived as socially incapacitating by others. Similarly some people can lose quite large volumes of urine but may see this as less of a problem than another person with much smaller but more frequent losses.

Prevalence studies

It is difficult to measure the prevalence of incontinence accurately because people have different perceptions of the severity of their own symptoms. If questions are directed to professionals or carers rather than the individual with incontinence the perceptions may be different again. The way the data are collected can also have a notable effect (Thom 1998) as people may underreport the problem because of associated embarrassment, particularly in an interview situation. By contrast, positive responses to a postal questionnaire which asks 'have you ever wet your underclothing' are likely to overinflate the prevalence figures by inclusion of individuals who admit to infrequent loss of very small quantities of urine. Depending on the ultimate way in which the prevalence figures are to be used it may be useful to distinguish between people who have an incontinence problem, which is managed effectively with aids such as a catheter, and those without satisfactory management.

Prevalence figures based on a summary of what is currently the best available evidence and published in the Guidance (DoH 2000a) are presented in Boxes 1.1–1.3. The results of a recent survey of over 10 000 adults aged over 40, which included a high response rate of over 70%, showed that more than 1 in 3 had clinically significant symptoms of bladder problems (Perry et al 2000). More than 20%

Box 1.1 Prevalence of urinary incontinence (DoH 2000a)

For people living at home:
- Between 1 in 20 and 1 in 14 women aged 15–44
- Between 1 in 13 and 1 in 7 women aged 45–64
- Between 1 in 10 and 1 in 5 women aged 65 and over
- Over 1 in 33 men aged 15–64
- Between 1 in 14 and 1 in 10 men aged 65 and over

For people (both sexes) living in institutions:
- 1 in 3 in residential homes
- nearly 2 in every 3 in nursing homes
- 1 in 2 to 2 in 3 in wards for the elderly and elderly mentally infirm

---

Box 1.2 Prevalence of nocturnal enuresis (DoH 2000a)

It is estimated that about 500 000 children in the UK suffer from nocturnal enuresis (persistent bedwetting). The prevalence decreases with age as follows:

- 1 in 6 children aged 5
- 1 in 7 children aged 7
- 1 in 11 children aged 8
- 1 in 50 teenagers.

The persistence of nocturnal enuresis into adulthood is frequently unacknowledged, but it is estimated that 1 in 100 adults continues to have lifelong bedwetting problems (ERIC 1995).

Box 1.3 Prevalence of faecal incontinence
(DoH 2000a)

Information about faecal incontinence is less extensive
than for urinary incontinence, but current best
estimates suggest:

Adults:
- 1 in 100 in adults at home
- 17 in 100 in the very elderly
- 1 in 4 in people in institutional care

Children:
- 1 in 30 children aged 4–5
- 1 in 50 children aged 5–6
- 1 in 75 children aged 7–9
- 1 in 100 children aged 11–12

Table 1.1 Perceptions of continence symptoms

Symptom severity	Women (%)	Men (%)	Total (%)
Bothersome	8.0	6.2	7.2
Want help	3.8	3.8	3.8
Socially disabling	3.2	2.2	2.8

Percentages of 10 226 adults over 40 whose symptoms
of urinary incontinence were a problem to them.
(Reproduced with permission from Perry et al 2000.)

of women and nearly 15% of men had incontinence
several times a month and approximately 20% of
both men and women had nocturia requiring them
to get up twice a night or more. Most people with
clinically significant symptoms did not find them
bothersome or want help but those who did are
shown, as percentages of the total sample, in
Table 1.1. Obesity has now been recognized as a
risk factor for incontinence in women, with a 4.2
times risk associated with stress incontinence and a
2.2 times risk associated with urge incontinence
(Abrams et al 2002) (see also Chapters 2 and 3).
Given that obesity now affects 20% of the population in the UK this factor needs greater attention.

Nocturnal enuresis is widespread in children
(Johnson 1998) and is more common in boys than
in girls (Chiozza et al 1998). Urinary symptoms
tend to decrease with age but are still experienced
by a significant number of healthy teenagers
(Swithinbank et al 1998).

Faecal incontinence affects people of all ages,
but its prevalence is more difficult to estimate

because it is seen by professionals and the public
to be more embarrassing, resulting in a reluctance by the former to ask questions and the
latter to seek help (Johanson & Lafferty 1996).
However it is more common in the general population than is often realized. Although prevalence
increases with advancing age and/or disability
there are also large numbers of younger people
who experience symptoms. A recent postal survey in the UK which included 10 000 respondents
(Perry et al 2002) found that 5.7% of women and
6.2% of men over 40 years living in their own
homes report some degree of faecal incontinence.
Overall 1.4% of adults reported major faecal
incontinence (at least several times a month) and
0.7% had disabling incontinence (with a major
impact on their life). The commonest cause of faecal incontinence in healthy women is childbirth
trauma (Kamm 1994). Different methods have
yielded different results and Box 1.3 shows the
summary of an analysis of prevalence data published by the DoH (2000a) in the Guidance.

Prevalence data are important in planning
service provision and resources but for those not
involved in such activities the meaning or useful-
ness of prevalence figures can often be quite difficult to grasp. The Continence Foundation (2000a)
make an interesting comparison between the
prevalence of incontinence and that of other
'common' conditions which helps to put the numbers into context. Urinary incontinence affects up
to 4 million people in the UK compared to asthma
(up to 3.4 million) and diabetes (up to 2.4 million).
Faecal incontinence affects up to 600 000 compared to dementia (700 000), epilepsy (420 000),
Parkinson's disease (120 000) and multiple sclerosis (85 000).

THE PSYCHOLOGICAL AND SOCIAL IMPACT OF INCONTINENCE

Incontinence is soul shattering. It can completely ruin
the lives of those of us who are affected by it.
Humiliation, degradation and shame are familiar
feelings that we experience when facing incontinence.
What is important for all of us to appreciate now is
that this suffering is not necessary. There are a great
many things that can be done to resolve incontinence.

The problem is finding people who are able to offer the help and advice required.

Written by an incontinent person to *In*contact

These words illustrate the depth of feeling and distress that can accompany incontinence but it is no longer the forbidden subject it once was. The powerful social taboos surrounding loss of bladder and bowel control are gradually being eroded, partly due to health promotion campaigns, media influence and society's changing attitudes to illness. Other previously unmentionable subjects, such as cancer, AIDS and child abuse, are now discussed openly and incontinence is also becoming easier to talk about. However, lack of understanding of the condition and embarrassment continue to be major factors stopping people seeking help. It is not easy for an adult to say 'I wet myself'. Symptoms like persistent headaches or vomiting will prompt people to seek medical help, whilst leaking urine or faeces is still often hidden.

The physical signs of incontinence are objectively demonstrable, but the effects on the quality of life of the individual, their understanding of the condition and ability to cope vary subjectively. An evaluation of a national helpline noted that almost a third of respondents never felt 'happy and healthy' (Joseph Rowntree Social Care Research 1991). Faecal incontinence carries an even greater stigma as it is more obvious. Smith & Smith (1987) describe faecal incontinence as one of the most humiliating problems a person can experience. It is easier to hide urinary loss than faecal loss. Information that is clear, factual and accessible to professionals and the public will help in reducing embarrassment and secrecy. However, this is not sufficient on its own and the effects of incontinence on quality of life must not be ignored or underestimated.

The British culture finds it difficult to cope with anything to do with bladders and bowels and the English language contributes to the problem. It is hard to find words that are both descriptive and easy to use. Professionals and public alike frequently resort to euphemisms which in themselves can be confusing, embarrassing and humiliating. Incontinence is not an easy subject to talk about. Referring to a person who is incontinent as 'a patient' can imply a powerlessness and issuing

appointment letters to attend an 'incontinence clinic' can inhibit people asking for time off work. *In*contact deliberately uses the word incontinence in its title and literature to encourage open discussion and the use of accurate words.

The day-to-day activities that the majority of people take for granted become a major planning exercise or just impossible for people with incontinence. Journeys on public transport are frequently out of the question for many people, making going to work, visiting places of public entertainment or socializing impossible. 'Being caught short' in a public place is a major concern. Finding accessible public toilets is a cause of anxiety for many people and coping strategies may include detailed mapping of public toilets and planning ahead for regular toilet stops. A study by Goldsmith (1992) highlighted the discrimination against women in public places. There was a higher ratio of toilets for men; toilets were not wide enough to accommodate a child's buggy and mother; travellers at main line stations had to struggle down flights of stairs with their luggage, and local authorities had closed public toilets on financial grounds. In addition, fears of odour detection or wetting the bed prevent many people staying away overnight.

Incontinence and enuresis can contribute to marital and family breakdown. People avoid making social contacts and lose their confidence in personal relationships. Disgust or fear of wetting or soiling partners can cause frigidity and impotence. Catheters and appliances can have a devastating effect on body image. Men and women have been known to refuse surgery because they were worried the consequences could have a detrimental effect on their sex life. Professionals rarely initiate advice on sexual activity and have been known to be uncertain whether sexual intercourse is possible for people with an indwelling catheter. (Advice on sexual activity in relation to incontinence is offered in several later chapters including with a catheter *in situ* – Chapter 9.)

Quality of life measures

People with incontinence have been found to be more depressed, have higher levels of anxiety, feel more stigmatized and have poorer life satisfaction compared to people who are continent (Shaw 2001). Although this can apply to all types of incontinence (see Chapter 2) people with urge incontinence or mixed incontinence appear to experience greater psychological distress than those with symptoms of stress incontinence (Sandvik et al 1993). Other studies have concurred with this and it is suggested that frequency, urgency and nocturia, which are all very common symptoms of urge incontinence, can be more troublesome than urine leakage. Many studies have identified the impact of incontinence on quality of life (see Research study 1.1) and there is evidence that some people become virtual recluses: 'I've not gone out for nine years for fear of wetting someone's chair or car seat' was a caller's sobbing answerphone message on the Continence Foundation Helpline (Continence Foundation 2000b).

Some key themes are recurrent in studies of psychological distress associated with incontinence (Button et al 1998). These include:

- distress
- embarrassment
- inconvenience
- threat to self-esteem
- loss of personal control
- desire for normalization.

The severity of symptoms is an important factor in promoting help-seeking behaviour but is strongly related to the individual's own perception of severity rather than direct measures of severity. For example, some people consider themselves continent if they wet on a pad but do not if they leak on to their clothing or the floor (Mitteness & Barker 1995). A number of studies have examined reasons for people not seeking treatment. One of the main reasons seems to be that incontinence is not viewed as a legitimate medical condition but rather as a normal part of the ageing process (Shaw 2001) or something which is somehow the individual's own fault, perhaps through being a woman and giving birth (Ashworth & Hagen 1993). In the absence of an 'illness identity' it is often not considered or recognized as appropriate for discussion with a health professional. This is illustrated in the first quotation above, written to *In*contact, where the author questions where to find help. Other common reasons include lack of knowledge of availability of treatment or not believing that treatment can help, being too embarrassed or being too busy.

Coping mechanisms

Coping mechanisms vary from person to person but are commonly directed towards concealing the problem. This has sometimes been described in terms of achieving 'social continence'. Failure to conceal results in social isolation and loss of self-esteem. As a consequence incontinence sufferers generally make strenuous efforts to prevent leakage by strategies including restriction of fluid intake, frequent toilet visits, wearing protective clothing and/or pads. If that fails efforts are directed towards controlling the aftermath of leakage by concealing visible signs or smell of leakage and avoiding social activities. A complex set of behavioural strategies can sometimes take up much of the individual's time and energy. Although a number of papers report on coping strategies there is less discussion of 'coping styles' (Shaw 2001). It could be helpful to health professionals to gain insights into a person's preferred coping style when planning an individualized care regime with them.

This approach has clear parallels with the concept of expert patient programmes (DoH 2001d) which is about developing the confidence and motivation of patients to work in partnership with health professionals and to use their own skills and knowledge to take effective control over their condition. There is evidence that self-management programmes for a number of chronic conditions can result in tangible benefits in terms of reduced severity of symptoms, improved life control and activity and improved resourcefulness and life satisfaction. The self-help book *Don't Make Me Laugh* (Asbury & White 2001) is a good example of effective partnership working (including active listening!). This book resulted from discussions during a series of focus groups with people experiencing continence problems. The group participants identified

---

Research study 1.1 Measuring quality of life

The work of Anderson & Burckhardt (1999) suggests that psychosocial variables such as self-esteem, social support and negative affect are at least as important as illness-related variables in demonstrating successful health outcomes. Quality of life (QoL) measures are becoming increasingly important in evaluations of treatment interventions and particularly in clinical trials for the comparison of treatments with little apparent difference in measurable clinical outcomes, but where patient morbidity is reduced or patient/carer satisfaction is increased (Kelleher 2000). As many studies are now multicentre and sometimes multinational it is essential to identify the most widely acceptable tool to facilitate comparisons between studies. QoL can also be an important outcome in economic evaluations of continence care and is the most obvious effectiveness measure from the patient's point of view.

A common approach for clinical trials is to include both a disease-specific and a generic questionnaire, such as the SF-36 or the Nottingham Health Profile that has been used successfully in similar studies. It is beyond the scope of this book to look at such measures in depth but some examples of disease-specific measures are indicated here.

One of the most recent developments in continence-specific QoL measures is the International Consultation on Incontinence Questionnaire, short form (ICIQ–SF) presented at the Paris conference in 2001. The questionnaire asks three simple questions: How often does leakage occur? How much is lost? How much does leaking interfere with everyday life? The respondent is asked to consider how they have been over the last 4 weeks and a score is assigned to each answer. The total score possible ranges from 0–21 and the ICIQ has been tested for validity (including comparison with other existing scales), for sensitivity to treatment outcomes and for reliability (i.e. stability over time when symptoms themselves are stable). It is anticipated that further modules of the ICIQ will be developed for specific groups (e.g. frail elderly, children, individuals with neurological impairment).

Other commonly used measures in studies of urinary incontinence include the Incontinence Impact Questionnaire and the Urogenital Distress Inventory (Shumaker et al 1994) and the Symptom Severity Index (Sandvik et al 1993). A QoL measure for faecal incontinence has been developed by Rockwood et al (2000). When selecting any QoL measure to use as part of a study or evaluation it is important to check what patient group (e.g. male, female or both), particular age group and particular continence problem (e.g. urge incontinence) it was originally designed for and whether it has been tested and validated for the group you wish to use it with.

---

important and common concerns, which were then addressed in the resulting user-focused book. Group members were invited to review the early drafts and contribute to the book's final content and format.

Professionals also have their own coping styles and strategies. It is generally assumed that nurses are comfortable with all aspects of care, but it can be as embarrassing assisting people to perform intimate tasks as it is for those receiving the help. It is important that we recognize we can feel disgusted at someone not able to control their bodily functions and resentful at having to deal with the mess and the smell, but it is equally important that we develop effective ways of managing our reactions. In 1995 a report on incontinence in residential care by the Royal College of Physicians (RCP) recommended that carers should be given the opportunity to share their own feelings with staff and to be aware of the effects of social and cultural differences in their own lives.

CONTINENCE EDUCATION

Lack of education and knowledge relating to continence within the health and social care professions is a limiting factor in service development and delivery. This deficit often results in avoidance of the subject of continence promotion, the use of inappropriate management methods (e.g. indiscriminate use of pads) or inappropriate referrals to more expensive services that are already overloaded (RCP 1995). Most nurses receive some formal educational input on managing incontinence in their preregistration programmes but often little on continence promotion. A study by Laycock (1995) showed that in some Schools of Nursing continence education was as low as 1–2 hours. The average time spent was 9.4 hours, with a high percentage taught in the clinical area.

A report by the Audit Commission (1999) found that assessment skills were inadequate and that 20% of district nurses had not received training in continence assessment. In a study of continence care in the community (Bignell & Getliffe 2001) continence training in general nursing training was only reported by 25% of 171 respondents. Similarly continence training as part of training for district nursing or health visiting qualifications was only reported by 25% of respondents. Only 7% had taken a formal postregistration course on Promotion of Continence (ENB 978). The RCP (1995) reported that a high percentage of staff nurses working in elderly care settings had received no formal education or training in continence since qualifying yet only 12% of nurses surveyed identified lack of knowledge as a problem. It is questionable how much change in attitudes and approaches to continence care can be expected when education input continues to remain low.

The changing educational needs of community nurses with regards to needs assessment were examined by Cowley et al (2000). Analysis of results from this multiple case study conducted in four different regions in England demonstrated the complex interactions between differing ideals (relating to policy, nursing and ascribed worth), various types of needs assessment (purpose, formality/specificity and complexity) and timing (in relation to client, service and practice needs). Clearly these issues need to be taken into consideration when planning services, in clarifying what is expected of community nurses and in providing appropriate educational support.

In a survey designed to measure attitudes of a range of health professionals to incontinence, GPs generally did not identify continence promotion as part of their role. They did not consider it necessary to assess continence in each patient and they believed it was a 'normal' part of ageing (Smith 1998). The RCP report (1995) recommends the inclusion of continence training as a core subject in medical schools and a more recent RCP report (2000) emphasizes the necessity for continence promotion and management to be included in training programmes for medical, nursing, social work and paramedical professions.

Health care support workers (HCSWs) are now encouraged to complete National Vocational Qualifications (NVQ) in Care and some employers insist on HCSWs holding at least the NVQ in Care Level II before employment. The Level II and III programmes contain comprehensive units on continence promotion for both urinary and bowel problems, but the potential benefit of these programmes is reduced by the fact that they are not compulsory for attainment of the award. However, the management of incontinence is often delegated to HCSWs and therefore it is important to encourage completion of this unit.

Continence organizations worldwide

Peer group support and self-help are strong in continence issues. In the UK, professionals took the lead in setting up organizations, whilst in North America similar groups were consumer led. A forum for non-profit-making continence organizations held in Amsterdam in 1990 found that organizations shared similar objectives and problems and were unanimous that a continued international exchange would benefit public and professional education worldwide. This led to the first gathering of continence organizations from around the world in Rome in 1993 (Gartley & Norton 1993). Fourteen organizations from ten countries focused their discussion on public awareness, fund raising and avenues for international collaboration. There are continence organizations in Australia, Austria, Canada, Denmark, Germany, Ireland, Japan, the Netherlands, New Zealand, Singapore, Sweden, the UK and the USA. The UK is well represented by interdisciplinary and consumer non-profit-making organizations, most having charitable status. Details of these organizations are available on the Internet at www.continenceworldwide.org. Representatives of these organizations continue to meet prior to the annual International Continence Society meeting and produce an annual newsletter. The International Continence Society (ICS) and its UK group (ICS UK) provide a forum for exchange of scientific data on continence at their regular conferences.

Information technology

Information technology and the Internet have opened unlimited opportunities to share continence information worldwide. There are around 15 000 websites across the world dealing with continence issues. All the major continence organizations and manufacturers have their own websites and many link in to other relevant sites. The content and quality of information may sometimes be variable but people of all ages are increasingly using this source of information. Helplines report calls from many people asking for further help and advice as a result of surfing the net.

The benefits to reticent consumers in providing an opportunity to take an active role in their own continence care are enormous. Sandvik (1999) describes a study carried out in Norway, which evaluated the Internet as a source of information using fictitious women with symptoms of stress incontinence. The author concluded that the Internet is a source of excellent information. Electronic information has become an essential tool for the public, professionals and industry. The Centre for Applied Special Technology (CAST) – an educational non-profit-making organization – uses information technology to expand opportunities for *all* people to access information through information technology. Websites such as www.cast.org/bobby advises on the most beneficial way to present information to people with special needs and www.31 offers guidance on accessing information for people with visual impairment.

CONCLUSIONS

Incontinence is a common condition but it is one that can be cured in around 70% of cases (RCP 1995) and significantly improved in the majority of others. Nationally and internationally, continence services are gaining a higher profile and there is an active collaboration and commitment by policy makers and professionals to reducing the prevalence of treatable incontinence. Some of the key UK government documents influencing the development of continence services are outlined in Box 1.4. The media are now more receptive to issues surrounding incontinence, helping to break down the myths and taboos that surround the subject.

Box 1.4   Some of the key government documents influencing development of continence services and cited in *Good Practice in Continence Services* (DoH 2000a)
• Better services for vulnerable people; EL(97)62/CI(97)24 • The New NHS: Modern, Dependable. A national framework for assessing performance: consultation document (DoH 1998) • Approach to quality as outlined in the document A First Class Service: quality in the new NHS (DoH 1998) • Inclusion of promoting independence in 'Modernising Health and Social Services' – the national priorities guidance for 1999/2000 to 2001/2002 (DoH 1998) • Health improvement programmes, HSC(98)167/LAC(98)23 • Modernising Health and Social Services: national priorities guidance (DoH 1999) • Fit for the Future? National required standards for residential and nursing homes for older people (DoH 1999) • Caring about carers: a national strategy for carers (DoH 1999) • First Assessment: a review of district nursing services in England and Wales. Audit Commission (1999) • National Service Framework for Older People (DoH 2001) • Valuing people: A new strategy for learning disabilities (DoH 2001a) • Policy directions set by other departments and cross-departmental initiatives including National Carers Strategy (1999) and the Green Paper 'Supporting families' (1998)

Current challenges are:

- to put into practice active consumer and carer involvement in planning services
- to utilize a common language which is understood and acceptable to the public and professionals alike
- to develop an integrated service which can be accessed by all people with continence problems and to treat them with the sensitivity and dignity they deserve
- to continue to develop treatments and products to promote an optimum quality of life
- to ensure that public places and services provide adequate and accessible toilet and changing facilities
- to keep continence as a key issue on health care agendas.

KEY POINTS FOR PRACTICE

- Consult and collaborate with users and carers.
- Aim for a common language for professionals and the public.
- Promote the availability of straightforward information on continence problems, treatments and management, in an accessible format to meet the needs of different clients, including ethnic and other minority groups.

- Professionals must take responsibility for ensuring they are appropriately knowledgeable about continence problems as part of their continuing professional development. Healthcare organizations must ensure that there are planned programmes of education and training (commonly in conjunction with higher education institutions) to support staff assessing and treating people with incontinence.

REFERENCES

Abrams P, Cardozo L, Khoury S E, Wein A J (eds) 2002 Incontinence. Report of the second International Consultation on Incontinence, 2nd edition. Health Publication Ltd.

Anderson K, Burckhardt C 1999 Conceptualization and measurement of quality of life as an outcome variable for health care intervention and research. Journal of Advanced Nursing 29(2): 298–306

Anthony B 1998 Provision of continence supplies by NHS Trusts. Middlesex University, London

Ashworth P, Hagan M 1993 The meaning of incontinence: a qualitative study of non-geriatric urinary incontinence sufferers. Journal of Advanced Nursing 18: 1415–1423

Asbury N, White H 2001 Don't make me laugh. Northumbria Healthcare NHS Trust, North Shields

Audit Commission 1999 First assessment: a review of district nursing services in England and Wales. Audit Commission, London

Bayliss V, Cherry M, Locke R, Salter L 2001 Pathways for continence care: background and audit. In: Pope Cruikshank J, Woodward S (eds) Management of continence and urinary catheter care. British Journal of Nursing Monograph. Quay Books, Dinton

Bignell V, Getliffe K A 2001 Clinical guidelines for promotion of continence in primary care: community nurses' knowledge, practice and perceptions of role. Primary Health Care Research and Development 2: 163–176

Brocklehurst J, Amess M, Goldacre M et al 1999 Health outcome indicators: urinary incontinence. Report of the working group to the Department of Health. National Centre for Outcome Development, Oxford

Brown J 2000 Urinary incontinence. Does it increase risk for falls and fractures? Journal of the American Geriatric Society 48(7): 721–724

Button D, Roe B, Webb C et al 1998 Continence: promotion and management by the primary care health team. Consensus guidelines. Whurr, London

Cheater F, Lakhani M, Cawood C 1998 Audit protocol: assessment of patients with urinary incontinence. Eli Lily National Clinical Audit Centre, Leicester

Chiozza M, Bernardinelli P, Caione R et al 1998 An Italian epidemiological multicentre study of nocturnal enuresis. British Journal of Urology 81(Suppl. 3): 86–89

CNO (1977) Standards of nursing care: promotion of continence and management of incontinence. CNO (SNC) (77)

Continence Foundation 2000a Making the case for investment in an integrated continence service. Continence Foundation, London

Continence Foundation 2000b Incontinence: a challenge and an opportunity for primary care. Continence Foundation, London

Cowley T 2001 The role of the occupational therapist in continence care: A comprehensive review. Disabled Living, Manchester

Department of Health 1996 Promoting clinical effectiveness: a framework for action in and through the NHS. NHSE, Leeds

Department of Health 1998 They look after their own don't they? DoH, London

Department of Health 1999a Saving lives: our healthier nation. DoH, London

Department of Health 1999b Making a difference. DoH, London

Department of Health 2000a Good practice in continence services. DoH, London

Department of Health 2000b The NHS Plan. DoH, London

Department of Health 2001a Valuing people: a new strategy for learning disabilities for the 21st century. DoH, London

Department of Health 2001b National Service Framework for Older People. DoH, London

Department of Health 2001c The essence of care. DoH, London

Department of Health 2001d The expert patient: a new approach to chronic disease management for 21st century. DoH, London

ERIC 1995 Incontinence promotional leaflet. Enuresis Resource and Information Centre, Bristol

Euromonitor 1997 World survey of incontinence products. Euromonitor, London

Euromonitor 1999 Disposable paper products: the international market. Euromonitor, London

Gartley C, Norton C 1993 A new forum for international exchange is launched. Continence Worldwide. Rome, September

Goldsmith R 1992 The queue starts here: a raw deal for women's access by design. Centre for Accessible Environments, London

Haggar V 1995 Working with ethnic minority communities. Nursing Standard 9(25) Suppl: 3–4

ICCC 1998 Interprofessional collaboration in continence care: nurses and physiotherapists working in continence care. Report of a consensus meeting at the King's Fund supported by an educational grant from Pharmacia & Upjohn. King's Fund, London

Johanson J F, Lafferty J 1996 Epidemiology of faecal incontinence. The silent affliction. American Journal of Gastroenterology 91: 33–36

Johnson M 1998 Nocturnal enuresis. Urological Nursing 18: 259–273

Joseph Rowntree Social Care Research 1991 Findings 17: Evaluating a helpline. JRSCR, London

Kamm M 1994 Obstetric damage and faecal incontinence. Lancet 344: 730–733

Kelleher C 2000 Quality of life and urinary incontinence. Clinical Obstetrics and Gynaecology 14(2): 363–379

King's Fund 1983 Paper 43: Action on incontinence. King's Fund, London

Laycock J 1995 Must do better. Survey of continence education in schools of nursing, medicine, physiotherapy and GP training. Nursing Times 91(7): 64

Mandlestam D 1990 The continence advisory service in the UK. In: ICS Pre-Congressional Symposium on Ethics and Urodynamics. Aarhus, Denmark

Mitteness L, Barker J 1995 Stigmatising a 'normal' condition: urinary continence in later life. Medical Anthropology Quarterly 9(2): 188–210

NHS Executive 1993 EL(93)54: Priorities and planning guidance 1994–5. NHSE, Leeds

Norton C 1995 Commissioning comprehensive continence services. Continence Foundation, London

Norton C, Christiansen J, Butler U et al 2002 Anal incontinence. In: Abrams P, Khoury S E, Wein A J (eds) Incontinence – Report of the second WHO International Consultation on Incontinence, 2nd edition. Health Publication Ltd.

O'Neale V 2000 Excellence not excuses: inspection of services for ethnic minority children and families. DoH, London

Perry S, Shaw C, Assassa P et al 2000 An epidemiological study to establish the prevalence of urinary symptoms and felt need in the community: the Leicestershire MRC Incontinence Study. Journal of Public Health Medicine 22(3): 427–434

Perry S, Shaw C, McGrowther C et al 2002 The prevalence of faecal incontinence in adults aged 40 years or more living in the community. Gut 50(4): 480–484

Rhodes P 1993 The sound of silence. Health Services Journal 21 Oct: 28–29

Rhodes P, Parker G 1993 The role of continence advisors in England and Wales. Social Policy Research Unit, Centre for Health Economics, University of York

Rockwood T H, Church J M, Fleshman J W et al 2000 Faecal incontinence quality of life scale. Diseases of the Colon and Rectum 43: 9–17

Roe B H 1990 Development of continence advisory services in the UK. Scandinavian Journal of Caring Sciences 4(2): 51–54

Roe B, Wilson K, Doll H, Brooks P 1996 An evaluation of health interventions by primary health care teams and continence advisory services on patient outcomes related to incontinence. Health Services Research Unit, Department of Primary Health and Primary Care, University of Oxford

Rooker J W 1992 Community continence services. House of Commons, London

Royal College of Physicians 1986 Physical disability in 1986 and beyond. RCP, London

Royal College of Physicians 1995 Report of a Working Party. Incontinence – causes, management and provision of services. RCP, London

Royal College of Physicians 1998 Promoting continence: clinical audit scheme for the management of urinary and faecal incontinence. RCP, London

Royal College of Physicians (RCP), Royal College of Nursing (RCN) and British Geriatrics Society 2000 The health and care of older people in care homes: A comprehensive interdisciplinary approach. Royal College of Physicians, London

Rudd A G, Irwin P, Rutledge Z et al 1999 The national sentinel audit for stroke: a tool for raising standards of care. Journal of the Royal College of Physicians 33: 460–464

Sanderson J 1991 Agenda for action for continence services. DoH, London

Sandvik H 1999 Health information and interaction on the Internet: a survey of female urinary incontinence. British Medical Journal 319: 29–32

Sandvik H, Hunskaar S, Seim A et al 1993 Validation of a severity index in female urinary incontinence and its implementation in an epidemiological survey. Journal of Epidemiology and Community Health 47: 497–499

Shaw C 2001 A review of the psychosocial predictors of help-seeking behavior and impact on quality of life in people with urinary incontinence. Journal of Clinical Nursing 10(1): 15–24

Shumaker S, Wyman J, Uebersax J, McLeish D, Forti V 1994 Health related quality of life measures for women with incontinence: the Incontinence Impact Questionnaire and the Urogenital Distress Inventory. Quality of Life Research 3: 291–306

Smith C 1998 Attitudes of healthcare workers to incontinence. Journal of Community Nursing 12(4): 8–14

Smith P S 1979 The development of urinary incontinence in the mentally ill. Unpublished PhD thesis, University of Newcastle upon Tyne

Smith P S, Smith L J 1987 Continence and incontinence: psychological approaches to development and treatment. Croom Helm, London

Swithinbank L, Brookes S, Shepherd A, Abrams P 1998 The natural history of urinary symptoms during adolescence. British Journal of Urology 81: 90–93

Thom D 1997 Medically recognised urinary incontinence and risks of hospitalisation, nursing home admission and mortality. Age and Aging 26: 367–374

Thom D 1998 Variations in estimates of urinary prevalence in the community: effects of differences in definition, population characteristics and epidemiological literature. Journal of the American Geriatrics Society 46: 1411–1417

2

Normal and abnormal bladder function

Kathryn Getliffe
Mary Dolman

'Knowledge is created only by additions: we are as children carried on the shoulders of a giant; and aided by the labours of our predecessors we see all they have seen and something beyond.'

Guy de Chauliac

INTRODUCTION

This quotation, which emphasizes the way in which knowledge about any subject is built up as a gradual process, is equally true for knowledge and understanding relating to normal and abnormal bladder function. Whilst a clear comprehension of the normal function of the bladder and lower urinary tract is important in order to understand the effects of abnormal function and to underpin approaches to the promotion of continence and management of incontinence, controversy and uncertainty still exist in certain areas such as precise physiological control mechanisms. This chapter begins by addressing the anatomy and physiology of the normal urinary system, including some discussion of changes that may occur during the normal ageing process. Later sections consider abnormalities that can result in problems of incontinence, providing a basis for the subsequent discussion of assessment of urinary incontinence.

NORMAL BLADDER AND LOWER URINARY TRACT FUNCTION

The bladder and lower urinary tract have two main functions: *storage* of urine, and periodic

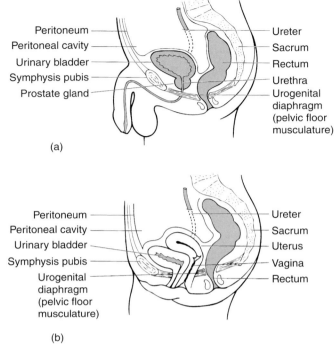

Peritoneum
Peritoneal cavity
Urinary bladder
Symphysis pubis
Prostate gland

Ureter
Sacrum
Rectum
Urethra
Urogenital diaphragm (pelvic floor musculature)

(a)

Peritoneum
Peritoneal cavity
Urinary bladder
Symphysis pubis
Urogenital diaphragm (pelvic floor musculature)

Ureter
Sacrum
Uterus
Vagina
Rectum

(b)

Figure 2.1 Anatomical location of the bladder and pelvic organs: (a) male, (b) female.

elimination of urine. The major anatomical structures involved in both functions are:

- the bladder and bladder neck
- the urethra, and urethral sphincter mechanism
- the pelvic floor.

The bladder

The bladder is a hollow muscular organ, which lies in the anterior part of the pelvic cavity, behind the symphysis pubis. It is outside the peritoneal cavity and extends upwards as it fills, between the peritoneum and the external body wall. In the male the rectum lies behind the bladder whilst in the female the vagina is situated between the bladder and the rectum (Fig. 2.1). In both sexes the rectum is separated from the bladder by a tough fascia of fused layers of peritoneum which provides an effective barrier against rectal invasion from tumours of the bladder or prostate. The upper surface of the bladder is covered by the peritoneum, which joins the anterior abdominal wall above the bladder. This structure allows surgical access to the bladder retropubically without incising the peritoneal cavity.

The bladder receives urine from the kidneys via the ureters. These are hollow muscular tubes, approximately 25 cm long and 0.5 cm in diameter, extending from the renal pelvis to the posterior surface of the bladder. Urine is transported away from the hilum of the kidney towards the bladder by peristaltic-like contractions of the ureters, assisted by gravitational influences. For most of their length the ureters lie outside the peritoneal cavity and enter the bladder near its base, in the small triangular area known as the trigone (Fig. 2.2). The ureters run obliquely through the bladder wall for approximately 1.5 cm to open into the bladder at the left and right ureteric orifices. The oblique angle formed effectively creates a *valve* which prevents retrograde reflux of urine by compressing the ureter when pressure inside

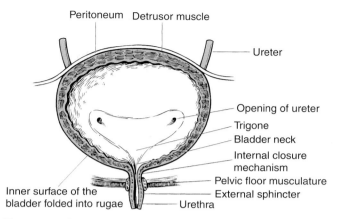

Figure 2.2 Cross-section of the female urinary bladder.

the bladder increases during filling, or when muscular contraction of the bladder occurs leading to expulsion of urine.

The area formed between the left and right ureteric orifices and the internal urethral meatus defines the trigone. This area undergoes little change in size during bladder filling and is very sensitive to stretch owing to the large number of sensory nerve endings it contains. The sensory impulses arise from bare nerve endings of the parasympathetic supply, not from sensory receptors (Gosling et al 1983). Impulses are transmitted to the spinal cord via the pelvic nerves, as the bladder fills.

The bladder wall is generally considered to have four distinct layers, although some controversy exists over the exact nature of the layers (Bullock et al 1991). The innermost *mucosal layer* is extensively folded into rugae when the bladder is not full, and is composed of mucus-secreting transitional cell epithelium which facilitates stretching. These two features allow considerable distension to take place as the bladder fills. The second layer, or *submucosa*, is formed of connective tissue linking the mucosa with the third layer. The muscle fibres of this third layer are collectively known as the *detrusor muscle* and include both circular and longitudinal fibres forming an interlacing meshwork. Contraction of the detrusor therefore causes the bladder to reduce in length and diameter so that it is emptied effectively. The fourth and outermost layer is the *serosa*, which in some respects is

not strictly a continuation of bladder tissue since it is composed of peritoneum and covers only the upper surface of the bladder.

The bladder neck

At the base of the bladder, the bladder neck 'closure mechanism' (not a true 'internal' sphincter in anatomical terms) leads into the urethra, through which urine is expelled to the external environment. The anatomical nature of the bladder neck appears to differ between the two sexes.

In the male there is a circular layer of smooth muscle around the bladder neck which extends down into the prostatic capsule below, together with longitudinal muscle fibres. Contraction of these muscle fibres, which are innervated with sympathetic nerves sensitive to noradrenaline (norepinephrine), prevents retrograde ejaculation of semen into the bladder during orgasm. However, their role in closure of the bladder neck for the maintenance of continence is less clear.

In the female there is no circular layer of smooth muscle. The smooth muscle fibres extend longitudinally into the wall of the urethra and are innervated by cholinergic parasympathetic nerves.

The position of the bladder neck is supported by ligaments arising from the pelvic bone and fascia (Hald 1984). The fascia is closely related to the *levator ani* muscles of the pelvic floor (see page 25), and the position of the bladder neck is influenced by the tonic contraction of the pelvic floor. In the female the bladder neck is also partially supported by the anterior vaginal wall since the urethra and anterior vaginal wall are not two separate adjacent structures, but are bound by connective tissue which unites them. Contraction of the levator ani supports the proximal urethra and also pulls the bladder neck anteriorly, compressing it closed against a band of fascia. Relaxation of the muscles allows the bladder neck to descend and facilitates its opening (DeLancey 1990). Therefore the position of the bladder neck is not static but mobile and under voluntary control.

Under normal conditions the location of the bladder neck at rest, during bladder filling, allows transient increases in abdominal pressure to be transmitted equally to the bladder and bladder neck such that continence is maintained. If, however, weaknesses of supporting structures allow the bladder neck to descend to a lower position, increases in abdominal pressure will exert pressure on the bladder to empty without a corresponding pressure on the bladder neck keeping it closed.

The urethra and the external sphincter

The anatomy of the urethra differs considerably between the sexes. The female urethra is straight and only 3–5 cm long, passing through the muscles of the pelvic floor (*levator ani*), with its external meatus opening anteriorly to the vagina, between the clitoris and the vagina. Its muscle structure comprises an inner longitudinal smooth muscle layer and an outer, circular, striated (voluntary) muscle layer, which forms the *external sphincter*.

By contrast the male urethra is S-shaped, is approximately 18–22 cm long and can be considered to be composed of the following four regions (approximate lengths shown in parentheses):

- The *prostatic urethra* (3–4 cm) passes through the prostate gland which lies below the bladder and attached to its base (Fig. 2.3), receiving ducts from the prostate. On the posterior wall of the lower part of the prostatic urethra is a pyramid-shaped structure called the *verumontanum* (true mountain). This is an important landmark during surgical resection of the prostate since it is close to the prostate and above the level of the external sphincter. Its identification, therefore, reduces the risk of damage to the external sphincter and subsequent incontinence.
- The *membranous urethra* (2 cm) passes through the pelvic floor musculature and includes the location of male external sphincter.
- The *bulbar urethra* (1.5 cm) is surrounded by the 'bulb' of *corpus spongiosum* (part of the erectile tissue extending along the length of the penis) and the contraction of this *bulbospongiosus* muscle assists in emptying of the urethra at the end of voiding.
- The *penile urethra* (15 cm) opens at the urethral meatus. Both the bulbar and penile urethra receive secretions from many periurethral glands via ducts located in the corpus spongiosum.

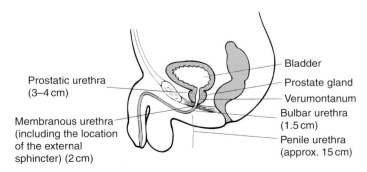

Prostatic urethra
(3–4 cm)

Membranous urethra
(including the location
of the external
sphincter) (2 cm)

Bladder

Prostate gland

Verumontanum

Bulbar urethra
(1.5 cm)

Penile urethra
(approx. 15 cm)

Figure 2.3 Anatomy of the male urethra.

Urethral pressure exerted by tonic contraction of the urethral smooth muscle plays an important role in the maintenance of continence. However, the vascularity of the closely closed folds of urethral mucosa may also be a contributing factor. Rud et al (1980) have suggested that vascular tissue contributes one-third of urethral closure pressure.

Although an external sphincter, which is under voluntary control, is recognized in both sexes, the precise anatomical structure and function in this area is subject to some controversy (Berne & Levy 1990). The external sphincter comprises circular striated muscle fibres, which are designed for prolonged contraction – the so-called *slow-twitch fibres*. These fibres are not easily fatigued and are capable of sustained contraction for long periods, with concurrent occlusion of the urethral lumen. Innervation of these fibres is via motor branches of spinal nerves (pudendal nerve) from the level of the sacral vertebrae S2–S4.

The pelvic floor

The muscles, ligaments and fascia which form the pelvic floor provide a sling-like support for the organs of the lower pelvis (Fig. 2.4). The pelvic floor is pierced by the rectum posteriorly and by the urethra and vagina anteriorly. In addition to the provision of support, the pelvic floor contributes

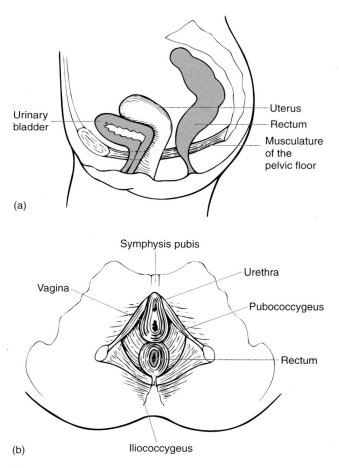

Figure 2.4 Pelvic floor musculature: (a) sagittal section of the female pelvis; (b) cross-section of the female pelvic floor.

to the action of the external sphincter in maintaining urethral closure.

Fibres of the *levator ani* and the *pubococcygeus* are particularly important in effective closure during events associated with a sudden increase in abdominal pressure such as coughing or sneezing. The *pubococcygeus* contains a mixture of both fast- and slow-twitch (70%) muscle fibres, with fast-twitch fibres comprising around 30% (Gilpin et al 1989). The fast-twitch fibres, which tire easily, are responsible for the fast reflex response associated with coughing and for providing a strong maximum contraction to suppress an urgent desire to void. The fibres of the *pubococcygeus* are not attached directly to the walls of the urethra but in females insert into the lateral walls of the vagina. Consequently digital vaginal examination can be used to evaluate muscle tone and strength of voluntary contraction.

Several reflexes appear to play a role in control of micturition and Laycock (1994) highlights two of these. The tone of the pelvic floor musculature promotes reflex inhibition (relaxation) of the detrusor through the perineodetrusor inhibitory reflex (Mahony et al 1977, 1980). Reduction in pelvic floor tone can result in an overactive detrusor and contribute to problems in maintaining continence (Mahony et al 1977). A second reflex, the detrusosphincteric inhibitory reflex, produces reflex inhibition (relaxation) of the pelvic floor and external urethral sphincter on detrusor contraction.

Innervation of detrusor and pelvic floor

The nervous control of the detrusor and sphincteric mechanisms is coordinated by complex nervous pathways that are not entirely understood (Fig. 2.5) (see also Chapter 11). The bladder and urethra are supplied by parasympathetic and

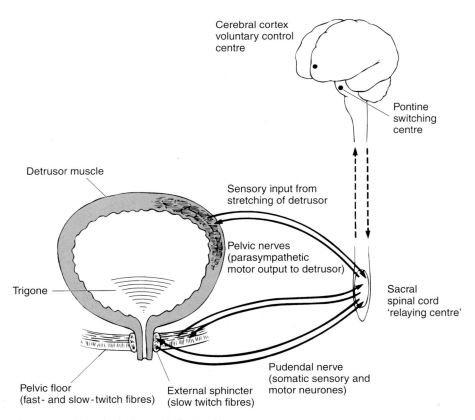

Figure 2.5 Neurological control of micturition.

sympathetic nerves. The pelvic nerves are the important parasympathetic nerves supplying the detrusor smooth muscle and bladder neck sphincter. These nerves originate at the S2–S4 level of the spinal cord and run ventrally to innervate the bladder, urethra and rectum. Arising at a higher level in the spinal cord are the hypogastric nerves from the thoracolumbar region, T2–L3. These are the sympathetic nerves which supply the smooth muscle of the base of the bladder and the bladder neck sphincter. They carry sensory messages from the bladder and urethra to the higher centres. Their main function is to promote detrusor relaxation and, in men, secure bladder sphincter contraction during ejaculation.

The pudendal nerves, which supply the striated muscle of the pelvic floor and rhabdosphincter, are somatic nerves originating at the sacral roots of spinal cord segments S2–S4. These provide voluntary control, which allows the individual the ability to perform pelvic floor muscle contractions. Sensory impulses are also relayed from the pelvic floor, bladder and urethra to the cortical centre.

Nerve impulses and muscle contraction

In order for a muscle to contract it must be activated by an impulse which travels down a motor neurone to stimulate muscle fibres. Neurones consist of a cell body and several extensions, which convey the nerve impulses to and from the cell body. The nerve impulse is a wave of electrochemical activity that passes along the nerve fibre using energy already stored as part of the membrane potential. A resting membrane potential is present across the membrane of the cell body and the whole length of the nerve fibres, the longest of which is the axon. The resting membrane potential occurs because there is a small build up of negative charge just inside the membrane and an equal build up of positive charge on the outside. Such a separation of positive and negative electrical charges is a form of potential energy, which is measured in volts or millivolts (mV). A cell that exhibits a membrane potential is said to be polarized. When the membrane potential changes from $-70\,mV$ (resting potential) to $+30\,mV$ it generates an action potential (impulse) and excitation

occurs. This involves a process of depolarization (with reversal of the membrane polarization from negative to positive) followed by repolarization and is controlled by sodium (Na^+) and potassium (K^+) pumps which control the permeability to these ions (Tortora & Grabowski 1993).

A nerve impulse is triggered only when depolarization reaches about $-55\,mV$ and once this threshold is reached the impulse, or action potential, is generated automatically and spreads along the nerve fibre at a rate characteristic for that particular type of nerve fibre. The speed of travel of the nerve impulse is not related to the stimulus strength. The diameter of the fibre and the presence or absence of an insulating cover (myelin sheath) are important: generally the larger the nerve fibre diameter in myelinated nerves, the lower the electrical resistance and faster conduction. The nerve impulse passes from one node to the next at the nodes of Ranvier where there is interruption to the myelin sheath.

Each muscle is composed of many individual muscle fibres and these are innervated by the motor neurones. There is only a single axon innervating a given muscle fibre; however, a single motor neurone axon may innervate an average of 150 muscles fibres (Fig. 2.6). At the neuromuscular junction a chemical neurotransmitter (acetylcholine) is released and crosses the synaptic gap to bind with receptors on the muscle fibre membrane and stimulate the muscle fibre to contract. Muscle relaxation occurs passively by the cessation of the transmission, there is no special

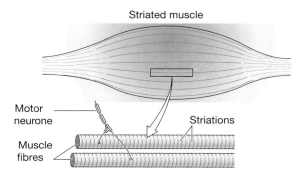

Figure 2.6 Skeletal muscle and a motor neurone innervating more than one muscle fibre with only one axon at a time.

message from the nerve to induce relaxation. The strength of muscle contraction is controlled by the number of muscle fibres contracting and the diameter of the fibres – large diameter fibres contract more forcefully than smaller ones. Muscle tone is generated by sustained small contractions, which give firmness to a relaxed skeletal muscle. At any instant a few muscle fibres are contracted while most are relaxed. Exercise increases muscle strength by increasing the number of fibres 'recruited' to contract and, over a longer period of time, by an increase in size in the individual muscle fibres. This is the aim of pelvic floor exercises (see later in this chapter and Chapter 3).

Control of micturition

Although the mechanisms of continence are not fully understood, a complex process of neuromuscular coordination is required to regulate switching between urinary storage and urinary elimination modes. Within the spinal cord between S2 and S4 is an area known as the *spinal micturition centre*. This acts as a relaying centre for incoming sensory nerve impulses providing information about bladder activity and for outgoing motor nerve impulses (Fig. 2.5). From the spinal micturition centre, nerve fibres also link to the micturition centres in the pons and cerebral

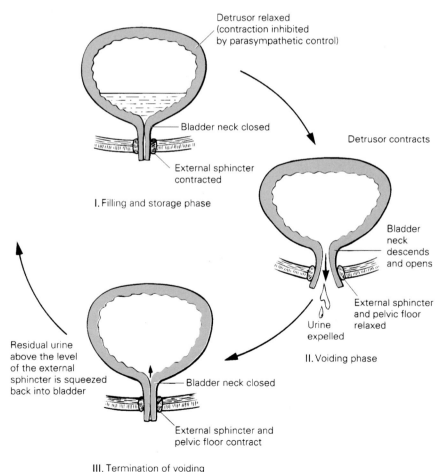

Detrusor relaxed
(contraction inhibited
by parasympathetic control)

Bladder neck closed

External sphincter
contracted

I. Filling and storage phase

Detrusor contracts

Bladder
neck
descends
and opens

Urine
expelled

External sphincter
and pelvic floor
relaxed

II. Voiding phase

Residual urine
above the level
of the external
sphincter is squeezed
back into bladder

Bladder neck closed

External sphincter and
pelvic floor contract

III. Termination of voiding

Figure 2.7　Bladder cycle of filling and emptying – muscular contraction and relaxation.

cortex, relaying information to higher centres and allowing voluntary inhibition of the micturition reflex. The pontine centre may be considered as a type of 'neural switch' between the storage and voiding functions of the bladder (de Groat 1994). Localized areas within the frontal lobes of the cerebral cortex appear to have a role in inhibiting detrusor contraction (Andrew & Nathan 1964). Potential roles in these central pathways have been proposed for a wide range of different neurotransmitters (de Groat 1990) but further clarification is required, particularly as many studies are based on animal models.

Control of micturition depends on learned behaviour occurring during maturation of the nervous system as well as on primitive reflexes present in the neonate. Such control mechanisms are commonly learned by the age of 3–4 years (see also Chapter 5). However, because of the very low location of the sacral spinal micturition centre, the control of micturition is very vulnerable to dysfunction resulting from damage to the spinal cord occurring anywhere above this level. Furthermore, since effective function is dependent on complex neural networks extending between the sacral spinal cord and the cerebral cortex, changes in lower urinary tract function are common early signs of a number of neurological diseases (see Chapter 11).

Bladder filling

Bladder function comprises cycles of filling and emptying (Fig. 2.7). Urine production by the kidneys is continuous and during the bladder filling phase the rugae flatten and bladder volume increases with very little change in internal (intravesical) pressure (Fig. 2.8). This is termed *compliance* and is possible because the lining layers of transitional epithelial cells can overlap and slip over each other as the volume increases (Laker 1994). As the bladder fills it first becomes spherical and then 'pear-shaped' as it rises up out of the pelvic cavity. However, the normal pressure rise on filling from around 10 ml of urine to 400 ml is only about 5–10 cmH$_2$O (Berne & Levy 1990). During filling the detrusor muscle is relaxed (parasympathetic control inhibits detrusor

contraction) but urinary leakage is prevented by contraction of the bladder neck and external sphincter. At approximately 150–250 ml capacity an awareness of distension and a mild desire to void is usually experienced which can be suppressed by conscious inhibitory control from the cerebral cortex until a suitable time and place for voiding occurs.

Voiding

The voiding phase is initiated voluntarily but the simultaneous relaxation of the external sphincter and the bladder neck, and the contraction of the detrusor, is coordinated via the 'spinal–pontine–spinal' reflex which involves the micturition centre in the pons. Relaxation of the external sphincter initially leads to a reduction in pressure within the urethra, and relaxation of the pelvic floor muscles allows the bladder neck to descend and to open (Harrison 1983). Simultaneous parasympathetic stimulation of the detrusor muscle results in its contraction, producing a rise in intravesical pressure (typically around 100 cmH$_2$O) and expulsion of urine under pressure. As emptying is completed and the urinary flow ceases, the external sphincter closes under voluntary control and the proximal urethra also contracts, forcing any urine above the level of the external sphincter back into the bladder. Finally the higher centre

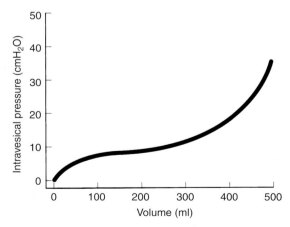

Figure 2.8 Intravesical pressure changes during filling, showing that minimal changes in pressure occur during the initial period of filling.

Box 2.1 Summary of control of micturition: effective storage

- Sustained contraction of the urethral external sphincter and urethral smooth muscle ensures urethral pressure is higher than intravesical pressure – *voluntary control of the sphincter by motor impulses from parasympathetic fibres in the pudendal nerves.*
- Relaxation of the detrusor muscle allows a low intravesical pressure to be maintained during filling (compliance). Detrusor contraction is inhibited by control via the parasympathetic system – *inhibition via parasympathetic fibres in pelvic nerves.*
- Unimpaired pathways between pontine and sacral centres are necessary to coordinate these activities.
- The bladder is supported by the muscles of the pelvic floor. Transitory increases in abdominal pressure are transmitted equally to the bladder and the urethra so that intravesical and urethral pressure differences are maintained.
- The tone of the pelvic floor musculature promotes reflex relaxation of the detrusor through the perineodetrusor inhibitory reflex.
- The bladder neck is closed at rest, but an effective watertight seal depends on a number of factors including competence of the external sphincter and pelvic floor muscles, the tone of the bladder neck and urethral smooth muscle component, and the vascularity of the closely closed folds of urethra mucosa.

Box 2.2 Summary of control of micturition: effective emptying

- Emptying of the bladder is initiated voluntarily, but relies also on involuntary contraction of the detrusor muscle – *response to sensory impulses from nerve endings in the bladder wall and trigone area providing conscious awareness of bladder filling.*
- Relaxation of the voluntary muscles of the pelvic floor allows the bladder neck to descend and open – *mediated by inhibition of motor impulses via pudendal nerves.*
- Sustained detrusor contraction increases intravesical pressure and is maintained to ensure bladder empties fully – *inhibition mediated via cortical, pontine and sacral centres is removed and muscle contraction is stimulated via parasympathetic motor fibres in pelvic nerves.*
- Concurrent relaxation of the urethral sphincter results in a lower urethral pressure compared with intravesical pressure – *mediated by inhibition of motor impulses via pudendal nerves.*
- The detrusosphincteric inhibitory reflex produces reflex relaxation of the pelvic floor and external urethral sphincter on detrusor contraction.
- Unimpaired pathways between pontine and sacral centres are necessary to coordinate these activities.

inhibition is again enforced, allowing the filling cycle to recommence. The control of micturition is summarized in Boxes 2.1 and 2.2.

ACHIEVING AND MAINTAINING CONTINENCE

Since the precise mechanisms involved in micturition are still unclear, it is not surprising that the acquisition of continence is also an area that is only partially understood. It seems likely that the coordination of this complex skill, which is usually achieved in early childhood, results from an interaction between maturational factors and learning (Smith & Smith 1987). In early infant life the development of the central nervous system is incomplete and bladder (and bowel) emptying occurs involuntarily via spinal reflexes. However, by about 2 years of age conscious inhibition becomes possible with development of the cerebral cortex. The child learns to interpret sensations of

bladder fullness and to briefly inhibit the desire to void. As bladder capacity increases, successful control develops with practice and continence becomes subconscious and automatic for most individuals.

Normal bladder function has been defined as: '…the ability to store and void urine at will in suitable places and at convenient times' (Feneley 1986). However, from a clinical viewpoint, bladder function should always be considered in the context of what is 'normal' for that particular individual, including what is *perceived* as 'normal' by the client or patient, since this may not necessarily be the same as the perception of a healthcare professional.

There are a variety of causes or circumstances that may contribute to failure to achieve or maintain continence. Whilst physiological difficulties or abnormalities are apparent in the majority of cases, psychological, environmental and social factors may also play an important part in determining continence or lack of it. For example, some patients with congenital abnormalities, including neurological problems or learning

Box 2.3 Basic skills required to achieve urinary continence

- The ability to initiate micturition voluntarily at an appropriate time
- The ability to delay voluntarily the onset of micturition temporarily
- The ability to recognize socially acceptable places and/or circumstances to micturate
- The ability to communicate needs and interpret oral/written signs necessary to get assistance or locate a toilet
- Possession of sufficient physical mobility and manual dexterity to reach a toilet, adjust clothing, maintain an appropriate body position during micturition, manage doors, flushing systems, seats and washing facilities

disabilities, may never achieve continence. Others experience deterioration in their ability to control their bladders owing to indirectly related factors such as poor mobility or manual dexterity, or mental illness such as severe depression. For some individuals (often elderly) or victims of disease such as stroke, symptoms of incontinence are likely to be multifactorial (e.g. limited mobility, physiological impairment of bladder control, cognitive disability, communication difficulties). Any or all of these factors may be compounded by multiple medications prescribed.

If one or more of the foregoing basic skills is lacking, for whatever cause, urinary incontinence is a likely consequence. Box 2.3 summarizes the basic skills required to achieve urinary continence.

'Normal patterns of micturition'

Normal patterns of micturition are difficult to define, particularly as the majority of studies that have considered frequency of micturition have been conducted on patients attending clinics for investigation of urinary dysfunction. Patterns of diurnal voiding vary from individual to individual and may change within the lifespan of each individual. However, two studies of healthy female populations (151 women and 33 women respectively) both demonstrated very similar mean frequencies of voiding during 24 hours (5.8 ± 1.4 and 5.63 ± 1.26 respectively) (Kassis & Schick 1993, Larson & Victor 1988), with no identifiable age-related changes in pattern in either study.

Under normal circumstances it is generally accepted that most adults will void at 3–5 hour intervals during the day and will have no need to void at night – but it is important to recognize that individual habits may vary when undertaking an assessment.

ALTERATIONS IN PATTERNS OF URINARY ELIMINATION

When alterations in patterns of urinary elimination occur, the characteristics of the symptoms expressed are often indicative of the type of underlying problem. The most commonly occurring symptoms are presented below.

- *Frequency* describes an abnormally frequent desire to void, often of only small quantities (e.g. less than 200 ml).
- *Urgency* describes an intense desire to void immediately. It often accompanies frequency.
- *Dysuria* is abdominal discomfort or pain, and a burning or smarting sensation accompanying voiding.
- *Residual urine* is urine retained in the bladder after micturition due to incomplete emptying. This stagnant urine can provide a focus for infection and for the formation of bladder stones or calculi. The actual amount can be measured by passing a catheter to withdraw the urine or by ultrasound scan. If the amount retained is 100 ml or more some action should be taken.
- *Nocturia* is disturbance of sleep by the need to void. Some degree of nocturia is accepted as 'normal' by many individuals.
- *Alterations in urinary stream* (e.g. hesitancy) are usually due to some obstruction in the bladder outlet region or in the urethra. Hesitancy occurs because more pressure within the bladder is required to force the urine past the obstruction, the muscles tire before the bladder is empty. After a few moments the bladder contracts again and voiding is resumed.
- *Retention of urine* describes an inability to void. It is not uncommon after surgical procedures or childbirth but is usually temporary. It also occurs as a result of obstruction and in neurological disease such as multiple sclerosis.

Acute distension of the bladder can be very painful, although chronic retention which develops more slowly over a period of time may not be. In any situation where retention is prolonged, including in those patients with lack of sensation due to neurological disease or injury, there is a risk of increased back pressure on the upper urinary tract and reflux of urine into ureters and kidneys, with further risk of upper urinary tract infection and/or stone formation.

- *Retention with overflow* is characterized by frequent voiding of small amounts (e.g. 25–50 ml). It may be possible to palpate a distended bladder.
- *Nocturnal enuresis* is urinary incontinence while asleep. It occurs most often in children but may continue into adulthood.

These alterations in patterns of urinary elimination are considered in further detail during the discussion of assessment of patients with urinary incontinence, and in subsequent chapters.

INCONTINENCE IN OLDER PEOPLE
(see Chapter 6)

Urinary incontinence is certainly not an inevitable part of the ageing process, but it is nevertheless a common problem for elderly people, occurring in 15–30% of those living in the community (Hellstrom et al 1990, Herzog & Fulz 1990) and in up to 50% of patients in institutional care (Nazarko 1994, Ouslander et al 1987). Incontinence may be associated with ageing because elderly people are perhaps more susceptible to physiological, pharmacological and psychological risk factors which may influence their ability to maintain continence. Environmental and social factors can also be important in promoting continence (see the later section on assessment) and are addressed as a continuing theme throughout this and later chapters.

Although age-related differences in patterns of micturition are not apparent in studies of healthy people (Kassis & Schick 1993, Larson & Victor 1988), the situation may be different when underlying pathological problems are present (Saito et al 1993) (Research study 2.1).

Research study 2.1   A comparison of frequency between elderly and adult patients

In the study by Saito et al (1993) which compared frequency of micturition in patients complaining of frequency, four significantly different factors were found between a group of 130 adult patients (16–64 years) and a group of 85 elderly patients (65–84 years). Although the mean urinary volume in 24 hours was very similar in both groups, in elderly patients:

- total urinary volume produced during sleeping hours was larger
- total urinary volume during waking hours was smaller
- tidal volume voided (per episode of micturition) during sleeping hours was smaller
- micturition frequency during sleeping hours was greater.

There was no difference between the two groups in sleeping hours (8.64 ± 0.96 h for the elderly and 8.46 ± 1.09 h for the adult patients). These results strongly suggest that both pathological conditions and age can influence patterns of micturition.

Transient incontinence

Older adults can also experience transient incontinence as a result of illness or change of environment. An illness such as a chest infection, accompanied by a severe cough, can raise intra-abdominal pressure, resulting in stress incontinence (Nazarko 1994).

PHYSIOLOGICAL BLADDER DYSFUNCTION

Bladder dysfunction can be classified into three main types:

- detrusor instability or overactive bladder[1]
- genuine stress incontinence
- voiding difficulties caused by outflow obstruction or by detrusor hypoactivity.

Detrusor instability: urge incontinence

Under normal circumstances the detrusor muscle is relaxed during bladder filling and contracts

---

[1]Current terminology recommended by the International Continence Society (ICS).

only when voluntary voiding is initiated. Detrusor instability (or 'unstable bladder') results in contractions which may occur spontaneously or on provocation (e.g. with coughing or vigorous exercise), or while the patient is attempting to inhibit micturition. Whilst the contractions may be sufficiently strong to cause incontinence, the bladder may not be emptied effectively and large residual volumes of urine (greater than 100 ml) are common. The bladder's capacity also decreases since it no longer has the opportunity to fill completely.

Patients with detrusor instability usually complain of urgency with little or no warning of the need to void, and may be incontinent of urine before reaching the toilet. In addition, they commonly experience persistent frequency and nocturnal enuresis. Detrusor instability can be objectively demonstrated by urodynamic studies, which measure pressure changes as they occur within the bladder and urethra during filling of the bladder. This assessment technique is discussed in detail later in the chapter.

Causes of detrusor instability

Causes of detrusor instability are varied. Neurological lesions resulting from conditions such as strokes, Alzheimer's disease, Parkinson's disease, multiple sclerosis, tumours and spinal cord lesions, may cause loss of inhibitory impulses from the brain, allowing inappropriate activation of the sacral reflex arc so that the bladder begins to contract before micturition is voluntarily initiated. Alternatively, symptoms may arise from increased sensory input from the bladder arising from local causes such as acute urinary tract infection (UTI), stones, tumours, faecal impaction or prostatic enlargement. Increased fluid intake, particularly of alcohol or drinks containing caffeine, can also cause local irritation. However, there are a number of cases of so-called *idiopathic detrusor instability*, where no detectable pathological cause can be identified.

Genuine stress incontinence

Genuine stress incontinence is characterized by a loss of a small amount of urine if there is any increase in abdominal pressure (exerted on the bladder) from physical exertion, such as coughing. It is defined as 'an involuntary loss of urine when the bladder pressure exceeds the maximum urethral pressure, *but in the absence of detrusor activity*'.

It is important to distinguish between genuine stress incontinence and urge incontinence since both can result in leakage with coughing, but a distinction can usually be made by urodynamic investigation. However, mixed incontinence can occur with symptoms of both stress and urge incontinence, and is most common in postmenopausal women. Stress incontinence is common in females but rare in males, although it can occur after prostatectomy. It is usually associated with bladder outlet incompetence because of weakness of the supporting pelvic floor muscles.

Voiding difficulties

Outflow obstruction

Outflow obstruction is far more common in males than in females and is most often associated with prostatic enlargement (which increases with age in men over 45 years), urethral stricture and chronic constipation. The bladder is emptied by frequent voiding of small amounts and micturition is associated with hesitancy, poor urine flow and postmicturition dribble. Frequency, urgency and nocturia or constant dribbling can occur if there is a large residual volume.

Detrusor hypoactivity

In detrusor hypoactivity the muscle is underactive and fails to provide a sustained or adequate contraction. This condition is usually caused by damage to peripheral nerves to the bladder, or by damage to the lower spinal cord, in conditions such as diabetic neuropathy, pelvic injury and multiple sclerosis. The sensation of bladder filling may be absent or reduced and the bladder often increases in capacity by overstretching. Large residual volumes (500–2000 ml) may accumulate, with overflow incontinence. This condition is considered more fully in Chapter 11.

ASSESSMENT OF INCONTINENCE

Assessment can be defined as:

An evaluation or appraisal of a condition; the process of making such an evaluation; an examiner's evaluation of the disease or condition based on the patient's subjective report of the symptoms and course of the illness or condition and the examiner's objective findings, including data obtained through laboratory tests, physical examination and medical history.

Mosby's Medical, Nursing and Allied Health Dictionary

Skills for assessment

Interviewing

Interviewing skills are essential in order to make a meaningful assessment, and these skills are not innate. The way questions are asked will evoke different answers, so asking the right questions is essential. Body language (posture, eye contact, tone of voice), the environment, space and privacy are all part of the interviewing process (Argyle 1982).

Observing the patient's behaviour at interview may also give the assessor an idea of the individual's attitude, feelings and coping mechanisms. Often the signals are non-verbal. Observations made by primary carers may provide further information, especially when the patient's cognitive powers are reduced or absent. However, the patient's permission to seek information from other people, such as family, friends and other carers, should be obtained if at all possible.

Accurate recordings

The skill to record an accurate history takes practice. It is all too easy to record what you think was said and not what was actually said. Patients have a tendency to say the same thing in different ways, and often this changes the meaning. Clarity and understanding must be established. There is nothing more off-putting for a patient than to watch the assessor writing notes while being asked so many questions. Notes should ideally be made immediately after the interview, which of course requires accurate recall.

Empathy and listening

Patients usually want empathy, not sympathy. Conveying understanding of the problems can stem only from a sound knowledge base. Professionals who have not been suitably trained in the subject of incontinence or in the assessment process will not be empathetic.

Listening skills are perhaps the most difficult to learn and they will develop only with familiarity of the subject and practice. For example, it is so easy to help someone to say a word you think they are searching for, but this interruption can put the person off their train of thought. Consequently the wrong information may be given.

Time

An assessment, done properly, takes time; a patient must not feel hurried or rushed. They must be helped to feel relaxed, comfortable in the presence of the assessor, and not embarrassed. An hour is the minimum time for an initial assessment, but it is unlikely that all the information will be obtained at the first meeting. Ongoing data collection may include laboratory tests, radiography, etc., as well as further verbal information from the patient or carers.

Data collection

There are many assessment 'forms' available to collect patient data in relation to bladder and/or bowel dysfunction. Indeed, most Trusts will have developed their own unique assessment form (Winder 2001) which in most cases will not have been fully validated and should only be considered on a face-validity basis. In today's context of clinical governance assessment forms must provide data for audit – therefore the information needed is a clinical baseline and intervention and outcome measures (subjective and objective) at discharge. Other auditable parameters are waiting time to first appointment, inappropriate referrals, waiting time in clinic and total numbers seen for type of incontinence. The use of evidence-based care pathways (Bayliss et al 2000) provides

KEY POINTS FOR INITIAL ASSESSMENT

History taking and recording
- Relevant medical, surgical and obstetric history
- Urinary symptoms and date of onset
- Related circumstances or events precipitating incontinence
- Current medication
- Bowel habit
- Attitude to problem (on the part of the patient, carer or staff)
- Support services used
- Environmental/living conditions
- Aids/appliances used

Frequency/volume charts
- How much urine is lost (see Fig. 2.9)
- Day/night frequency
- Baseline chart of frequency of continent and incontinent episodes
- Fluid intake

Physical examination and tests
- Mobility
- Dexterity
- Hearing and eyesight
- Mental alertness
- Abdominal, rectal and vaginal examinations
- Residual urine (postvoiding via Nelaton catheter or ultrasound)
- Urinalysis
- Pad test (if indicated)

opportunities for unified assessment for all patients (see Appendices for examples of assessment forms). The care pathway was validated by a panel of experts in the field of continence and is well based on evidence referenced from the literature. The resultant data collection forms have been evaluated for their ability to accurately predict the causes of incontinence in a range of patients, ensuring that patients have appropriate referrals, investigations and subsequent treatments.

A frequency/volume chart is an extremely useful way of identifying a patient's usual pattern of voiding. Many patients find a relatively simple chart such as that illustrated in Figure 2.9 easy to use and it can also be used as a bladder training chart. However, it is a matter of personal preference as all charts achieve the same objective of recording an individual's frequency and volume per day. Five days of baseline charting is sufficient to indicate the patient's voiding pattern. The charting can be repeated at a later stage during treatment and used as feedback to demonstrate improvement in both frequency (reduced) and voiding volume (increased). Such a chart can also be used to determine a patient's timed voiding

DAY	DAYTIME Time/volume (millilitres)	NIGHTIME	Number of pads used in 24-hour period
1	Example: *7 am/200* *1 pm/at work* *6 pm/400* *11 pm/300*	*3 am/200* *6 am wet*	
2			
3			
4			
5			
6			
7			
AVERAGE DAILY INTAKE (in cups)			

Figure 2.9 A typical frequency/volume chart to be filled in by a patient (day 1 completed: note that the patient could not measure urinary output at work).

patterns, as in an elderly person with dementia or in children with learning disabilities (see Chapter 10). In these cases frequency and wet episodes can be recorded and the times for voiding adjusted to try to achieve continence.

Whatever information is required, it is essential to include clear, simple instructions at the top of the chart, especially if it is to be used in a ward situation where multidisciplinary carers will be doing the recording.

An example of an assessment form for urinary and bowel dysfunction is reproduced in Figure 2.10. This indicates the various questions that need to be asked and the components an assessment should cover. This is an assessment form whereas a full care pathway is intended to provide a structure to the process of 'service delivery' of which assessment is a critical part. The algorithms in Figures 2.11–2.13 can be used as a guide to assess and treat patients by symptom.

Measuring outcomes

In today's climate of clinical audit, the outcomes of intervention must be fully recorded. This can be done on the assessment form (Fig. 2.10) by using outcome measures at discharge.

Section 12 of the assessment form uses a score system from the *Barthel Index*. This index, developed by Mahoney & Barthel (1965), is based on observed function and measures functional ability before and after interventions. Its use in this context is for elderly persons in hospital, where it is hoped that a low score on initial assessment would be higher on discharge. It must be emphasized that this is only one possible scale for scoring intervention and has not yet been fully validated. Using a *discharge code* in clinic is another way of measuring outcomes. For example:

- D/5 = dry
- D/4 = greatly improved
- D/3 = minimal improvement
- D/2 = referred to another discipline (GP, district nurse, physiotherapist, psychologist, etc.)
- D/1 = surgery

- D/0 = DNA (did not attend) or self-discharge.

This measurement is, of course, a subjective evaluation by the assessor, as is the *Oxford Grading System* for improvements in pelvic floor muscle strength (see Chapter 3).

Objective measures

An objective measure of continence improvement can be made by a pad weighing test. A dry pad is weighed and then weighed again after a set time of wearing. The increased weight is an indication of urine loss. From the initial assessment to the discharge date, it is hoped that the loss will be reduced. Urodynamic investigations (see later in this chapter) before and after intervention can also provide an objective measure of outcome. If the assessor is familiar with the use of a perineometer for measuring pelvic floor muscle strength, then the discharge reading would again be expected to be higher than that at initial assessment, demonstrating an increase in pelvic floor strength.

A record of the referral date and the date of the first appointment will measure waiting time to be seen in a clinic and provide statistics for managers concerned with resource planning. This can be useful in making a case for more staff to be recruited.

The above components of an assessment form are guidelines only and readers are encouraged to design a form relevant to their own workplace that conforms to their Trust's philosophy.

INTERPRETATION OF THE ASSESSMENT

Duration

If the onset of incontinence is recent it may be due to a transitory state such as urinary tract infection, anxiety, stress, bereavement or depression. If the symptoms have existed for a number of years, the underlying cause must be investigated, but it is never too late to improve the situation.

ASSESSMENT FORM FOR ELIMINATION PROBLEMS

PATIENT DETAILS:

SURNAME: .... FORENAME: ....

TITLE: .... DATE OF BIRTH: ....

ADDRESS: ....

....

POSTCODE: .... TELEPHONE NUMBER: ....

GENERAL PRACTITIONER: .... GP TEL. NO: ....

ASSESSMENT DATE: .... ASSESSED BY: ....

WHERE ASSESSED: .... CONSULTANT: ....

MAIN COMPLAINT:

Urinary incontinence: ☐   Faecal incontinence: ☐   Both: ☐

1. ONSET OF PROBLEM   When? ....

  If related to an event, please state: ....

2. URINALYSIS

  Labstick: NAD ☐
       Abnormality ☐   Please state: ....

  Urine sample to laboratory: Yes ☐   Date: ....
                              No ☐

  Result: ....

  Treatment: ....

3. FREQUENCY OF MICTURITION (in 24 hours)

  Continence chart commenced: ....

  Less than 4 times ☐   Urgency: Yes ☐
  4–7   ☐   No ☐
  8–10   ☐
  11+   ☐

  Nocturnal enuresis: Yes ☐   No ☐

  Nocturia: State number of times: ....

  FLUID INTAKE (24 hours) .... ml

Figure 2.10 Assessment form for elimination problems.

4. PHYSICAL EXAMINATION/HISTORY

Not done ☐   Done by Doctor ☐   Done by Nurse ☐

FEMALE:	Yes	No		MALE:	Yes	No
A Prolapse	☐	☐		A Post-voiding		
B Vaginal discharge	☐	☐		dribble	☐	☐
C Atrophic vaginitis	☐	☐		B Recent TURP	☐	☐
D Constipation	☐	☐		C Constipation	☐	☐

5. STRESS INCONTINENCE

Leakage on exertion/movement, cough, sneeze, etc: Yes ☐
                                                          No ☐

If Yes, is leakage: Slight   ☐
                        Moderate
                        Severe

6. VOIDING DIFFICULTIES

	Yes	No
Straining	☐	☐
Hesitancy	☐	☐
Poor stream	☐	☐
Terminal dribble	☐	☐

7. RESIDUAL URINE
(after voiding)

Done: Yes ☐   Amount ....
      No

8. URGE INCONTINENCE

Sudden leakage with, or just after, urge to void?   Yes ☐
                                                          No ☐

If Yes, is leakage: Slight ☐   Moderate ☐   Severe ☐

9. OVERFLOW INCONTINENCE

Dribbling leakage with occasional gushes	Yes ☐	No ☐
Is patient continually wet?	Yes ☐	No ☐
Is patient unaware of leakage?	Yes ☐	No ☐
Has a residual urine been taken?	Yes ☐	No ☐

10. PASSIVE INCONTINENCE

Does bladder empty without warning?	Yes ☐	No ☐
Has patient cognitive difficulties?	Yes ☐	No ☐
Is pad or appliance used for incontinence?	Yes ☐	No ☐

Figure 2.10   *(continued)*

11. PATIENT'S RESPONSE TO PROBLEM

Apathy ☐   Denial ☐   Coping well ☐   Distress ☐

12. CONTRIBUTORY FACTORS

MOBILITY: Independent (2) ☐
Walks with aid (1) ☐
Chair/bed bound (0) ☐

TOILET USE: Independent (2) ☐
Needs help (1) ☐
Dependent (0) ☐

DRESSING: Independent (2) ☐
Needs some assistance (1) ☐
Dependent (0) ☐

TRANSFER: Independent (2) ☐
Needs major help (1) ☐
Unable (0) ☐

INITIAL SCORE: ☐   DISCHARGE SCORE: ☐

13. OTHER INFORMATION

Date   Results

.... Pad test   ☐   Weight preuse............................ gm
                                                                Weight postuse......................... gm
.... Plain abdominal X-ray ☐   ....
.... Ultrasound   ☐   ....
.... Urodynamics   ☐   ....
.... IVP   ☐   ....
.... Cystoscopy   ☐   ....

14. BOWEL ASSESSMENT

Frequency of bowel action .... day(s)

Spurious diarrhoea ☐   Diarrhoea ☐   Constipation ☐

Does patient feel sensation to defaecate?   Yes ☐   No ☐
Special diet for bowels?   Yes ☐   No ☐

Foods to be avoided ....
Daily fluid intake .... ml

Use of laxatives (state) ....
Bulking agents (state) ....
Stool softeners ....

Rectal examination: Done ☐   Not done ☐
If done, result: ....
....
....
....

Figure 2.10   *(continued)*

15. **RELEVANT CONTRIBUTORY FACTORS, MEDICAL HISTORY, OPERATIONS AND URINARY TRACT INVESTIGATIONS**

....
....
....
....

16. **PRESENT MEDICATION**

....
....
....
....

17. **NURSING DIAGNOSIS**

....
....
....
....

18. **PLANNED GOALS**

....
....
....
....

19. **MANAGEMENT OF PROBLEM**

State size and type:

Catheter	....
Urinary drainage sheath	....
Bodyworn appliance	....
Reusable bed pad	....
Reusable bodyworn pad	....
Disposable bed pad	....
Disposable bodyworn pad	....
Other	....

DATE OF REASSESSMENT	
SIGNATURE OF ASSESSOR	
BASE/WARD	....
DATE	....

Figure 2.10 *(continued)*

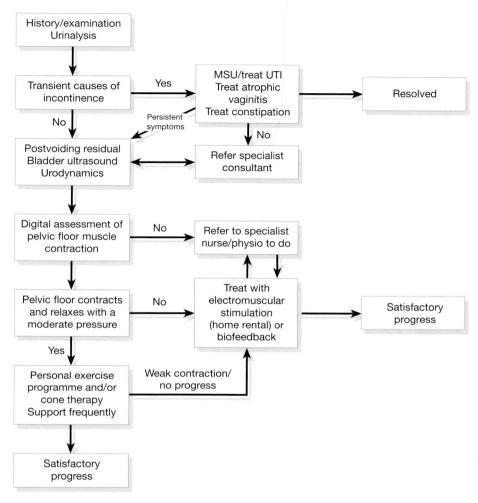

Figure 2.11 Assessment by symptom and approaches to care. MSU, midstream specimen of urine; UTI, urinary tract infection.

Medical history

Many medical conditions can affect the normal functioning of both the bladder and bowel, and these underlying causes need to be treated. Examples are neurological conditions, multiple sclerosis, diabetes (mellitus and insipidus), spinal injuries, learning disabilities, stroke, dementia and back pain. Conditions which exacerbate incontinence include asthma and chronic chest conditions, because continual strain is exerted on the urethral sphincter mechanism by coughing, which increases abdominal pressure.

Surgical history

Previous surgical interventions need to be noted. Gynaecological and urological types are important, but also note any surgery where a Foley catheter was inserted because this may have initiated a long-term problem of outflow obstruction caused by scarring or necrosis of the urethral lining. Retention of urine is another cause of bladder dysfunction following surgery. Prostatectomy may leave a man with a postvoiding dribble, possibly due to a weak detrusor contraction or a weak sphincter; 'milking' the urethra (see Chapter 4)

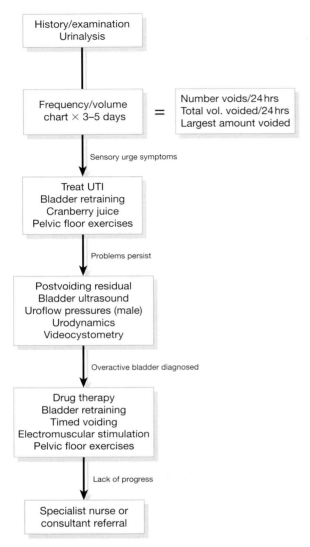

Figure 2.12 Assessment of urge incontinence and approaches to care. UTI, urinary tract infection.

and pelvic floor exercises are conservative treatments for this problem.

Urological history

- *Incontinence*
  —Onset: When did it start?
  —Duration: How long has the problem existed?
  —Degree: Mild, moderate, severe?
  —Type: Stress, urge, overflow, enuresis?
- *Irritative symptoms*
  —Frequency: How often in 24 hours?
  —Urgency: Able to reach toilet in time?
  —Nocturia: Need to get up for toilet at night?
  —Dysuria: Does it hurt to pass urine?
- *Voiding difficulties*
  —Poor stream: Is the urine flow slow/intermittent?
  —Hesitancy: Trouble starting urine flow?
  —Straining: Straining to empty the bladder?
  —Residual: Is the bladder emptying completely?
- *UTI (urinary tract infection)*
  —Urinalysis/midstream specimen of urine: Confirmed or suspected?
- *Suprapubic pain*
  —Interstitial cystitis: Pain, discomfort remains after emptying bladder, frequency?

Urinary symptoms and possible causes

- *Frequency*: detrusor instability, sensory urgency, UTI, cystocele, urinary residual.
- *Urgency*: all the above, plus pregnancy, small bladder capacity, menopause, pelvic mass, radiation, lesions, obstructions, habit, excess fluid intake, anxiety.
- *Stress incontinence*: weak pelvic floor, bladder neck open, detrusor instability, retention.

Mobility and dexterity

An individual who has difficulty with mobility often fails to reach the toilet in time, and so regular, timed toileting may be useful to try to maintain continence. Similarly, reduced manual dexterity may prevent someone from managing their clothing or performing intermittent self-catheterization (ISU), so alternative techniques need to be considered.

Medications

Many drugs can disturb bladder and bowel function (see Chapters 7, 8 and 9). A constant review

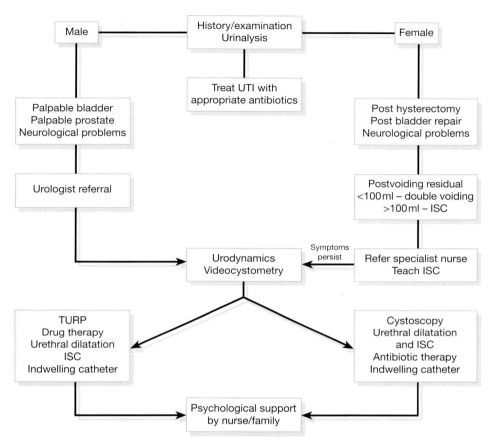

Figure 2.13 Assessment of voiding difficulties. Patient complains of difficulty emptying the bladder. There is usually a poor stream, slow and often intermittent. ISC, intermittent self-catheterization; MSU, midstream specimen of urine; TURP, transurethral resection of the prostate gland; UTI, urinary tract infection.

of medications is necessary to see whether dosages can be reduced, stopped or taken at different times of the day. Polypharmacy often occurs in the elderly when medications are not reviewed regularly in this way.

Physical examination

Pelvic floor muscle assessment and vaginal assessment are discussed in Chapter 3. Other physical examinations include observation of the abdomen for surgical scars, and palpating the abdomen for bladder distension and constipation. A rectal examination may be used for palpating a prostate or to feel for a faecally loaded rectum. Observation of skin condition around the symphysis pubis and

groin may reveal soreness from urinary incontinence or the wearing of pads. Vaginal dryness or atrophic vaginitis can be observed by parting the labia. It is essential that physical examinations are carried out by a fully trained assessor in digital palpation of the pelvic floor and digital rectal examinations.

Social history

This is a most important part of assessment. The impact of incontinence on working life, sexual relationships, family and friends may be dramatic. Embarrassment may lead to someone becoming virtually housebound and unable to continue working. Attitudes towards incontinence will often determine a person's motivation to comply with treatment or management. Box 6.6 (p. 155) illustrates some of the psychological, environmental and social factors influencing continence in older people, but some factors may be equally applicable to younger people, particularly those with physical or learning disabilities.

DIAGNOSTIC INVESTIGATIONS

Diagnostic investigations include urodynamics, ultrasound, X-ray of kidneys, ureter and bladder (KUB), cystoscopy or biopsy. These are usually ordered by the medical team but may also be ordered by other members of the integrated continence team (DoH 2000).

Urinalysis

A simple reagent strip can detect abnormalities in the urine, and this test should be done for every patient at the initial assessment. Only if abnormalities are detected should a specimen of urine be sent for culture and sensitivity (see Fig. 2.14). Urine analysis has three principal applications:

- screening – for disease, both systemic and renal
- diagnosis – to confirm or refute a suspected condition
- management – to monitor the progress of an established disease.

Reading a reagent strip

- *Specific gravity.* The normal range is 1.002–1.035. Very low values represent water diuresis and very high values indicate dehydration.
- *pH.* This represents the acidity/alkaline balance. The normal range varies between 4.5 and 8.0. At low values the urine is more acidic, which may predispose to formation of calculi in the kidney or bladder.
- *Appearance and odour.* The colour of urine is normally yellow, but the intensity of colour varies inversely with the rate of urine formation. 'Concentrated' urine has a relatively strong yellow colour while 'dilute' urine is pale. Colour can change due to food pigments,

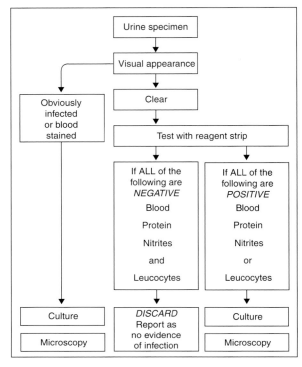

Figure 2.14 'Think negative in UTI': based on a wallchart from Bayer Diagnostics.

colouring agents and drugs. Urine is normally odourless, but in patients with a urinary tract infection it may smell foul or of ammonia.
- *Protein.* This indicates possible renal disease. Further investigations, including urine culture, should be carried out.
- *Nitrites.* Positive nitrite test on a reagent strip indicates bacterial infection. If the patient is asymptomatic, antibiotics are not normally required. If systemic symptoms are present, full microbiological analysis is needed to establish sensitivity and to aid prescription of antibiotics.
- *Glycosuria and ketones.* A positive reagent strip indicates possible diabetes mellitus. Blood tests should also be taken for diagnosis of other conditions, such as thyrotoxicosis.
- *Blood.* Further investigations are essential if blood is detected in the urine. It can indicate impaired renal function or bladder papillomas. However, it may also be detected in the urine of female patients during menstruation.

A simple urine test performed with reagent strips can reveal conditions that would remain undetected if not included as part of an assessment for urinary incontinence. It is an essential part of a nurse's assessment.

URODYNAMICS

Urodynamic investigations study the dynamics of the lower urinary tract – the bladder and urethra. They comprise uroflowmetry, cystometry and urethral pressure profile (UPP). Some patients will require a videocystometrogram, whereby the filling and voiding phases can be observed on a screen and the information stored on videotape.

The purpose of urodynamic studies is to define the pathophysiology of the bladder and urethra, and the investigations provide information about the way the bladder accommodates to increasing volumes, central nervous system control over the detrusor reflex and sensory qualities. There are now many urodynamic centres throughout the UK and a few satellite community centres run by specially trained nurses. These investigations are not appropriate for all patients because of their invasive nature, but they are essential prior to any surgical intervention, for both men and women. These studies form just one part of a range of investigations required for diagnosis.

Uroflowmetry

Uroflowmetry measures the rate at which the urine is voided, in millilitres passed per second (peak flow rate should be at least 15 ml/s for a volume of at least 150 ml). The patient sits on a commode or, if male, can void directly into a funnel of the machine.

The most common method for measuring the flow rate is by a rotating disc at the bottom of the funnel, which spins continuously as urine is voided onto it. As this happens, the motor demands more power in order to keep the disc rotating at a constant speed. The change in power required is then used to calculate the flow rate (Laker 1994). The patient is asked to attend the clinic with a full bladder, so this investigation can take place prior to cystometry. Ideally a series of flow rates should be taken, but this is not always

possible. It is essential, therefore, to ask the patient whether the flow and volume were 'normal'. If not normal for the patient, this should be noted on the recording. Privacy is important for this test as hesitancy and slow urine stream may be due to the embarrassment of someone else being in the room. Figure 2.15 shows some typical flow rate profiles.

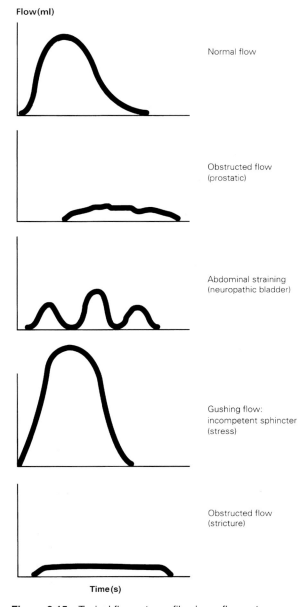

Flow(ml)

Normal flow

Obstructed flow (prostatic)

Abdominal straining (neuropathic bladder)

Gushing flow: incompetent sphincter (stress)

Obstructed flow (stricture)

Time(s)

Figure 2.15 Typical flow rate profiles in uroflowmetry.

Cystometrogram (CMG)

The patient may be investigated in the supine, sitting or standing position, and various provocative manoeuvres may be applied. Here the bladder pressure is recorded both during filling and when voiding. A straightforward CMG does not outline the bladder neck; this is where videocystometry is required to see whether the bladder neck stays closed or opens inappropriately.

It is not yet established how much patient information is advisable prior to an appointment because there is quite a high non-attendance rate. However, a suggested patient handout (Box 2.4) explaining the procedure is provided here.

Box 2.4 Urodynamic investigations: a patient's guide

1. Urodynamics investigates the functioning of your bladder.
2. The test takes about 40–60 minutes.
3. Try to drink 500 ml (1 pint) of water prior to the test so that you arrive with a fairly full bladder. You will not have to wait long for the test to begin.
4. You will undress and put on a gown which is provided.
5. You will be asked to empty your bladder into a commode-like toilet which is electronically connected to a recording machine. This measures the rate of the flow of urine.
6. You will then lie on a couch (or X-ray table, if pictures are to be taken) so that two small catheters can be put into the bladder. One fine catheter measures the pressure inside the bladder, another is for filling the bladder with water.
7. A small rubber balloon is placed just inside the rectum. This measures the pressure in your abdomen.
8. Water enters your bladder slowly and any bladder activity is recorded on the machine.
9. When you feel full the water flow is switched off and the filling catheter is removed. You will be asked to cough while still lying down so that any leakage can be noted.
10. When you stand up you will be asked to give a series of coughs and/or gentle movements to see whether leakage occurs.
11. Finally, you empty your bladder again on the commode-like toilet before the pressure catheters are removed.
12. The way your bladder is functioning will have been recorded and a diagnosis of the problem can be made.

The procedure

After the patient has emptied the bladder for the flowmetry test, the next part of the investigation is cystometry.

With the patient in a supine position and using a strictly aseptic technique, a Nelaton urethral catheter is inserted into the bladder. This is for filling the bladder with saline or radiopaque contrast. An intravesical pressure catheter – a polythene cannula 1 mm external diameter – is inserted at the same time. Any residual urine will be noted and measured and if necessary a specimen taken for culture. Next a rectal plug is inserted into the rectum, using a 2 mm external diameter water-filled polythene cannula, protected by a finger cot against faecal contamination. This measures the intra-abdominal pressure. The computer will subtract the intra-abdominal pressure from the intravesical pressure, thus giving the intrinsic intravesical pressure or detrusor pressure (see Fig. 2.16). The two pressure lines are connected to the cystometer and flushed with water to allow the recordings to take place.

The patient is asked to cough; this raises the abdominal pressure and therefore the total bladder pressure, but the detrusor pressure should show no rise. Bladder filling can then commence while the patient remains in the supine position or moves to a standing position with the pressure lines securely fastened to the leg with micropore tape.

Normal physiological filling of the bladder occurs at approximately 1 ml/min, but this is too slow for practical cystometry. A 'medium-fill' rate of between 10 and 100 ml/min is generally used. In patients with a suspected neuropathic bladder the filling rate is reduced to 10–20 ml/min because filling too quickly may give an abnormal rise in bladder pressure. 'Rapid-fill' rates (above 100 ml/min) are rarely used as they may initiate spurious detrusor contractions.

Cystometric recording

1. The infusion is started via an intravenous giving-set. Saline should be at body-warm temperature.

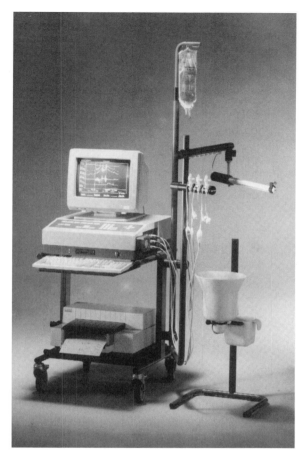

Figure 2.16 Dantec cystometry recorder. Courtesy: Dantec Electronics Ltd.

2. The patient is instructed to report the first sensation of bladder filling. This is marked FS (= first sensation) on the cystometrogram.
3. The patient is asked to suppress the desire to void and report when the urge is so strong that the bladder feels entirely filled. This volume is marked on the recording (maximum cystometric bladder capacity), and the infusion is stopped. The filling Nelaton catheter is then removed.
4. For provocative tests for detrusor instability or stress incontinence, the patient may now be asked to cough repeatedly and strongly, and to do on-the-spot star-jumps or walking.
5. The patient then empties the bladder as for uroflowmetry, but the pressure transducers

are brought in line with the symphysis pubis to prevent artificial pressure rise. During the voiding phase the patient is asked to try to stop the urine flow thus suppressing detrusor contraction. Voiding then continues to completion. The voided volume should equal the infused volume.
6. The pressure catheters are removed and the patient can dress before discussing the results.

Interpretation of cystometry recordings

Residual urine

Normally the bladder empties completely. In cases with residual urine, the amount may vary considerably from day to day in the same patient. A normal urinary residual is less than 50 ml.

Bladder resting pressure

The bladder resting pressure is often 5–15 cmH$_2$O in the supine position and 20–50 cmH$_2$O in the standing position, depending primarily on the weight of the intra-abdominal organs. Normally the detrusor pressure on filling is less than 10 cmH$_2$O for 300 ml or 15 cmH$_2$O for 500 ml.

First sensation to void

The first sensation (FS) reflects the functioning of the sensory pathways from the bladder. In a normal bladder, the first desire to void occurs at volumes between 150 and 250 ml, depending on the filling rate. If the detrusor is decompensated or the sensory nerve function is deficient, the first sensation to void occurs at larger volumes, and it may even be difficult for the patient to report any desire to void.

Maximal cystometric bladder capacity

The maximal cystometric bladder capacity depends on the filling rate, the sensory nerve function and the detrusor function. Normal capacity is 400–600 ml. In patients with an overactive detrusor or contracted bladder the capacity may vary from 50 to 250 ml. In hypotonic or 'floppy' bladders the capacity may be 500–1000 ml. A cystometric recorded maximal bladder capacity differs from the functional capacity as measured by voided volumes in micturition diaries or charts.

Bladder pressure during filling

The normal bladder accommodates to rapid changes in volume, from empty to maximal cystometric capacity, with a pressure increase of less than 10 cmH$_2$O for 300 ml or 15 cmH$_2$O for 500 ml. Abnormal increases in bladder pressure during filling may be due to fibrosis in the bladder wall (contracted bladder, low compliance), to detrusor contractions, or to movements during the investigation (e.g. talking, laughing or coughing). Straining causes abrupt pressure variations, with steep pressure increases and steep decreases. Detrusor contractions are seen as more gradual, bell-shaped increases in the bladder pressure. An overactive detrusor function is characterized by involuntary detrusor contractions during filling of the bladder, either spontaneous or after provocative manoeuvres, which cannot be suppressed by the patient.

Summary

Detrusor functioning reflects the integrated functioning of the central and peripheral neuromuscular control of the lower urinary tract. Peripheral efferent and afferent neuronal pathways connect the muscular and sensory structures in the bladder and urethra with the central nervous system (CNS).

An overactive detrusor function may be due to lesions in the CNS or to disease in the bladder or the urethra. An overactive detrusor function may also be diagnosed in normal, asymptomatic patients. This reflects the fact that all diagnostic investigations have a certain proportion of false-positive and false-negative test results in relation to a given symptom or diagnosis. Hence there is a need for more than one diagnostic approach: cystometry is often done in conjunction with bladder ultrasound.

Figures 2.17–2.21 show some urodynamic line graphs to show normal filling cystometry, stress incontinence, sensory urge, detrusor instability and an underactive (hypotonic) bladder.

Videocystometry

The procedure is essentially the same as a plain CMG, except that it needs to be carried out in an X-ray department and a radiopaque contrast is used for the filling medium. Radiographs can be taken intermittently throughout the procedure as requested by the investigator while viewing on a screen monitor. On the monitor the bladder neck and urethra can be observed during filling and

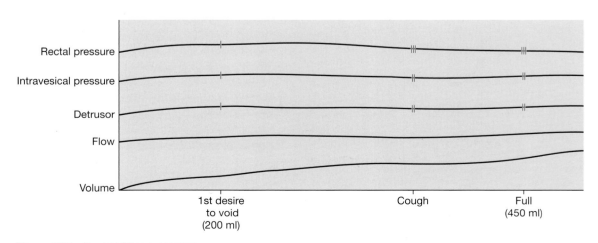

Figure 2.17 Normal filling cystometry.

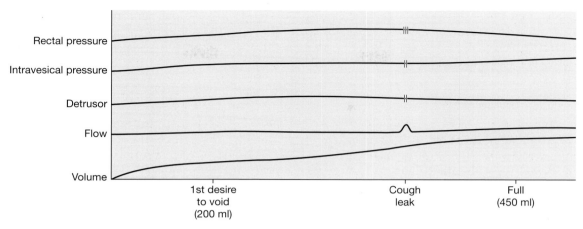

Figure 2.18   Cystometry recording for stress incontinence.

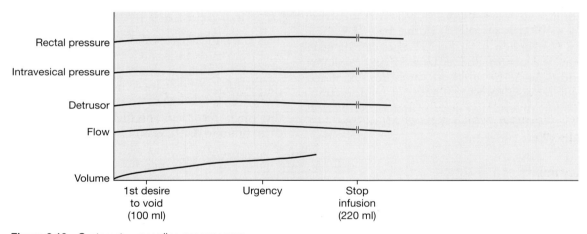

Figure 2.19   Cystometry recording sensory urge.

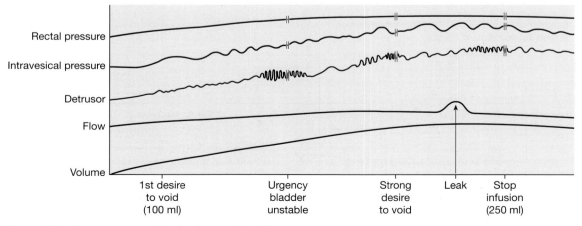

Figure 2.20   Cystometry recording for detrusor instability.

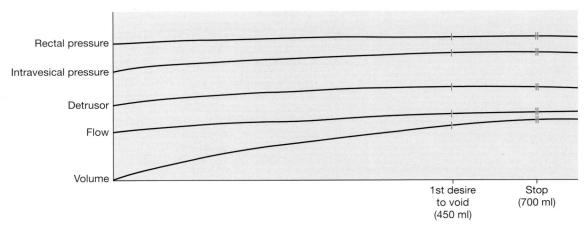

Figure 2.21 Cystometry recording for an underactive bladder (hypotonic).

voiding. The information is stored on a videotape. This method is preferable in the male if an outflow obstruction is suspected as it can be seen where the obstruction is located (i.e. prostatic, bladder neck or urethral stricture). A video screening also shows evidence of bladder trabeculation, diverticulae and/or ureteric reflux, and this significantly enhances the diagnostic capability of the procedure.

Urethral pressure profile (UPP)

This is the measurement of the intraurethral pressure from the bladder neck to the external meatus. It involves passing a catheter along the urethra into the bladder, and then mechanically withdrawing it at a constant rate so that the pressure along the urethra can be recorded. This test needs to be repeated three times to reach an accurate recording.

KEY POINTS FOR PRACTICE

- Clear understanding of the normal function of the bladder and lower urinary tract is important in order to recognize and understand abnormal function and to underpin care strategies.
- Careful and thorough patient assessment takes time and empathy (not sympathy). It may require more than one session to complete.
- Symptomatology can provide good indications of underlying problems but further diagnostic

investigations may be needed and clear protocols and pathways for referral should be established.
- Not all symptoms of incontinence are due to abnormal bladder and lower urinary tract function. Coexisting problems can affect capacity to achieve and maintain continence.

REFERENCES

Andrew J, Nathan P W 1964 Lesions of the anterior frontal lobes and disturbances of micturition and defaecation. Brain 87: 233–262

Argyle M 1982 Verbal and nonverbal communication. In: The psychology of interpersonal behaviour. Penguin, Harmondsworth

Bayliss V, Cherry M, Locke R, Salter L 2000 Pathways for continence care: development of the pathways. British Journal of Nursing 9(17): 1165–1172

Berne M R, Levy M N 1990 Principles of physiology. Wolfe, St Louis

Bullock N, Sibley G, Whitaker R 1991 Essential urology. Churchill Livingstone, Edinburgh

De Groat W C 1990 Central neural control of the lower urinary tract. In: The neurobiology of incontinence (Ciba Foundation Symposium). John Wiley, Chichester, pp 27–56

De Groat W C 1994 Neurophysiology of the pelvic organs. In: Rushton D N (ed) Handbook of neuro-urology. Marcel Dekker, New York

DeLancy J O 1990 Functional anatomy of the female lower urinary tract and pelvic floor. In: The neurobiology of incontinence (Ciba Foundation Symposium). John Wiley, Chichester, pp 57–76

Department of Health 2000 Good practice in continence services. DoH, London

Feneley R C L 1986 Normal micturition and its control. In: Mandelstam D (ed) Incontinence and its management, 2nd edn. Croom Helm, London

Gilpin S A, Gosling J A, Smith A R B, Warrell D 1989 The pathogenesis of genito-urinary prolapse and stress incontinence of urine: a histological and histochemical study. British Journal of Obstetrics and Gynaecology 96: 15–23

Gosling J A, Dixon J S, Himpherson J A 1983 Functional anatomy of the urinary tract: an integrated text and colour atlas. Churchill Livingstone, Edinburgh

Hald T 1984 Mechanisms of continence. In: Stanton S (ed) Clinical gynaecologic urology. Mosby, St Louis

Harrison S M 1983 Stress incontinence and the physiotherapist. Physiotherapist 69: 144–147

Hellstrom L, Ekelund P, Milsom I, Mellstrom D 1990 The prevalence of urinary incontinence and the use of incontinence aids in 85-year-old men and women. Age and Ageing 19(6): 383–389

Herzog A R, Fulz N H 1990 Prevalence and incidence of urinary incontinence in community dwelling populations. Journal of the American Geriatrics Society 38: 273–281

Kassis A, Schick E 1993 Frequency-volume chart pattern in a healthy female population. British Journal of Urology 72: 708–710

Laker C 1994 Urological nursing. Scutari Press, London

Larson G, Victor A 1988 Micturition patterns in a healthy female population studied with a frequency/volume chart. Journal of Urology and Nephrology (Suppl.) 114: 53–57

Laycock J 1994 Pelvic floor reeducation for the promotion of continence. In: Roe B (ed) The promotion and management of continence. Prentice Hall, Hemel Hempstead

Mahoney F I, Barthel D 1965 Functional evaluation: the Barthel Index. Maryland State Medical Journal 14: 61–65

Mahony D T, Laferte R O, Blais D J 1977 Integral storage and voiding reflexes. Urology 1: 95–105

Mahony D T, Laferte R O, Blais D J 1980 Incontinence of urine due to instability of micturition reflexes (Parts 1 and 2). Urology 3: 229–239, 379–388

Nazarco L 1994 Drugs, continence and elderly people. Primary Health Care 4(1): 19–22

NIH Consensus Conference 1989 Urinary incontinence in adults. JAMA 261: 2685

Ouslander J G, Uman G C, Urman H N, Rubenstein L Z 1987 Incontinence among nursing home patients: clinical and functional correlates. Journal of the American Geriatrics Society 35: 324–330

Rud T, Andersson K E, Asmussen M 1980 Factors maintaining the intraurethral pressure in women. Investigative Urology 17: 343–347

Saito M, Kondo A, Kato T, Yamada Y 1993 Frequency-volume charts: comparison of frequency between elderly and adult patients. British Journal of Urology 72: 38–41

Smith P S, Smith L J 1987 The role of maturation and learning. In: Roe B (ed) Continence and incontinence. Croom Helm, London

Tortora G, Grabowski S 1993 Principles of anatomy and physiology. Harper Collins, New York

Winder A 2001 Continence assessment in primary care: what is the next step? British Journal of Community Nursing 6(10): 520–524

3

Mostly female

Mary Dolman

---

*'There is no English soul
More stronger to direct you, than
yourself.'*

William Shakespeare

INTRODUCTION

Should one's quality of life be impaired by urinary incontinence just because of being a woman? Stories about bladder problems following childbirth have abounded for generations. Now in the 21st century the myths about accepting such problems have almost been dispelled as women have better information and educational advice before and during pregnancy. They now know how and where to seek help as soon as any changes in bladder function are noticed.

Although both men and women can experience incontinence, the prevalence studies mentioned in Chapter 1 indicate that women are much more susceptible to this condition. According to Cardozo & Cutner (1993), 15–30% of women in all age groups are affected. It is not difficult, therefore, to understand that the psychological, occupational, physical and sexual aspects of women's lives can be affected. This chapter focuses on women and will discuss why urinary incontinence is more prevalent in females.

Although women can suffer from any of the types of incontinence discussed in Chapter 2, stress incontinence occurs almost exclusively in females and will form a major focus of this chapter. Urge incontinence or conditions which show mixed elements of both urge and stress incontinence are also common in women and will be addressed later in the chapter, although it should be recognized that this problem also occurs in men (see Chapter 4).

A preventative approach for reducing the risk of incontinence, by the use of pelvic floor exercises, will be highlighted, as will the other conservative, non-surgical nursing interventions.

Although surgery has been a primary treatment for stress incontinence, its success lies in the competencies of the surgeon. Types of surgery will be explained, but the main emphasis of the chapter is on the prevention of incontinence plus the conservative treatments that primary healthcare members of a multidisciplinary team should be able to initiate when a woman asks for advice.

EMBRYOLOGICAL DEVELOPMENT OF THE VAGINA AND URETHRA

It is important to know that between the eighth and twelfth week of intrauterine life, the urogenital membrane forms the distal part of the urethra, the upper bladder and the vagina in the female (Fig. 3.1). Therefore, the urethra and trigone muscle of the bladder have the same hormone-dependent tissue as the vagina. The submucosal folds along the urethra help to provide a 'watertight' seal for maintaining continence. The mucosal folds are sensitive to oestrogen and when fully oestrogenized provide the watertight seal. When there is oestrogen depletion or deficiency – at the

menopause or lowered oestrogen levels immediately prior to menstruation – the mucosal folds become less effective. This may explain why so many women say their incontinence is worse during the week before a period.

DEFINITION OF STRESS INCONTINENCE

The International Continence Society defines stress incontinence as 'the involuntary loss of urine when the intravesical pressure exceeds the maximum urethral closure pressure in the absence of detrusor activity'. Stress incontinence occurs due to the deficiency in the urethral closure mechanism during episodes of raised intra-abdominal pressure such as coughing, sneezing, running, etc. (Fig. 3.2).

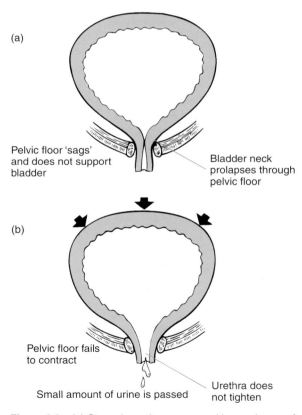

(a)

Pelvic floor 'sags' and does not support bladder

Bladder neck prolapses through pelvic floor

(b)

Pelvic floor fails to contract

Small amount of urine is passed

Urethra does not tighten

Figure 3.2 (a) Stress incontinence caused by weakness of pelvic floor muscles. (b) Coughing, laughing, running, etc. cause a rise in intra-abdominal pressure which results in leakage of urine. Reproduced with kind permission of Coloplast Ltd.

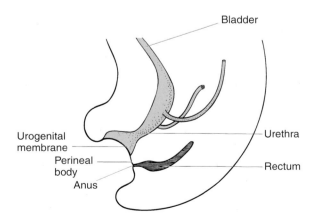

Bladder

Urogenital membrane

Perineal body

Anus

Urethra

Rectum

Figure 3.1 Diagram showing the fetal urogenital membrane at about the eighth week of intrauterine life.

POSSIBLE CAUSES OF STRESS INCONTINENCE IN WOMEN

Causes of stress incontinence are to be found when there is an incompetent bladder neck closure with weakened smooth urethral muscle, atrophic changes in urethral mucosa, weakened supporting ligaments and striated pelvic floor muscles. These changes may be due to primary injury of the tissues concerned, such as in multiple parity, prolonged difficult labours, forceps-assisted deliveries and additional perineal trauma. Degenerative changes occur due to hormonal deficiency or age-related atrophy of the tissues. Neurological defects affect the pudendal nerve serving the pelvic floor striated muscles (Hald 1975).

Urinary stress incontinence is a common symptom in women and is associated with pregnancy, vaginal delivery, previous surgery for incontinence, congenital weakness of the pelvic floor muscles and the menopause (Tapp et al 1988).

Research study 3.1 The role of pregnancy and childbirth in partial denervation of the pelvic floor

A study by Allen & Warrell (1987) on 40 primigravid women showed a dramatic change in urinary symptoms during and after pregnancy compared with pre-pregnancy urinary control. A questionnaire was completed at 36 weeks' gestation recording urinary control, and pelvic floor function was measured by a perineometer. At between 2 and 6 days postpartum, any changes in urinary control since delivery were recorded and the pelvic floor squeeze measured. This was repeated 2 months later. Stress incontinence rose from 13% pre-pregnancy to 69% during pregnancy and 43% postnatally. It was found that the vaginal squeeze pressure fell significantly after delivery and although there was some recovery at the 2-month postnatal examination, the pressures did not return to the antenatal level.

According to Snooks et al (1985), patients with stress incontinence have abnormal conduction in the perineal branch of the pudendal nerve which innervates the periurethral striated muscle. Injury to the nerve supply may occur at childbirth and the pudendal nerve terminal motor latency (electrical conduction) is prolonged 24–72 hours after delivery. Damage to the innervation of the striated urinary and anal sphincter muscles can be detected by an increase in the pudendal nerve terminal latency after delivery, by electromyography (EMG) studies of the *pubococcygeus* and *puborectalis* muscles. The severity of this abnormality can be detected by electrophysiological techniques (EMG) and can be related to the duration of the second stage of labour. Other factors suggesting difficult labour are forceps delivery and multiparity.

Donald (1979), in writing about practical obstetric problems, refers to stress incontinence in both early and late stages of pregnancy as well as the stresses in labour, which may weaken the fascial supports of the bladder neck. He states that 'disability' results, if not straight away, at least in years to come, particularly at the time of the menopause.

There is still some confusion between oestrogen deficiency in postmenopausal women and changes in urethral tissue due to ageing (Carlile et al 1987), although Guthrie (2001) states that natural menopause is not a significant risk factor for urinary incontinence but women who have had a hysterectomy were more likely to experience incontinence than their counterparts. Histological examination along the length of the urethra shows it to be lined with epithelium: stratified squamous, pseudostratified columnar and very occasionally transitional. With advancing age, there is a gradual change from squamous to columnar epithelium. As age increases there is a decrease in the volume of connective tissue but there is no change in the smooth muscle components. The age-related changes in some parts of the female urethra may result in impaired urethral function. However, Benness et al (1991) found that oestrogen deficiency after the menopause did not seem to be an important factor in the pathogenesis of symptoms of urinary incontinence.

Surprisingly, stress incontinence and voiding difficulty symptoms were more common in women on hormone replacement therapy (HRT). It was suggested by Benness et al (1991) that the progesterone phase of HRT increased urinary frequency, nocturia and urgency. Burton & Dobson (1993) investigating this possibility further found that if the symptoms of frequency, nocturia and urgency were increased in the progesterone phase, then the urine flow rates would be increased and this could be a method of treating women with voiding difficulties. They concluded that progesterone appears to increase the urine flow rate on 'normal' bladder function in women during the progesterone phase of HRT. However, they are uncertain why this happens other than by relaxing the urinary sphincter.

It has been suggested that obesity can weaken the pelvic floor muscles supporting the bladder owing to the increased strain of extra weight, and thus precipitate stress incontinence (Bump et al 1992). Clinical experience has shown that women have a reduction in their stress incontinence symptoms with the loss of only a few kilograms in weight. A chronic cough, as seen in women with chest complaints, also puts continued strain on the pelvic floor musculature, as does chronic constipation or occupations requiring heavy lifting.

INCONTINENCE RELATED TO PREGNANCY AND CHILDBIRTH

About 46% of women complain of urinary incontinence during pregnancy (Chiarelli 1991), but Cardozo et al (1993) state that up to 55% of pregnant women have stress incontinence depending on the gestation. When it occurs antenatally it is normally transient and usually resolves postnatally; but when it occurs for the first time postnatally, it is likely to be more severe and permanent owing to a weakened urethral sphincter closure pressure.

During pregnancy the role of the hormone *relaxin* also needs to be taken into account. The normal physiology of the menstrual cycle causes relaxin to circulate in the bloodstream even before the ovum is fertilized in the fallopian tube. This hormone is responsible for softening all the ligaments and muscles of the pelvic outlet so that the baby's head can be pushed out at delivery. When the ovum is fertilized, the levels of relaxin continue to rise and reach a peak at about the twelfth week of pregnancy. The tissues continue to soften and the growing fetus acts as a stretching force.

Allen & Warrell (1987) found stress incontinence in pregnancy to be significantly increased due to partial denervation of the pudendal nerve which supplies the striated muscle of the pelvic floor along with pelvic branches of the sacral plexus. This partial denervation results in reduced postural tone of the sphincter mechanism, but is usually resolved postpartum.

Labour and delivery

According to Cardozo et al (1993) 'Intrapartum events which may have a profound effect on postpartum lower urinary tract function include: the method of delivery, the length of time of the labour, and the weight of the baby'. A long first stage and a long active second stage (pushing) have both been shown to result in urethral sphincter damage. Changes in the position of the bladder neck during labour may result in the stretching of supporting muscles and ligaments which can also cause damage to the urethral sphincter closure mechanism.

Poor bladder management during labour can result in voiding difficulties such as overflow incontinence, particularly if an epidural anaesthetic has been administered. Labour causes a decrease in bladder sensation and combined with epidural analgesia may result in an overdistension of the bladder unless urine output is carefully monitored (Dolman 1992). It has been shown by Weil et al (1983) that a single overdistension of the detrusor muscle can result in long-term voiding difficulties because the detrusor cannot be contracted for long enough or strongly enough to empty the bladder completely.

Women who have caesarean section will not be at risk of damage to the pudendal nerve supplying the pelvic floor muscles, but the hormonal changes in pregnancy which may affect continence will still apply.

Perineal trauma: episiotomy and forceps-assisted delivery

Trauma to the perineal body, perineum and layers of the pelvic floor muscles, which results from overstretching with additional use of forceps, tearing or episiotomy, causes damage to the pudendal nerve. Denervation causes loss of sensation and the ability to move the pelvic floor muscles.

HEALTH PROMOTION FOR CONTINENCE

Health promotion for continence must surely start in higher education when teenagers are receptive to information. Using an anatomical model, the position of the pelvic floor muscle, its role in maintaining continence and all the issues around a healthy pelvic floor muscle can be discussed. The awareness of pelvic floor muscle function is most important for this age group. For younger age groups, it can be the role of the school nurse to help children realize the difference between good and bad toileting habits; eat healthy, balanced diets to avoid constipation; understand the reasons for having an adequate fluid intake; and ensure plenty of exercise.

Box 3.1 shows a health promotion checklist for women which will contribute to the promotion of continence.

History of pelvic floor exercises

An American gynaecologist, Arnold Kegel (1948), was the first to report on an uncontrolled study of 500 women doing pelvic floor exercises. Consequently in America they are referred to as 'Kegel exercises'. He reported a 'cure' rate of 84%, but 'cure' was not defined. He recommended 300 contractions a day plus the use of a perineometer twice daily for resistance exercises and for giving the woman biofeedback. Kegel described the weak muscles as a 'syndrome of lack of awareness of function and coordination of the pubococcygeus

---

Box 3.1 Health promotion checklist – a woman's guide

1. *Diet*:
   Eat balanced nutritional foods.
   Eat 18–20 g fibre daily to avoid constipation.
   Lose weight if necessary.
   Drink semiskimmed milk for calcium intake to help prevent osteoporosis.
2. *Chronic cough*:
   Treat underlying chest condition to reduce coughing episodes. (Chronic coughing causes additional strain on the pelvic floor muscles but should not stop women from trying to strengthen them.)
   Stop smoking as this causes coughing, as the increased pressure is transmitted to the pelvic floor muscles.
3. *Fluid intake*:
   Daily fluid intake should be approximately 1–2 litres (2–4 pints).
   Limit alcohol intake: it stimulates bladder contraction.
   Coffee, tea and drinks with caffeine stimulate the bladder: try alternative fluids.
4. *Medications*:
   Review medications that affect the bladder/bowel directly or indirectly, and discuss with GP. (Sometimes medications can be stopped or dosages reduced, or the time of day that medication is taken can be changed.)
5. *Toileting habits*:
   Allow the bladder to fill properly (350–500 ml).
   Do not 'hold on' for more than 5–6 hours.
   Make sure the bladder empties completely.
6. *Before pregnancy*:
   Regular pelvic floor exercises to obtain maximum strength in the muscle for and during pregnancy.
7. *After childbirth*:
   Restart pelvic floor exercises when the perineum is no longer sore.
8. *Professional advice*:
   Ask a skilled professional to assess the pelvic floor muscle function about 6–8 weeks postnatally.
   Seek professional advice as soon as any prolonged change in bladder/bowel function is noticed.

Research study 3.2 Continence advisor demonstrates value of education about pelvic floor exercises in older teenagers

Dolman (1994a) reported on two schools' participation in pelvic floor muscle education for girls aged 13–16 years. It was found that the younger teenagers were 'giggly', 'embarrassed' and 'shy' about the subject, but the older teenagers (15–16 year olds) were receptive to the information. Overall, the girls evaluated the session as 'important knowledge to have' and 'more of this sort of thing should be introduced into schools'. The results of a short questionnaire distributed 6 weeks following the educational session indicated that 85% had tried pelvic floor exercises more than three times within a month. The educational session included:

- Where is the pelvic floor muscle?
- What is its function?
- Why is it important to exercise these muscles?
- How are these muscles exercised?

Ten schools were approached, but only two agreed to the pelvic floor educational session for the girls. This was made possible because of the two enthusiastic school nurses and the teachers. The cooperation of school nurses and teachers is essential for this subject to be introduced as an aspect of 'health' promotion for this age group.

muscle'. He also noted that 30% of women could not elicit a contraction on command.

Little activity in this field followed the American presentation, but in recent decades there has been renewed interest in pelvic floor exercises as a method of treatment for stress incontinence and bladder control. Gomer-Jones (1963) adopted Kegel's method of exercises and emphasized the importance of teaching awareness of the pubo-coccygeus muscle and its ability to draw in, draw up and retract the perineum. Emphasis was also placed on the need to hold the muscles in this contracted state and then relax the muscles completely during half-hourly exercise sessions. Gomer-Jones maintained that more than ten contractions at each session would cause fatigue and would therefore be counterproductive.

Pelvic floor exercises – the evidence-base

The purpose of pelvic floor exercises is to increase *muscle volume* (Bø et al 1991). Theoretically, increased bulk of the pelvic floor muscles will result in an increase of urethral closure pressure and stronger reflex contractions following a quick rise in intra-abdominal pressure. The goal for exercising these muscles is therefore to increase their strength, endurance and power, thereby enhancing postural tone and the reflex activity when the intra-abdominal pressure is raised as in coughing, lifting, running, etc. (see Box 3.2).

The striated muscle comprises both slow-twitch fibres (Type I) and fast-twitch fibres (Type II) and when exercising the muscle both fibre types must be exercised. According to Doughty (1994), this muscle group should be treated in the same way as any other striated skeletal muscle which is exercised.

Studies on pelvic floor exercises, however, differ in terms of grading the muscle function, intensity, duration, frequency and compliance with the exercises, which can sometimes make comparisons of their effectiveness difficult.

There is substantial written evidence to demonstrate that pelvic floor exercises reduce the incidence of incontinence, both urinary and faecal (Bø et al 1991, Glavind et al 1996, Glazener et al 2001, O'Brien & Long 1995).

Box 3.2 How to do your pelvic floor exercises

1. Sit comfortably with knees slightly apart. Without moving your tummy muscle or bottom, try to squeeze the muscle around the back passage. Pretend you are trying to stop wind from escaping!
2. Now try the same with the front part of the muscle. Again, without moving the tummy or bottom, squeeze and lift the muscle into the vagina. Moving this front part of the muscle is harder than that mentioned above and takes time to practise.
3. Once you can tighten and lift the muscles (lifting is as though you are taking the muscle up steps one at a time), pull as hard as you can and hold for as long as you can (e.g. 5 seconds), then relax. Repeat this 5–10 times with a good 'rest' between each contraction. Do the group of 5–10 exercises as many times a day as you can without making your muscle ache.
4. Also try to squeeze your muscle quickly like a one-second 'flick', then relax. Repeat this five times. Only do this once before your group of slow contractions.
5. These two actions of moving your muscle – i.e. slowly and then fast – will strengthen the pelvic floor muscle so that you will be able to do more repetitions and hold the squeeze longer. This will make the muscles strong and powerful.
6. To help you identify the correct muscles, you may wish to try placing two fingers into your vagina and then squeezing around the fingers with the pelvic floor muscles only. This could be tried when you are in the bath.
7. If in doubt about exercising properly, then do not hesitate to contact your healthcarer who should be able to advise you.
8. Pelvic floor exercises are an important aspect of health promotion for life for all women.

Women have often measured their own improvement after a pelvic floor exercise programme by saying there is a reduction in pad wearing, or their quality of life has improved. Clinicians can add more clinical data when digitally assessing the pelvic floor muscle as supported by Brink et al (1989) in conjunction with a graded scale proposed by Laycock (1987). This is known as the *Oxford Grading Scale* (Fig. 3.3). Digital assessment has the advantage of being readily available to a clinician, whereas a perineometer or biofeedback devices are not always available to all clinicians. Isherwood & Rane (2000) compared the results of measuring the strength of the pelvic floor muscle using a digital assessment and perineometer assessment, and concluded a good agreement between the two methods of assessing.

0 = nil	3 = moderate
1 = flicker	4 = good
2 = weak	5 = strong

Figure 3.3 The Oxford Grading System for assessing pelvic floor strength.

Digital assessment of the pelvic floor

The woman should be put at ease as much as possible and a clear explanation of the examination will help to achieve this. When she is lying in the crooked supine position notice her body language for any resistance to the examination and reassure once again. Observe the condition of the skin in the genital area and signs of prolapse or haemorrhoids. Ask for the perineum to be tightened and drawn upwards towards the pubic bone. This will give an indication of pelvic floor contraction or not. With a gloved hand part the labia and ask the patient to cough. Note if there is any urine leakage, perineal descent or obvious prolapse. (A prolapse of the bladder is a cystocele, prolapsed rectum is a rectocele and a prolapsed womb is an enterocele.) Place a lubricated gloved index finger into the vagina about 2.5 cm and palpate around 360° to detect areas of sensitivity, pain, discomfort or any irregularities. Support the bladder neck with the tip of the index finger and ask the patient to cough. Note if there is palpable descent of the bladder or bladder neck hypermobility. Then sweep the index finger at 4 and 8 o'clock of the pelvic floor muscle, noting any differences in bulk and sensitivity. Ask the patient to cough again and try to determine if there is any reflex activity of the muscle. The next stage of the assessment is to place the index and middle fingers into the vagina no more than 4 cm and part the fingers slightly (this may not be possible if the introitus is narrow). By stretching the pelvic floor muscle this might be enough stimulation for it to contract and it also gives the patient a better awareness for isolating the muscle. Ask the patient to squeeze around the fingers with the pelvic floor muscle and note the strength of the contraction using the Oxford Grading Scale shown in Figure 3.3.

Once the patient has understood what she is supposed to be doing and can comply, determine the length of the contraction and number of repetitions of the slow contractions and then the number of possible fast contractions.

An easy way to remember the full assessment of the pelvic floor examination is to use the mnemonic PERFECT (Box 3.3) as suggested by Laycock (1994).

Box 3.3 Pelvic floor examination – PERFECT	
P = POWER	(Using the Oxford Grading Scale, Fig. 3.3) Both fast- and slow-twitch muscle fibres are being used. 'Nil' indicates there is no movement in the muscle whereas flicker describes a fluttering of the muscle. Weak contraction shows a weak pressure around the fingers but is not fluttering. Moderate, good and strong contractions are steady increases in pressure around the examining fingers. All subjective measurements but with experience the grading becomes obvious.
E = ENDURANCE	The length of time in seconds the pelvic floor muscle can hold a contraction; this is using the slow-twitch fibres.
R = REPETITIONS	The number of repetitions of the specific contractions that can be done with a 5-second rest between without the muscle fatiguing.
F = FAST	After a 2-minute rest, determine the contractibility of the fast-twitch fibres. A quick contraction with no holding is required and note the number attainable up to ten times. These muscle fibres fatigue easily as they are for reflex activity and not for endurance.
E = EVERY **C = CONTRACTION** **T = TIMED**	All this reminds the assessor to monitor progress by timing all contractions. A summary of the above can be seen in Box 3.4, A nurse's guide to pelvic floor muscle assessment.

Box 3.4 A nurse's guide to pelvic floor muscle assessment

With the woman lying in a supine position, hips flexed and abducted:

Observe
- skin excoriation in pubic and groin areas
- scar tissue in perineum from suturing
- alignment of perineal body to vaginal opening
- vaginal tissue for vaginitis by parting the labia with the index and middle fingers and observing colour
- for prolapsing of urethra, bladder, rectum or cervix into the vagina, by asking the woman to cough repeatedly.

Assess
- Place a gloved and lubricated index finger 2.5 cm into the introitus and palpate the rim of the 4 o'clock and 8 o'clock positions for muscle bulk.
- Check the resilience of the triangular ligament by asking the patient to squeeze.
- Introduce the index and middle fingers into the vagina and palpate for prolapsing of the urethra, bladder, rectum or cervical descent.
- With the fingers spread laterally in an anterior–posterior position, ask the woman to squeeze and lift the examining fingers as hard as possible. Grade the muscle strength as per the Oxford Grading System. Check for power difference on right and left sides of muscle (skill comes with experience).
- Assess muscle fatigue by counting, in seconds, the length of time the muscle is able to stay contracted. Ensure this is 'isolated' pubococcygeal activity.
- Count the number of repetitions the woman can do to evaluate endurance, ensuring an 'active' relaxation phase of the muscle.
- Record the number of quick, one-second contractions (flicks) the woman can perform.

Example of assessment recorded:

4	6	5	4
Good contraction	Held 6 seconds	Repeated 5 times	4 flicks

Now you can set a personalized target for a daily home exercise programme provided the woman has recorded a grade 3 or above.

Research studies 3.3 and 3.4 Long-term effects of pelvic floor exercises

Study 3.3
The long-term effects of pelvic floor exercises and bladder retraining were evaluated by O'Brien & Long (1995) on 229 women, 4 years after their first randomized controlled trial of the management of incontinence in primary care. Using a similar questionnaire they asked the women about their continence status in respect of pad usage, exercises or other treatments in the intervening 4 years. The results showed 69% of the women had either maintained their original improvement or cure or had improved further, although 16% had deteriorated and a further 15% neither benefited from the original programme nor had further change. They noted that only 27% of women did their exercises for more than a year and 61% exercised for less than a year while 12% stopped exercises immediately. In conclusion it was felt that pelvic floor exercises for 1 year or more was strongly associated with improvement or maintenance (56/61) of benefit compared with exercises for less than a year (102/168).

Study 3.4
Bø & Talseth (1994) conducted a long-term follow-up on women who had had a 6-month intensive pelvic floor exercise programme 5 years earlier; they reported 70% ($n = 20$) of participants as satisfied with their condition. These 'satisfied' women avoided surgery, but in both studies the 'improved' or 'cured' had, initially, relatively mild incontinence. Although the outcomes were self-reports, the objectivity was confirmed by pad tests and palpation for pelvic floor strength.

These long-term results indicate that exercises to maintain an effective urethral closure pressure, thus preventing, reducing or eliminating urinary incontinence symptoms, are needed for at least 3–6 months. To date there is no research to show what a lifetime maintenance programme *should* entail, but without doubt an ongoing exercise regime requires each individual to have motivation and compliance. Some patients find a maintenance regime of 2 or 3 days a week beneficial but it is unknown if this continues for life.

Verbal instruction for pelvic floor exercises: is it enough?

Bump et al (1991) assessed women's performance of pelvic floor exercises following brief verbal instruction. The results confirmed that this method of instruction did not adequately prepare a woman to start an exercise programme, and endorsed the need for a digital pelvic floor muscle assessment.

Many women require some method of *performance feedback* in order to isolate the muscle function and muscle behaviour. To re-educate the correct muscle action, a woman must be able to squeeze, lift, hold and relax the pelvic floor (Laycock 1994). Some women are unable to contract the proper muscles when given verbal instruction; they often 'bear down' or contract the gluteal and abdominal muscles exclusively or in combination with contraction of the pelvic floor. A digital palpation will give a woman awareness of the muscles to contract and identify the correct action required for successful pelvic floor exercises. Dolman (1994b) found that 71% of women who had been examined vaginally were doing pelvic floor exercises, compared with 59% who had not been so examined. However, it is not always possible or desirable for a woman to have a digital pelvic floor assessment, so in these cases verbal or written instructions will have to suffice. There are many leaflets available to patients on how to perform pelvic floor exercises (Continence Foundation or commercial companies) and most specialist continence units have their own leaflets to hand out.

The stop–start test: a question of validity

Bump et al (1991) state: 'the worst way to instruct women is to ask them to interrupt the urinary stream repeatedly during micturition'. Reasons for this statement are, first, that most women are unable to interrupt their urinary flow; second, the bladder's storing ability is not improved by interfering with the emptying function; and third, contracting the sphincter in the middle of normal micturition encourages vesicosphincter dyssynergia.

It has also been noted in clinical practice that some women can stop the flow of urine even when there is no palpable contraction of the pelvic floor muscles. A possible explanation for this may be the inhibitory factor on detrusor contraction from the cortical centre, i.e. it is inhibited detrusor contraction that stops the flow of urine, rather than the contraction of the pelvic floor muscles. This is an unsupported speculation but often seen in practice.

Sexual benefits of pelvic floor exercises

The pubococcygeus has often been referred to as the 'love muscle'. Women with strong pelvic floor muscles seem to enjoy the bonus of good sexual response, as found in a study of orgasm by Graber & Kline-Graber (1979). They reported that orgasm was significantly related to maximum pubococcygeal squeeze pressure. The pelvic floor muscles are directly reponsible for the amount of sensation that women feel during intercourse (Chiarelli 1991). The vaginal mucosa is not well endowed with sensation and most vaginal sensations come from the pelvic floor muscles that loop around and behind the vagina. The pubococcygeus also directly affects the amount of sexual sensation male partners feel – by tightening these muscles the woman is able to exert a firmer grip.

The nerve endings in the muscles respond to being stretched, so the firmer and stronger the muscle is, the more it responds to the erect penis. As the glans of the penis moves back and forth during intercourse, the firm muscles rhythmically stretch and relax, thus heightening vaginal sensations. The pubococcygeus is also responsible for helping to lubricate the vaginal walls during foreplay and intercourse, so, sexually speaking, these muscles play a vital role.

To summarize, a strong pelvic floor muscle will:

- increase vaginal lubrication during foreplay and intercourse
- enhance sexual sensation vaginally
- increase orgasmic response
- enhance the maintenance of urinary continence.

Compliance with exercises

Helping women to remember to do the exercises is an important part of the education process. In a study by Dolman & Chase (1996) it was suggested that in order to maximize compliance with pelvic floor exercises, health professionals need to provide women with more information and to develop techniques that help women to remember to perform them. A suggestion is to incorporate the exercises into their daily routine where the activity is repetitive, i.e. after each visit to the toilet, having a drink, taking and picking up children from school. Some women like to keep a diary and tick off how many times they have done the exercises each day (Fig. 3.4). Conversely, this can also put women off when they see that days have elapsed without doing any pelvic floor exercises!

Week/date	Mon	Tues	Wed	Thurs	Fri	Sat	Sun
1							
2							
3							
4							
5							

Figure 3.4 An example of a weekly diary to record the total number of exercises per day.

In the report by O'Brien & Long (1995) they demonstrated the advantages of even a short 3-week course of training in continence assessment and management in primary care. In their 4-year follow-up of women who had been assessed by a suitably trained nurse, who taught them pelvic floor exercises and/or bladder re-education, 69% (158/229) had either maintained their original improvement or cure or had improved further (see Research study 3.3). These authors concluded that training in assessment techniques in primary care can offer a practical, accessible and acceptable service for all women with urinary incontinence. This service provision would also benefit secondary care by ensuring that patients requiring further treatment are appropriately referred.

There has been further development for continence assessment at a first level in both primary care and acute Trusts, and pathways for continence care (Bayliss et al 2000) are being implemented, or an adaptation, in many primary care trusts. Nurses are trained at a basic level of knowledge regarding continence symptoms, urinalysis testing and first-line interventions (e.g. pelvic floor exercises, bladder retraining and fluid/dietary intake). If there is a variation from normal parameters measured by evidence-based symptomatology (a symptom chart is provided) the assessor knows where to refer on for more experienced assessment and treatment. This saves the patient having an unnecessary or inappropriate referral when treatment and advice can be given at first level. The forms used are one page, user friendly and are accompanied by charts showing normal values, i.e. normal amount of daily fluid intake required according to the person's body mass index. An audit can be carried out on the assessment forms by the continence services to show that: the system is working; there is no duplication of tests; care is consistent and within existing resources; and care is given in partnership with the patient. Ultimately care pathways in continence should help reduce the cost in pad and drug usage, thus monetary savings can be reinvested to improve continence services. A sample of the forms used for care pathways can be found in the Appendices.

DETRUSOR INSTABILITY

Chapter 2 describes the underlying causes of detrusor instability, a condition that can be found in both sexes and at all ages. Whether or not detrusor instability results in incontinence depends on the efficiency of the urethral sphincter mechanism. The actual cause of instability is often unknown and in most women it is idiopathic. The presenting symptoms are urgency, frequency and nocturia, sometimes including nocturnal enuresis, but emotional and other psychosomatic factors are often associated with urge incontinence.

In some women the symptoms may be due to long-term bad toileting habits, such as going to the toilet 'in case' rather than waiting for bladder signals to indicate that it needs emptying. This behaviour does not allow the bladder to fill properly to accommodate holding reasonable amounts of urine.

There is an increased incidence of detrusor instability following surgery for stress incontinence (Cardozo 1991). Often detrusor instability coexists with stress incontinence and diagnosis depends on evidence of failure to inhibit detrusor contractions during urodynamic investigations.

Up to 10% of the population may have detrusor instability, most of whom do not seek help. Affected women learn to cope by knowing where all the public toilets are situated on a shopping route, and often withdraw from social activities.

Treatment is aimed at reducing the bladder instability and increasing the length of time between voiding, thus increasing bladder functional capacity. Women with mild or intermittent symptoms may require only reassurance and advice on normal bladder functioning, so that bad habits can cease. Simple measures such as decreasing excessive fluid intake (over 2 litres daily) and avoiding bladder stimulants such as tea, coffee and alcohol often reduce frequency. However, most women require combination therapy using bladder retraining and electromuscular stimulation, and/or behavioural techniques such as biofeedback (to improve cortical control over the sacral reflex arc), or modifying detrusor innervation by using drugs and, in severe cases, surgery (Fig. 3.5).

When using electromuscular stimulation a probe using a stimulation frequency of 10 Hz is inserted into the vagina. This specific stimulation frequency is believed to reduce detrusor instability by direct inhibition of the micturition centre in the sacral part of the spinal cord. The treatment is applied for 20 minutes each day. A reduction in frequency symptoms has been reported after just seven treatments, but 15–20 treatment sessions produce better reductions in frequency, urgency and nocturia.

Bladder re-education

Before a process of bladder re-education is commenced, charting the frequency and volume for 5 days to obtain a baseline of the bladder's behaviour is necessary (see Chapter 2). The patient is then asked to increase the time between voiding, so the urine outputs when measured for another 5 days should show greater volumes with a reduced frequency pattern. This practice continues until the patient reaches her optimum frequency (4–8 times daily is considered normal) and nocturia occurs only once, or not at all. A simple handout to help patients is shown in Box 3.5.

When the instability is severe as diagnosed on urodynamic investigations, electromuscular stimulation plus or minus anticholinergic drugs may have to be used with the bladder re-education. It is considered wise to prescribe a low dose of oxbutynin (2.5 mg once or twice daily) and slowly increase the dose if necessary. This is thought to minimize side-effects (see Chapter 8). Frequent follow-up appointments are needed to support the patient as treatment usually takes 3–6 months, sometimes even longer.

Non-invasive approaches in the form of bladder re-education, biofeedback (Cardozo 2000), electrical stimulation (Lewey 1999), hypnotherapy or acupuncture (Kelleher 1998) have been used successfully to treat idiopathic detrusor instability and improve symptoms in up to 80% of women. Unfortunately these treatments are time consuming and require the patient to be highly motivated.

Timed voiding in the elderly, confused woman can help to maintain continence. A baseline chart of her voiding habits and/or wet episodes is first recorded for 5–7 days. If a pattern emerges, times to void can be set, thus pre-empting the wet episodes. If no pattern emerges, then regular times for voiding should be considered (e.g. 2–3 hourly during waking hours) to try for continence (see Chapter 6).

Non-surgical approaches	Bladder re-education Biofeedback Hypnotherapy Acupuncture
Medication Drugs to inhibit bladder contractions	Anticholinergics Musculotrophic Calcium-channel blockers Tricyclic antidepressants
Drugs to increase outlet resistance	Alpha-adrenergic stimulators Beta-adrenergic blockers
Drugs affecting local tissues	Oestrogen
Drugs to reduce urine production	Desmopressin
Phenol injections	
Surgery	'Clam' ileocystoplasty

Figure 3.5 Selected treatments for detrusor instability.

Box 3.5 Your guide to bladder retraining

Bladder retraining is a form of self-help for people with certain types of bladder problems. These include:

- *Urgency*: having to rush to pass urine with little or no warning
- *Urge incontinence*: not making it to the toilet in time and so becoming wet; this may be a few drops or a whole bladder full of urine
- *Frequency*: having to pass urine more often than 5–7 times in 24 hours (adults pass urine every 3–5 hours depending on their fluid intake)
- *Nocturia*: getting up more than once at night to pass urine.

Bladder retraining
1. Keep a record of how often you pass urine, or get wet, for 2–3 days. It would also be a good idea to measure the amount of urine each time you go to the toilet. This will show you how much the bladder will hold 'at its best', how many times the bladder is emptied during the day and night, and how much urine is produced in 24 hours.
2. Look at the pattern and then attempt to 'hold on' once you feel the urge to go. Wait 1 minute, then 5 minutes, then 10 minutes, etc. Gradually increase the time interval between visits to the toilet. If you are passing urine every 2 hours, try to wait at least 2½ hours; if you go ten times a day, aim for nine times the next day.
3. Tighten the pelvic floor muscles at the time of feeling 'the urge' as this will help relax the bladder and the urge feeling will disappear. This will help you to hold on.

The purpose of the retraining programme is to increase the bladder capacity for holding on to the urine, *and for you to gain confidence that your bladder can behave*. It may take weeks or even months to overcome the urge to pass urine, but you will succeed. **It is not always easy and you need to be determined to make it work – so don't give up!**

Bladder re-education programmes

- **Promoting continence** by re-educating the bladder to an improved pattern of voiding (requires good motivation and active participation by the patient)
  Approach: gradual increase in interval voiding
  Suitable patients: well-motivated, physically and mentally able to manage own clothing

- **Habit training**
  Approach: assigned toileting schedule (e.g. 2-hourly) but based on baseline chart

Suitable patients: those with some mental awareness

- **Timed voiding**
  Approach: fixed times which may include techniques to trigger voiding
  Suitable patients: those with spinal cord lesions; physical/mental disability

- **Prompted voiding**
  Approach: prompted to void at regular intervals; only taken to toilet if response is positive
  Suitable patients: those with severe mental/physical disabilities (see Chapters 10 and 11).

Case study 3.1

Joan is aged 60 years. Her obstetric history is: parity three, none over 8.5 lb, no forceps; one tear with suturing of perineum and internal sutures.

Patient's perception of problem: Always going to the toilet and sometimes not getting there in time. Having to get up at least three times during the night, and this is getting her down as she is tired all day.

Medical history: Irritable bowel several years; anxious lady, a worrier. Prone to coughs and colds. HRT for 5 years.

Surgical history: Abdominal hysterectomy 10 years ago. Fusion of L3 and L4, 5 years ago. Still suffers back pain from muscle spasm, for which she takes analgesics.

Assessment: Pelvic floor muscle grade 3, hold 5 seconds, repetitions 8, quick contractions × 5.

Investigations: Urinalysis – NAD. Urodynamics – detrusor instability confirmed.

Treatment implemented: Bladder re-education using frequency/volume charting for 1 week (see Chapter 2 for details of bladder charting). Pelvic floor exercises to strengthen muscle. Informed how to contract muscles when feeling the urge to go to the toilet so that the feeling fades away and patient holds-on for a further 15 minutes.

Four weeks later: Joan found it difficult to hold on for the extra 15 minutes and was disappointed in herself and the lack of progress. Plenty of support was given as well as a description of the working of the bladder and the need to control the unstable bladder activity. Another weekly bladder chart was commenced so that Joan could monitor her own frequency pattern and measure some volumes to record increased voiding volumes. It was important for Joan to have professional support so another appointment was agreed for 2 weeks later.

(continued)

Case study 3.1   *(continued)*

Two weeks later: Still not much progress in Joan's view, but while reflecting the past 2 weeks she realized the nocturia had reduced to two occasions and sometimes only once. The anticholinergic drug, oxybutynin, was discussed and a quick telephone call to the GP was made. The urodynamic results and the slow progress to date with bladder retraining were discussed. The GP agreed to a small dose of 2.5 mg twice a day and for the continence advisor to monitor its use. This was duly done on three weekly appointments.

Two months later: Frequency reduced to seven times a day and once or less at night. Side-effect of the drug was a dry mouth but not too unbearable. The oxybutynin was reduced by taking it every morning and alternate evenings. Joan was beginning to feel better about herself as she had learnt to control the urgency and had more confidence to 'hold on'.

One month later: Noticeable progress, daytime frequency down to six times with larger urine volumes voided; nocturia occasionally once only. A further reduction in oxybutynin dosage was instigated by stopping the nighttime dose and taking one 3 mg dose on alternate mornings. This is the dose Joan remained on to maintain the improved bladder control. A postvoiding residual urine measurement was arranged every 6 months.

Six months after the first assessment Joan was discharged from the continence clinic a much happier lady as she was in control of her bladder. The thought of a 6-monthly residual urine test meant she still had contact and support.

ELECTROMUSCULAR STIMULATION

Digital examination will reveal whether or not a woman has the ability to contract the pelvic floor muscle. When there is no voluntary movement, treatment should begin with *electromuscular stimulation*. In the past this was the domain of physiotherapists, but now, with such treatment available as preprogrammed home devices, it is necessary for clinicians in the field of continence promotion to be more familiar with this concept of pelvic floor rehabilitation.

Neurophysiologists have opened up new horizons in re-education of the neuromuscular system. A clearer understanding of the normal mechanism of control which exists between nerves and muscles makes it possible to take over this control of muscle metabolism by the appropriate application of precise electronic signals.

It has been shown (Gibson et al 1988) that nerves control muscle by transmitting a neurological code. This code occurs in two frequency bands according to the type of muscle fibre. Postural fibres (slow-twitch) require a tonic feeding at the rate of 10 pulses per second (pps), if given for periods of 1 hour or more a day. Using this technique, it is possible to maintain a baseline muscle tone until voluntary contraction can be controlled. Muscles treated in this way are able to preserve bulk, capillary bed density and their essential ability to utilize oxygen (Fall 1984). Using a stimulation frequency of 10 Hz for 20 minutes a day is believed to reduce detrusor instability (Lewey 1999) by direct inhibition of the micturition centre in the sacral part of the spinal cord (S2–S4). A reduction in frequency of symptoms can often be seen after 2 weeks of treatment but up to 6 weeks of daily treatment can produce better results when the woman has regained self-control. Because there are no side-effects it should be a first-line option over the use of anticholinergic medication.

The second frequency band occurs at 30 pps, and feeds information to the fast-twitch contracting muscle fibres which give the power to a movement. This feeding occurs naturally in a phasic way and, therefore, treatment to promote these fibres is given for shorter periods of time.

This physiological approach to stimulating the muscles also requires pulses that are shaped like the naturally occurring nerve signals, and with very brief pulse widths. By mimicking nature as accurately as possible, electrical stimulation has been used for prolonged periods without causing any undesirable side-effects. Neuromuscular electrostimulation is increasingly the primary approach towards the re-education of pelvic floor muscles in the absence of any contraction or a weak non-sustaining contraction, for stress and urge incontinence (Blowman et al 1991, Lewey 1999).

For electrical stimulation to be effective the pulse width (measured in milliseconds), along with the intensity (measured in amps), must be sufficient to overcome the excitation threshold of the nerve fibres to be stimulated (Haslam 1998). If pulse widths are too long a duration the sensory nerve fibres are stimulated and this can cause pain and discomfort. The most frequently used pulse width is a range between 0.2 and 0.5 milliseconds. The intensity output from the machine must be sufficient to cause an adequate stimulation. The principal rule for this therapy to be effective is:

> **The intensity of the current pulse and its duration must be adequate to meet or exceed the threshold excitability of the tissue being stimulated.**

Patients using home devices (Fig. 3.6) must have supervision and instruction to understand this principle (training in the use of stimulators is referred to in Chapter 12). If the intensity is too low it will not have any therapeutic effect. Care must be taken not to fatigue the muscle being stimulated and to prevent this there is an on/off cycle – known as the duty cycle – where pulses and rest times are set. Very often weak muscles are treated with a rest time twice as long as the pulsating period of time and this can be altered as the muscle improves. As stimulation improves cortical awareness of the pelvic floor muscle and its contraction, treatment can progress with the woman doing voluntary contractions with the stimulation and prolonging the contraction even after the stimulation has ended.

Regular appointments are essential to monitor progress and to gradually increase the workload of pelvic floor exercises until there is an acceptable reduction in urinary incontinence symptoms, or preferably a cure. Dolman (2000), having used electromuscular stimulation for treating incontinence in 63 patients for only 3 months, found over 70% of women were satisfied with the treatment and 48% were symptom free.

Suggested treatment guidelines for pelvic floor muscle rehabilitation using electromuscular stimulation can be found in Figure 3.7. A patient guide in the use of eletromuscular stimulation is summarized in Box 3.6.

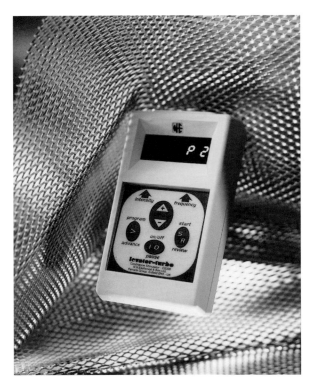

(a)

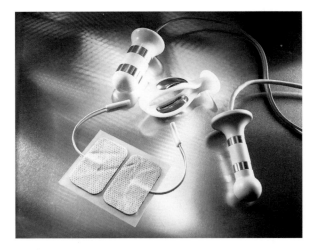

(b)

Figure 3.6 (a) Home-use electromuscular stimulator: Levator 200. (b) Typical probes for electromuscular stimulators. (Photographs courtesy of Ferraris Medical Ltd.)

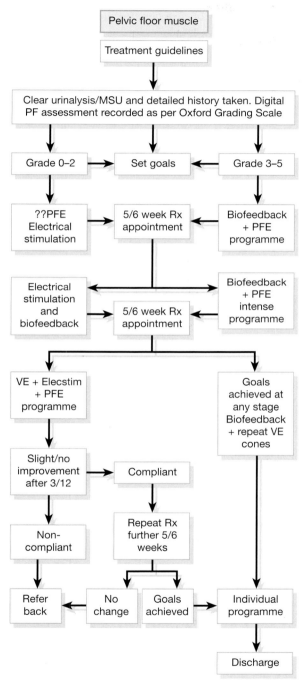

Figure 3.7 Treatment guidelines for rehabilitation of the pelvic floor muscle using electromuscular stimulation. Elecstim, electromuscular stimulation; PF, pelvic floor; PFE, pelvic floor exercises; VE, vaginal examination.

Box 3.6 How to use an electromuscular stimulator: a patient guide

- Insert the detachable lead into the socket of the unit. Moisten the vaginal electrode with water or KY-jelly and insert it into the vagina.
- Switch the unit 'on'.
- Select the chosen programme to treat symptoms. Select from a full 'workout' to specific symptoms of stress or urge incontinence or pain.
- Start the machine.
- With the intensity button increase intensity to a tolerable level but as high as possible. This can be adjusted by the operator pressing the plus or minus button as required.
- If the pulsing cannot be felt initially this indicates a loss of normal sensation. The numbness should rectify with treatment, but care should be taken with the early application. The electrode should be inserted to within a centimetre or so from the mouth of the vagina and the treatment intensity increased until a deep tingling sensation is felt on the lips of the vulva.
- The electrode is then inserted a further centimetre or so. Treatment will now be effective although the woman may not feel it.
- During any of the chosen programmes there will be changes in frequencies and pulse widths for specific time periods relevant to each frequency band. At each change the frequency is briefly displayed in hertz or pulses per second. The unit will automatically switch off at the completion of the treatment programme.

Basic guidelines for using electromuscular stimulation

Before using this type of treatment some questions should be considered:

- What effect is intended and can this be achieved? Sometimes this is not known until treatment is tried and often any effect will take a number of weeks to be recognized. However, an experienced clinician can usually judge effectiveness following the assessment.
- Is it safe? For most electromuscular therapy, treatment risks are negligible. Some important contraindications are: patient with a cardiac pacemaker; pregnancy (no evidence but do not put patient at risk); retention of urine; pelvic masses and fistulae; urinary tract infections; vaginal discharge or severe prolapse; recent

postoperative status and local inflammation/ recent radiotherapy.

- Can this treatment complement other modalities from which the patient will benefit and be cost-effective, i.e. used with biofeedback therapy? Sometimes a referral to a physiotherapist is required to achieve this.

BIOFEEDBACK THERAPY

Biofeedback simply means giving the patient immediate information about a physiological state of a bodily process, for example heart beat (ECG), brain electrical activity (EEG) or striated muscle activity (EMG). Although biofeedback is a relatively new therapy in the UK in the field of incontinence, it has been used successfully in the USA for more than 20 years. It is used to teach the patient how to isolate the pelvic floor muscle without using accessory muscle groups such as the abdominals or gluteals and it assists in monitoring the rehabilitation progress of the pelvic floor muscle towards maintaining continence. Biofeedback is an important behavioural component of pelvic floor rehabilitation even in its simplest form of digital palpation. Other biofeedback mechanisms specific to the pelvic floor muscle include: manometric pressure measured by a perineometer; sensory input via probes; assessor's tone of voice; vaginal cones and electromyography (EMG) biofeedback.

Several studies have reported on the efficacy of biofeedback in continence training (Burgio 1990, Glavind et al 1998, Smith & Newman 1994) but most conclude it is best used in combination with other treatment modalities. The advantage of this therapy is that there are no side-effects and the immediate information not only shows the muscle dysfunction but also helps the patient to isolate the muscle. An assessment of the functional capability allows the assessor to set an accurate training programme. It provides an objective assessment of the muscle function and records accurately the progress of muscle rehabilitation. The muscle bioelectricity can be recorded by using a vaginal periform probe or rectal anuform probe, or by using surface electrodes placed externally either side of the anal sphincter at 3 and 9 o'clock or needles in the perineum. The reference lead is attached to the thigh or a bony prominence such as the hip. Surface electrodes for monitoring abdominal muscle contraction are placed in an arc around the umbilicus about 2.5 cm apart, with the reference electrode between the positive and negative electrodes. The skin should be dry and clean for the pre-jelled electrodes to adhere properly to make a good contact.

Biofeedback education and its use with patients is a great stimulant for motivation and compliance to do a home exercise programme (Smith & Newman 1994). Patients who are actively involved in their therapy are more motivated to do well and therefore respond quickly to the treatment. An example of the use of biofeedback is demonstrated in Figure 3.8.

Phases of pelvic floor development using biofeedback

- *Phase 1*. Gives an awareness, identification and coordination of the muscle groups.
- *Phase 2*. Transition – muscle control develops and strengthening begins.
- *Phase 3*. Muscle strengthening completed and pelvic innervation improves with symptoms decreasing.
- *Phase 4*. Muscle tone good – palpation finds a firmer, bulkier and broader muscle.

The principles of biofeedback

Muscle strengthening is done with maximal contractions which are held for 5–10 seconds at a time, with 10 second rest periods in between. These work/rest cycles are repeated several times until the contraction begins to show fatigue or when the patient begins to compensate with accessory muscle groups. Endurance training is done with submaximal contractions held for increasingly longer periods of time (Fig. 3.9). For example, 50% contraction held for 30 seconds can be held longer at each repetition. This is working on the slow-twitch muscle fibres. Speed of recruitment is practised with several repetitive contractions without holding the contraction, i.e. a quick flick, which works the fast-twitch muscle fibres.

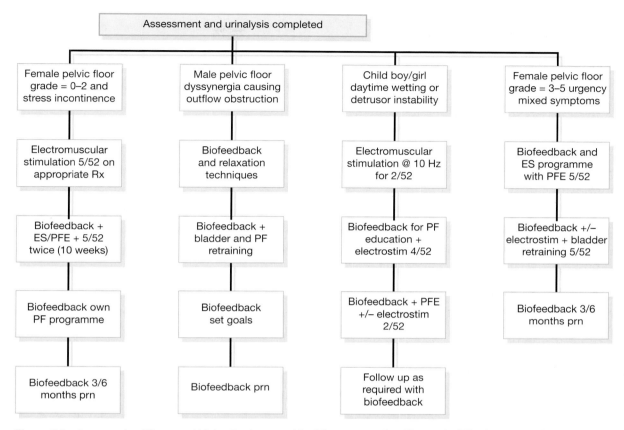

Figure 3.8 An example of the use of biofeedback as used in different scenarios. Electrostim/ES, electromuscular stimulation; PF, pelvic floor; PFE, pelvic floor exercises; prn, when required.

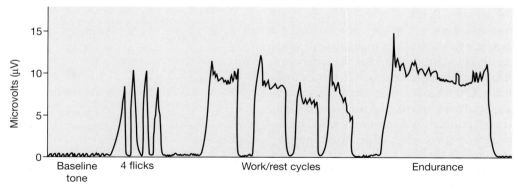

Figure 3.9 Sample EMG line graph.

As these fatigue easily, ten successive contractions performed within 10 seconds is usually sufficient. A progressive contraction can also be done by asking the patient to contract and relax the muscle gradually. The time spent on each type of training depends on the patient's problem and response.

Patients who have a high postural tone reading of 6 microvolts or more need to learn to relax the pelvic floor muscle. This can sometimes be done following a strong contraction but relaxing techniques will also have to be employed. Conditions that often show a high resting tone included unstable bladder, constipation (see Chapter 7), dyssynergia and idiopathic pelvic floor contractions.

There are several choices of equipment available for both home use and more sophisticated computerized systems for clinic use. Some are referenced in Chapter 12.

WEIGHTED VAGINAL CONES

Another conservative therapy which can be added to the treatment programme when a patient has attained grade 3 of the Oxford Grading Scale is a weighted vaginal cone. The idea of the cone is to place it in the vagina and the creation of a sensory feeling of something slipping out causes the pelvic floor muscle to contract to keep the cone in place. This treatment is ideal for women who wish to maintain a healthy muscle but have low compliance with the exercises. By using the cone for 5–10 minutes 2 or 3 days a week will help the non-complier to do a pelvic floor workout. There have been several studies in the past two decades testing the efficacy of this treatment but cones are not suitable for women with weak pelvic floor contractions so alternative therapy is first required, i.e. electromuscular stimulation.

The Cochrane Review (2001) on the use of vaginal cones concluded there was limited evidence of the benefits of their use in women with stress incontinence. The results are tentative as a much larger scale study is still needed to measure relevant outcomes and therefore cones are only useful to those who find them acceptable. The cones are best recommended by a clinician but patients can buy these without any clinical supervision which is why they are not always used correctly and give no benefit to the user. When they are used properly cones provide a positive feedback of muscle progress (weights can be added or cones go up in weight by 12.5 g each), thus giving a sense of achievement. Contraindications for cone usage are summarized in Box 3.7.

Box 3.7 Contraindications for cone usage

- Pelvic muscle strength below grade 3 of the Oxford Grading Scale
- No perineal sensation (sensory deficit)
- Severe uterine, bladder or rectal prolapse
- Very lax vagina
- Vaginitis or discharge

Case study 3.2

'Being incontinent makes me feel as though I have lost my femininity.'

Anne is 32 years old. Her obstetric history is as follows: Parity one; twin girls with use of Kielland's forceps for delivery of second baby. Third-degree tear of perineum and breakdown of suturing within 48 hours. Resutured, slow healing of haematoma. Six months after the birth of the twins, Anne started aerobic classes and found she could not take part in anything that required her to jump or move quickly as she leaked urine and was very embarrassed. This was the reason she asked for the continence advisor's help. However, on further history taking it was revealed that Anne could not keep a tampon *in situ* and sexual intercourse was not very stimulating as she could not feel much sensation.

Examination of the pelvic floor muscle showed a very weak contraction with a hold time of 2 seconds and only four repetitions. There was a slight cystocele but no other abnormalities noted. There were no medical or surgical problems, nor was Anne on any medication. Apart from being absolutely distraught that she was incontinent at her age, she was also very upset that she could not do pelvic floor exercises either.

Urinalysis: NAD.

Diagnosis: stress incontinence.

Treatment programme:
Electromuscular stimulation was explained and Anne agreed to commence the treatment; she was desperate to try anything! Other than not using the stimulator during menstruation, Anne chose to 'plug in' for an hour while watching the television in the evenings and a follow-up appointment was made for 6 weeks later. A contact telephone number was available for Anne during the 6 weeks. At this appointment Anne felt she was more aware of the pelvic floor muscles but there had been no change in the urinary incontinence symptoms. Support was given to stimulate motivation and it was suggested that she try to contract the pelvic floor muscles voluntarily with the pulses on the machine for the second half of the programme. At the 12-week appointment Anne was much

(continued)

Case study 3.2 *(continued)*

more positive and hopeful as she felt there was an improvement in the incontinence. A vaginal examination showed improvement in the muscle strength to grade 3 and a longer increased hold time of 5 seconds. At this stage an individual exercise programme was implemented and this included five quick contractions followed by slow endurance contractions with lifting technique to 5 seconds. Anne was encouraged to do groups of five contractions with 10 second rest time, 4–5 times a day and to use the stimulator for another 4 weeks.

At the *16th week assessment*, the use of the stimulator was discontinued and Anne increased the number of daily pelvic floor exercises to groups of ten with a hold time of 8 seconds and rest 5 seconds. The quick contractions were also increased to ten. Anne confessed that remembering to do her own exercises was proving difficult as she had a busy lifestyle, and asked if there was anything else she could use. The weighted vaginal cones were discussed as the muscle strength had reached a good grade 3 and Anne was suitable to use them. She was delighted to be able to give herself this therapy twice a day with cone number one and this also helped her to remember to do some exercises herself.

Six months later, Anne was able to return to her aerobic classes, do all the activities without incontinence and her self-esteem had been restored. She realized that pelvic floor exercises must be part of her life and she continued to do them in the car on the way to the aerobic classes twice a week. She bought the set of three vaginal cones for use in the future as she did not want to be incontinent again and the cones would help her to continue treating herself.

SURGICAL TREATMENTS FOR STRESS INCONTINENCE

When conservative therapies fail, surgery must be considered. The mere fact that there are over 100 different operative procedures for urinary stress incontinence is evidence of the desperation surgeons face in this difficult condition (O'Dowd 1993). Some surgical treatment in women has been carried out by gynaecologists with a verbal 'I'll just put a few stitches in to pull up your bladder and you will be alright again'. The final choice to have surgery must lie with the patient, and it seems increasingly evident that women now only choose surgery as a last resort.

Vaginal repair

Anterior colporrhaphy may be performed for a cystourethrocele (bladder and urethral prolapse), but this procedure works best for anterior vaginal wall prolapse and is not always successful for stress incontinence.

The technique involves making a longitudinal midline incision down the anterior vaginal wall, mobilizing the bladder neck, and inserting one or two Kelly or Pacey sutures. The pubovesical fascia is then approximated and the anterior vaginal wall closed. A vaginal hysterectomy, amputation of the cervix (Manchester repair) or posterior wall repair may be performed at the same time if indicated.

Although there are few complications with anterior colporrhaphy, haemorrhage or trauma to the bladder or urethra may occur (Cardozo et al 1993). Later problems that seem to recur are further prolapse, urinary incontinence, dyspareunia or urethral stricture. The success rate for this surgery, based on objective assessment, is reported to be 36–60% (Hilton 1987).

Abdominal surgery

The Marshall–Marchetti–Krantz procedure

This procedure, used for primary or recurrent stress incontinence (Krantz 1986), takes a double bite of tissue from the bladder neck which is hitched up to the periosteum on the back of the pubic bone with non-absorbable suture material. In about 5% of cases *osteitis pubis* has been reported as a complication. The main problem with this operation is that it does not correct a cystocele, but as a treatment for stress incontinence the results are good.

Colposuspension

The Burch colposuspension is used for both primary and recurrent stress incontinence with or without prolapse. According to Hilton (1987), there is an 80–90% success rate with this procedure, provided it is the first line of surgical treatment.

The operation is carried out through a transverse suprapubic incision. Retropubic dissection

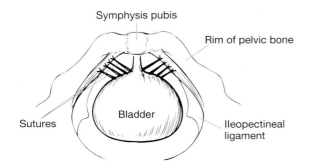

Figure 3.10   Diagram to illustrate a colposuspension.

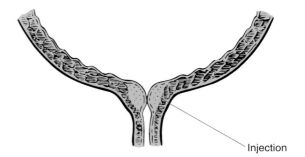

Figure 3.11   Diagram to illustrate a collagen implant.

is performed to mobilize the bladder and bladder neck medially off the underlying fascia, and two to four long-term absorbable or non-absorbable sutures are inserted from the paravaginal fascia to the ileopectineal ligament (Fig. 3.10).

Although the aim of most operations of this type is to elevate the bladder neck, different approaches by individual surgeons vary in the extent to which this is achieved. The higher the bladder neck is raised, the better the chance of reducing incontinence symptoms, but also the greater the risks of inducing outflow obstruction with postoperative voiding difficulties. Women with preoperative voiding problems should be operated on with caution, but most are taught intermittent self-catheterization prior to surgery.

Collagen implant

With the availability of new, more biocompatible materials, injectable implant therapy for urinary incontinence in women is becoming a viable surgical option. Contigen (Bard Ltd) is highly purified bovine dermal collagen, lightly cross-linked with glutaraldehyde. It is sterile and non-pyrogenic.

Contigen is usually injected under local anaesthesia around the neck of the bladder. The procedure is carried out as a day case in an outpatient department. Under direct cystoscopic vision, Contigen is injected submucosally at or near the bladder neck until tissue bulking closes the lumen across the midline of the urethral opening (Fig. 3.11). The injection procedure is repeated on the opposite side until the urethral lumen is

occluded and urethral outflow resistance is achieved.

This treatment should be attempted only by specially trained surgeons. Patients must have a skin test at least 28 days prior to the procedure to determine any hypersensitivity to bovine dermal collagen. Patients should be evaluated urodynamically following treatment, and follow-up visits should be at least once within the first 3 months, then depending on the individual's circumstances.

Patients should be warned that Contigen implant is not necessarily a permanent therapy and additional injections may be needed to achieve and maintain improvement of the condition. In a 2–3 year follow-up of 60 women who had periurethral collagen implants, Stanton (1994) concluded that collagen injections may continue to be effective at 2 years, although there is some decline with time. He also proposed that functional urethral length and clinical assessment of bulking may be more useful than maximum urethral closure pressure for predicting success. However, there was no significant decrease in peak flow rate and no long-term complications. Collagen is appropriate in women with urethral hypermobility who wish to avoid surgical risks and in those for whom surgery is ill advised (Bent et al 2001).

Tension-free vaginal tape (TVT)

Studies are emerging on the use of tension-free vaginal tape in women with occult stress incontinence and severe prolapse, being used as a prophylactic procedure during surgery to pre-vent the development of postoperative stress incontinence. A preliminary study by Gordon et al (2001) is showing encouraging results when following up 30 women 1 year later and not one had developed stress incontinence. Clinical evaluation of this new method using TVT is currently being researched.

MANAGEMENT WITH OCCLUSIVE DEVICES
Bladder neck support

When urinary incontinence cannot be controlled by the various treatment options, then manage-ment options have to be considered. For the active woman, occluding the urethra mechanic-ally is a method to restore pressure and the anatomical angle by lifting and supporting the bladder neck and urethra.

The easiest device available on the market for women to purchase is a tampon-like sponge which can be inserted into the vagina. It is first moistened with water and squeezed to reduce its size for easy insertion. Once inserted it expands, thus applying external pressure to the urethra and bladder neck. It should be used for short periods only as the absorbable properties tend to make the vagina dry and sore. Some women use it as a method of managing incontinence when playing sport or going to aerobic classes. This allows them to participate in activities which they would otherwise cease to do. A similar device but made of a firm material is Contiform (Bard). It is easy to insert and supports the blad-der neck comfortably. Removing the device using the index finger can be very difficult. It is only available to purchase but should have a clin-ician's recommendation.

Urethral plug

A multicentre trial has been conducted on women to test the the efficacy and safety of an expandable urethral occlusion device (Fig. 3.12; see Staskin et al 1994). The sample size was small, with only 33 women completing the 4-month trial, but the

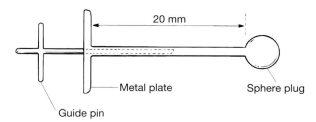

Figure 3.12 A urethral plug as described by Nielsen et al (1993).

results seem promising with reported ease and safety of use.

The same group of researchers (Staskin et al 1995) reported on a sample of 213 women at 4-month and 8-month intervals to test the efficacy and safety of a single-use urethral insert with an expandable balloon tip. Average use of the device was 2–3 times a day with a range of 1–6 hours per device. The subjective effectiveness was 95%, with 81% claiming to be completely dry. There was a 32% recording of urinary tract infections, of which 24% were treated with antibiotics before resuming the use of the intraurethral device. The FemSoft insert is available in the UK and the trials were similar to other studies regarding urinary infections. The material is soft and pliable, being made from liquid and silicone. It is latex free and is easily inserted once the woman has been taught how to do it. The trial showed a high satisfaction rate with ease of use, comfort and dryness, thus improving the quality of life for the 150 women.

Redesign of the intraurethral plug continues with ongoing trials, but long-term management with such a device may be the option women will choose in preference to surgery.

Disposable and washable pads

There is a wide range of disposable incontinence pads for women which manufacturers are contin-ually improving for comfort and efficacy. These are far too numerous to mention and the reader should refer to Chapter 12 to find a list of some suggested manufacturers. Visiting professional exhibitions to see the latest developments in disposable pads is a good method for keeping up-to-date.

The debate over reusable versus disposable products for incontinence continues. Cost, and environmental issues such as the actual disposal of used pads and the number of trees required to make pulp, are strong arguments for using washable products.

Philp & Cottenden (1993) looked at consumers' views on reusable products, and 17 people in their study rejected reusables altogether. There were four main reasons for this:

* unacceptable leakage
* increased workload and/or high cost of laundry and tumble-drying
* organization of washing and using the product
* carrying and changing pads around while out.

Washable products are therefore an option but will only be cost-effective if the right product is selected for appropriate patients. It must be remembered that each incontinent person is an individual who deserves individual assessment and attention. Women (and men) who have a mild degree of incontinence and need some protection to save embarrassing moments can purchase from a number of sources very nice almost 'designer' pants (see Chapter 12).

Medical and surgical treatments

Some patients do not respond to any medical intervention or cannot tolerate the side-effects of drugs. They may have had cystodistension or phenol injections, or intravesical instillation of anticholinergic therapy without success. If symptoms remain severe, a 'clam' ileocystoplasty may be a last resort. This operation involves augmenting the bladder with a section of the ileum. The bladder is bisected along the coronal plane anterior to the ureteric orifices to within 1 cm of the bladder neck. The distance is measured and a corresponding length of ileum is isolated, opened along its antimesenteric border, and sutured as a patch into the bisected bladder.

A postoperative complication may be voiding difficulties caused by diminished voiding pressures of the ileum section. Mucus production is another complication and the patient may need to learn to strain down to void the mucus plugs. Most patients will need to learn intermittent self-catheterization to empty the bladder and it is recommended that all should drink 200 ml of cranberry juice daily to help reduce mucus viscidity (Rosenbaum et al 1989).

OTHER CAUSES OF INCONTINENCE
The menopause

The embryological development of the vagina, trigone and urethra was explained earlier in this chapter. From this it can be understood how oestrogen affecting the vagina will also influence the lining of the urethra.

In premenopausal women, when the oestrogen level is depleted just prior to menstruation, the resting urethral pressure falls. Women often say that their incontinence and frequency are worse the week before their period. The urethral wall is soft and convoluted (forming many folds) and when fully oestrogenized creates a watertight seal. When the hormone level falls the urethral walls become less soft, the folds less pronounced and the closure less efficient.

In postmenopausal women, it may take about 10 years before the oestrogen level is inadequate, but some women will remain well oestrogenized into old age. The lowered level of oestrogen after the menopause, combined with weak pelvic floor muscles and perineal trauma from childbirth, can lead to stress incontinence. Lack of oestrogen may cause urethritis and trigonitis often associated with atrophic vaginitis. This is easily recognized by looking at the vulva which will appear red, inflamed and often dry. Vaginal dryness means there is a loss of sexual lubrication and intercourse can be uncomfortable and painful.

Some women experience discomfort whilst passing urine owing to the urine being in contact with the inflamed vulva. They are often treated with antibiotics for a urinary infection, when in reality they have atrophic vaginitis. Treatment for this condition is simply to replace the deficient oestrogen level in the vagina by means of application of topical oestrogen cream, oral oestrogen or Estraderm patches (best for women who have had a hysterectomy). Oestrogen supplementation improves the vaginal, urethral and trigonal epithelium and leads to a restoration of the premenopausal vaginal flora (Cardozo et al 1993).

Hysterectomy

In effect, hysterectomy can be considered as a surgical menopause, particularly if accompanied by bilateral oophorectomy. If hormone replacement therapy is not commenced, the symptoms described above will occur.

In addition to the oestrogen depletion following a hysterectomy, postoperative scarring and infection were suggested by Smith et al (1970) as aetiological factors for urinary symptoms following a hysterectomy. Women often state: 'I was all right until I had my hysterectomy'. Urethral obstruction due to periurethral fibrosis and damage to the bladder base and proximal urethra during a total hysterectomy results in scar formation. Women experience voiding difficulties, and when the bladder is not emptied completely 'needing to go again only 2 minutes after voiding' is a common complaint.

The symptom of frequency may be caused by a urinary infection, but investigations are required. Often a simple dilatation of the urethra will resolve the problem, or a woman can be taught to self-dilate the urethra using a Nelaton intermittent catheter (see Chapter 9).

Cystitis and urinary tract infection

Many women experience a urinary tract infection (UTI) during their lifetime and 3% experience recurrent infections (Nicolle & Ronald 1987). It is possible that the majority of infections in adult women are asymptomatic and clear up spontaneously. However, many women will be troubled by recurrent symptomatic infections which affect the quality of their life, including the enjoyment of sexual relationships. Box 3.9 provides a summary of approaches to dealing with recurrent UTI.

For women who do experience recurrent UTI, the frequency of episodes is highly variable. After any one infection, approximately two-thirds will experience another infection within 6 months (Kraft & Stamey 1977). Factors which precipitate infection are poorly identified, but sexual intercourse and the chosen method of birth control (e.g. diaphragm) are two well-documented associations (Nicolle et al 1982).

According to Cardozo et al (1993), there is a double peak in the prevalence of UTI in women, one occurring in the 30–40 age group and the other between 55 and 65 years. In the younger group, it is thought that intercourse predisposes women to UTI by micro-organisms readily entering the bladder from the vagina and perineum. In the postmenopausal group, the incidence of recurrent UTI may be related to the reduced oestrogen status, or it may be an age-related phenomenon.

Urinary pathogens

Indigenous intestinal bacterial flora are the primary source of urinary pathogens. These organisms contaminate the vagina and perineum and ascend into the bladder. The most common organism is *Escherichia coli*, which accounts for up to 85% of acute infections. Less common pathogens are *Proteus mirabilis*, *Klebsiella pneumoniae*, *Aerobacter aerogenes* and, rarely, Gram-positive cocci.

A UTI can affect any part of the urinary tract, but it is the 'adherence' of the bacteria that is an important factor in the pathogenesis of infections. The urinary tract has a natural ability to resist bacterial colonization and the intruding bacteria are efficiently eliminated by the interaction of multiple mechanisms. Urine acidity, osmolality, organic acids and urea have a role in inhibiting bacteria adherence and growth. The bladder mucosa has intrinsic antibacterial properties and destroys those bacteria remaining on its surface after micturition. However, if women do not empty their bladder completely and leave a residual urine, it reduces the host defence and makes them susceptible to urinary tract infections (Iravani 1988).

Symptomology

The woman complains of frequency of micturition, but dysuria may be absent or only minor with a UTI. When *cystitis* is the problem, the woman complains of frequency of micturition, urgency, dysuria and suprapubic discomfort. Between 20 and 30% of women presenting with classical symptoms of cystitis will *not* have a urinary tract infection.

Investigations

A midstream specimen of urine (MSU) is essential for diagnosis, and antibiotic treatment should be commenced only according to the results of the culture and sensitivity. It is unsound practice to treat a woman with a presumptive diagnosis as many cultures are negative and antibiotics will not be required.

Upper-tract pathology may be adequately investigated by renal ultrasound and X-ray of kidneys, ureters and bladder (KUB). Cystourethroscopy may be performed and a bladder biopsy may show evidence of chronic inflammation. Cystourethroscopy is more relevant in the elderly, as recurrent UTI could be the presenting symptom of a transitional-cell carcinoma.

Women under 40 years old should have a urodynamic investigation to eliminate the diagnosis of detrusor instability as this condition also gives rise to urgency symptoms. Urodynamic studies will also reveal mechanical outflow obstruction which may have resulted from previous bladder neck surgery. These women may not be emptying the bladder completely, thus suffering from symptoms of cystitis, but will have negative urine cultures.

Interstitial cystitis

Frequent episodes of cystitis do not inevitably lead to interstitial cystitis (IC) but if a condition becomes chronic it must be investigated further. Women are affected more commonly than men but it can occur at any age. The cause of IC is still unknown, hence the difficulty in treating the condition. The main symptoms present as frequency, which may be up to 60 times a day in severe cases, urgency and pain. Pain can be in the abdomen, urethra or vaginal area, thus pain is associated with sexual intercourse.

Box 3.8 Differences between IC and bacterial cystitis

Interstitial cystitis	Bacterial cystitis
Long term frequency	Frequency during attacks
Clear urine specimen	Urine cloudy and odorous
No bacteria present in urine	Bacteria shown in urine
Symptoms not relieved by antibiotics	Symptoms relieved by antibiotics
Temporary relief when voiding	Pain during voiding
Pain/discomfort with bladder filling	No symptoms with bladder filling
Continuous/permanent symptoms	Attacks last a few days

Differences between IC and bacterial cystitis are shown in Box 3.8.

Symptoms vary between patients and many self-help coping mechanisms are learnt from other sufferers via the Interstitial Cystitis support group (icsg) (details in Chapter 12). Because of the time it takes to get a diagnosis and then exploring the different approaches to treatment, the support group plays an important role and offers educational literature and information.

A urologist is likely to include some or all of the following investigations which are essential for any urological problem: Urine and blood tests; cystoscopy usually followed by a cystodistension; urodynamic studies; ultrasound; bladder biopsy; voiding cystourethrogram, X-ray of kidneys, urethra and bladder and, of course, a full physical examination.

Treatments offered

There is not one effective treatment to suit all patients but the most common approaches which try to alleviate the symptoms include:

- *Bladder distension*. This is stretching the bladder with water while the person is under general anaesthetic.
- *Oral medications*. These include anti-inflammatory, antispasmodic, antihistamines, muscle relaxants and antidepressants (amitriptyline which appears to have anti-pain properties).

- *DMSO (dimethyl sulfoxide)*. A medication which is instilled into the bladder and is believed to have an anti-inflammatory effect thus reducing pain.
- *Cystistat*. Also a bladder instillation to restore defective bladder lining.
- *TENS units*. A unit which supplies a low electrical current via surface electrodes attached over the bladder to relieve pain. Can be administered continuously or intermittently.
- *Diet and nutrition*. Eliminating certain foods may decrease the severity of the symptoms.

The debilitating effect of this condition cannot be understated as the quality of life is eroded. People become isolated and fear going out in public, the pain is often too great for socializing. Repeatedly getting up at night to go to the toilet results in severe tiredness and going to work is difficult.

Research continues to search for effective treatments but until the cause is known this is difficult. Patients with this condition require a lot of support and should be given the contact number of the icsg.

Effects of cranberry juice

As early as the 19th century, American Indians used crushed cranberries as a herbal remedy for the treatment of urinary infections (Bodel et al 1959). Many studies have focused on the anti-adherence activity of cranberry juice and its alteration of the urinary pH (Blatherwick & Long 1923, Schmidt & Sobata 1988). Research continues to investigate the benefits and contraindications of cranberry juice for UTI and cystitis, but many women benefit from it and find it pleasant to drink (see also Chapter 9).

SUMMARY

This chapter has highlighted 'mostly female' problems and tried to give practical advice for professionals involved in the care of women with bladder dysfunctions. Management of incontinence is a financial burden to individuals and to the NHS and so it is incumbent upon all healthcare professionals to help women prevent urinary

---

Box 3.9 Treatment and advice for cystitis/UTI

1. Check for an incorrectly fitted diaphragm which may be causing pressure during intercourse. This could cause dysuria and sometimes the onset of infection.
2. Spermicidal preparations or spermicidally treated condoms may cause dysuria secondary to a vaginitis due to an allergy.
3. Establish if there has been a change in sexual partner or sexual practice.
4. Treat UTI with appropriate antibiotic according to urine culture.
5. Treat any underlying condition which predisposes to recurrent UTI (incomplete bladder emptying or detrusor instability).
6. Treat atrophic vaginitis with oestrogen supplements.
7. Increase daily fluid intake by at least 1 litre. The diuresis will help wash out low-grade infections.
8. Take cranberry juice daily (at least three 250 ml glasses) during the acute phase. A glass a day may help as a prophylactic measure.

KEY POINTS FOR PRACTICE

- Preventing incontinence in women should be attempted through educational programmes aimed at teenagers, adolescents and young women.
- Detailed assessment – obstetric, gynaecological, medical and surgical – is required so that accurate treatment and advice can be given.
- Healthcare professionals should recognize their limitations and know when to make appropriate referrals (care pathways).
- Practitioners must learn the skills for assessing pelvic floor muscle behaviour.
- Practitioners should always assess a woman's pelvic floor muscle behaviour before commencing a treatment.
- Pelvic floor exercises are essential, not only for women with stress incontinence but also sensory/motor urgency.
- Treatment modalities must not be recommended unless the practitioner has knowledge and training in the treatments.

---

incontinence symptoms rather than manage the problem. Increased education on the subject from health professionals has helped eliminate the taboo subject and with the Internet many www. addresses have information on all incontinence subjects (Chapter 12). Women are now better informed than in the past two decades but research must continue to give professionals the evidence from which to practise.

REFERENCES

Allen R E, Warrell D W 1987 The role of pregnancy and childbirth in partial denervation of the pelvic floor. Neurourology and Urodynamics 6(3): 183–184

Bayliss V, Cherry M, Locke R, Salter L 2000 Pathways for continence care: background and audit. British Journal of Nursing 9(9): 590–596

Benness C, Gangar K, Cardozo L, Cutner A, Whitehead M 1991 Do progestogens exacerbate urinary incontinence in women on HRT? Neurourology and Urodynamics 10(4): 316–317

Bent A E, Foote J, Siegel S et al 2001 Collagen implant for treating stress urinary incontinence in women with urethral hypermobility. Journal of Urology 166(4): 1354–1357

Blatherwick N R, Long M L 1923 Studies of urinary acidity: the increased acidity produced by eating prunes and cranberries. Journal of Biological Chemistry 57: 815–818

Blowman C, Pickles C, Emery S et al 1991 Prospective double blind controlled trial of intensive physiotherapy with and without stimulation of the pelvic floor in treatment of genuine stress incontinence. Physiotherapy 77(10): 661–664

Bø K, Talseth T 1994 Five-year follow-up of pelvic floor muscle exercise for treatment of stress urinary incontinence: clinical and urodynamic assessment. Neurourology and Urodynamics 13(4): 374–376

Bø K, Hagen R H, Kvarstein B et al 1991 Effects of two different degrees of pelvic floor muscle exercise. Journal of the Association of Chartered Physiotherapists in Obstetrics and Gynaecology 6: 12–17

Bodel P T, Cotran R, Kass E 1959 Cranberry juice and the antibacterial action of hippuric acid. Journal of Clinical Medicine 56(4): 881–887

Brink C A, Sampselle C M, Wells T J et al 1989 A digital test for pelvic muscle strength in older women with urinary incontinence. Nursing Research 38(4): 196–199

Bump R C, Hurt W G, Fantl J A, Wyman J F 1991 Assessment of Kegel pelvic muscle exercise performance after brief verbal instruction. American Journal of Obstetrics and Gynecology 165(2): 322–329

Bump R C, Sugerman H J, Fantl J A, McClish D K 1992 Obesity and lower urinary tract function in women: effect of surgically induced weight loss. American Journal of Obstetrics and Gynecology 167: 392–399

Burgio K L 1990 Behavioral training for stress and urge incontinence in the community. Gerontology 36: 27–34

Burton G, Dobson C 1993 Progesterone increases urinary flow rates: a new treatment for voiding abnormalities. Neurourology and Urodynamics 12(4): 398–399

Cardozo L 1991 Urinary incontinence in women: have we anything new to offer? British Medical Journal 303: 1453–1457

Cardozo L 2000 Biofeedback in overactive bladder. Urology 55(Suppl.): 24–28

Cardozo L D, Cutner A 1993 Is disturbed bladder function after pregnancy normal? Maternal Child Health June: 180–183

Cardozo L, Cutner A, Wise B 1993 Basic urogynaecology. Oxford Medical Publications, Oxford

Carlile A E, Davies I, Farragher E, Rigby A, Brocklehurst J C 1987 Ageing in the human female urethra. Neurourology and Urodynamics 6(3): 149–150

Chiarelli P E 1991 Women's waterworks: curing incontinence. Neen Healthbooks, Dereham, Norfolk

Cochrane Review Abstracts 2001 http://www.medscape.com/cochrane/abstracts

Dolman M E 1992 Midwives' recording of urinary output. Nursing Standard 6(27): 25–27

Dolman M E 1994a Continence advisor demonstrates value of education about pelvic floor exercises in older teenagers. Innovations in Continence Care (2): 1–3

Dolman M E 1994b Remedial action. Nursing Times 91(24) (Continence supplement)

Dolman M E 2000 Electromuscular stimulation for urinary incontinence: Levator 100. British Journal of Community Nursing 5(5): 214–220

Dolman M E, Chase J 1996 Comparison between the health belief model and subjective expected utility theory: predicting incontinence behaviour in post-partum women. Journal of Evaluation in Clinical Practice 2(3): 217–222

Donald I 1979 Practical obstetric problems. Lloyd-Luke, London

Doughty M 1994 Pelvic floor exercise. Cited in: Laycock J, Wyndaele J J (eds) Understanding the pelvic floor. Neen Healthbooks, Dereham, Norfolk

Fall M 1984 Does electrical stimulation cure urinary incontinence? Journal of Urology April: 131

Gibson J N A, Smith K, Rennie M J 1988 Prevention of disuse muscle atrophy by means of electrical stimulation: maintenance of protein synthesis. Lancet 2(8614): 767–770

Glavind K, Nohr B, Walters S 1996 Biofeedback and physiotherapy versus physiotherapy alone in the treatment of genuine stress incontinence. International Journal of Urogynecology 7: 339–343

Glavind K, Laursen B, Jaquet A 1998 Efficacy of biofeedback in the treatment of urinary stress incontinence. International Journal of Urogynecology 9: 151–153

Glazener C M, Herbison G P, Wilson P D et al 2001 Conservative management of persistent postnatal urinary and faecal incontinence: randomized controlled trial. British Medical Journal 323: 593–596

Gomer-Jones E 1963 Nonoperative treatment for stress incontinence. Clinics in Obstetrics and Gynaecology 6: 220–235

Gordon D, Gold R S, Pauzner D, Lessing J B, Groutz A 2001 Combined genitourinary prolapse repair and prophylactic tension-free vaginal tape in women with severe prolapse and occult stress incontinence: preliminary results. Urology 58(4): 547–550

Graber B, Kline-Graber G 1979 Female orgasm: role of pubococcygeus muscle. Journal of Clinical Psychiatry 40: 348–351

Guthrie J R 2001 Natural menopause not a significant risk factor for urinary incontinence. Obstetrics and Gynecology 98: 628–633

Hald T 1975 Problem of urinary incontinence. In: Caldwell K P S (ed) Urinary incontinence. Sector Publishing, London

Haslam J 1998 Treating urinary incontinence using biofeedback and neuromuscular stimulation. Journal of Community Nursing 12(2): 23–25

Hilton P 1987 Urinary incontinence in women. British Medical Journal 295: 424–432

Iravani A 1988 Causes, diagnosis and treatment of bacterial infections of the urinary tract. Comprehensive Therapy 14(11): 49–53

Isherwood P J, Rane A 2000 Comparative assessment of pelvic floor strength using a perineometer and digital examination. British Journal of Obstetrics and Gynaecology 107(8): 1007–1011

Kegel A H 1948 Progressive resistance exercise in the functional restoration of the perineal muscles. American Journal of Obstetrics and Gynecology 56: 238–248

Kelleher C 1998 Acupuncture and lower urinary tract dysfunction. ACA Continence Journal 18(3): 12 (Conference abstract)

Kraft J K, Stamey T A 1977 The natural history of symptomatic recurrent bacteriuria in women. Medicine 56: 55–60

Krantz E K 1986 The Marshall–Marchetti–Krantz procedure. In: Stanton S L, Tanagho E A (eds) Surgery of female incontinence, 2nd edn. Springer Verlag, Berlin, pp 87–93

Laycock J 1987 Graded exercises for the pelvic floor muscles in the treatment of urinary incontinence. Physiotherapy 73(7): 371–373

Laycock J 1992 Pelvic floor re-education for the promotion of continence. In: Roe B H (ed) Clinical nursing practice. Prentice Hall, Englewood Cliffs, NJ, p 102

Laycock J 1994 Clinical evaluation of the pelvic floor. In: Schüssler J, Laycock J, Norton P, Stanton S (eds) Pelvic floor re-education: principles and practice. Springer Verlag, Berlin, Chapter 2.2

Lewey J 1999 Electrical stimulation of the overactive bladder. Professional Nurse 15(3): 211–214

Nicolle L E, Ronald A R 1987 Recurrent UTI in adult women: diagnosis and treatment. Infectious Disease Clinics of North America 1(4): 793–806

Nicolle L E, Harding G K, Preiksaitis J, Ronald A R 1982 The association of UTI with sexual intercourse. Journal of Infectious Diseases 146: 579–583

Nielsen K K, Walter S, Maegaard E, Kromann-Andersen B 1993 The urethral plug II: an alternative treatment in women with genuine urinary stress incontinence. British Journal of Urology 72: 428–432

O'Brien J, Long H 1995 Urinary incontinence: long-term effectiveness of nursing intervention in primary care. British Medical Journal 311: 1208

O'Dowd T C 1993 Management of urinary incontinence in women. British Journal of General Practice 43: 426–429

Philp J, Cottenden A 1993 Continence consumer test. Elderly Care 5(5): 27–30

Rosenbaum T P, Shaw P J R, Rose G A, Lloyd W 1989 Cranberry juice and mucus production in enterouroplasty. Unpublished work: presented to British Association of Urological Surgeons, June 1989

Schmidt R D, Sobata A E 1988 An examination of the anti-adherence activity of cranberry juice on urinary and non-urinary bacterial isolates. Microbias 55: 173–181

Smith D A, Newman D K 1994 Basic elements of biofeedback therapy for pelvic muscle rehabilitation. Urologic Nursing 14(3): 130–135

Smith P, Roberts M, Slade N 1970 Urinary symptoms following hysterectomy. British Journal of Urology 42: 3–9

Snooks S L, Badenock D F, Tiptaft R C, Swash M 1985 Perineal nerve damage in genuine stress incontinence: an electrophysiological study. British Journal of Urology 57: 422–426

Stanton S 1994 Periurethral collagen for female genuine stress incontinence: results at 2–3 year follow-up. Neurourology and Urodynamics 13(4): 449–450

Staskin D, Bavendam T, Sant G et al 1994 A multicenter experience using an expandable urethral occlusion device for management of urinary stress incontinence. Neurourology and Urodynamics 13(4): 380–381

Staskin D, Sant G, Bavendam T et al 1995 Use of an expandable urethral insert for GSI: long-term results of multicenter trial. Neurourology and Urodynamics 14(5): 420–421

Tapp A, Cardozo L, Versi E, Montgomery J, Studd J 1988 The effect of vaginal delivery on the urethral sphincter. British Journal of Obstetrics and Gynaecology 95: 142–146

Weil A, Reyes H, Rottenberg R D et al 1983 Effect of lumbar epidural anaesthesia on lower urinary tract function in the immediate postpartum period. British Journal of Obstetrics and Gynaecology 90: 428–432

4

Mostly male

Tracey Heath
Roger Watson

'Incontinence can be sometimes cured, often relieved, always made more tolerable.'

Isaacs (1986)

INTRODUCTION

It is estimated that between 2.5 and 4 million adults experience continence problems in the United Kingdom alone (Continence Foundation 2000a). Although figures vary considerably depending upon data collection methods, samples and operational definitions used within published prevalence studies, certain trends are apparent. Incontinence is less prevalent in males than in females at all ages (except early childhood – see below) and this may to some extent explain the relative dearth of studies focusing specifically upon the male populous. This said, the issue of incontinence in the male population cannot and should not be ignored. Incontinence in both sexes is more prevalent with advancing years and as our population ages it would seem fair to assume that at the very least this issue will not go away. Whilst many of the causes of incontinence are not specific to either sex and the principles of continence promotion and incontinence management are generally common to both, the male urinary tract and associated structures do present some very specific issues of causality and management. An increasing focus and interest in men's health should result in further research being undertaken in this area in the future. As discussed elsewhere in this book, the potential impact of urinary incontinence on the life of an individual, male or female, should not be underestimated and much can currently be done to assist males experiencing continence problems. This chapter builds upon the principles covered earlier in this publication and focuses specifically upon those aspects of care that are considered to be 'mostly male'.

BACKGROUND
Prevalence

It is appropriate, before embarking upon any discussion of the treatment and management of urinary incontinence in males, to explore the prevalence, causes and impact of this symptom within this group. A variety of operational definitions have been used in published research and this undoubtedly accounts for some of the wide variation in prevalence estimates. Nonetheless, whilst attention needs to be paid to the definition of incontinence used in the study and the instruments involved in data collection, some estimate of the size of the 'problem' and the extent to which males are affected can be gleaned.

Following systematic reviews of the literature pre- and post-1990 respectively Mohide (1992) and Button et al (1998) cite a plethora of studies that estimate the overall prevalence of incontinence in the adult population. Whilst actual figures vary, differences in the relative numbers of males and females experiencing this symptom and the relationship between the age of the study group and the proportion with urinary incontinence appear to be fairly consistent throughout. This is illustrated by one slightly dated though oft-quoted study, (perhaps because it is still viewed as one of the most reliable), that of Thomas et al (1980). Defining incontinence as 'the involuntary loss of urine on two or more occasions per month',

the prevalence of incontinence amongst respondents of a postal survey was found to be 8.5% in females and 1.6% in males, aged 15–64 years, and 11.6% in females and 6.9% in males aged 65 years and over (Thomas et al 1980).

Table 4.1 provides a summary of the findings of some of the more recent prevalence studies that have included males in their sample. Whilst it is virtually impossible to compare individual studies directly for the reasons cited earlier, it is well established that the prevalence of urinary incontinence is lower in men and increases in both sexes with advancing age. This is further reinforced by the data provided in Table 4.2 representing what the Department of Health (2000a) describes as 'currently the best' available.

The prevalence of urinary incontinence amongst both males and females residing in residential and nursing homes is consistently greater than in the general population (DoH 2000a, Royal College of Physicians (RCP) 1995). Evidence specifically relating to the prevalence of incontinence in acute care is less abundant than that for long stay or community settings; however, although more research is undoubtedly required, those studies that do exist suggest that its prevalence is far from insignificant (Mohide 1992). Given the potential sequelae of delayed discharge and repeated readmissions that may ensue, this area is beginning to attract more attention (DoH 2000a). However, here again prevalence rates for men are reported to be less than those for women – of the order of 44% in women and 23% in men (Stott et al 1990).

The figures described above relate to the adult population and figures for childhood incontinence show a slightly different picture. Most children are toilet trained by the age of 3–4 years, usually becoming dry in the day then at night (RCP 1995).

Table 4.1 Prevalence of urinary incontinence: comparison of figures for males and females

Study	Population (sample)	Methodology	Prevalence males (%)	Prevalence females (%)
Hellstrom et al (1990a)	Aged 85 years ($n = 954$)	Face to face interviews	24	43
Ju et al (1991)	Aged 65 years and over ($n = 1143$)	Face to face interviews	4.4	4.8
O'Brien et al (1991)	Aged 35 years and over (UK) ($n = 10\,300$)	Postal questionnaire	4.4	16.4
Brocklehurst (1993)	Age 30 years and over (GB) ($n = 4007$)	Face to face interviews	6.6	14.0
Wolfs et al (1994)	Males aged 55 and older ($n = 2734$)	Postal questionnaire	10.5	–

Table 4.2 Prevalence of urinary incontinence: people living in their own homes

Age range (years)	Males	Females
15–64	Over 1 in 33	Between 1 in 20 and 1 in 14 (aged 15–44 years) Between 1 in 13 and 1 in 7 (aged 45–64 years)
65 and over	Between 1 in 14 and 1 in 10	Between 1 in 10 and 1 in 5

Figures taken from Department of Health (2000a).

Table 4.3 Age-related disorders of the lower urinary tract associated with incontinence in males

Age group	Disorder
Childhood/youth	Anatomical abnormalities Detrusor instability Neuropathic bladder Bladder neck weakness
Middle age	Detrusor instability Neuropathic bladder Bladder neck obstruction Underactive bladder disorders
Older men	Outflow tract obstruction —uncomplicated —associated with instability Neuropathic bladder Detrusor instability Underactive bladder states Extraurological causes: —constipation —pharmacological agents —environmental difficulties

Reproduced with permission from the Royal College of Physicians (1995).

Primary nocturnal enuresis is most prevalent in children aged between 5 and 7 years old. The incidence of primary nocturnal enuresis in males aged 5–7 years is approximately 50% greater than in females of the same age (Hellstrom et al 1990b); however this difference in incidence is much less in adolescent bed-wetters (Devlin 1991) (see also Chapter 5).

Thus it would appear that urinary incontinence in men tends to occur at the extremes of life and that disorders of the lower urinary tract associated with incontinence in males are to some extent age related (RCP 1995), an observation illustrated by Table 4.3.

Research studies 4.1 and 4.2 Patterns of urinary incontinence in community dwelling populations

Study 4.1
Herzog et al (1990) interviewed a sample of 1956 people aged 60 years and over in their own homes at annual intervals. Incidence rates at 1 year were approximately 20% for women and 10% for men. Remission rates for previously incontinent persons were 12% for women and 30% for men.

Study 4.2
Ouslander et al (1993) studied the incidence of incontinence by following its course in 430 people aged 65 and over admitted to eight nursing homes. Incidence was found to be greater in men than in women at both 2 month and 1 year follow-up points (21% females, 51% males, and 16% females, 46% males respectively). Furthermore, female incontinence was more likely to have ceased during the study period, with 23% of women's urinary incontinence having resolved after 1 year compared with only 14% of men's. The authors of this study proposed that the development of urinary incontinence was associated with male sex, a diagnosis of dementia, immobility and faecal incontinence.

GENDER-RELATED DIFFERENCES IMPACTING ON CONTINENCE

Micturition does not conform to a standard pattern and exhibits wide variation between individuals (Cheater 1992). There are few studies that have examined differences in voiding patterns between the two sexes but further research on the voiding patterns of healthy volunteers, both males and females, is required to provide baseline data. There appears to be little difference at least in frequency of voiding (Abrams et al 1983).

It is equally difficult to obtain clear and meaningful figures that permit a comparison of the different types and causes of urinary incontinence occurring in men and women. Nevertheless differences do appear to exist, and these will be discussed in relation to the key structures of the lower urinary tract and the points of divergence between males and females.

The characteristics associated with three structures – the urethra, the pelvic floor and the prostate gland – offer some explanation for the differing prevalence figures and patterns of incontinence between males and females. This section is not intended to provide a comprehensive review of this area, only to offer some insight into the key factors that influence the different patterns of development in these two groups.

The urethra and pelvic floor

Males have an 'S' shaped urethra which is 18–22 cm in length, whilst females have a straight urethra which is 3–5 cm long (Colburn 1994). These characteristics are associated with a lower incidence of urinary tract infections in men compared to women. Urinary infections are in turn frequently cited as causing or predisposing to transient urinary incontinence by increasing sensory input from the bladder and contributing to urgency and detrusor instability (Cheater 1992). Urinary infection may also exacerbate other types of bladder dysfunction. However, whilst the length and shape of the male urethra may have a protective function with regard to infection, these characteristics can contribute to other problems such as the 'post-micturition dribble' experienced by many men and discussed later in the text.

Stress incontinence primarily results from a failure of the external urethral sphincter to accommodate increases in intra-abdominal pressure. The external (voluntary) sphincter is formed by the pelvic floor muscles; any factor contributing to a reduction in the strength of these muscles or in the patency of the seal formed by the urethra is therefore likely to predispose an individual to stress incontinence. Falls in oestrogen with advancing age (during the menopause) and the physical trauma of pregnancy and childbirth have all been associated with diminished capacity to sustain increases in intra-abdominal pressure (Cardozo et al 1993, NHMRC 1994, RCP 1995), although evidence in this area is far from conclusive. Clearly, once more these are predisposing factors that are not a concern for males. In fact, genuine stress incontinence is rare in neurologically normal males, although it may arise as a result of prostate surgery or chronic retention (Abrams et al 1983, RCP 1995). In contrast, genuine stress incontinence is the commonest cause of urinary incontinence in women (Cardozo et al 1993). Interestingly,

Stanton (1984) suggests a further contributing factor which increases women's predisposition towards stress incontinence. Women are described as anatomically weaker in the pelvic region and that this is at least in part associated with the evolutionary change from the horizontal to the vertical position such that the urethra leaves the bladder at the point of maximum gravitational force.

The prostate gland

The prostate gland is a structure that lies directly below the bladder in males. It forms part of the male reproductive system, is attached to the base of the bladder and surrounds the initial 3–4 cm of the urethra.

One of the main roles of the prostate gland is to secrete a lubricant into seminal fluid for the passage of sperm from the testes to the urethra during sexual intercourse. Enlargement of the prostate through disease processes and age-associated changes can, due to its position, serve to obstruct the outflow of urine. The most common cause of this is benign prostatic enlargement. The absence of a similar structure in women places them less at risk of outflow obstruction and associated difficulties in maintaining continence (Cheater 1992).

Urge incontinence also increases with age in men. This symptom too is sometimes associated with the prostate. Approximately 66% of men investigated for 'prostatic' outflow disorders will be unstable on cystometry before operation and one-third of men will remain so postoperatively despite relief of obstruction (RCP 1995). Although outflow obstruction and detrusor instability sometimes coexist, in severe cases of obstruction bladder contractions may be unsustained resulting in a progressive increase in residual volume.

A recent study supported by the Medical Research Council (Perry et al 2000) serves to demonstrate that both men and women experience a whole array of significant urinary symptoms (frequency, urgency, incontinence, nocturia, straining) and that none is the preserve of either one sex. This work appears to add weight to the argument that whilst some types and causes are more prevalent in males than others, incontinence in males can present in a variety of ways and be caused by any one or a combination of a range of underlying conditions or associated factors.

Impact of incontinence

Despite its potentially devastating impact upon the lives of individual sufferers and their carers, urinary incontinence is a condition for which few people seek help (Egan et al 1991). There is some evidence that the relative responses of men and women can differ. Both sexes display psychological distress in terms of reductions in mental well-being, ability to cope with domestic chores, social life, relationships with the family, intimate relations and work (McCormick & Palmer 1992), but as the severity of symptoms increases, this appears to have less overt impact on men than women.

The work of Herzog et al (1989) explores help-seeking behaviour and self-care activity amongst community-residing older adults. Significantly, only 20% of men compared with 69% of women had tried some means of self-management for their incontinence, and although not statistically significant, more women (65%) compared with men (48%) had talked to their doctor about their continence problems. Although the majority of sufferers do report that incontinence has a negative impact upon their lives, this is clearly not the case for all. In a study by Hunksaar & Sandvik (1993) 24% of men responding to an advertisement for incontinence aids felt that their urinary incontinence was a minor problem. However, Roe & May (1997) refer to the lack of impact studies focusing on or including men and believe this needs further attention.

Promoting continence

It is tempting to conclude that all attempts to improve continence promotion and incontinence management for males should focus upon the prostate. However, the causes of incontinence in males are varied and, as Table 4.3 illustrates, not all continence problems can be attributed to differences in anatomy. Just as in women, urinary incontinence, particularly in older men, can be multifactorial in nature and its treatment and management require consideration of the whole person. For example, not all individuals with bladder symptoms associated with benign prostatic hypertrophy (BPH) will become incontinent; it may be a change in environment necessitating a lengthier journey to the toilet, or the simultaneous presence of a urine infection that tips the balance. The importance of a thorough assessment of the patient's continence problem cannot be underestimated.

Prevention

Several studies have demonstrated positive links between risk factors and urinary incontinence. Button et al (1998) provide a useful overview of this area and identify smoking, body mass index (BMI) and exercise as issues that are also important from a general health promotion stance. There is evidence which is indicative of a relationship between smoking and deterioration in lower urinary tract symptoms in men. Although obesity is associated with increased risks of both stress and urge incontinence in women, similar risks for incontinence in men have not been shown (Abrams et al 2002).

Over recent years health promotion for males has gained far greater attention. For example, aside from the more conventional sources of health education, such as practice nurses, general practitioners and men's health clinics, several websites have emerged (Box 4.1). Mention of the prostate clearly forms an important part of overall health education strategies directed at males. For example, one website (mens-care.co.uk) includes a do-it-yourself international prostate symptom score (Fig. 4.1). It is clearly important that men should have knowledge of the signs and symptoms of early (as well as more advanced) prostate disease, and by implication potential bladder and continence problems if prevention of more serious complications is to be avoided and early treatment instituted. Billington (1999) proposes three simple questions (Box 4.2), which could easily be included as part of a broad-based patient/client health assessment. Answers to these questions will provide an indication of those most likely to benefit from more in-depth enquiry.

Patient Name Date		Not at all	Less than one time in five	Less than half the time	About half the time	More than half the time	Almost always	Your score
1.	*Incomplete emptying* Over the past month how often have you had the sensation of not emptying your bladder completely after you finish urinating?	0	1	2	3	4	5	
2.	*Frequency* Over the past month how often have you had to urinate again less than 2 hours after you finished urinating?	0	1	2	3	4	5	
3.	*Intermittency* Over the past month how often have you found you stopped and started again several times when you urinate?	0	1	2	3	4	5	
4.	*Urgency* Over the past month how often have you found it difficult to postpone urination?	0	1	2	3	4	5	
5.	*Weak stream* Over the past month how often have you had a weak urinary stream?	0	1	2	3	4	5	
6.	*Straining* Over the past month, how often have you had to push or strain to begin urination?	0	1	2	3	4	5	
		None	1 time	2 times	3 times	4 times	5 times or more	
7.	*Nocturia* Over the past month, how many times did you most typically get up to urinate from the time you went to bed at night until the time you got up in the morning?	0	1	2	3	4	5	

Total I-PSS score

The total score can range from 0–35 (asymptomatic to very symptomatic). Although there are at present no standard recommendations on grading patients with mild, moderate or severe symptoms, patients can be tentatively classified as follows:

1–7 = mildly symptomatic   8–19 = moderately symptomatic   20–35 = severely symptomatic

	Delighted	Pleased	Mostly satisfied	Mixed – about equally satisfied and dissatisfied	Most dissatisfied unhappy	Terrible	
Quality of life due to urinary symptoms							
If you were to spend the rest of your life with your urinary condition just the way it is now, how would you feel about that?	0	1	2	3	4	5	

Figure 4.1 International prostate symptom score (I-PSS). (Reproduced with permission from Barry et al 1992.)

Box 4.1 Continence resources – useful websites

Websites orientated towards the patient/client(s)
http://www.incontinencenet.org/www.mens-care.co.uk
http://www-continence-foundation.org.uk/index.html
http://www.UroSupport.com
http://medweb.bham.ac.uk/cancerhelp/public/specific/
prostate/index.html

**Websites orientated towards the healthcare
professional**
http://www.urohealth.org/index.shtml
http://www.pslgroup.com/enlargprost.htm
http://www.bui.ac.uk
http://urology.about.com
http://www.esir.com
http://www.uroweb.org
http://www.uronet.org
http://www.incontinencenet.org

Note: Information from websites – like that from other
sources – needs to be critically appraised before use.

Many websites provide access to others of a similar
nature; the British Association of Urological Surgeons
website (http://www.baus.org.uk) is very useful in this
respect.

Box 4.2 Highlighting continence problems: three
useful questions

- Have you noticed a deterioration in your flow of
  urine?
- Are you bothered by urinary symptoms?
- Do you have to get up at night to pass urine?

Based upon Billington (1999).

Nurses are often viewed as front-line workers
in continence care (DoH 2000a, Hagan 1990)
although this role is not exclusively theirs.
However, school nurses, practice nurses, occupational health nurses, midwives, community- and
hospital-based nurses, in addition to continence
advisors, are often presented with the opportunity
to educate people of all ages about the prevention
and treatment of continence problems (Cheater
1996). Given that so few seek help it is important
that such opportunities are not overlooked and
that proactive identification of need is pursued.
Innovative locations for clinics, such as in leisure
centres or in workplaces, can provide further
opportunities for men to come forward for information and advice.

Although many symptoms of incontinence are
common to men and women there are some
methods of urine collection that are more conducive to use by men than women including the
use of urine bottles, non-spill adapters and hydrophilic gel. Although urinals are available for
women, they are much easier to design and use
for men. Urinals are relatively inexpensive and are
particularly useful if an individual is experiencing
difficulty reaching the toilet or is suffering from
urgency. Whilst standard models are basically a
bottle (usually with a lid), versions with a handle
and fitted with non-spill adapters are also available and can prove particularly useful if difficulty is experienced in positioning or holding the
product. Sachets of gel powder, which can be
emptied into urine bottles to soak up most of the
fluid, are helpful in reducing the risk of spillage,
and collapsible and disposable urinals may prove
useful when travelling. Case study 4.1 presented
later in this chapter provides an example of how
the simplest of solutions can sometimes make a
profound difference to the life of an individual.

Treatment of urinary incontinence in males

Some distinction between treatment and management is necessary before discussing these aspects
of urinary incontinence in males. Treatment implies
some kind of intervention that is aimed at reducing or altogether 'curing' the urinary incontinence
(Long 1991). The management of incontinence
on the other hand implies the use of measures
designed to achieve social continence and will be
discussed later in the chapter.

Various strategies are currently employed to
promote and restore continence, including both
surgery and drug therapy. The use of treatments
specifically related to the male with urinary incontinence will be explored in the following sections
entitled 'Focus on the prostate' and 'Focus on
postmicturition dribble'.

FOCUS ON THE PROSTATE

As discussed earlier the prostate gland, or rather its
enlargement, particularly in later life, plays a major
role in the development of urinary incontinence.

Non-malignant enlargement of the prostate

Prostate disease and benign prostatic hypertrophy (BPH) (also referred to as benign prostatic hyperplasia) are now so common among older men that their absence could be regarded as abnormal (Webb & Simpson 1997). BPH is said to affect a third of men over the age of 50 years and the majority of those over 80 years (Billington 1999).

Many of the symptoms of BPH stem directly from obstruction of the urethra and resultant incomplete bladder emptying. The symptoms of BPH can vary but the most common ones include:

- a hesitant, interrupted, weak stream of urine
- urgency and leaking or dribbling
- more frequent urination, especially at night.

Severity of symptoms does not necessarily correlate with the degree to which the prostate gland is enlarged (Billington 1999), thus the first symptom for some men may be a complete inability to pass urine and consequent urinary retention. Since these symptoms are not disease specific, patients require objective assessment so that the most appropriate course of action can be taken. As the population ages it seems inevitable that the number of men presenting with BPH will increase and the recent advances in prostate assessment clinics are a response to this perceived trend in demand. The clinics aim to reduce waiting times, lead to prompt referral of those with severe symptoms and to provide better continuity and quality of care (Webb & Simpson 1997).

Malignant enlargement of the prostate

Prostate cancer is the second most common cancer among men in Britain (DoH 2000b). Every year in England and Wales in the region of 19 000 men are diagnosed with prostate cancer and approximately 8000 men die from it, characteristically around 4 or 5 years after diagnosis. Prostate cancer accounts for approximately 4% of all male deaths each year (DoH 2000c). In terms of prevalence it shows a similar pattern to BPH, in that it is generally a disease of older men and is rare in the under-50 age group. By the age of 80 about half of men will have a focus of cancer in their prostate, although only 1 in 25 males will actually die from it (DoH 2000b).

Recently there has been concern that for too long not enough has been done to detect prostate cancer or to improve the treatment and care of men diagnosed with it (DoH 2000b). This form of cancer is described as the 'most mysterious' (DoH 2000b) and may be more accurately referred to as cancers since anecdotal evidence suggests that prostate cancer behaves differently in different individuals. The cause of prostate cancer is unknown. However, a recent Department of Health report (DoH 2000b) has identified several factors associated with the disease's development:

- Having relatives who have had cancer of the prostate
- Belonging to certain ethnic groups (African Caribbean/African American)
- Eating a diet high in animal fat and protein.

The symptoms of BPH and prostate cancer are often similar; thankfully the majority of men with these symptoms do not have a malignancy. However, some individuals who have cancer may not experience symptoms at all and if they do it may not be until the late stages of the disease. Clearly diagnosis is important and will be discussed later.

Assessment of individuals with suspected prostate disease

The international prostate symptom score is a recognized tool used to assess the severity of an individual's symptoms (see Fig. 4.1). The use of a frequency volume chart can prove a helpful adjunct and will provide an indication of drinking patterns, maximum functional bladder capacity, frequency and the presence and degree of nocturia experienced. Any assessment should include reference to the impact that the individual's prostate problem is having on their life in general. Although the single question recommended in Figure 4.1 will not capture the total impact of symptoms on quality of life, it may serve as a valuable starting point on which to base further conversation between the practitioner and the patient.

Clearly other causes of urinary symptoms (such as infection) need to be excluded and a comprehensive baseline assessment in keeping with that currently recommended by the Department of Health (2000a) applies equally to those presenting with prostate symptoms. Urodynamic studies are used to assess the degree of obstruction experienced. If the maximum flow rate is less than 10 ml/s there is a 90% chance of prostatic obstruction (Abrams 1997). However, when an individual presents with acute urinary retention its immediate relief is an urgent priority if backpressure on the kidneys is to be prevented. Creatinine level investigation is commonly included as part of the initial assessment to check renal function (Blandy 1998).

Diagnosis

In view of the non-specific nature of prostatic symptoms, careful diagnosis is important and there are three recognized methods of distinguishing prostate cancer from BPH: prostate-specific antigen, digital rectal examination and transrectal needle biopsy.

Prostate-specific antigen (PSA)

Prostate-specific antigen is measured by taking a blood sample. Serum PSA levels are raised not only in prostate cancer, but also in several other conditions that affect the prostate gland such as prostatitis (infection). Although the precise threshold level indicative of cancer remains the subject of debate, some guidance does exist (Table 4.4).

Digital rectal examination (DRE)

Although the prostate is readily palpated by DRE, in its early stages prostate cancer is seldom detectable. Overall DRE in isolation is less than 50% accurate in detecting prostate cancer and is usually done in conjunction with PSA (DoH 2000b). The size, consistency and mobility of the prostate are key characteristics (Table 4.5). A normal prostate is approximately the size of a chestnut, smooth and elastic. A hard, nodular prostate, especially if fixed to adjacent tissue, may be malignant. A tender prostate suggests prostatitis (Billington 1999). The patient's general practitioner usually performs DRE, but as with other aspects of the assessment, a specialist nurse within a nurse-led clinic sometimes undertakes the procedure.

Transrectal needle biopsy

In this technique an ultrasound probe is inserted into the rectum enabling the specialist to 'see' the prostate and biopsy different parts for histological examination. There is a risk of infection with this procedure, as a result of which patients are usually prescribed a course of antibiotics.

BPH and prostate cancer: treatment options

The treatments of BPH and cancer do have some similarities, but also marked differences. They are therefore considered separately for ease of

Table 4.4 PSA testing – interpreting the PSA

PSA value	Interpretation
0.5–4 ng/ml	Normal
4–10 ng/ml	20% chance of cancer
>10 ng/ml	50%+ chance of cancer
Rise of >20% a year	Refer immediately for consideration of biopsy

PSA, prostate-specific antigen.
Reproduced with permission from Kirby et al (2000).

Table 4.5 Assessment through digital rectal examination

Characteristic	Appearance
Size	The normal prostate gland is the size of a chestnut, enlargement occurs in both BPH and prostate cancer
Consistency	A normal prostate is smooth or elastic. The lateral lobes are symmetric and divided by a palpable sulcus A tender prostate may indicate prostatitis A hard, nodular prostate may indicate prostate cancer
Mobility	A malignant prostate gland may be fixed to adjacent structures

Based on Billington (1999) and Lazzaro & Thompson (1997).

discussion. The main treatment options are discussed within this section. For a more comprehensive and detailed account the reader is referred to more specialist texts.

In males with BPH, if there is no urgent reason to refer, a period of conservative treatment of 3 months is recommended (Abrams 1997, Feneley et al 1999). Conservative treatment in this case consists of bladder training, advice on fluid intake, pelvic floor exercises, plus or minus an anticholinergic drug if the patient is thought to have detrusor instability. It is not unknown for older men to experience a year or more during which their prostate irritates them, only for symptoms to get better without any treatment (Blandy 1998).

Men can be taught how to carry out pelvic floor exercises in the same way as women (see Chapter 3 for further details), but have the added advantage that by practising in front of a mirror they can observe muscle contraction at the base of the penis and a scrotal lift. They can also learn to palpate muscle contraction at the perineum 2 cm medially and 2 cm anteriorly to the ischial tuberosity (Dorey 2001). This is useful when teaching and learning the correct technique but the frequency and intensity of the exercise regime are determined by individual assessment and digital rectal examination. It is advantageous for patients to receive education about the use of pelvic floor exercises and to have begun to practise them prior to surgery.

Drug therapy exists predominantly in the form of alpha-blockers and 5-alpha reductase inhibitors. Surgery is also an option for those individuals with BPH who are experiencing persistent, moderate or severe symptoms. Surgical prostate ablation, by transurethral resection of the prostate (TURP) or less frequently open prostatectomy, is still the 'gold standard' and produces the greatest measurable and long-term reduction in both symptoms and bladder outlet obstruction (Feneley et al 1999). Other methods of ablation (e.g. laser techniques) are newer and evidence of their efficacy is currently limited.

The treatment and care of men diagnosed with prostate cancer depends upon the extent of the disease although the evidence base for these decisions is limited. For early stage cancer the options include 'watchful waiting' (to determine whether the cancer is active or slow growing), radical prostatectomy and radiotherapy. For cancer that has spread beyond the prostate radiotherapy and hormone therapy remain the main treatment options (DoH 2000b).

Treatment of BPH

As suggested earlier, conservative treatment or 'watchful waiting' is the preferred option for men with mild symptoms as disease progression is uncertain and often slow (Billington 1999). The Bristol Urological Institute suggests that if the patient wishes to try drug therapy an alpha-blocker (e.g. prazosin, indoramin) is the treatment of first choice for BPH, since its effects, if any, are immediate (Feneley et al 1999). These drugs improve both filling and voiding symptoms in BPH, by relaxing smooth muscle and reducing urethral resistance. Caution is advised in the treatment of older men or those on antihypertensives using this method. However, some drugs are now said to be more urospecific or selective and therefore to have fewer side-effects (e.g. alfuzosin). Nonetheless, patients using these drugs should be advised of potential side-effects such as postural hypotension and dizziness.

The use of 5-alpha reductase inhibitors to shrink the epithelial part of the gland is another option. The action of drugs such as finasteride is to reduce the size of the prostate by suppressing plasma levels of dihydrotestosterone (DHT), the principal agent causing prostatic enlargement. However, it is suggested that these drugs benefit only a minority of men, with maximum effect taking at least 6 months to be achieved (Feneley et al 1999). Men receiving alpha reductase inhibitors need to be warned of potential side-effects such as impotence, reduced ejaculate volume and loss of libido (Billington 1999).

Surgical treatment of BPH most commonly involves transurethral resection of the prostate (TURP). An instrument is passed along the urethra to the prostate gland and the enlarged prostate is 'pared' away from inside the urethra (Fig. 4.2). The process can be easily visualized if you imagine the coring of an apple. The aim of this technique is to relieve the obstruction at the bladder neck

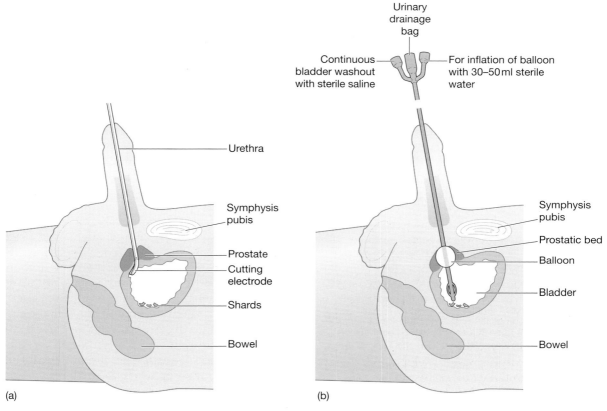

Figure 4.2 (a) Transurethral resection of prostate (TURP). (b) Three-way catheter allowing continuous irrigation of the bladder to remove shards of prostate tissue.

and thereby relieve the retention of urine. The process of TURP may have to be repeated several times as the prostate continues to enlarge and the frequency at which surgery has to be repeated varies between individuals. The procedure is usually performed under general anaesthetic and is a relatively successful option for those who are fit enough to undergo surgery.

Other forms of prostate ablation such as transurethral incision of the prostate and laser therapy are becoming increasingly popular, although TURP is still the more usual procedure. Other alternatives such as the use of radiowaves, microwaves and prostatic stent insertion (a coil-like catheter that is placed in the prostatic urethra) are also used (Downey 2000). However, even when enlargement is benign an open prostatectomy (whereby an incision is made into the abdomen and the whole prostate gland is removed) is occasionally necessary (Game & Farrer 1989).

Complications following surgery

All surgery carries risks; prostate surgery can result in urinary incontinence and/or retrograde ejaculation, aside from the possibility of immediate postsurgical complications such as haemorrhage and hypovolaemic shock (Morrison et al 1994). Postsurgical urinary incontinence is attributed to the trauma associated with surgery in the area of the bladder neck, dilatation of the urethral sphincters and the insertion of large gauge urinary catheters to facilitate irrigation (Laker 1994). Newer treatments such as radiowave (transurethral needle ablation) and laser therapy tend to be associated with less incontinence (Downey 2000).

Box 4.3 Prostatectomy: helpful hints following surgery

1. After your operation do not be too disappointed if you find everything is not perfect immediately. Your bladder is going to take a little time to adjust to both the problems you had before, and the operation itself. So be patient! You may have problems with controlling the bladder and may even be wet occasionally, but this should improve with time. Here are some hints which can help you to help yourself.
2. Drink plenty of fluids, 2 litres (3–4 pints) a day. Do not restrict your fluid intake because you are afraid of being wet. Concentrated urine will irritate the bladder and cause urgency when you do have to pass water. It may also lead to a urinary infection. Plenty of fluids will also help you from being constipated.
3. For a while, you may find that sitting down to pass urine will help empty the bladder completely. If this does not seem to be a problem, then stand to urinate in the usual way.
4. Do try to 'hang on' for a few minutes before passing water, particularly if you have to go frequently. This will help your bladder to get used to going for longer periods between emptying.
5. Every time you pass water, try to stop the stream. The muscles to do this are the pelvic floor muscles and once you have identified them, try tightening them when you are not urinating. Another way to locate your pelvic floor muscle, is to sit on a chair and try to lift your scrotum off the chair. Frequent tightening and relaxing of the pelvic floor muscles will help to strengthen them and thus prevent leakage from your bladder. A suggested number to do each day is 75–100, in groups of ten. Do not overexercise the muscle at any one time as it will get tired and the exercise will be counterproductive. Soon you will regain control of the unwanted urinary leakage.
6. If a few drops of urine leak out after you think you have finished passing water, it may be that some urine is 'trapped' in the outlet where your prostate used to be. This can often be overcome by pushing up behind the scrotum and massaging the base of the penis with your thumb. This helps to expel the last few drops of urine *before* you leave the toilet!
7. A very common problem after a prostatectomy is for semen to go back into the bladder during intercourse rather than come out through the penis. You will notice that your urine looks cloudy after intercourse when you first pass water. However, this should not affect your ability to have an erection or impair enjoyment of sexual relationships.
8. If for some reason involuntary urine leakage continues, ask a specialist for advice about a suitable collecting device. There are many to choose from and most are discrete and available on prescription.

Nearly all men who have undergone TURP experience retrograde ejaculation. Small numbers of men also suffer from impotence. Both impotence and urinary incontinence are associated with open prostatectomy (Downey 2000). It is therefore particularly important that consent to surgery is informed and that men are aware of the potential urinary and sexual problems that may follow.

A programme to assist the achievement of full continence should be instigated as soon as possible (see the patient handout on 'Helpful hints following surgery' – Box 4.3). Several options exist to promote postsurgical urinary continence, including pelvic floor re-education and bladder training programmes. A recent review by Moore et al (2000) of the conservative management of postprostatectomy incontinence concluded that its value remains unclear and that men's symptoms tended to improve over time irrespective of treatment. Nonetheless some support for the benefit of pelvic floor re-education and bladder retraining in treating urinary incontinence does exist although more trials are clearly indicated (DoH 2000a). Insertion of an artificial urethral sphincter (Fig. 4.3) may be an option for a small proportion of men with intractable postprostatectomy incontinence (Cheater 1996). Venn et al (2000) reviewing long term outcome following sphincter

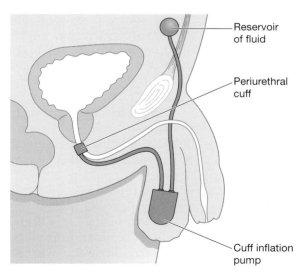

Figure 4.3 An artificial sphincter.

Reservoir of fluid

Periurethral cuff

Cuff inflation pump

Box 4.4 Bladder training chart

BLADDER TRAINING CHART

Week Commencing: _____ Name: _____

Please tick in the **plain** column each time you pass urine

Please tick in the **shaded** column each time you are wet

	Monday		Tuesday		Wednesday		Thursday		Friday		Saturday		Sunday	
6.00 am														
7.00 am														
8.00 am														
9.00 am														
10.00 am														
11.00 am														
12.00 am														
1.00 pm														
2.00 pm														
3.00 pm														
4.00 pm														
5.00 pm														
6.00 pm														
7.00 pm														
8.00 pm														
9.00 pm														
10.00 pm														
11.00 pm														
12.00 pm														
1.00 am														
2.00 am														
3.00 am														
4.00 am														
5.00 am														
Totals														

Comments:

implantation conclude that male postprostatectomy incontinence seemed especially amenable to such treatment. Fluid volume or specifically designed bladder training charts such as that reproduced in Box 4.4 can be useful in helping both the patient and the healthcare professional assess and monitor the improvement of urinary symptoms.

Sexual problems such as impotence can sometimes be the result of anxiety rather than a direct consequence of the surgery. Even so, whatever the underlying cause of the problem, referral to a specialist clinic is the main course of action. The impact that a loss of potency and incontinence can have on an individual in terms of self-image should not be ignored and is considered in more detail later.

Treatment of prostate cancer

As mentioned earlier in the chapter the treatment of prostate cancer is largely dependent on the stage of the cancer at the time of diagnosis. Treatment options for prostate cancer, aside from watchful waiting, include surgery, radiotherapy and drug therapy. As indicated earlier radical (total) prostatectomy is a major operation and whilst there are no precise figures for the United Kingdom, impotence and urinary incontinence are possible sequelae.

Radiotherapy treats cancer by using high-energy rays that destroy cancer cells. For prostate cancer this may be achieved in two ways: using an external beam that produces X-rays that focus on the prostate from outside of the body or using brachytherapy. The latter involves the insertion (under a general anaesthetic) of small radioactive seeds that release radiation slowly over time. Both forms of radiotherapy have side-effects, but the newer technique of brachytherapy appears to

---

Research study 4.3 Early localized prostate cancer

The Centre for Reviews and Dissemination Reviewers (2000), in reviewing the management and treatment of early, localized prostate cancer, concluded that there was only a 10% difference in survival rate between radical and conservative treatment for early localized prostate cancer. Conservative management they suggest is a reasonable option for men with localized disease. However, they also indicate that in the absence of evidence from randomized controlled trials concerning the relative benefits of treatments, informed patient choice should be a major consideration. Furthermore, they also indicate that the potential costs of screening programmes are huge, and that there are limited economic evaluations available to provide this practice, especially as the efficacy and effectiveness of treatments remains unresolved.

---

result in less damage to the bowel and less impotence (DoH 2000b).

For cancers that have spread beyond the prostate, radiotherapy and hormone therapy are the options. Hormone therapy relies upon the fact that most prostate cancers depend on a continuing supply of male hormones, mainly testosterone. Reducing the amount of testosterone by removing the testicles (orchidectomy) or by pharmacological means can help to control prostate cancer and relieve symptoms for months or years. Pharmacological treatment may often be used as an adjunct to surgical intervention where cancers have spread outside the prostate (DoH 2000b).

There are two main types of pharmacological therapy: luteinizing hormone releasing hormone (LHRH) analogues and total androgen ablation or blockade. LHRH analogues act directly on the pituitary gland to inhibit the release of follicle stimulating hormone and luteinizing hormone, thus blocking production and release of testosterone. Total androgen blockade is used when a patient no longer responds to other hormonal treatments. Some antiandrogens are given in conjunction with a LHRH analogue or bilateral orchidectomy. This regimen blocks the effect of all circulating testosterone, including that produced by the adrenal glands (Greifzu 2000). These treatments are not without side-effects, the main ones being hot flushes, decreased libido and impotence.

Cytotoxic chemotherapy using drugs such as methotrexate to prevent growth of the malignant cells may also be employed, but this is not considered a treatment of choice. However, none of the above non-surgical treatments is shown to be superior and none is wholly effective (DoH 2000b, Marsh 1992).

To screen or not to screen?

There is pressure to introduce screening for prostate cancer but, to date, there is no high-quality evidence that screening reduces mortality (National Screening Committee 2000a,b). The prostate-specific antigen (PSA) test has a limited accuracy and could therefore lead to a false-positive result for those without the disease. The United Kingdom National Screening Committee states emphatically

---

Case study 4.1

Bill is a 72-year-old retired government employee. Three years ago he had a prostatectomy for malignant enlargement of the prostate gland; there was no evidence of metastases. Postoperatively he had frequency and urgency and underwent some undefined physiotherapy. His surgery was performed 'out of area' in a private hospital. General health is good, but he does have high blood pressure and arthritis. Medications include hypertensives and diuretics. Occasionally he takes analgesics if the arthritis is painful. He loves his garden, walking and is active in the Church. He has regular appointments with the urologist for PSA blood tests and to date all is clear.

He was referred to the Community Continence Advisor by the consultant, as he was complaining of urgency, frequency and nocturia. It was the disturbed sleep that worried him and his wife most of all. They were both getting very tired and felt they could no longer put up with this situation. He also admitted that on a few occasions he had wet himself while out walking and he 'dribbled' before reaching the toilet most mornings, once he had taken the diuretic.

He said he had done some pelvic floor exercises after the 'op' but had not done them for a long time now as he found them difficult to do. He felt the muscle was very weak.

The specialist nurse talked about the pelvic floor exercises but realized this was not a viable treatment at this stage. Instead, electrical stimulation with the use of an anal plug was suggested and it was explained that the daily treatment could be done in the comfort of his own home. Bill was very willing to try this as he woke up early every day and could do it before breakfast. It was suggested that he waited until after his bowel movement and he agreed. He understood that the length of time for the treatment was 12–16 weeks and that he might not see much improvement until after 6 weeks. Meanwhile he was given two pairs of washable men's pants with an integral pad to stop him from worrying about wetting his trousers. He was so thrilled with these that he bought four more pairs himself.

At the 6-week follow-up, he reported that using the device was no problem, but he was not feeling much benefit from it. He was given time to express all his feelings and then encouraged not to give up yet. Six more weeks was a different story! He said his morning frequency was less, he did not 'dribble' and he only got up three times in the night. More encouragement from the specialist nurse and also praise that he had done well. At the final appointment, 6 weeks later again, he felt a new man. Daytime frequency was seven times and his wife reported 'he sleeps through the night now, it's wonderful'. He had been trying his own pelvic floor exercises with the machine, so now that the treatment period is over he continues with the exercises himself. He also wears the pants as he says that gives him peace of mind when he is out. He has a direct contact with the continence service and can ring anytime if the symptoms return. He knows that it is possible to have a 4-week 'top-up' with the electrical therapy whenever he feels he needs it.

As the consultant said in his letter after seeing Bill in the outpatient clinic 'Long may this last'.

---

that it should not be used for screening. Further ethical issues surround those correctly identified as having prostate cancer as it is often impossible to distinguish between slow-growing tumours that cause no harm and fast-growing tumours that kill (DoH 2000c). If screening were to be introduced many men would be subjected to traumatic treatment with the unpleasant side-effects of impotence and incontinence, who might never have suffered any ill effects from prostate cancer in their lifetime.

At present prostate screening is not recommended for routine use, on evidence provided in two systematic reviews of the literature undertaken in 1997 (Chamberlain et al 1997, Selley et al 1997). Further work is being funded in this area however, but this does not affect the clinical management of men with symptoms of prostate cancer.

For those men concerned about the possibility of prostate cancer, the PSA test is still available. However, it is stressed that clear information should be provided to patients to ensure that they are fully informed of the reliability of the test before giving consent. The impetus for improvement in this area of care comes from the Prostate Cancer Risk Management Programme and is accompanied through the National Prostate Cancer Programme by a substantial (20-fold) increase in research funding directed towards all aspects of prostate cancer diagnosis and treatment (DoH 2000b).

FOCUS ON POSTMICTURITION DRIBBLE

Postmicturition dribble – the loss of a small amount of urine after voiding is completed – is

---

Box 4.5 Reflection point – other causes of urinary problems in men

As indicated earlier, urinary retention, resulting predominantly but not solely from outflow obstruction, is a significant cause of continence problems in men. However, enlargement of the prostate, either benign or malignant, is not the only cause of urinary retention (Bullock et al 1994). Other causes include:

- previous surgery involving the neck of the bladder (which may lead to stenosis in this area)
- bladder neck dyssynergia (the cause of which is not always discernible, but which leads to a functional retention of urine whereby the sphincters either fail to relax or contract as urine is voided)
- urethral strictures (which occur when a part of the urethra narrows, either for no apparent reason or as a result of previous catheterizations, resulting in a slower urine flow, leading to other urinary symptoms such as urinary tract infection).

It is important, with men as with women, not to arrive at hasty conclusions about the underlying cause/causes of incontinence. The symptom of urinary retention alone serves as a useful reminder of the importance of thorough assessment and the need to appreciate that continence problems may be the result of one or more of a whole plethora of causes.

Research study 4.4 Pelvic floor exercises as a treatment for postmicturition dribble

Paterson et al (1997) undertook a study on 49 men aged 36–83 years in Australia. The men were randomly assigned to one of three treatment groups: pelvic muscle exercise, urethral milking or counselling. Participants in each group followed the treatment specific to their group for 3 weeks. Using the outcome measure – improvement in pad weight gain – the authors concluded that both pelvic floor exercises and urethral milking were effective treatments for postmicturition dribble compared with counselling alone. Pelvic floor exercises were more effective in reducing urine loss than urethral milking in this study.

MANAGING INCONTINENCE

The management of incontinence implies the use of measures designed to achieve social continence and in so doing make incontinence more tolerable. Alleviating the often unpleasant and undesirable consequences of urinary incontinence may be a short-term measure (during treatment) or a long-term strategy when other options have been exhausted. Management options for males can be grouped into two major categories: containment aids and conduction aids. Examples include small pouches for dribbling incontinence and urinary sheath drainage systems respectively.

Urinary incontinence can be cured or alleviated in up to 70% of cases (RCP 1995), implying that it is rarely acceptable to adopt conservative management strategies without also addressing the underlying cause of the problem. Other courses of action need to be explored and urinary incontinence should not be considered irreversible until it has been demonstrated to be so (Gooch 1991).

The aim of management is to restore social continence, prevent secondary problems such as skin excoriation and odour and to make incontinence more tolerable. In cases where treatment is not an option (or where the individual chooses not to pursue this route), the more quickly a suitable form of management can be found, the better. Even when further investigation is being carried out or treatment instituted, management strategies are often still an appropriate short-term measure in order to promote the individual's dignity.

unique to men and is a common and troublesome condition in later life. It is a symptom that can affect quality of life and is an important factor in motivating men to consult their doctor. Milliard (1989) suggested that postmicturition dribble that is not associated with obstruction might be caused through the urethra being emptied incompletely by the muscles surrounding it. Denning (1996) suggests that it is caused by pooling of urine in the bulbar urethra which for some reason is abnormally lax and wide.

A technique called 'milking' the urethra is sometimes helpful. This involves putting the ball of the thumb behind the testicles and pushing up and forwards to exert pressure on the urethra causing urine to be expelled. There is much anecdotal evidence that milking the urethra or pelvic floor exercises are effective methods of treating this problem.

Other causes of urinary problems in men are reflected on in Box 4.5.

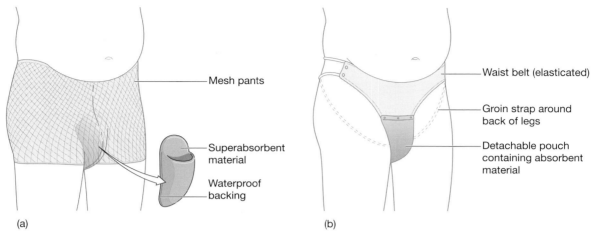

(a)   (b)

Figure 4.4   Absorbent pouches.

There are a great variety of options to select from in order to aid the management of urinary incontinence in men. Some strategies such as the use of absorbent pads are common to both sexes, others strategies such as the use of urinary sheaths are designed specifically for men. Again discussion will focus on those options that are 'mostly male'.

Containment aids

There are two types of product classed as containment aids: body worn pads/pants and underpads. The Continence Foundation publishes a useful directory of those available (Continence Foundation 2000b) and some sources are provided in Chapter 12.

Cottenden (1992) provides a useful review of research undertaken on containment aids. However, product comparison is difficult to undertake. Shirran & Brazzelli (2000) conclude that data are too few and of insufficient quality to provide a firm basis for practice, although disposable products may be more effective than non-disposables in reducing the incidence of skin problems and super-absorbents may be better than fluff pulp. However, whilst it is generally agreed that large bulky nappy pads are best avoided unless all other alternatives have been tried unsuccessfully, Cottenden's (1992) conclusion that 'no one product suits everybody' appears to hold true and

serves to emphasize the importance of individual assessment, patient choice and review.

There are some absorbent products for low levels of incontinence, which are specifically designed for males. The 'dribble pouch' is designed to fit over the penis and absorb small amounts of incontinent urine (Norton 1987) (Fig. 4.4). These pouches are usually disposable and they are held in position by means of a washable jockstrap or tight-fitting underpants.

Conduction aids

Urinary sheath

One method of managing urinary incontinence, which is unique to males, is the urinary sheath. The history of the urinary sheath begins with the use of modified contraceptive sheaths and also 'Paul's tubing', neither of which was specifically designed for the management of urinary incontinence. In recent years, however, the development of urinary sheath systems has greatly improved. Sheaths – also sometimes referred to as condom or external catheters (Cottenden 1992) – are available in a variety of materials and a range of different sizes (Fig. 4.5).

Sheaths are supplied as one- or two-piece systems, and some of those available come complete with their own applicator. A number of problems

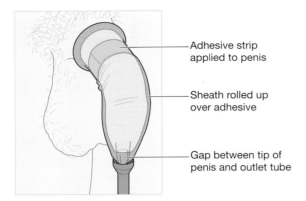

Adhesive strip applied to penis

Sheath rolled up over adhesive

Gap between tip of penis and outlet tube

Figure 4.5 Application of a penile sheath.

have been associated with the use of urinary sheaths such as the sheath becoming detached, irritation of penile skin and difficulty in self-application if manual dexterity is poor (Cheung 1989). Many can be avoided through proper patient assessment, correct fitting and review. It is doubtful whether there is one universal best sheath system and it may be advisable to provide the patient with a selection to try.

A number of criteria must be satisfied in order for an individual to be fitted with a urinary sheath, whether it is a two-piece or a one-piece system. The nurse or person fitting the sheath should check that:

- the penis is not retracted
- the skin is not broken or inflamed (although a barrier cream may be used)
- the individual is not confused and at risk of pulling the sheath off
- the individual has sufficient manual dexterity if self-caring, or alternatively that the sheath can be applied by a carer or health professional.

Despite the fact that these devices come in a variety of designs and that most manufacturers provide a range of sizes, it is essential that the penis is not too retracted for the attachment of a sheath. If the penis is retracted in any way, if the man is obese or there is herniation around the base of the penis, then it is unlikely that this technique can be applied. It is possible to try a sheath over a

---

Box 4.6 Fitting a penile sheath

When a decision has been made to try a penile sheath for managing urinary incontinence, part of the success for the wearer is selecting the right size, type and fitting of the sheath. Most manufacturers offer a one- or two-piece system in a range of sizes from 22 mm to 35 mm.

1. Firstly, the size of the penis can be measured using a specially designed measuring device provided by the manufacturer. The circumference is estimated by placing the device at the base of the penis so that the fit is not too tight or too big. The size of the sheath required is shown on the measuring device at that position.
2. Once the size is chosen, some samples of different makes of sheath should be given for the patient to choose from.
3. Wash and dry the penis but do not apply talc or creams as this may prevent the sheath from forming a secure seal against the skin.
4. Take the sheath from the packet and using the packet, cut a hole in the middle which can go over the penis to keep the pubic hair away from the shaft of the penis. Make sure the foreskin is kept forward.
5. If using the one-piece self-adhesive sheath, place the penis into the sheath leaving a small gap (about 1 cm) at the bulbous end and then gently unroll the sheath the length of the penis and secure firmly by pressing on the penis.
6. If using the two-piece system, carefully stretch the adhesive strip before winding it around the shaft of the penis. This allows for any change in penis size while wearing the sheath. Roll the sheath over the adhesive strip in the same way as described above.
7. Remove the protective 'collar' made from the packet and discard. Attach the drainage bag securely making sure that the tube's connector goes past the 'waist' of the outlet tube and then strap to the leg (straps are provided with bags).
8. Sheaths are durable for 24 hours' wear, but sometimes they remain in place for a longer period.
9. To remove a sheath, simply roll it off over the tip of the penis and discard.
10. Wash and dry the genital area thoroughly after removing the sheath and before replacing it with a fresh one.

5-day period as described by Watson (1991) to test if this approach is suitable for the individual. If the sheath can be kept in place for more than 12 hours then it is probably an appropriate technique. Confused men are very likely to pull off a urinary sheath and this method of management may be unsuitable for such clients (Irvine 1991).

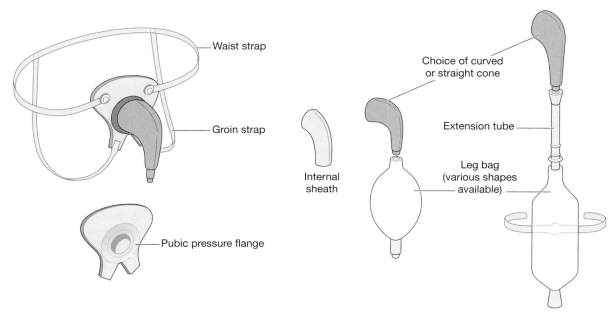

Figure 4.6 A pubic pressure urinal.

This may account for the very low use of urinary sheaths in psychogeriatric units (Stott et al 1990). Sheaths are generally not suitable for men with obstruction, or with symptomatic urinary infection (Button et al 1998).

Some research into the use of urinary sheaths has demonstrated that different sheath systems vary in their effectiveness, but that when clear protocols for their application are used, they can be very effective (Watson 1989, Watson & Kuhn 1990). Cheung (1989) and Playford (1991) have published guidelines for their proper use. Guidance on fitting a penile sheath is provided in Box 4.6.

Drainage systems for use with a sheath are similar to those used with an indwelling catheter (see Chapter 9). These include free-standing and smaller body-worn drainage bags. Urine bags are made by several manufacturers and come in a variety of sizes and colours, with different methods of attachment and a variety of tap fittings. As with other products patient assessment (including leg length and manual dexterity) and individual patient preference are vital considerations when selecting a product.

Pubic pressure device

A second group of male conduction aids are those generally termed body-worn urinals or pubic pressure devices. This form of appliance is most often used in men who are unable to wear either a dribble pouch or urinary sheath because they have a retracted penis – the penis is effectively too small to hold the appliances in place. Pubic pressure devices work by exerting pressure around the base of the penis and are fitted by an experienced appliance fitter (a service often supplied by the manufacturer – see Chapter 12). The device consists of a rubber cone held in place by means of waist and groin straps and attached to a leg drainage bag (Fig. 4.6).

Cottenden (1988) records that users sometimes complain of discomfort such as sweating and soreness, which is perhaps not surprising given the bulkiness of the device. In suggesting this option, consideration needs to be given to the individual's ability to apply the product and its acceptability.

Indwelling catheterization

Catheterization is usually considered a last resort in the management of incontinence, and indwelling catheters are usually only chosen when other strategies have failed. However, catheterization may be absolutely the right choice for some individuals. Furthermore in cases of acute retention catheterization may be vital if further problems of ureteric reflux and backpressure to the kidneys are to be avoided. When obstruction is the cause of retention suprapubic catheterization may be the option of choice. Neither technique is without its problems. Difficulties associated with indwelling catheters include infection, leakage, pain, encrustation and blockage (Chapter 9) and although suprapubic catheterization has been associated with less urinary infection in a 3-year follow-up study of men with acute retention resulting from prostate enlargement, frequent dislodgement was a problem (Horgan et al 1992).

Whilst long-term catheterization carries significant risks, particularly in patients with urinary retention who are unfit for surgery, it may still be the best option for some patients. The decision to catheterize brings with it the responsibility to ensure that the individual (or his carer) can manage the device when at home. Education should not only include general maintenance (e.g. the importance of good hygiene and adequate fluid intake, maintaining a closed system and applying, positioning and changing drainage bags) but also the action to be taken in the event of blockage, leakage or the catheter falling out. The principles of choosing a drainage/leg bag apply equally when an indwelling catheter is *in situ*, although in some individuals a catheter valve may be the preferred option.

Intermittent self-catheterization (ISC)

ISC has replaced long-term indwelling catheterization for many individuals in certain patient groups including those with a neurogenic/hypotonic bladder (Winder 1992). However, it is not a strategy to be adopted lightly. A thorough assessment of the patient and the acquisition of specialist skills on behalf of the healthcare practitioner are required before proceeding. Whilst the advantages of this 'clean' technique are self-evident (reduced risk of infection and that a private problem is prevented from becoming public) the individual must find the procedure acceptable, have sufficient cognitive abilities to understand instruction and sufficient dexterity to carry out the task.

Occlusive devices

Although the two categories of product described above are those most frequently employed, Button et al (1998) identify a third smaller category of appliance also intended to promote effective continence management – 'occlusive devices'. Apart from artificial sphincters, which are inserted surgically and mentioned above, the only other form of device aimed at preventing outflow of urine is the penile clamp. Penile clamps are not recommended and rarely used, so they are given brief consideration only in this chapter. The problem lies in the fact that, in order to prevent outflow of urine, the clamp has to be reasonably tight and if the clamp is sufficiently tight to prevent outflow of urine it is also tight enough to restrict blood flow in the penis. This may lead to skin breakdown similar to a pressure sore, pain, oedema and also to ischaemia in the tip of the penis.

Choice of product

Continence appliances are not without their problems and the decision to use/choice of product should be carefully considered. Five key principles for using an aid or appliance are identified by Button et al (1998). Although forming part of a set of consensus guidelines aimed at the primary healthcare team, these principles are equally applicable to other settings:

- The restoration of continence should be the aim for all persons.
- Assessment should precede any issue of aids or appliances.
- Individual patient/client choice should be a key consideration in determining a suitable management strategy.
- Care should include education in the correct use of any aid or appliance issued.
- Product suitability and requirements should be reviewed regularly.

When choosing a product, the National Prescribing Centre (1999) suggests the use of the EASE mnemonic:

- How **E**ffective is the product? (At containing odour and urine?)
- How **A**ppropriate is the product for this patient? (Can they manage it easily, is it comfortable and discreet?)
- How **S**afe is the product? (Is it environmentally friendly, easy to dispose of?)
- Is the prescription cost **E**ffective?

In addition to comprehensive patient assessment and careful choice of product (which includes incorporation of patient views) it is essential that products are used effectively and according to the manufacturer's instructions. Education and effective communication are important determinants of the proper use of appliances. Table 4.6 is intended to provide guidance and uses catheter care as an example, although the framework would appear equally applicable to patient education in the use of body-worn pads or urinary sheaths.

The importance of effective communication in relation to the use of aids and appliances is an issue also worthy of separate mention. On discharge from hospital or transfer to another setting it is important that details of appliances are forwarded (in addition to a short-term supply if applicable). This will facilitate continuity of care and prevent the individual being subjected to problems resulting from the use of inappropriate products. Patient records should contain clear and unambiguous details of product use. In relation to urinary drainage systems, this should include not only the make and type of sheath but also the size required, and details of the drainage system used. Failure to document such details accurately can lead to inconsistent care and unnecessary disruption to the patient. Similar principles apply to the use of other products.

Table 4.6 Using appliances: a framework for patient education

A framework for patient education	Example: What does the patient need to know about catheter care?
Why (and why not)? How the appliance was selected and what problems or complications may arise	Why the products were selected (to allow informed choice), including the function and location of the catheter The risk of the catheter falling out The risk of infection, blockage and bypass Potential impact upon sexuality
What? What is required to ensure that maximum benefit is gained from the appliance and potential problems avoided?	The importance of hand washing and hygiene The importance of meatal cleansing (males) The importance of avoiding constipation Instructions with regard to fluid intake Instructions on observing colour/volume of urine
Who? Who is the most appropriate person to provide care related to the appliance on a day-to-day basis? Who should be contacted if problems occur?	Expectations of patient/carer Support to be provided by the healthcare team Who to contact should problems arise
How? What is involved in ensuring that appliances are used safely and effectively? How do I care for myself? What will be done in the event of problems occurring?	How to empty, change and dispose of urine bags How to obtain new supplies of urine bags
When? How often does care related to my appliance need to be carried out? How often does the appliance need to be changed?	How often bags require emptying How often catheter will need to be changed

Based on Roe (1989).

Case study 4.2 Examining the effectiveness of continence care

Mr Harold Mumby was a 76-year-old gentleman of previous good health. He was admitted to an acute medical ward following a cerebrovascular accident (stroke).

He had recovered well from his stroke and was hoping to return home in the near future. However, he was still experiencing problems with his bladder. Although continent during the day, Harold wet the bed most nights.

The nurses on the ward had fitted Harold with a urinary sheath after his attempts to use urine bottles had proved unsuccessful. Harold was unable to fit the sheath himself and even when fitted by the nurses it rarely stayed on all night.

Harold had lived alone prior to admission but planned to live at his daughter's on discharge from hospital. However, his daughter felt that that she could not take her father home until he was completely continent of urine. There were two main issues as she saw them:

- Who would apply the sheath?
- How would they deal with the washing and the spoiling of bed linen/mattress when the sheath fell off?

The continence nurse was asked to help.

Harold explained his distress, frustration and embarrassment. A core care plan was found in the nursing notes which referred to the need to ward test the patient's urine, assess his constipation risk and do a 3-day continence chart. The evaluation column of the care plan mentioned the use of a urinary sheath ('Conveen applied') and made reference to a 'wet bed'.

The notes indicated that the urine test was 'NAD' and that 'bowels' had been 'well opened' on several occasions. A 3-day fluid volume chart had been partially completed 2 weeks previously and filed in the notes. There was no evidence that the doctor had been informed of the patient's continence problem.

In your view was the nursing care for Harold's continence problem clinically effective?
What factors may have influenced the effectiveness of Harold's care?
What would you do as the continence nurse to ensure that Harold's care was effective in future?

Points for reflection
Was the right thing done right? Did it lead to the right outcome?
It may help in arriving at a decision to consider the following issues:

- Why was urine bottle use unsuccessful? Had his stroke or another coexisting complaint affected Harold's grip?

- Why wasn't the sheath staying on? There was no reference to the size of the appliance in the care plan. Had Harold's sheath size been determined and communicated to everyone who was involved in assisting him to change the appliance?
- Was a sheath appropriate? Harold could not fit it himself and no one was available to help at home. Harold did not like the sheath. Had Harold been given a choice? Was that choice informed?
- Was Harold's incontinence really intractable? What was really causing it? The fluid volume chart was incomplete. The standard (core) care plan had no name on it; had it been tailored to Harold's needs? Medical staff were not aware of the continence problem. Would Harold's incontinence problem have benefited from the knowledge of other members of the multidisciplinary team?

What would have constituted a desirable outcome for Harold?
Option One: Continence.
Option Two: A management solution that was acceptable to Harold, manageable by him and left minimal risk of a wet bed with resultant distress on his part and that of his daughter.

What was the outcome?
Harold's continence problem was thoroughly assessed and an individual plan of care established.

Harold's continence assessment revealed a high urine output at night. Nighttime was when Harold was least capable of reaching the toilet/using a bottle because he was tired and having to take sleeping pills whilst in hospital. (He had been unable to sleep through worry.)

Following consultation with the medical staff Harold was given furosemide (frusemide) at 6 o'clock each evening to eliminate his urine load and reduce the high volume of urine produced at night when he was least able to cope with it. He was provided with a urine bottle with non-spill adapter, as his grip was weak especially when tired. He was also weaned off his sleeping pills as these had been started during his hospital stay and had added to his drowsiness when he did need to awaken to pass urine.

The result – Harold was continent on discharge (but bought a protective bed sheet and took the continence nurses contact number just in case!).

Effective care had been achieved based upon a comprehensive assessment of the problem, goals that were patient focused and negotiated with Harold and his daughter, and an individualized plan of care which served to ensure that all those involved knew of Harold's requirements.

Sexuality and the use of appliances

The potential impact of urinary incontinence in general and the use of appliances in particular on the individual should not be underestimated. Alterations in body image, relations and sexual activity are issues that it would be all too easy to overlook (Royal College of Nursing 2000a). Although these are arguably not subjects to be broached until a sufficiently trusting relationship

---

Case study 4.3

Samuel McCarthy is a 70-year-old gentleman who resides in a residential home. When visiting the home to see another client the district nurse was asked whether there was anything that could be done about the sore, broken skin at the base of Samuel's penis. Samuel was using a urinary sheath system as a result of occasional incontinent episodes (which his family associated with his move into residential care earlier in the year).

Further enquiry suggested that Samuel's continence problem had not been fully assessed but that, with the best of intentions, the care staff had fitted the sheath from a supply held on the premises, thinking that this would at least help to preserve Samuel's dignity.

The district nurse could not attribute the soreness directly to the sheath, although on examination the sheath did not appear to fit properly. Samuel went on to explain that it was uncomfortable, but that he had been willing to 'put up with it' as most of the time it 'did the job'.

The district nurse suggested to Samuel and the care staff that a thorough assessment of the gentleman's continence problem would be the best course of action. She explained that there were many options available other than sheaths and that there was even a possibility that the urinary incontinence could be cured. In the meantime it was agreed that alternative management strategies would be explored as the broken skin precluded the application of sheaths (at least until it had healed).

The district nurse discussed the provision of continence information and education with the home's manager. Study sessions were arranged for all the care staff focusing upon not only how they could avoid developing continence problems of their own (!) but also how sometimes attention to the simplest things (such as the accessibility of the toilet facilities) could prevent long-term difficulties. The care and management of clients with urinary sheaths was also discussed, but in the context of the need for individualized assessment and review and the very real possibility that urinary incontinence could be cured.

---

has been established between healthcare practitioner and patient/client, they are important considerations.

One of the problems arising from the use of devices to manage urinary incontinence is that of altered body image and this is particularly the case where an appliance is being worn (Wheeler 1991). Essentially the message regarding sexuality is that a great deal can be done to maintain sexual image and also to maintain sexual activity. When a man is wearing a urinary sheath or a urinary catheter, provided that the collecting bag has been fitted correctly to the inside of the leg, there is no need for anyone else to know that a device is being worn. On the other hand, the use of pads may be more obvious as many of these are bulky. With improved products, which are smaller and more absorbent, the situation is improving. As with any kind of appliance, good skin hygiene is essential in order to prevent odour and discomfort. These measures will reduce the impact of urinary incontinence on sexuality.

Sexual activity is possible even with an indwelling urinary catheter *in situ*. The catheter can be taped back along the shaft of the penis, or alternatively it can be removed altogether and replaced after intercourse. Replacement is usually done by the man himself or a partner/carer who has been taught the technique. The outlet to the bladder is blocked during erection of the penis so it is unlikely that urine will leak during intercourse.

Involving a partner in the care of an individual – whether directly, in terms of changing catheter bags or continence pads, or indirectly, as a source of support – must not be done without careful consideration. Blannin (1987) suggests that where a partner adopts the role of 'nurse' this may produce conflicts in the relationship resulting in a loss of self-esteem and sexual desire. It may also be prudent to emphasize here that age is no barrier to experiencing a close sexual relationship (Duffin 1992).

Obviously, consideration of sexuality and sexual function requires a sensitive approach and discussion between partners (Wheeler 1991). It is possible that specialist advice may need to be sought. Any sexual dysfunction as a result of urinary incontinence should be brought to the attention of an appropriate therapist, such as a specifically trained counsellor, a continence advisor or general practitioner who may be able to offer help and advice. It may also be appropriate to inform individuals and their carers of the existence of local support groups and services, as well as national organizations such as the Continence Foundation (see Chapter 12).

CONCLUSION

In the nursing strategy document *Making a Difference* (DoH 1999) continence is identified as one of eight 'fundamental and essential aspects of care' that sometimes fall 'below acceptable standards'. Yet incontinence is a significant cause of morbidity associated with considerable personal and economic costs. Recent government policy initiatives provide the impetus for further development in this area (Royal College of Nursing 2000b). In order to be able to 'make a difference', nurses and other health and social care professionals need not only to believe that something can be done to help those who experience urinary incontinence, but also to have the necessary knowledge and skills to effect such help when required.

KEY POINTS FOR PRACTICE

- Overall prevalence of urinary incontinence is less in males than in females.
- Male urinary incontinence tends to occur at the extremes of life.
- Anatomical differences provide some explanation for the different patterns of cause and effect found when comparing urinary incontinence in males and females.

- Many of the general principles of effective continence care apply equally to both sexes.
- Various 'male only' options exist to promote continence and manage urinary incontinence.
- There is a relative dearth of research specifically addressing the impact of urinary incontinence and associated bladder problems in males.

REFERENCES

Abrams P 1997 Urodynamics, 2nd edn. Springer, London
Abrams P, Feneley R, Torrens M 1983 Urodynamics. Springer, Berlin
Abrams P, Cardozo L, Khoury G F, Wein A S (eds) 2002 Incontinence, 2nd International Consultation on Continence, 2nd edn. Health Publication Ltd.
Barry M J, Fowler F J, O'Leary M P et al 1992 The American Urological Association symptom index for benign prostatic hyperplasia. Journal of Urology 148: 1549–1557
Billington A 1999 Prostate disease. Nursing Standard 13(25): 49–53
Blandy J 1998 Lecture notes on urology. Blackwell Science, Oxford
Blannin J 1987 Incontinence: men's problems. Community Outlook February: 27–28
Brocklehurst J C 1993 Urinary incontinence in the community: analysis of a MORI poll. British Medical Journal 306: 832–834
Bullock N, Sibley G, Whitaker R 1994 Essential urology, 2nd edn. Churchill Livingstone, Edinburgh
Button P, Roe B, Webb C et al 1998 Consensus guidelines: continence promotion and management by the primary healthcare team. Whurr, London
Cardozo L, Outner A, Wise B 1993 Basic Urogynaecology. Oxford University Press, Oxford
Centre for Reviews and Dissemination Reviewers 2000 Diagnosis, management and treatment of early localised prostate cancer. Database of Abstracts of Reviews of Effectiveness, Volume 1, September 2000
Chamberlain J, Meilia J, Moss S, Brown J 1997 The diagnosis, management, treatment and costs of prostate cancer in England and Wales. Health Technology Assessment 1: 3

Cheater F 1992 The aetiology of urinary incontinence. In: Roe B H (ed) Clinical nursing practice: the promotion and management of continence. Prentice Hall, New York, Chapter 2
Cheater F 1996 Promoting urinary continence. Nursing Standard 10(42): 47–54
Cheung NF 1989 Incontinence sheaths: when are they necessary? Professional Nurse 4(6): 280–281
Colburn D 1994 The promotion of continence in adult nursing. Chapman & Hall, London
Continence Foundation 2000a Making a case for investment in integrated continence services: a source book for continence services. Continence Foundation, London
Continence Foundation 2000b Continence product directory, 5th edn. Continence Foundation, London
Cottenden A M 1988 Incontinence pads and appliances. International Disability Studies 10: 44–47
Cottenden A M 1992 Aids and appliances for continence. In: Roe B H (ed) Clinical nursing practice: the promotion and management of continence. Prentice Hall, New York
Denning J 1996 Male urinary incontinence. In: Norton C (ed) Nursing for continence, 2nd edn. Beaconsfield Publishers, Beaconsfield, Buckinghamshire
Department of Health 1999 Making a difference – strengthening the nursing, midwifery and health visiting contribution to health and health care. DoH, London
Department of Health 2000a Good practice in continence services. DoH, London
Department of Health 2000b The NHS prostate cancer programme. DoH, London
Department of Health 2000c The NHS cancer plan: a plan for investment, a plan for reform. DoH, London

Devlin A L 1991 Prevalence and risk factors for childhood nocturnal enuresis. Irish Medical Journal 84: 118

Dorey G 2001 Male patients with lower urinary tract symptoms 2; treatment. In: Pope Cruikshank K, Woodward S (eds) Management of continence and urinary catheter care. British Journal of Nursing Monograph. Mark Allen, Dinton

Downey P 2000 The prostate. In: Downey P (ed) Introduction to urological nursing. Whurr, London

Duffin H 1992 Assessment of urinary incontinence. In: Roe B H (ed) Clinical nursing practice: the promotion and management of continence. Prentice Hall, New York, Chapter 3

Egan M, Thomas T, Meade T W 1991 Incontinence: who cares? In: Garrett G (ed) Healthy ageing: some nursing perspectives. Wolfe, London, pp 118–123

Feneley R C L, Gingell J C, Abrams P et al 1999 Urology guidelines for GPs. Urological Institute, Bristol

Game C, Farrer H 1989 Disorders of the male reproductive tract. In: Game C, Anderson R E, Kidd J R (eds) Medical–surgical nursing: a core text. Churchill Livingstone, Melbourne, pp 644–653

Gooch J 1991 Care of the urinary incontinent patient. In: Garrett G (ed) Healthy ageing: some nursing perspectives. Wolfe, London, pp 131–136

Greifzu S P 2000 Prostate cancer. Registered Nurse 63(6): 26–32

Hagan T 1990 Nurses take the lead in continence work. Nursing Standard 4(40): 24–28

Hellstrom L, Ekelund P, Milsom I, Mellstrom D 1990a The prevalence of urinary incontinence and the use of continence aids in 85 year old men and women. Age and Ageing 19(6): 383–389

Hellstrom L, Hanson E, Hansson S et al 1990b Micturition habits and incontinence in 7-year old Swedish school entrants. European Journal of Pediatrics 19(61): 383–389

Herzog R, Fultz N H, Normolle D P, Brock B M, Diokno A C 1989 Methods used to manage urinary incontinence by older adults in the community. Journal of the American Geriatrics Society 37: 339–347

Herzog A R, Diokno A C, Brown M B, Normolle D P, Brock B M 1990 Two year incidence, remission and change patterns of urinary incontinence in community dwelling populations. Journal of Gerontology 45(2): 67–74

Horgan A F, Prasad B, Waldron D J, O'Sullivan D C 1992 Acute urinary retention: comparison of suprapubic and urethral catheterization. British Journal of Urology 70: 149–151

Hunksaar S, Sandvik H 1993 One hundred and fifty men with urinary incontinence. Scandinavian Journal of Primary Health Care 11: 193–196

Irvine L M 1991 Continence in later life. In: Garrett G (ed) Healthy ageing: some nursing perspectives. Wolfe, London, pp 124–130

Ju C C, Swan L K, Merriman A, Choon T E, Viegas O 1991 Urinary incontinence among the elderly people of Singapore. Age and Ageing 20: 262–266

Kirby R, Fitzpatrick J, Kirby M, Fitzpatrick A 2000 Shared care for prostatic diseases, 2nd edn. ISIS Medical Media, Oxford

Laker C 1994 Urological nursing. Scutari Press, London

Lazzaro M, Thompson M 1997 Update on prostate cancer screening. Lippincott Primary Care Practice 1(4): 408–420

Long M L 1991 Managing urinary incontinence. In: Chenitz W C, Stone J T, Salisbury S A (eds) Clinical gerontological nursing. Saunders, Philadelphia, pp 203–215

Marsh M 1992 Malignant disease of the prostate gland. Nursing Standard 6(36): 28–31

McCormick K A, Palmer M H 1992 Urinary incontinence in older adults. Annual Review of Nursing Research 10: 25–53

Milliard R J 1989 After dribble. In: Bladder control – a simple self help guide. William & Wilkins, NSW, Australia

Mohide E A 1992 The prevalence of urinary incontinence. In: Roe B H (ed) Clinical nursing practice: the promotion and management of continence. Prentice Hall, New York

Moore K N, Cody P J, Glazener C M A 2000 Conservative management of post prostatectomy incontinence. Cochrane Database of Systematic Reviews, Issue 2

Morrison M, Shandran T, Smithers F, Fawcett J N 1994 The urinary system. In: Alexander M, Fawcett J N, Runciman P J (ed) Nursing practice: hospital and home. Churchill Livingstone, Edinburgh, pp 291–324

National Health and Medical Research Council 1994 Incontinence and the older person – series on clinical management problems in the elderly, No. 5. NHMRC, Canberra

National Prescribing Centre 1999 Prescribing Nurse Resource Pack: urinary incontinence. National Prescribing Centre, Liverpool

National Screening Committee 2000a Second report of the UK National Screening Committee. DoH, Wetherby

National Screening Committee 2000b Information sheet on screening for prostate cancer. DoH, Wetherby

Norton C 1987 Selecting incontinence aids. Geriatric Nursing Home Care 7(11): 11–15

O'Brien A M, Sethi P, O'Boyle P 1991 Urinary incontinence: prevalence, need for treatment and effectiveness of intervention by nurse. British Medical Journal 303: 1308–1312

Ouslander J G, Palmer M H, Rovner B W, German P S 1993 Urinary incontinence in nursing homes: incidence, remission and associated factors. Journal of the American Geriatrics Society 41: 1083–1089

Paterson J, Pinnock C B, Marshall V R 1997 Pelvic floor exercises as a treatment for post micturition dribble. British Journal of Urology 79: 892–897

Perry S, Shaw C, Assassa P et al 2000 An epidemiological study to establish the prevalence of urinary symptoms and felt need in the community: the Leicestershire MRC Incontinence Study. Journal of Public Health Medicine 22(3): 427–434

Playford V 1991 Management of male incontinence using a sheath. In: Garrett G (ed) Healthy ageing: some nursing perspectives. Wolfe, London, pp 137–140

Roe B H 1989 Study of information given by nurses for catheter care to patients and their carers. Journal of Advanced Nursing 14: 203–210

Roe B H, May C 1997 Effective and ineffective management of incontinence: a qualitative study with implications for health professionals and health services. Clinical Effectiveness in Nursing 1: 16–24

Royal College of Nursing 2000a Sexuality and sexual health in nursing practice: a discussion document. RCN, London

Royal College of Nursing 2000b Continence is everyone's business: how to influence the HimP. Research, Education and Development, Truro

Royal College of Physicians 1995 A report of the Royal College of Physicians – Incontinence: causes, management and provision of services. Royal College of Physicians, London

Selley S, Donovan J, Faulkner A, Coast J, Gillat D 1997 Diagnosis, management and screening of early localised prostate cancer. Health Technology Assessment 1: 2

Shirran E, Brazzelli M 2000 Absorbent products for containing urinary and faecal incontinence in adults. Cochrane Database of Systematic Reviews, Issue 4

Stanton S L 1984 Sphincter incompetence. In: Mundy A R, Stephenson T P, Wein A J (eds) Urodynamics: principles, practice and application. Churchill Livingstone, Edinburgh

Stott D J, Dutton M, Williams B O, MacDonald J 1990 Functional capacity and mental status of elderly people in long-term care in West Glasgow. Health Bulletin 48: 17–24

Thomas T M, Plymat K R, Blannin J, Meade T W 1980 Prevalence of urinary incontinence. British Medical Journal 281: 1243–1245

Venn S N, Greenwell T J, Munday A R 2000 The long-term outcome of artificial urethral sphincters. Journal of Urology 164(3): 702–707

Watson R 1989 A nursing trial of urinary sheath systems. Journal of Advanced Nursing 14: 467–470

Watson R 1991 Incontinence in perspective. Nursing 4(39): 7–10

Watson R, Kuhn M 1990 The influence of component parts on the performance of urinary sheath systems. Journal of Advanced Nursing 15: 417–422

Webb V, Simpson R 1997 Older man's burden. Nursing Times 93(5): 77–80

Wheeler W 1991 A kind of loving? The effect of continence problems on sexuality. In: Garrett G (ed) Healthy ageing: some nursing perspectives. Wolfe, London, pp 144–149

Winder A 1992 Intermittent self-catheterisation. In: Roe B H (ed) Clinical nursing practice: the promotion and management of continence. Prentice Hall, New York, Chapter 7

Wolfs G G, Knottnerus J A, Janknegt R A 1994 Prevalence and detection of micturition problems among 2734 elderly men. Journal of Urology 152: 1467–1470

FURTHER READING

Button P, Roe B, Webb C et al 1998 Consensus guidelines: continence promotion and management by the primary healthcare team. Whurr, London

Department of Health 2000 Good practice in continence services. DoH, London

Downey P (ed) 2000 Introduction to urological nursing. Whurr, London

Royal College of Physicians 1995 A report of the Royal College of Physicians – Incontinence: causes, management and provision of services. Royal College of Physicians, London

5

Mainly children: childhood enuresis and encopresis

Diane Lukeman

'Bad Habits. – Most children have some bad habit, of which they must be broken; but this is never accomplished by harshness without developing worse evils. Kindness, perseverance and patience in the nurse, are here of utmost importance.'

**Mrs Beeton's Book of Household Management,
1906 (Ward, Lock & Co Ltd)**

INTRODUCTION

Bedwetting was certainly included in Mrs Beeton's definition of bad habits. It is, however, encouraging to know that progress has been made in our understanding of the developmental and learning processes involved in acquiring toileting skills and that there is now a sound basis of evidence about the efficacy of treatments when these tasks are not accomplished at an appropriate time.

This chapter addresses the importance of setting the issues of incontinence and its treatment in children and adolescence in a developmental and social context. The period of childhood is characterized by marked developmental change. While the changes can be described in physical terms, it is acknowledged that these are influenced by family, social and environmental factors. It is helpful to acknowledge that, through studies of childhood, we can learn about the normal process of the development of continence, which serves to inform us about this process throughout the whole life cycle.

The organization of this chapter is as follows:

- Development of continence and toileting skills
- Nocturnal enuresis
  —definitions
  —epidemiology
  —assessment
  —aspects of intervention
- Nocturnal enuresis through adolescence to adulthood
- Diurnal enuresis
- Encopresis
  —definitions
  —epidemiology
  —assessment
  —aspects of intervention
- Referral guide for enuresis and encopresis.

THE DEVELOPMENT OF TOILETING SKILLS

The acquisition of toileting skills is part of normal development. Most children become clean and dry between the ages of 18 months and 3 years, with night dryness following after. The oft-used expression at development checks – 'clean and dry by day and at night' – indicates that a child appears to be aware of a full bladder and bowel and is able to retain urine and faeces until the opportunity arises or is created so that voiding can be carried out in the appropriate place.

Children become clean and dry when they have learned to respond to both physiological and environmental cues. They need to have attained the appropriate level in the following areas:

- *Physiological maturity* – linking of the message of a full bladder to the action required.
- *Communication skills* – the child can tell an adult that there is a need.
- *Mobility* – the child needs to be able to move to toilet or potty.
- *Social skills* – the child needs to know where and when action can be taken.

The development of toileting skills is usually a combination of the readiness of the child in the above areas, together with parental awareness and

Table 5.1 Development of bladder and bowel control

Age	Stage in bladder control	Stage in bowel control
First year	Reflex activity	Reflex activity
Second year	Gradual awareness of full bladder and need to take action	Gradual awareness of need to void bowel
Third year	Ability to tense muscles of pelvic floor and 'hold'; increase in bladder capacity	Ability to stop defecation for long periods
Fourth year	Ability to initiate urine stream as well as to stop process	Ability to hold on to faeces and let go voluntarily

responsiveness. Many parents are unable to recall the process in detail – unless there have been problems. With bladder and bowel control, as with most issues considered in childhood, there appears to be a developmental progression (Buchanan 1992, MacKeith et al 1973; see Table 5.1).

According to Erikson (1950), in the first 18 months approximately, the child develops 'basic trust' – the expectation that needs will be met by parents/carers and a developing sense of self. This is followed by a shift towards some independent behaviour, signalled by the beginnings of mobility. The child can move away from the parents/carers and explore the outside world. The child is also beginning to develop recognizable language and is, therefore, able to communicate needs to others outside the family. Prior to this stage, the parent/carer role can be primarily one of interpretation:

- interpreting the outside world to the child ('that loud noise is thunder up in the sky – no need to be frightened')
- interpreting the child to the outside world ('she always cries a bit like that when she is doing poo').

Now the child can move (often crawling or shuffling before 'toddling') and is, therefore, able to reach the potty or toilet. Instructions can be followed and items fetched – 'Bring the potty in here'.

The development of toileting skills is an important part of the stage of autonomy. While there is a drive to develop independence, the child at this

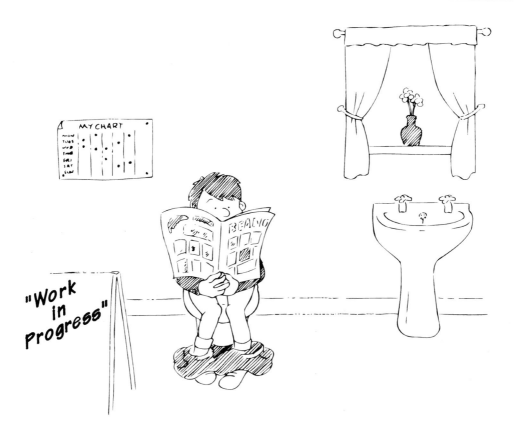

age has few ways in which to express this. Indeed, few decisions are actually within the child's control. There is still dependence on parents/carers for the meeting of basic needs. Life is challenging and there are times when the environment and what is going on can be overwhelming for the toddler. At such times, the toddler may need to be 'babied' and if this is not on offer may show this need by reverting to behaviour more appropriate to a younger age. In the face of a separation from a familiar carer or with the arrival of a new baby, the child may stop (as a form of protest) using the newfound skill of sitting on potty or toilet and may wet or soil in clothes or may request a nappy.

Some parents may be unprepared for the start of independent behaviour in their children and can feel threatened. They may find it difficult to accept that children can be unpredictable in their behaviour at this time, and toileting can become a focus of tension. We will return to this theme later when discussing assessment.

NOCTURNAL ENURESIS

'How can I stop doing it? I'm sleeping when it happens' said an indignant Joe, aged 4 years.

DEFINITIONS

Nocturnal enuresis is usually defined as the involuntary discharge of urine during sleep in a child aged above 4 or 5 years, in the absence of congenital or acquired defects of the nervous system or urinary tract (Shaffer 1994).

Primary or *persistent nocturnal enuresis* describes the situation when a child has never been dry for a significant period.

Secondary or *onset enuresis* is loss of control after a significant period of being dry. The significant period is generally accepted as being 12 months or more beyond the age of 3 years.

EPIDEMIOLOGY

Nocturnal enuresis is not an uncommon problem but, as would be expected, the frequency decreases with age (Shaffer 1994). In the literature there are variations in the figures reported. This may be connected with the definitions used for nocturnal wetting: how many nights per week or month; at what age this is being considered; how long a period there has been without any incidents. Parental definition of a problem may differ from the clinical view: there may be a family history of bedwetting; comparisons may be being made with other children (Butler 1991, Shaffer et al 1984). This is evident in surveys that have investigated the prevalence of the problem and consultation for help which may be as low as 50% (Rona et al 1997).

On the basis of the figures in Table 5.2, approximately a quarter of a million children between the ages of 6 and 16 years in England and Wales have nocturnal enuresis. After the age of 5 years, approximately twice as many boys as girls are enuretic, until around the age of 13 years when the numbers are more evenly divided (Verhulst et al 1985).

ASSESSMENT

There may be many factors involved in the development and/or maintenance of bedwetting. We have not differentiated here between causal and maintaining factors, because by the time a family

Table 5.2 Frequency of nocturnal enuresis throughout childhood

Age	Frequency (%)
5 years	15–20
7 years	7
10 years	5
12–14 years	2–3
15 years+	1–2

requests help it may not be possible to distinguish between these. It is possible that a child is delayed in becoming dry because of maturational factors. That may interact with a parental expectation of early dryness; tensions can arise which lead to behaviour, on the part of both parent and child, which serves to maintain the problem. A thorough assessment is vital as the relative significance of different factors leads to the choice of method of intervention and indicates its likely success. This section will consider physical factors, child factors, family factors, and the history of the problem.

Physical factors

Genetic factors

There seems to be strong evidence for a genetic component in the presence of nocturnal enuresis (Shaffer 1994), but there are no clinical features relevant to the course or prognosis of the condition. There may appear to be a genetic link because of similarities in toileting behaviour within a family. However, an apparent genetic link may be, to a great extent, due to the transmission of attitudes and interactions within the family. This, in turn, may perpetuate a myth about the problem of enuresis being 'in the family' and, indeed, could be one of the maintaining factors in its continuation.

Bladder capacity and function

The relationship between bladder size, functional capacity and nocturnal enuresis has been considered in detail in many studies (Butler 1998, Geffken et al 1986, Shaffer 1994). (It should be noted, however, that bladder size is measured by its functional capacity.) It would appear that many enuretic children have an urge to pass urine when their bladders are holding a relatively small amount of fluid. Children who have been treated successfully by behavioural methods do not appear to develop an increased functional bladder capacity; children with a small functional bladder capacity do have dry nights; some non-enuretic children have small bladder capacities. While Shaffer (1994) notes that this has been linked to the presence of speech and language delay as well as of behavioural problems, the relationship is not clear and no studies are quoted. He suggests that having a small functional bladder capacity together with some developmental delay may slow down the process of bladder control in some children.

Urinary tract abnormalities

The definition of nocturnal enuresis does preclude the presence of organic factors in the urinary tract. Urological investigation is not usually justified when there is nocturnal enuresis. It is, however, important when there is diurnal enuresis, with or without nocturnal enuresis, to seek a medical opinion to exclude the rare conditions that could be connected with this. There are likely to be other symptoms, such as difficulties with urine flow, lack of control or pain.

Urinary tract infection

There is a need to be aware of the possibility of this occurring in children, particularly when there is the onset of secondary enuresis. In the years of middle childhood, the occurrence of urinary tract infections is more common in girls, whereas enuresis tends to occur more frequently in boys. There are likely to be other symptoms associated with this, such as sudden-onset day and night wetting and a tendency to frequent episodes of wetting at night. It is important to consider that children with nocturnal enuresis may be more prone to infection because of lying in bed during the night in wet bedclothes.

We need to take into consideration also that the child who has had repeated urinary tract infections may develop a dysfunctional bladder. There may be a residual anxiety because of frequency of need and difficulty in micturition during the infections. If a child is wetting at night, the discomfort and aftermath of a urinary tract infection may delay improvement in the enuresis.

Sleep patterns

There appears to be a contradiction between parental report of their bedwetting children as being deep sleepers and the research findings which do not confirm this (Butler & Brewin 1986, Butler et al 1986, Sorotzkin 1984). There seems to be no difference in sleep patterns of enuretic and non-enuretic children nor, for the enuretic children, on wet and dry nights. Wetting seems most likely to occur approximately 4 hours after sleep or a previous wetting incident. There does, however, appear to be an issue of arousability – children with nocturnal enuresis are unable to wake when their bladders are full (discussed in Butler 1998, von Gothard 1998).

Child factors

Developmental factors in the process of toilet training have already been mentioned. When assessing a referral, it can be useful to consider the different aspects of a child's development. However, it has to be borne in mind that there is close interaction between these different areas.

Chronological age

One of the first stages in the assessment process, particularly with referrals of young children, is to establish whether the expectations of the parents/carers of the child are consistent with what might be expected at a particular age. With older children and adolescents, there are clear expectations that continence is under control and the significant factors are likely to be found in other areas of the assessment.

Physical development

It is important to assess whether the child may have physical limitations such as mobility or dealing with clothing which would prevent or slow down the attaining of dryness at night. For the child with physical disability, special furniture may need to be considered so that a child can be seated appropriately on the toilet. The child may also need a signalling device so that others can be alerted to the need if the child is not able to reach the toilet unaided.

We need to know whether any physical condition (illness) the child has is related to enuresis.

We may also need to consider that the child or adolescent has particular difficulties because of a previous condition which has led to a dysfunctional learned pattern.

Cognitive development

This clearly is linked to chronological age, but there may be some indication of developmental delay affecting learning which could slow down the process of becoming dry.

Emotional/social factors

Shaffer (1994) reviews the literature that has considered the relationship between enuresis and anxiety, and whether it can be considered to be a psychiatric disorder. While many children with enuresis who are referred to mental health services do present with anxiety and/or behavioural problems, there are reasons why this may be brought about by the enuresis rather than causing it. This may be an important factor when assessing a child (and family) where the enuresis is long standing or secondary.

When assessing this area, there is a need to consider several questions:

- Are there particular stresses in the child's life, such as illness requiring hospitalization of the child or parent, another reason for separation, or major events in the family? This is particularly pertinent with a secondary nocturnal enuresis.
- Were there any stressful events around the age when the child would have been becoming dry?
- Are there particular tensions or negative attitudes around the child who is wetting? Are these because of the wetting or are there other factors in the child's behaviour or role in the family? Are there issues of significant harm to the child either as part of the cause of the enuresis or resulting from it?

Behavioural

Observation of the child as well as information from parents/carers and school can give an indication of behavioural problems which may be contributing towards the enuresis: difficulties in sleep patterns or eating and drinking patterns; lack of cooperation with parents/carers; or self-esteem issues.

The child's understanding of the condition

Part of the assessment needs to take account of the child's understanding of the condition. Whatever their level of understanding, it is not surprising that children with enuresis lack self-confidence. For the most part, they do not wish to be wet. They wish to wake up dry and not have to deal with the practicalities of washing and changing beds. They become aware that there are limitations on activities – not being able to stay away overnight or, indeed, have friends to stay.

Butler et al (1990) have explored children's attitudes to their enuresis by the use of a structured interview prior to treatment. It seems that understanding of the practical difficulties arising from bedwetting is not sufficient to bring about change. When children begin to understand psychological outcomes, such as the effect of a change on their lives and on those around them, they are more likely to be treated successfully. This is a very important finding and may be crucial in the treatment of children who have appeared to be resistant to any form of intervention.

Family factors

Family history

We have already considered the fact that enuresis is more common in some families than in others. There is some evidence of genetic influence. It may also reflect attitudes of parents: 'I was late in becoming dry so there is not much point pushing the toilet training'. We know, too, that there are cultural differences which reflect differing expectations of children (De Jonge 1973). When carrying out developmental assessments or where advice is sought about toileting, it is important to establish on what parents' expectations are based, including the expectations learned from their own childhood and from their own parents' views.

Environmental factors

It is important to be aware of the physical situation at home. How possible is it for the child to reach the toilet safely at night? Is it dark? Are there obstacles in the way? Fears of the dark are common in young children, as are fears about the toilet – the noise of the flushing mechanism and the disappearance of what goes into the toilet.

It has been found that the prognosis for any method of treatment is reduced where there are poor housing conditions (Dische et al 1983).

Stressful life events

Events at a crucial age in toilet training may influence progress. The events themselves may now be in the past but they have helped establish patterns or interactions within the family which may maintain the pattern of wetting.

Jarvelin et al (1990) compared enuretic and non-enuretic children and confirmed earlier work on the influence of environmental factors on nocturnal enuresis. They found that divorce and separation increased the risk in children. This may be a result of changes or deterioration in living conditions as well as the psychological effects of separation from a parent.

Family attitudes and expectations

There can be a tendency to assume that, in the absence of physical factors, there are psychological factors and these may be within the child or within the family. By the time that the problem comes to the notice of a professional, there is often an atmosphere of tension within the family and negative attitudes towards the wetting child have developed. These clearly need careful exploration and we need to be aware that the effect on the family of a child who is wetting can be considerable.

It can often be difficult for a parent or sibling to feel positive towards a child when their first contact each day is with wet sheets and pyjamas and a strong smell of urine. Time must be taken every morning for sheet changing and washing as well as for thorough washing by or for the child.

Researchers have, however, identified another aspect of maternal attitude, in particular the extent of tolerance towards the enuretic child (Butler 1987, Butler et al 1988). Using the maternal tolerance scale (Morgan & Young 1975), there are indications that where maternal tolerance is low this can precipitate action for help. It can, unfortunately, also lead to anger and dropout from treatment. However, where there is low maternal tolerance and engagement in treatment, outcome is more likely to be successful. The converse is true – where parents (mothers, in particular) do not complain about the enuresis, change the sheets themselves as a matter of course, protect the child from the need to spend nights away, there is little motivation to seek treatment. This would indicate (as in Case study 5.2) that a high level of maternal tolerance might prolong the problem.

There may be a lack of knowledge or understanding of the condition. In some families the child may be seen as 'sick', 'disturbed', 'wetting deliberately'. In other families where enuresis is seen as 'not a problem', the issue may be ignored. In both situations, the child may be left feeling unsupported.

The parent–child relationship

It can be important to assess the quality of the relationship between parents and child. This can be particularly important with children in middle childhood and adolescence. Parents may feel that they have, somehow, not succeeded in toilet training their child. There may be a sense of low self-esteem or other factors that are undermining parental skills. This sense of failure may be being reinforced by critical others, such as the extended family.

While enuresis alone is unlikely to be an indication of abuse of the child, we know that there can be an increased risk of abuse when there are negative attitudes towards a child (Browne et al 1988). Bedwetting could be a provocation in families where there may be existing tensions.

While a parent continues to take responsibility for the problem, there may be little motivation to accept treatment. This can sometimes be related to the need or wish of a parent to continue with the practical tasks of parenthood and an unwillingness to see a child as an independent individual.

History of the problem

It is necessary to have as clear a picture as possible of the development of the problem. This can be difficult to obtain initially. Sometimes, having sought and found access to a professional, families can feel that 'maybe things are not too bad' or, on the contrary, they may feel compelled to present the worst picture ('if we need help, things must be bad'). It is important to surmount these attitudes by taking as 'matter of fact' an approach as possible. Among the questions that need to be asked are:

- When has the situation been at its best?
- When has the situation been at its worst?
- Is it worse in particular seasons, related to particular events, days of the week?
- What methods of treatment or management have been used?
- What methods have worked/not worked?
- How is it now compared with 6 months/ 12 months ago? You may be seeing a gradual improvement with 'ups and downs'.

Summary of assessment

Assessment has been considered under the four headings: physical factors, child factors, family factors and the history of the problem. The objectives of the assessment are to try to understand what factors are salient in each individual family referred with an enuretic child. It is often helpful to formulate this with the family as this will lead into the next stage – the choice of treatment. The assessment may indicate that other issues need to be dealt with before treating the nocturnal enuresis.

KEY POINTS FOR IMPLEMENTING TREATMENT

- Engage both parents and child.
- Ensure that improvement is seen as a possibility.
- Ensure that parent and/or child take an active part and responsibility for the treatment.
- Set in place some practical help.
- Ensure that there is regular monitoring by the professional reducing in frequency as improvement occurs.
- Focus on the gains, however minimal these are initially.

INTERVENTIONS
General issues

Before considering each method of intervention in turn, there are general issues that need to be considered.

Practical tips

It can be helpful, at the start of contact with a family with a child who is bedwetting, to ensure that they have some practical measures in place to minimize the distress. The following are some suggestions:

- Use a cover on the mattress. There are suitable sheets, commercially available, which cause minimal distress from noisy rustling. Having a cotton sheet on top reduces the risk of perspiration.
- Have easy access to dry sheets.
- Make suitable arrangements for wet sheets.
- Set a regular routine so that the child is able to wash properly in the morning.
- Ensure obstruction-free access to potty or toilet with adequate lighting.
- Encourage use of the toilet before going to bed or if awake for any reason during the night.

Measurement

In order to start any intervention programme, it is necessary to establish baseline measures against which to assess any improvement. This can also be useful when there is a relapse or lack of progress, as the information collected can inform us how to proceed. The action of asking parents/ carers and child to keep a record can often be helpful in itself and plays a vital role in the process of engaging them in treatment (Fig. 5.1). It indicates that the problem is being addressed and it gives a definite task. The approach to the collection of the data can be instructive in exploring attitudes further within the family.

Rewards and star charts

Rewards and star charts are usually used as part of any intervention programme and help to fulfil the

CHART FOR BLADDER TRAINING

Date	Bedtime	Time checked	Wet or dry	Time woke to use toilet	Alarm time and notes	Alarm time and notes

Notes for parent/child: Try to fill in as much as possible. Refer, in space under alarm, to size of patch, what done in toilet, who woke.

Figure 5.1 Chart for bladder training.

criterion of focusing on the gains (see below). Implementing a reward system is more demanding than simply putting up a star chart and giving a child a star for each dry night. While it is part of the measurement and monitoring of the situation, it has to be considered separately.

At the risk of stating the obvious, rewards must be rewarding. Gold stars may mean nothing to one child but may be valued by another. For an older child, a token system may be more appropriate. Some examples of this are: one token equals half an hour extra staying up, two tokens equals being taken swimming. It is often asked 'At what age can you start using stars?' or 'At what age are children too old for stars?'. The answers to these questions involve knowing and listening to the child. It often helps to ask parent and child for suggestions themselves and recommend that they make a chart together as a shared activity. This part of the treatment programme is similar to setting up a contract (Douglas & Richman 1984).

Parents often assume that if the child is responding to a reward, this means that laziness is the cause of the problem or that wetting is being done deliberately. This is very rarely the case. We know that behaviour can be changed by rewarding it, whatever the underlying cause. The rewards may not be initially for a dry night, because the child may not yet be able to achieve that. There are other signs of progress which can be reinforced, such as:

- spontaneous waking to use the toilet
- fewer wet episodes
- smaller wet patches
- wetting occurring later in the night, indicating an increase in holding capacity.

The following points need to be considered when implementing a star chart:

- Do not mix together record sheets (for assessment and monitoring) and star charts.
- Record only *positive gains* on a star chart.

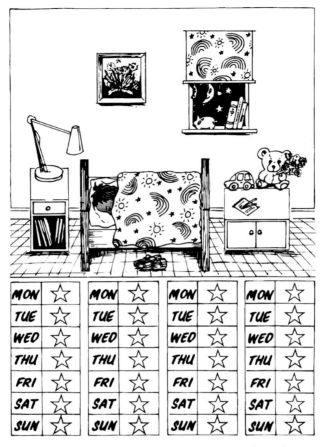

MON	☆	MON	☆	MON	☆	MON	☆
TUE	☆	TUE	☆	TUE	☆	TUE	☆
WED	☆	WED	☆	WED	☆	WED	☆
THU	☆	THU	☆	THU	☆	THU	☆
FRI	☆	FRI	☆	FRI	☆	FRI	☆
SAT	☆	SAT	☆	SAT	☆	SAT	☆
SUN	☆	SUN	☆	SUN	☆	SUN	☆

Example of a star chart – the child receives a star for each dry night.

- A blank chart is a record of failure. Create a situation where *some* reward is achieved by referring to the list above.
- Instructions must be clear and precise and understood by both parents and child.
- Rewards and their timing should be specified.
- Goals and rewards can and should be altered as progress is made – or, indeed, if there is no progress.
- Parents need the support of the professional to enable them to praise and encourage their child.

Information and reassurance

This will be part of any treatment intervention for children with nocturnal enuresis and their families. Following the assessment, the professional will give feedback to the family. This will set the problem in its context: developmental, child factors, family issues and the history of the problem. In addition, information on how the bladder works and why things go wrong can be an essential part of the treatment process (see Box 5.1).

Families often find it helpful when their professional helper is able to discuss the following statements about nocturnal enuresis:

- 'It will get better.'
- 'Other people have this problem.'
- 'It does not mean you have some incurable illness or condition.'
- 'Children do not wet deliberately.'

Box 5.1   Enuresis: information sheet for parents

You have asked for advice because your child is not yet dry at night. It may be that you have just begun to think that it is time that the wetting stopped. It may be that you are fairly desperate as the wetting has been a problem for years, because trips away from home are difficult and because you have tried everything. You may be somewhere between these stages.

The reasons why your child is not yet dry at night may be straightforward or more complex.

It may be one of the following or a combination of these:

- Age
- Developmental level
- Physical ability or maturation
- Emotional state
- Events relating to school or family
- Practical difficulties.

In order to implement a plan of action tailored to your child's individual needs and to the family, it is important to consider all possible factors and to form a clear picture of the pattern of wetting. Treatment plans may include star charts and enuresis alarms. All involve record-keeping.

Remember
- Wetting is not usually deliberate.
- Irregular patterns of wet and dry nights can be quite normal.
- As with any developing skill, children vary in the age and stage when they become dry.
- Restricted drinking will not help develop control and may impede the process.
- Research studies do not confirm the view of many parents that deep sleep is the cause.
- Lifting helps to keep beds dry but the child needs to be awake when urinating.
- Most children grow out of it eventually.

It is important to start keeping a record of the pattern of night wetting even before your referral to someone who can help. The person giving you this sheet can advise you.

Name .... Profession ....
Can be contacted at ....

- 'You may have tried some ways of improving the situation but it is worthwhile considering what you can try again.'
- 'Improvement takes time.'
- 'Failure with one approach does not mean that all is lost. The information collected can direct us to a more successful approach.'

Intervention methods
Enuresis alarm

Forsythe & Butler (1989) summarized the history and progress of the enuretic alarm over a period of 50 years. There seems little doubt that it has been the most successful method of treating bed-wetting (Houts et al 1994) but it is not without its disadvantages.

Alarms are usually suitable for children aged over 7 years who want to be dry and, with help, can take responsibility for the alarm. The purpose of an enuresis alarm is to alert and to sensitize the body to respond quickly and appropriately to a full bladder during sleep. The child generally reacts to the noise of the buzzer which occurs as urination begins. As the child wakes up in reaction to the alarm, there is tightening of the muscles of the pelvic floor thus stopping the urine flow. The child reaches the toilet (with or without parental help) and completes urination. The child then learns to respond to the sensation of a full bladder and tightening of the pelvic floor muscles.

There are two main types of alarm: buzzer or pad and bell alarm; a mini or body-worn alarm. These are placed on the bed with an appropriate arrangement of sheets (or attached to the child's pyjamas) according to instructions given with the apparatus. It is important to follow these exactly and to carry out all the procedures with the child present. The whole family will need to agree on a suitable starting date and make a commitment to carry out the programme for the required time. Choose a time for starting that is suitable and convenient for the family, i.e. not when there is some other change or stress. A school holiday may be a good time to start.

While it is important to have the support and cooperation of the family, there are circumstances when a child or adolescent may be encouraged to take on this responsibility because of a strong motivation to solve the problem which is not shared by parents or other family members.

After assessment and measurement, a reward system can be set up. The professional who is managing the programme may find it useful to visit the home at some point to discuss the full implications of using the alarm and to assess practical issues: who will hear the alarm, how is the toilet reached, are extra sheets available? Where possible, written information should be left with the family. There is often material available locally. If not, that available from ERIC (the Enuresis Resource and Information Centre) is very useful (see Chapter 12).

Overlearning. The failure rate of the alarm can be reduced by overlearning. This is done by stretching muscles by drinking extra fluids before bedtime. If this is tolerated, bladder control is progressively strengthened. Overlearning should not take place before the child has had 14 consecutive dry nights using the alarm. The procedure is as follows:

- Give the child as much drink as is comfortable to take – usually ½–1 litre (1–1½ pints) spread over the hour before bedtime.
- Use the alarm in the usual way.
- Continue until 14 consecutive dry nights are achieved. Discontinue extra fluid intake at this point.
- If the number of wet nights increases to more than four per week, abandon extra fluid intake and continue to use the alarm until 14 dry nights are achieved again.

Common problems in using alarms, and some solutions.

- Family members may find this method too disruptive. There are practical ways of minimizing this, but an additional approach is to stress the short-term nature of the problem and the advantages for the child and the family to be free of it.
- The child may see it as a punishment to be disturbed at night in this way. This requires further explanation and acknowledgement of the problem for the child and family. Ensure that there are positives for the child during the day.
- The child may not wake to the alarm. If this is a problem, there is a need for preparation for an assigned parent or carer to do so.
- The child may have difficulty in stopping in midstream. This problem would point to practice in 'holding on' during the day.

- The alarm may fail to go off or go off for no reason. If this happens, help is needed in checking the equipment and being able to find a substitute quickly if repair is needed.

Lifting or waking

This approach can be useful to try when a child seems to be gaining control or when an alarm is not acceptable at that time. The procedure is as follows.

- The child is wakened to go to the toilet. It is important that the child is properly awake and is not emptying the bladder while asleep.
- A 'staggered' waking schedule can be used to decrease the possibility of 'automatic' wetting occurring.
- If there is evidence from record keeping that the child wets during the later part of the night, a schedule of waking to an alarm clock may be more appropriate. Again, a younger child may have to be awoken by a parent or carer; an older child might wish and be able to take on this responsibility.

Bladder training

It has been found helpful to encourage children to practise 'holding on' during the day before urinating to increase bladder capacity. Sometimes an explanation and the encouragement of pelvic floor exercises can be helpful. Paediatric physiotherapists can give appropriate advice about this. Bladder training has been found helpful as an adjunct to treatment with the alarm, particularly for those children with small functional bladder capacity (Geffken et al 1986).

Medication

Two main types of medication are used:

- antidiuretic hormone (ADH) in the form of desmopressin (Desmospray or Desmotabs)
- a tricyclic antidepressant (e.g. Imipramine, Tofranil) which inhibits micturition.

These drugs can alleviate the problem in the short term but do not effect a 'cure'. When a child stops taking them, bedwetting usually returns (Houts et al 1994, Shaffer 1994, Wille 1986). Pharmacological issues are dealt with in more detail in Chapter 8.

There are some gains to be made by a trial of medication:

- for holidays and trips away from home when a child may otherwise be prevented from taking part in these activities
- for helping a child to have the experience of being dry
- for starting off a behavioural programme.

Dry bed training

This treatment, which includes a reward system, an enuresis alarm and an all-night training procedure, has been developed for use in institutional settings. It is based on the work of Azrin et al (1974) and involves a fairly complex training programme either in hospital or with a trained professional in the home to initiate it. Griffiths et al (1982) describe such a study, based on modifications to the work of Azrin. They recommend further evaluation, as the results were inconclusive. Butler et al (1988) compared this with treatment using an alarm and found outcomes to be similar.

This method is not likely to be readily available in normal clinical practice for children and adolescents, and it may be advisable to use the more common interventions. It would be important to seek an expert in the use of this treatment only if all else is failing.

Other psychological interventions

In the literature there are descriptions of interventions for bedwetting based on more general psychological treatments. This is likely to be the case where there appear to be associated behavioural or family difficulties (Graham 1973). Psychotherapy alone has not been found to be effective. However, with an overall change in the psychological state of the child, together with a possible shift within the family dynamics, there is often more acceptance of symptomatic treatment by one of the methods described.

Hypnotherapy alone has been found to be effective (Edwards & van der Spuy 1985). Butler (1993) describes the successful use of visualization techniques to help a boy with persistent enuresis which had been resistant to most methods; he became dry without the alarm.

There are indications that, where children are not responding to standard methods of treatment, attention needs to be given to their understanding and motivation as well as to attitudes within the family (Butler et al 1986).

Summary of interventions

General principles and specific techniques of intervention have been discussed. Houts et al (1994) reviewed the literature and analysed information from 78 reports of treatment for enuresis and Murphy & Carr (2000), using recently developed techniques for reviewing evidence-based practice, have established that urine alarm-based programmes are the most effective treatment for enuresis with improvement in up to 80% of patients. They suggest that the focus should now be on the development of packages of treatment for those who do not respond to the alarm. The choice of method or combination of methods depends on the many factors that may have been considered during the assessment. Table 5.3 presents a summary taking into account the age of the child which would guide the practitioner.

NOCTURNAL ENURESIS THROUGH ADOLESCENCE TO ADULTHOOD

There is little to find in the literature on the frequency or treatment for adolescents and adults with nocturnal enuresis. Feehan et al (1990) followed a large group of enuretic children from age 11 to 15 years; at age 15 there was no significant association between enuresis and behaviour disorder. The Enuresis Resource and Information Centre (ERIC) has produced a booklet, *Bedwetting: a Guide for Teenagers* (1991), which is a useful source of information and support for adolescents.

Adolescents who are enuretic are, indeed, a hidden group. They are likely to be unwilling to

Table 5.3 Summary of intervention practices for nocturnal enuresis at different ages

Action	Under 4s	5–7	8–12	13+
Information and support	Setting in developmental context	Understanding the problem	Understanding involvement in treatment	
Practical help		Routines for washing, sheet-changing, mattress protection		
Measurement		Frequency, timing, amount of wetness, association with other factors		
Alarm		?✓	✓	✓
Bladder training	✓	✓	✓	✓
Lifting/waking	✓	✓		
Medication			✓ For events away from home	✓
Dry-bed training			?Possible if a major problem	
Psychological intervention	If symptom is causing concern, may be other significant family factors	Could be linked to family stress, especially if secondary		Individual help for associated self-esteem issues

identify themselves and there are no routine medical checks that include a question about enuresis. The symptoms may be intermittent; patients may have tried most treatments without success at a younger age and therefore be reluctant to ask for help; they may not know where to turn; there may be high family tolerance for the symptoms (see Family attitudes and expectations, p. 113). Continence advisers can be a useful source of help and do see some teenagers and adults who have a long history of the problem. School health sisters (school nurses) may need to be alerted to this problem in their contact with children at secondary school. A useful web search on www.bedwetting.co.uk can help adolescents and adults who still wet the bed; the email facility for questions is an excellent way to get help, support and information.

The forms of treatment are those already outlined. If symptoms are predictable in certain circumstances, or interfere with trips away from home, desmopressin could be useful. Acceptance of an alarm may be difficult but is likely to be the most effective long-term method of reducing symptoms.

DIURNAL ENURESIS

This is a less common problem and is often associated with infection or organic conditions (Fielding & Doleys 1988, von Gothard 1998).

Many children have occasional 'accidents' when excited or anxious in strange situations. They may be in an unfamiliar place and have difficulty in indicating their need. Some children lose control when they sneeze or giggle. It does also happen that, following a urinary tract infection, the establishment of the sensation of a full bladder is disrupted. The child may respond by frequent visits to the toilet not matched to need and may lead to reduced control, to urgency and to difficulty in 'holding on'.

If episodes of day wetting are more frequent than the occasional accident, it is clearly important to seek medical advice. In the absence of pathology, it is useful to assess the situation in the way that is done for nocturnal enuresis. Monitoring the frequency of the problem, as described above, can be helpful. This may help to identify where and when the problem is occurring. Children who seem to be having difficulties are often encouraged by adults to go frequently to the toilet. However, this can encourage the sensation of need to void when the bladder is far less than full. While it may be tempting, also, to advise cutting down on fluid intake, this is not to be recommended because the urine could become stronger and more irritant.

There may be practical help that can be offered to a child. Discussion with staff at school may be important to ensure that the child feels safe to go to the toilet at school. There may need to be encouragement to go at the appropriate breaks.

The above pointers can be used to design a 'relearning' programme. Reassurance and information for child, family and school is needed. The child should be encouraged to have longer gaps between visits and to learn the sensation of having a full bladder. A timetable for the child's visits to the toilet may be helpful. There should not be any attempt to cut down on fluids. Using a star chart for reinforcing an appropriate gain (e.g. a reduction in wetting incidents in a given period of time, rewards for holding on for a fixed time after requesting to go to the toilet) is often successful.

There is an increasing interest in treating nocturnal enuresis and daytime wetting in children with maximal electrical stimulation (see Case study 5.1). Studies have shown that the cause of

---

Case study 5.1

Becky, aged 12 years, attended a private continence clinic with a diagnosis of detrusor instability as seen on cystometry, which had been performed by a consultant. The suggested non-intervention was 'you will grow out of it'. Becky did not have enuresis but she was very embarrassed by wetting her pants and carried several spare pairs to school each day. She told no one at school of her problem and she rarely participated in activities – not surprising, therefore, that she was quiet and reserved. After taking a full history and seeing her bladder charts (she had done these for the consultant) it was evident she had a small bladder capacity with frequency, urge and urge incontinence.

Most children are computer literate so it did not take much persuading to use surface electrodes attached at 3 and 9 o'clock of the anal sphincter and use biofeedback to teach Becky to locate and use her pelvic floor muscle correctly. Mum was present at all times and encouraged her too. When this was achieved, in about 2 minutes, an explanation on how to use the muscle functionally was then given (i.e. on feeling the urge to go to the toilet, contract the pelvic floor muscle to maximal strength and hold for 3–5 seconds).

Treatment at home comprised the use of electrical stimulation using surface electrodes placed on S2–S4 levels of the spinal cord for 20 minutes a day using 10 Hz stimulation. This was usually done while Becky did her homework each evening. After 4 weeks Becky was in total control of her urgency which was slowly diminishing, and because she had so much more confidence at not having urge incontinence, she started participating in after-school activities. Six months later Becky was absolutely fine and no longer had wet episodes. **Editor's note (MD).** This intervention is not used by clinical psychologists but some paediatric specialists are getting more involved with this form of teatment.

Research study 5.1   Effectiveness of psychological and pharmacological treatments for nocturnal enuresis

There has been a search over the years for a 'cure' for the problem of nocturnal enuresis. Houts et al (1994) reviewed the literature and analysed information from 78 published reports of treatment of enuresis in children in order to compare the effectiveness of psychological and pharmacological treatments.

The authors found that children who receive treatment (either psychological or pharmacological) are more likely to stop bedwetting than those who do not – an important finding for those who often advise parents and children that they will grow out of it. Psychological treatments are more effective than pharmacological treatments. The use of an enuresis alarm was the most effective treatment. The results did not support the view that using behavioural procedures together with the alarm increased its effectiveness, but the authors state that there were too few observations to make reliable inferences. There was evidence that desmopressin was more effective than other medications.

Other factors which appeared to influence successful outcome were length of treatment, quantity of professional contact and longer follow-up period. In order to facilitate successful outcome, longer treatment time with regular professional contact appears to be important. A longer follow-up time with an allowance for a slow reduction in wet nights was predictive of a greater probability of cessation of the problem.

This review is instructive in bringing together research findings since 1960. It highlights some of the methodological problems which need to be considered in comparing treatments and in measuring outcome. The enuresis alarm appears still to be the most effective intervention but the current view of desmopressin as a useful treatment is borne out. See also Murphy & Carr (2000).

Case study 5.2

Jamie, aged 14 years, was referred to a clinical psychologist for advice about his nocturnal enuresis by the school health sister. She described him as being of a shy, nervous and anxious disposition, not making friends easily and struggling at school. The enuresis was long standing and affected his functioning and that of the family. His father had been enuretic as a child and his two older siblings had been late in becoming dry at night but had been so by this age.

There had been successful attempts in the past at treatment using an enuresis alarm. However, relapse had occurred within a short time and there was unwillingness to go back to the professionals involved. Currently, desmopressin was being used.

Jamie came to the meeting with the psychologist with his mother who did most of the talking. Jamie seemed uninterested and seemed to consider any discussion of change 'too much of a hassle'. The mother did the bed changing and sheet washing and, while on the one hand expressing concern, showed a high degree of tolerance

(as measured on the maternal tolerance scale developed by Morgan & Young 1975).

Jamie stopped taking the desmopressin and a diary showed him to be wet about four times each week. The psychologist met with Jamie alone during part of the sessions to explore issues of his independence and to identify his strengths. Initially, he showed low self-esteem together with helplessness. As the sessions progressed, there appeared to be a shift towards more independent thinking on Jamie's part. His feelings of helplessness diminished and he began to express enthusiasm for having a further trial of the alarm.

Continuing observation indicated that wetting was likely to occur in the second part of the night. The mother began to expect help from Jamie in sheet changing. An enuresis alarm was implemented with regular supervision and support from the psychologist. There was a gradual and steady reduction in night wetting over 8 weeks. The overlearning procedure was carried out and Jamie still remains dry 6 months after this.

---

these conditions may be detrusor instability (Butler & Holland, 2000, Medel et al 1998), which can be treated with maximal electrical stimulation (Trsinar & Kraij 1996) and/or biofeedback (Yamanishi et al 2000). Both studies reported a cure rate of over 75%.

ENCOPRESIS

DEFINITIONS

Encopresis is the persistent voluntary or involuntary passage of formed motions of normal or near-normal consistency into places not intended for that purpose in the individual's own sociocultural setting.

Primary encopresis is defined when a child has never achieved appropriate bowel control.

Secondary encopresis is defined when a child passes motions inappropriately after having achieved appropriate use of the toilet at an earlier age.

A distinction has been made in the literature (Fielding & Doleys 1988) between *retentive* and *non-retentive* encopresis. Retentive encopresis with 'overflow' may occur secondary to the physical condition of constipation. This can lead to an enlarged colon (megacolon) and loss of sensation of the need to defecate. At this stage, there may be frequent soiling, which is 'overflow' around the blocked mass. While this may appear to be a soiling problem, the emphasis needs to be on treating the constipation (see also Chapter 7).

EPIDEMIOLOGY

Examination of the literature shows varying frequencies reported for the presence of encopresis. It is clearly much less frequent than enuresis and the problem appears to be about four to six times more likely to occur in boys than in girls (Table 5.4).

Table 5.4 Frequency of encopresis throughout childhood

Age (years)	Boys (%)	Girls (%)
3	11	5.2
5	3.5	1.0
7	2.4	0.7
10–12	1.2	0.3

ASSESSMENT

As with nocturnal enuresis, there are likely to be many factors involved in the development of encopresis and its maintenance. There are, however, some important differences in the development of the two processes of bladder and bowel control:

- There are strong bodily sensations attached to defecation and, therefore, more awareness for the child.
- Bowel movements are more discrete events, on the whole, than bladder activity.
- Constipation can have a major part in a soiling problem. There is potential for pain and discomfort associated with passing of motions where there is a tendency to constipation.
- There are more emotive issues and negativity surrounding faeces than for urine.
- Bowel training can become a battleground for control between child and parent.

It is clear that there is unlikely to be one causal factor in the development of encopresis. Detailed assessment is vital in each case so that the clinician can understand the individual circumstances and intervention can be tailored accordingly. This section will consider physical factors, child factors, family factors and the history of the problem.

Physical factors

Genetic factors

There is little support for a genetic or constitutional basis for encopresis (Hersov 1994). However, where constipation is a factor, this may be familial. Again, this link could be genetic or environmental with diet and attitudes playing a part (see below).

Bowel function

Studies of the physiology of defecation (Fielding & Doleys 1988) inform us that the process is an active one: there needs to be physical awareness and a degree of coordination between muscle contractions to push and external anal sphincter relaxation. Figure 5.2 illustrates how function

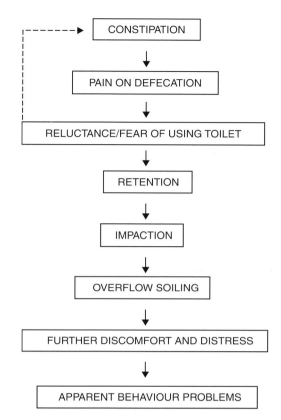

Figure 5.2 Sequence leading to retentive soiling.

may be disrupted leading to megacolon and lack of sensation of the need to defecate.

Organic pathology

A child who is showing bowel dysfunction must be examined medically. The presence and amount of faecal matter can indicate whether constipation is a factor. Hirschsprung's disease, a rare condition present in 1 in 25 000 births, is the most common organic cause for bowel dysfunction and is characterized by constipation from early infancy. There are likely to be other symptoms present such as anaemia and failure to thrive.

Diet

Constipation is common in those children who are encopretic. It is important to assess dietary factors, and it can be useful to know whether the child has particular problems with feeding such as faddiness or irregular appetite. In addition, it can be helpful to have an overview of the family's diet.

Child factors

Developmental factors in the process of toilet training have already been described. Although different areas have been separated out, it must be borne in mind that there is a close interaction between them. The development of bowel control is a significant stage in childhood. Voluntary retention of urine is difficult; voluntary retention of faeces is possible and is a more common problem at the time when a child is trying to become independent. Young children have a strong wish to be independent but they have little control over their environment. Refusing to defecate can be a symptom of this battle for control.

Chronological age

We have seen that the acquisition of bowel control is a developmental process. It follows daytime control of the bladder and may precede or occur around the same time as nocturnal bladder control.

It is important to assess whether parental expectations are appropriate. There was in the past a tendency to put infants on the pot immediately after meals (some readers may remember baby feeding chairs and tables where the chair had a potty inserted). Reflex action led to faeces in the pot and a view that the infant was 'toilet trained'. There was often great surprise when, at 18 months or so, the toddler was no longer responding in that way and defecating only in a nappy.

Physical development

It is important to be aware of physical factors that may be interfering with mobility or balance. Children with physical disabilities may be more prone to constipation because of their lack of mobility, positioning difficulties and dietary restrictions. The act of defecation is preferably a private activity; those with handicaps often need

to be assisted in the toilet and that can inhibit the process.

The greater incidence of boys with encopresis has been noted. It has been suggested that a contributory factor at a younger age may be that boys do not learn early to sit on the toilet. They may rush to copy their fathers and stand up to urinate (Anderson et al 1991).

Constipation can lead to conditions such as an anal fissure which can cause pain on passing faecal material. This can set up a pattern of toileting refusal and retention of faeces.

Cognitive development

Children who are delayed in overall development are likely to be late in gaining bowel control. There is the requirement for coordination of the sensation of needing to defecate and the action to be taken. Development of such coordination may be slow as are other tasks of learning. Delay in the ability to communicate is also a factor.

Emotional/social factors

For the older child, there is more likelihood that encopresis is a symptom of other issues going on within the family (Anderson et al 1991).

For all age groups, there is the negative effect that the soiling has on others, leading to rejection and low self-esteem. Soiling can clearly have an effect on social relationships.

As in the section on enuresis, it is important to consider the occurrence of stressful events in the child's life and in the family: in particular stressful events around the time when bowel control was being established and tensions or negative attitudes around the soiling child, either because of the problem or preceding it.

Behavioural factors

There are contradictory findings about the association between encopresis and behavioural problems. The experience of soiling is clearly a negative one. For the young child with constipation and overflow, there may be issues of control and this will affect other areas of behaviour (see Case study 5.3).

Information on a child's behaviour in general is important. Is the child generally uncooperative? Are there battles in other areas? Are relationships variable: good with some members of the family, difficult with others?

The child's understanding of the condition

The process of bowel control can be a difficult one for the child to understand. It can lead to unusual (and unhelpful) ideas of what is going on inside. One child was overheard to say: 'I think I won't eat, then poo won't come in my pants'. The discomfort felt on passing faeces may provoke anxiety, as can the whole process of flushing away something solid from the body.

It is important to assess the child's attitude to the problem and his/her desire for change. The child may be reluctant to talk about the problem; name-calling may have occurred at school; there is awareness that others notice the smell; self-esteem may be low – why can the child not achieve what everyone else manages with ease?

Family factors

Family history

It is helpful to know whether there is a family history of bowel dysfunction, as this may need to be discussed before consideration of a treatment programme for the child. Also, if constipation and laxative taking is a usual occurrence, this may be providing a model for the child.

It may be important to help some parents to understand that a problem encountered by one member of the family may be different for another.

Environmental issues

It is helpful to know the physical situation at home in terms of access to the toilet. Children who are anxious about separation may be reluctant to go far for a bowel movement when they are already worried about that.

Is the toilet at a height for the child to sit comfortably? It is preferable for feet not be left dangling but for there to be the support of a box.

The child's normal pattern may be to go at a time that is not convenient for the family – for example when everyone is rushing out in the morning.

Stressful life events

Because encopresis is a less frequent occurrence than enuresis, we do not have available the same amount of information on the link between it and stressful events. However, clinical experience indicates that the encopresis in itself is a stressful factor for families and can cause social isolation (Hersov 1994). Children who are prone to problems of bowel dysfunction are likely to be affected by other major life stresses around them.

Family attitudes

For many families, the subject of soiling is not one that is easily discussed. While wet sheets can be dealt with relatively discreetly, soiling which is more likely to occur during the day is, practically, more difficult. The smell and mess can cause negative reactions towards the child and to the parents/carers.

There are often myths in families, based on experience, about what is the normal frequency of bowel movements and at what time they should occur. This may shape the attitude towards the encopretic child. Attitudes may not be a causal factor in the problem; they may, nonetheless, be a factor in maintaining it.

In the equivalent section dealing with nocturnal enuresis, the development of negative attitudes was reviewed; similar processes are likely to occur with encopresis. If a negative attitude has developed towards the child, there may be little chance for positive viewing of strengths and successes and this could lead to a continued lowering of self-esteem. Help may not be sought because the child and the situation are seen as 'hopeless'.

The parent–child relationship

There is a need to assess the quality of parent–child relationships. It may be that there is a better relationship with one parent than the other and this could be important in intervention.

The sense of failure which the child may feel could be a reflection of feelings of parental failure. The risk of abuse is then increased – the soiling can be interpreted as a deliberate action attacking the parents/carers. Buchanan (1989) discusses the issues of confusion which have arisen following the Cleveland Report (Butler-Sloss 1988) between the symptoms of the constipated, soiling child and the child who has been sexually abused. In both conditions, there are other signs and symptoms that need to be considered before diagnosis.

History of the problem

It is necessary to have as clear a picture as possible of the current symptoms as well as of the development of the problem. A matter-of-fact approach is best, with a view that it can be the first stage in treatment. The following should be ascertained where possible:

- number of bowel movements per day
- sizes of bowel movements
- times of bowel movements
- consistency of faecal material
- spontaneous visits to the toilet
- prompted visits to the toilet
- timing of soiled pants
- what happens to soiled pants
- situations when soiling might be likely to occur
- use of medication and its effect
- the child's attitude to sitting on the toilet
- the child's understanding of defecation, awareness of sensation, need to 'push', level of anxiety, etc.
- what happens when there is soiling – the reactions of others (punitive or rewarding?)
- changes over time in all the above.

Summary of assessment

As in the earlier section on nocturnal enuresis, assessment has been considered under the four headings: physical factors, child factors, family factors and the history of the problem. It should be possible now to have a formulation of the problem which can lead towards appropriate intervention.

INTERVENTIONS
General issues

The guidelines for implementing treatment for enuresis (see Keypoints, p. 114) apply here also. There may be even more reluctance on the part of families to approach professionals about this problem, and the child may be embarrassed.

Practical tips

It can be helpful to discuss matters of cleanliness and hygiene – appropriate places for soiled underwear (a bucket with a disinfecting solution), the availability of clean underwear and routines for washing.

Measurement

In order to start any intervention programme, it is necessary to establish baseline measures against which to assess any improvement. The keeping of a diary (Fig. 5.3) is a useful indication of overall motivation. It can often signify for parents and child that the problem is being addressed. In addition, discussion of the diary is a further stage in the assessment process. The chart allows space to record observed soiling (at the time the child is taken to the toilet) as well as bowel movements wherever they occur. It is also designed to encourage a regular toileting pattern.

Rewards and star charts

Refer to the relevant paragraphs in the first section of this chapter (pp. 114–116). The same issues apply about focusing on the gains which, initially, may not be clean pants all the time. As an example of this, some 3- and 4-year-olds who are dry by day request a nappy 'to do poo'. This can be acceptable practice in order to prevent retention. However, suggest that the child should so defecate in the bathroom/toilet area rather than in the kitchen or living areas. This can become part of a gradual approach – sitting on the potty/toilet

CHART FOR BOWEL TRAINING

Name ....

Date	Soiling*				Toilet visiting**				Comment
	1	2	3	4	1	2	3	4	

Take child to toilet after each meal and any occasion he/she asks.

*Check pants:
S   if stained
S+   if small amount of soiled matter
S++ if a large amount of solid matter

** Mark
A   if child asks
T   if taken
BM   if bowel movements in toilet

Figure 5.3 Chart for bowel training.

with the nappy on, partial removal of nappy, and then complete removal. For children showing reluctance to approach the toilet through fear or anxiety, this gradual approach is also appropriate with the goals shifting with progress.

Information and reassurance

This is an essential part of any treatment programme. Feedback on the assessment is part of this. Information on the development of bowel control is important both for parents/carers and child. For children, drawings and play material (such as Plasticine and plastic tubes) can be helpful in illustrating the process.

It is often important for the helping professional to describe to the parents how the situation might feel from the child's point of view, and to promote positive discussion and cooperation between parents and child. An example of an information sheet for parents is provided in Box 5.2.

Intervention methods

It is likely that intervention will involve a combination of the approaches described below (Sprague-McRae et al 1993, Thapar et al 1992, Wakefield et al 1984).

Medication clearly has a central role where constipation is present. It has also been seen as a useful adjunct to behavioural work. However, in the controlled trial of Berg et al (1983), attenders at a soiling clinic were allocated to one of three groups. All children and their families received behavioural treatment. One group received senna (Senokot), one was given a placebo and the third had no medication. The medication appeared to make no contribution to improvement. The choice of intervention will depend on which factors appear to be causing/maintaining the problem.

Resolving constipation

If the problem is diagnosed as one of constipation with overflow, there may be impacted faeces which need to be removed (Levine 1975). This may require medical intervention from a GP or paediatrician (see Chapter 7). Stool softeners and

---

Box 5.2 Encopresis: information sheet for parents

Your child is having difficulties with bowels and going to the toilet. There might be great difficulty or discomfort when trying to pass a motion (faeces). There may be refusal to sit on the pot or toilet and there may be soiling of underwear.

Your doctor may have examined your child and said that there was no disease or obstruction. You may be puzzled as to what is going on: 'Why is my child not able to do what everyone else does naturally?' It may seem at times that it is caused by naughtiness or wilful disobedience.

What is more likely is that, for whatever reason, your child is trying not to let out the faeces. There may be a history of constipation. Discomfort from hard faeces may have caused fear of sitting on the toilet. Your child may now be so constipated that no amount of trying will bring a result. Sometimes, the soiling is 'overflow' – runny matter seeping around the hard faeces. Your child probably does not feel this coming because he has temporarily lost the sensation of passing a motion. Sometimes children develop a habit of ignoring the signals which the body sends that mean 'I need to go to the toilet' and then it comes in the underwear.

Your child is probably anxious too. Children can develop strange ideas about how their body works and may feel muddled.

It is advisable to consult your GP or health visitor if your child is under school age. They can advise on medication and behavioural management to help things on.

If your child is of school age, there may be a slightly different pattern of soiling. There may not be constipation and 'overflow' but soiling may occur. There may be other stresses around which are contributing to this. Your GP and/or school health sister may be able to make an appropriate referral.

Whatever the age of your child, it is helpful to keep a record of the soiling incidents until an appointment is offered. This can be useful in indicating a way forward. The person giving you this sheet may be able to supply you with a suitable chart.

The person giving you this sheet is:

Name ....
Profession ....
Can be contacted at ....

---

laxatives will be required. It is likely that their use will be continued for a considerable period of time while other behavioural and psychological treatments are in progress. Their use can then be gradually reduced. Parents/carers often raise concern about the long-term use of medication ('Will the child ever manage without?'). Explanation and reassurance are important.

Diet

Together with medication for resolving constipation, there needs to be attention to diet (Houts et al 1988). Roughage is important as well as an increase in fluid intake. This is not as difficult as it may seem as there are reasonably acceptable high-fibre cereals on the market as well as bran crisps. With a young child where there are issues of control between parent and child, there may also be a battle about eating (see Case study 5.3). It is important not to have more than one 'battlefront' at a time or to substitute a feeding battle for a toileting one.

Physiotherapy

For some children, particularly those with chronic constipation, advice from a physiotherapist about abdominal and general exercise prior to sitting on the toilet can be useful. The physiotherapist can teach the child and/or parents the appropriate way of carrying out abdominal massage which can be helpful when the child is on the toilet. Wakefield et al (1984) have incorporated this into their treatment programme and teach parents. They suggest it is useful for several reasons:

- It allows the detection of retention.
- It helps to stimulate the gut.
- It teaches parents what is going on inside their child's gut and gives them a means of dealing with it.
- It gives the child confidence that parents know how to help rather than criticize or blame.
- It gives a positive interaction over bowel issues between parent and child.

Work at their clinic also included yoga exercises and hydrotherapy – acknowledging that for children who soil, lack of exercise can compound the problem. They often avoid physical education at school because of embarrassment about changing in public.

Biofeedback

This method is described in Chapter 7 and has been used in some studies with children. The evidence (Murphy & Carr 2000) seems to indicate that this may not be more effective than behavioural management and psychoeducation. However, research continues to be carried out in this field and may prove an alternative non-invasive treatment in children with faecal soiling.

Behavioural management

The aim of this is to establish bowel functioning in appropriate places and at suitable times. It involves regular sitting on the toilet at times when a bowel movement is likely. The preparation of charts will indicate the most appropriate times, but 20 minutes or so after meals is the most likely time for defecation. Pants should be checked for soiling and changed if necessary.

The child should be encouraged to sit for about 5 minutes, reading or being read to, listening to music or being chatted to in a generally relaxing atmosphere. If there is a bowel movement, this should be noted and rewarded as agreed. If there is no action, there should be no comment. As the child starts to cooperate with this programme, there should be encouragement to take responsibility for it.

With children who have become fearful of using the toilet, an anxiety management programme may need to be implemented. This could involve relaxation training and desensitization and/or a graded approach to the situation, carried out with a system of rewards.

Brown & Doolan (1983) present a case description where behavioural techniques, particularly a backward-chaining procedure, were used successfully. They made an analysis of a 4-year-old girl's toileting behaviour and considered the focus of the difficulties. The child could accomplish the final stages of cleaning herself and dressing. This was encouraged during the five prescribed daily toilet visits and reinforced (regardless of whether defecation had taken place). The next stage was where defecation in the toilet was encouraged and reinforced. Mother and child moved then to a new stage where the child was asked at regular intervals whether or not she needed to go to the toilet. The programme continued until all soiling stopped and toileting behaviour became 'age appropriate'. This is a fairly complex procedure with regular supervision by a clinical psychologist to adapt the programme and the level of reinforcement. The authors highlight the importance of handing over the procedures from therapist to parents/carers.

Family therapy

There have been few controlled studies evaluating different approaches to treatment. Anderson et al (1991) describe the importance of different approaches matched to the assessed problems. An understanding approach to family dynamics appeared to be important in those children with encopresis aged 6 years and over. Phillips & Smith (1986) took a behavioural approach but describe how they needed to build in flexibility to take account of family variables which could have impeded the intervention programme.

Summary of interventions

Murphy & Carr (2000), using recently developed techniques for reviewing evidence-based practice, indicate that successful treatment approaches are family based and multimodal. This includes standard medical care (laxatives and dietary considerations), together with behavioural management. With encopresis, treatment takes time. The treating of constipation when it is present often involves a change of diet, together with long-term medication. Retraining of bowel function and toileting behaviour is also a vital factor. Children who have never developed or have lost the habit of responding to inner sensations – or, indeed, of recognizing these as associated with the need to defecate – need the opportunity and information to learn or relearn. There is more likely to be a need for a psychotherapeutic approach because the effect of the encopresis can be a cause of considerable family stress. With older children, there are likely to be underlying family issues which are maintaining the encopresis.

SERVICES FOR CHILDREN WITH ENURESIS AND ENCOPRESIS

In some areas, the way in which children are referred to the various agencies can be haphazard.

Some of the issues involved in setting up a service for children with nocturnal enuresis are discussed by Street & Broughton (1990). Hunt (1997) outlines a model of good practice and describes setting up a Enuresis Audit.

General practitioner

Parents and child may consult a GP initially. When any physical cause has been eliminated, the GP may offer information and support or refer on if it appears that further psychological help is required.

Health visitor

With younger children, many referrals are dealt with appropriately by health visitors. They also play an important role in prevention of problems in the area of wetting and soiling. They provide information to parents and may become aware of family anxieties around such issues.

School nurse

In many districts, a school nurse carries out the initial health interviews on children entering school. Parents can use this opportunity to discuss bedwetting and soiling. School health sisters often run enuresis clinics and are the source of enuretic alarms and information leaflets.

Staff grade paediatrician

The comunity doctor's role supports the school nurse and treats uncomplicated medical problems.

Paediatrician

Referral is made when organic factors are suspected. This would include children where there is:

- intermittent daytime wetting or dribbling
- dysuria or urgency
- problems with lower limbs

- excessive drinking
- increased appetite with weight loss
- chronic constipation
- soiling.

Continence Advisory Service

There is now an increase in continence services for children by specialist nurses but not in all health trusts. Parents and professionals are advised to ask locally if this service is available or contact ERIC (Enuresis Resource Information Centre; see Chapter 12) for more information.

Child mental health services

The referral could be to a clinical psychologist, psychiatrist, child psychotherapist, family therapist or psychiatric social worker. This would be usual when:

- nocturnal enuresis is present in the context of other behavioural, emotional or family problems

---

Research study 5.2 Children who soil: a review of referrals to a clinical psychology service

This review by Anderson et al (1991) highlights some of the important issues for those in primary care faced with referrals of children who soil. The psychologists in the service reviewed referrals over the previous 5 years and identified a total of 43 children and adolescents who had been referred with soiling as their main problem. Clinical information was summarized under several headings: age, gender, length of soiling problem, significant family problems, psychological formulation and type, length and outcome of intervention.

There was a clear division on most of the features and the group divided into two subgroups: those under 6 years and those over this age. These subgroups did not differ in the ratio of boys to girls (3:1) nor in length of treatment from a few months to nearly 2 years.

In the younger subgroup, about one-third had a history of constipation; the rest showed difficulties around accepting use of the toilet. The majority suffered from retentive, overflow soiling. Behavioural approaches were found to be successful in most cases.

In the older subgroup, the soiling appeared to be related to other psychological factors within the family. Intervention needed to be more flexible to allow for the complex interactions that were operating and involved the use of other psychotherapeutic techniques with or without behavioural management.

Although this survey was based on referrals to a mental health service, there is the implication that older children who soil are likely to be in more need of specialist services.

Case study 5.3

Tom, aged 4 years, was referred to the clinical psychologist by a paediatrician because of constipation and soiling as well as an eating problem. Tom had been constipated since infancy (no family history of this). When he had become dry by day and was out of nappies, he refused to sit on a potty or toilet to defecate; he did pass a motion as soon as his bedtime nappy was on. He was on medication – Senokot and lactulose – with some improvement. There was now refusal to go to the toilet and increasing episodes of soiling.

Tom had always been a lively child and not easy to manage. He was the oldest of three boys – James (2.5 years) and Nicholas (8 months) – and, indeed, was expected to be the 'big boy' although only 4. The younger boys had been more placid and easier to establish in a routine. The father worked shifts and the mother had some early morning part-time work.

Mealtimes were also an area of difficulty. Tom was reluctant to sit with the family and his appetite was variable – depending on his level of constipation and the amount of in-between snacks. Charts were kept by his mother and Tom and a pattern was identified: voluntary visit to toilet with large bowel movement; period of non-soiling during which Tom takes himself to the toilet; soiling starts and increases. Although it was recommended that Tom be taken regularly by a parent and encouraged to sit, this proved to be difficult in the hectic family schedule. On his own, Tom was passing only small amounts in his quick visits. This led to a build up of faecal material and hence to soiling.

The clinical psychologist had met on two occasions with both parents and explored the conflict between them over management of Tom. This stemmed from their own very different backgrounds. Some compromise was reached and they began to understand the importance of working together. At follow-up, there had been improvements and periods of relapse. Charts had continued to be kept. Tom very much took part in the discussion and was clearly anxious to 'get things right'. It was pointed out to the family that establishing a pattern takes time. Focus was placed on the gains that had been made which reduced parental irritation. Over the next 6 months, contact was maintained with the family and there was continued liaison with the paediatrician. There were some setbacks but a gradual overall behavioural improvement, appropriate toileting behaviour, a reduction in soiling and a reduction in medication.

- a child aged 10 years or over is still bedwetting
- there is secondary enuresis
- previous interventions have not succeeded or improvements are not maintained
- soiling in a younger child is causing family stress and disturbance in parent–child relationships

- for older children with long standing or secondary encopresis, there is likely to be behavioural and emotional stress within the family.

ACKNOWLEDGEMENT

I wish to acknowledge the constructive comments received from Nicholas Grey, Clinical Psychologist who, as a trainee on placement, read earlier drafts of this chapter.

REFERENCES

Anderson S, Charnock S, Mandelstam A, Youngson S 1991 Children who soil: a review of referrals to a clinical psychology service. Newsletter: Association of Psychology and Psychiatry 13(3): 10–14

Azrin N H, Sneed T J, Foxx R M 1974 Dry-bed training: rapid elimination of childhood enuresis. Behaviour Research and Therapy 12: 147–156

Berg I, Forsythe I, Holt P, Watts J 1983 A controlled trial of Senokot in faecal soiling treated by behavioural methods. Journal of Child Psychology and Psychiatry 24: 543–549

Brown B, Doolan M 1983 Behavioural treatment of faecal soiling: a case study. Behavioural Psychotherapy 11: 18–24

Browne K, Davies C, Stratton P (eds) 1988 Early prevention and prediction of child abuse. Wiley, Chichester

Buchanan A 1989 Soiling and sexual abuse: the dangers of misdiagnosis. Newsletter: Association of Psychology and Psychiatry 11(5): 3–8

Buchanan A 1992 Children who soil: assessment and treatment. Wiley, Chichester

Butler R J 1987 Nocturnal enuresis: psychological perspectives. Wright, Bristol

Butler R J 1991 Establishment of working definitions in nocturnal enuresis. Archives of Diseases in Childhood 66: 267–271

Butler R J 1993 Establishing a dry run: a case study in securing bladder control. British Journal of Clinical Psychology 39(4): 453–463

Butler R J 1998 Annotation: Night wetting in children: psychological aspects. Journal of Child Psychology and Psychiatry 24: 543–549

Butler R J, Brewin C R 1986 Maternal views of nocturnal enuresis. Health Visitor 59: 207–209

Butler R J, Holland P 2000 The three systems: a conceptual way of understanding nocturnal enuresis. Scandinavian Journal of Urology and Nephrology 34: 270–277

Butler R J, Brewin C R, Forsythe W I 1986 Maternal attributions and tolerance for nocturnal enuresis. Behaviour Research and Therapy 24: 307–312

Butler R J, Brewin C R, Forsythe W I 1988 A comparison of two approaches to the treatment of nocturnal enuresis and the prediction of effectiveness using pre-treatment variables. Journal of Child Psychology and Psychiatry 29: 501–509

Butler R J, Redfern E J, Forsythe W I 1990 The child's construing of nocturnal enuresis: a method of inquiry and prediction of outcome. Journal of Child Psychology and Psychiatry 31: 447–454

Butler-Sloss, Lord Justice E 1988 Report of the enquiry into child abuse in Cleveland 1987. HMSO, London

De Jonge G A 1973 Epidemiology of enuresis: a survey of the literature. In: Kolvin I, MacKeith R C, Meadow S R (eds) Bladder control and enuresis. Spastic International Medical Publications/Heinemann, London

Dische S, Yule W, Corbett J, Hand D 1983 Childhood nocturnal enuresis: factors associated with the outcome of treatment with an alarm. Developmental Medicine and Child Neurology 15: 67–80

Douglas J, Richman N 1984 Coping with young children. Penguin, Harmondsworth

Edwards S D, van der Spuy H J J 1985 Hypnotherapy as a treatment for enuresis. Journal of Child Psychology and Psychiatry 26: 161–170

Erikson E H 1950 Childhood and society. Norton, New York. (Reprinted in paperback by Triad/Paladin, London, 1977.)

Feehan M, McGee R, Stanton W, Silva P A 1990 A 6-year follow-up of childhood enuresis: prevalence in adolescence and consequences for mental health. Journal of Paediatrics and Child Health 26: 75–79

Fielding D M, Doleys D M 1988 Elimination problems: enuresis and encopresis. In: Mash E J, Terdal L G (eds) Behavioural assessment of childhood disorders. Guilford Press, London

Forsythe W I, Butler R J 1989 Fifty years of enuretic alarms: a review of the literature. Archives of Disease in Childhood 64: 879–885

Geffken G, Johnson S B, Walker D 1986 Behavioural interventions for childhood nocturnal enuresis: the differential effect of bladder capacity on treatment progress and outcome. Health Psychology 5(3): 261–272

Graham P 1973 Enuresis: a child psychiatrist's approach. In: Kolvin I, MacKeith R C, Meadow S R (eds) Bladder control and enuresis. Spastic International Medical Publications/Heinemann, London

Griffiths P, Meldrum C, McWilliam R 1982 Dry bed training in the treatment of nocturnal enuresis: a research report. Journal of Child Psychology and Psychiatry 23: 485–495

Hersov L 1994 Faecal soiling. In: Rutter M, Taylor E, Hersov L (eds) Child and adolescent psychiatry: modern approaches. Blackwell, Oxford

Houts A C, Mellon M W, Whelan J P 1988 Use of dietary fiber and stimulus control to treat retentive encopresis: a multiple baseline investigation. Journal of Paediatric Psychology 13: 435–445

Houts A C, Berman J S, Abramson H 1994 Effectiveness of psychological and pharmacological treatments for nocturnal enuresis. Journal of Consulting and Clinical Psychology 62: 737–745

Hunt S 1997 Setting up an Enuresis Audit. ERIC, Briston

Jarvelin M R, Moilanen I, Vikevainen-Tervonen L, Huttunen NP 1990 Life changes and protective capacities in enuretic and non-enuretic children. Journal of Child Psychology and Psychiatry 31: 763–774

Levine M D 1975 Children with encopresis: a descriptive analysis. Paediatrics 56: 412–416

MacKeith R C, Meadow S R, Turner R K 1973 How children become dry. In: Kolvin I, MacKeith R C, Meadow S R (eds) Bladder control and enuresis. Spastic International Medical Publications/Heinemann, London

Medel R, Ruarte A C, Castera R et al 1998 Primary enuresis: a urodynamic evaluation. British Journal of Urology 81(Suppl 3): 50–52

Morgan R T T, Young G C 1975 Parental attitudes and the conditioning treatment of childhood enuresis. Behaviour Research and Therapy 13: 197–199

Murphy E, Carr A 2000 Enuresis and encopresis. In: Carr A (ed) What works with children and adolescents? A critical review of psychological interventions with children, adolescents and their families. Routledge, London

Phillips G T, Smith J E 1986 The behavioural treatment of faeces retention: an expanded case study. Behavioural Psychotherapy 14: 124–136

Rona R J, Li L, Chinn S 1997 Determinants of nocturnal enuresis in England and Scotland. Developmental Medicine and Child Neurology 39(10): 677–681

Shaffer D 1994 Enuresis. In: Rutter M, Taylor E, Hersov L (eds) Child and adolescent psychiatry: modern approaches. Blackwell, Oxford

Shaffer D, Gardner A, Hedge B 1984 Behaviour and bladder disturbance of enuretic children: a rational classification of a common disorder. Developmental Medicine and Child Neurology 26: 781–792

Sorotzkin B 1984 Nocturnal enuresis: current perspectives. Clinical Psychology Review 4: 293–316

Sprague-McRae J M, Lamb W, Homer D 1993 Encopresis: a study of treatment alternatives and behavioural characteristics. Nurse Practitioner 18: 52–63

Street E, Broughton L 1990 The treatment of childhood nocturnal enuresis in the community. Child: Care, Health and Development 16: 365–371

Thapar A, Davies G, Jones T, Rivett M 1992 Treatment of childhood encopresis: a review. Child: Care, Health and Development 18: 343–353

Trsinar B, Kraij B 1996 Maximal electrical stimulation in children with unstable bladder and nocturnal enuresis and/or daytime incontinence: a controlled study. Neurourology and Urodynamics 15(2): 133–142

Verhulst F C, van der Lee J H, Akkerkuis G W et al 1985 The prevalence of nocturnal enuresis: do DSM-III criteria need to be changed? Journal of Child Psychology and Psychiatry 26: 989–993

Von Gothard A 1998 Annotation: Day and night wetting in children – a paediatric and child psychiatric perspective. Journal of Child Psychology and Psychiatry 39(4): 439–451

Wakefield M A, Woodbridge C, Steward J, Croke W M 1984 A treatment programme for faecal incontinence. Developmental Medicine and Child Neurology 26: 613–616

Wille O 1986 Comparison of desmopressin and enuresis alarm for nocturnal enuresis. Archives of Disease in Childhood 61: 30–33

Yamanishi T, Yasuda K, Murayama N et al 2000 Biofeedback training for detrusor overactivity in children. Journal of Urology 164: 1686–1690

FURTHER READING

Blackwell C 1989 A guide to enuresis. Enuresis Resource and Information Centre, Bristol

Blackwell C 1989 A Guide to Encopresis. Enuresis Resource and Information Centre, Bristol
These two guides have been developed from clinical practice and are an excellent resource for both topics, including questionnaires for interviewing both parents and children. They are obtainable from ERIC.

Butler R J 1987 Nocturnal enuresis: psychological perspectives. Wright, Bristol

This is an easy-to-read book which contains useful research background as well as a wealth of information on clinical practice.

Douglas J, Richman N 1984 Coping with young children. Penguin, Harmondsworth
This is referred to in the sections on measurement and star charts. It is also useful for information on toilet training in general.

Exploring parenthood. Latimer Education, London
Latimer Education Centre (194 Freston Road, London W10 6TT) sells copies of its leaflets on different

aspects of children's behaviour. One is available on toilet training.

Morgan R 1988 Help for the bedwetting child. Mandarin, London
A useful self-help book for parents of enuretic children.

Nocturnal enuresis.
A strategy for management report of a working group on enuresis, produced for Ferring Pharmaceuticals by the publishers of Update *and* Hospital update.

Smith P S, Smith L J 1987 Continence and incontinence: psychological approaches to development and treatment. Croom Helm, London
A good overview of both topics with an historical introduction as well as a useful section on adults.

6

Focus on older people

Lesley Wilson

'The fact that an opinion has been widely held
is no evidence whatsoever that it is not utterly
absurd. Indeed, in view of the silliness of the
majority of mankind, a widespread belief is
more likely to be foolish than sensible.'

Bertrand Russell 1929, **Marriage and Morals**

INTRODUCTION

Incontinence is *not* an inevitable part of the ageing
process despite the widespread belief of many
health professionals and the general public that it
is. Perpetuation of the myth that incontinence is
inevitable with advancing years, and that little or
nothing can be done to relieve symptoms or effect
a cure, has been responsible for shaping many of
the negative attitudes and beliefs held by society
about older people and incontinence.

The causes of incontinence in healthy older
people are little different from those in younger
age groups but the elderly are more susceptible to
physiological, pharmacological and psychological
risk factors that may affect their continence status
(Fonda et al 1999, Malone-Lee 2000, Royal College
of Physicians 1995). Older people are more vulnerable to illness and the effects of even minor
illnesses are often more debilitating than in a
younger adult. Older people often take longer to
recover and when incontinence is a symptom, continence is not always fully restored with recovery.
However, continence is achievable in the majority
of cases with correct management and support.

Frail older people can present different problems. Fonda et al (1999) define frailty as being

Table 6.1 Scale and levels of frailty

Scale	Level of frailty
0	Able to walk without help Can perform basic activities of daily living (eating, dressing, bathing, bed transfers) Continent of bowel and bladder Cognitively intact
1	Urinary incontinence only
2	Needing assistance with at least one activity of daily living or mobility (two if incontinent) Has cognitive impairment without dementia Urinary or faecal incontinence
3	Totally dependent in at least two activities of daily living or transfers (three if incontinent) Combined urinary and faecal incontinence Diagnosed with dementia

After Rockwood et al (1999).

homebound or living in an institution as a result of multiple medical conditions and disabilities (comorbidity). A scale to define and classify frailty was devised by Rockwood et al (1999) as the term previously had no accepted definition (Table 6.1). Implicit in the term 'frail' is the acceptance that such individuals may neither wish nor be fit enough to be considered for the full range of therapies likely to be offered to healthy incontinent individuals. However, every person should be given the opportunity to achieve continence irrespective of their frailty or disability. According to Fonda et al (1999) this can be:

- independent continence
- dependent continence – dry with assistance from a carer
- social continence – dry with the use of continence aids or appliances.

Stages and levels of incontinence are discussed more fully later in the chapter in the section on management.

This chapter explores the following aspects of continence in the context of older people:

- prevalence
- attitudes, beliefs and expectations
- coping strategies
- causes of incontinence
- consequences and complications
- assessment
- management

- incontinence in residential care settings
- service provision
- prevention.

PREVALENCE OF INCONTINENCE IN OLDER PEOPLE

Prevalence studies are important in order to understand the magnitude and distribution of problems and to guide service development and resource management. However, the prevalence of urinary incontinence is difficult to measure accurately as discussed in Chapter 1 and by Button et al (1998) and Hunskaar et al (1999). A further question to be considered is the degree to which a prevalence rate reflects the extent to which incontinence is perceived as a problem by the individual.

The Royal College of Physicians (RCP) (1995) and Fonda et al (1999) reviewed existing prevalence studies of urinary incontinence and found ranges of prevalence between 10 and 70% in adults of 65 years or more. For older people who live at home, prevalence of urinary incontinence ranges between 5 and 41% with women having twice the prevalence of men (Pfister 1999, Roberts et al 1999, RCP 1995). A recent survey has suggested that 34% of adults over the age of 40 have significant symptoms of bladder problems with 15% reporting incontinence (Perry et al 2000). For older people in residential or nursing home care, the prevalence of urinary incontinence rises to between 25 and 55% (Roberts et al 1999, Robinson 2000, RCP 1995). In long-term hospital care it is reported to be as high as 70% (RCP 1995).

Reports of the prevalence of faecal incontinence vary depending on the definition of incontinence and the population studied. Urinary incontinence is unpleasant but faecal incontinence is a devastating symptom with underreporting being a substantial problem. Even people with bowel symptoms are unlikely to report incontinence to a hospital consultant as one of their symptoms (Norton 1996a).

Nelson et al (1996) reported 2.2% prevalence of anal incontinence with 0.8% incontinent of solid stool, 1.2% of liquid stool and 1.3% of flatus in a survey of 2570 households in North America. Of those with anal incontinence, 30% were over 65 and 63% were female. Although the study excluded residents in nursing homes, separate data enabled the authors to calculate that 1.1% of the total population of the USA were incontinent of solid stool and 2.6% had some form of anal incontinence.

In a review of existing studies by Kamm (1998), it was found that 2% of the adult population have daily or weekly episodes of faecal incontinence with 7% of healthy independent adults over 65 and a third of older people in residential or hospital care being incontinent of stool. Other studies suggest prevalence rates of between 3 and 17% for older people living in the community, between 10 and 30% in older people living in residential care and up to 60% of patients in long-stay facilities (Alessi et al 1993, Chassagne et al 2000, RCP 1995). Roberts et al (1999) found the prevalence of faecal incontinence was more likely to increase with age in men than in women, from 8.4% in men in their fifties to 18.2% among men in their eighties. In women the prevalence rose from 13.1% in 50-year-old women to 20.7% in women 80 years or older.

There are fewer data on prevalence of combined urinary and faecal incontinence. Nakanishi et al (1997) report prevalence rates of 5.3% in community-dwelling older people. Roberts et al (1999) looked at people with faecal incontinence and found that in this group concurrent urinary incontinence was present in 51.1% of men and 59.6% of women. These findings suggest that combined incontinence is relatively common in older men and women living at home, ranging from 5–9%, being higher in women than in men. This study also found that despite the higher prevalence rates of urinary and faecal incontinence in women than in men, the association between the two conditions was stronger in men than in women. In nursing home populations the prevalence is, not surprisingly, higher. Chiang et al (2000) found that 54% of 413 nursing home residents (mean age of 84 years and 75% females) had combined urinary and faecal incontinence.

The reason for widely varying prevalence rates for both urinary and faecal incontinence is at least partially due to underreporting of the problem in some studies. There is evidence that less than half of individuals with urinary incontinence consult healthcare providers (Burgio et al 1994a, Mitteness 1990, Perry et al 2000) and only approximately 36% of those with faecal incontinence consult a doctor about it (Norton 1996a, b).

ATTITUDES, BELIEFS AND EXPECTATIONS

People of all ages who are incontinent commonly have feelings of embarrassment, shame, low self-esteem and frustration. Shame and the feelings of loss of control are often associated with lower self-esteem although not necessarily so. Simons (1985) found no difference in self-esteem between incontinent and continent elderly women. Mitteness (1990) suggests the belief that incontinence is normal with ageing may protect self-esteem by normalizing incontinence in older people. However, many individuals experience significant anxiety and depression related to their incontinence with negative effects in self-perception (Lagro-Janssen et al 1992, Morison 1998, Wyman et al 1990). A recent study provided clear evidence that urinary incontinence is commonly related to depressive symptoms. The findings demonstrated that physical and mental health, life satisfaction and the perception that urinary incontinence interfered with daily life were significant predictors of depressive symptoms in older adults (Duggan et al 2000). Lagro-Janssen et al (1992) found that urge incontinence in women had a greater impact on their psychological health than stress incontinence, probably because of the higher degree of lack of control and predictability associated with urge incontinence.

A study by McNeil (1995) demonstrated that 55 adults with a mean age of 79 years had limited knowledge of their incontinence condition, with 50% reporting they had not had any explanation about their condition. However, despite being asked if there were any questions they wished to ask, all responses were negative. Of the participants, 40% restricted fluid intake and 23% perceived an improvement following assessment despite no reduction in pad usage. Proactive strategies such as pelvic floor exercises and bladder retraining were being carried out by only 6%. A further study in Massachusetts, USA, found that older adults considered the psychological consequences of incontinence more burdensome than functional disability (DuBeau et al 1998). Many individuals with incontinence choose to restrict their activities and hobbies with resultant social isolation. Incontinent elderly housebound women have been found to have less social interaction, especially with family, than continent housebound women (Wyman et al 1990). Some people even experience social exclusion from their peers due to their incontinence (Mitteness 1990). A fear of odour which can be detected by others is of overriding importance and may be a major factor in reduction of social activities.

Older people who are incontinent are more likely than continent individuals to consider their health as being poor despite being otherwise healthy and able to perform the activities of daily life (Johnson et al 1998). The measures used in this large survey of community-dwelling adults of 65 years or older were the responses from interviewer-administered questionnaires. These included questions on urinary incontinence, activities of daily living, age, gender, place of residence, race, education, need for proxy response to the questionnaire and number of medical conditions.

Underreporting of incontinence is a problem in all ages (DoH 2000) and there is evidence that up to 70% of older people with continence problems do not seek help for their problem (Branch et al 1994). Some of the probable reasons for underreporting are shown in Box 6.1.

Box 6.1 Reasons for underreporting of incontinence

- Embarrassment
- Being unaware of help available
- Hoping the problem will improve without intervention
- Low expectations of the benefits of treatment
- Believing that incontinence is a normal part of ageing
- Believing nothing could be done
- Fear of surgery
- Perception that the problem is not serious enough
- Belief that they are too old for treatment

Attitudes and beliefs about incontinence are still largely governed by 'folk knowledge' or old wives' tales, particularly in older populations. Although there is greater awareness, the subject is still taboo to many and those who are affected feel stigmatized. Sources of information may not be readily accessible for the older individual; for example, women's magazines are often cited as a major source of information but they are targeted at the younger age groups.

The experience of incontinence is unique to each individual and it is important that the spectrum of potential psychological effects is considered and examined during any assessment process. This will help to identify the degree of commitment from the incontinent person and confidence in proposed treatment or management regimes.

The recent Department of Health guidance, *Good Practice in Continence Services* (DoH 2000), usually referred to as the Guidance, places key responsibility for first-line assessment in primary care. However, not all nurses working in primary care have the appropriate knowledge base and skills to perform comprehensive assessment and to plan and implement programmes of care (see also Chapter 1). Erroneous beliefs that little can be done for older people with continence problems can be reinforced if the nurse provides the person with incontinence aids after a limited assessment, and opportunities for continence promotion are missed. The Guidance recognizes the need for all health organizations to develop and provide in-service programmes of education in partnership with local education and training consortia. In conjunction with higher education institutes, health organizations should ensure that pre- and postregistration training are in line with local service policy, reflect contemporary practice and fulfil local needs.

COPING STRATEGIES

The majority of older people cope with incontinence by managing their problem as best they can in the belief that it is 'normal' to become incontinent as part of growing older. This approach is perpetuated by lack of awareness of the many treatments and strategies that can be used to improve or even cure their condition. People have individual ways of coping with their incontinence and it is important for the health professional to understand the ways people cope in order to give the most effective help and support.

Robinson (2000) found that residents of nursing homes engaged in a process of 'managing their incontinence' and identified six main coping strategies (Fig. 6.1). Robinson suggests that by managing the problem the individual protects physical, psychological and social integrity by ensuring physical comfort, preserving dignity and privacy and maintaining social position and standing. Management of incontinence was described in the study as a dynamic process in which the consequences are dependent on the degree to which strategies are used with satisfaction by the person with incontinence and supported by others.

Although Robinson's research describes coping mechanisms used by nursing home residents, most people with incontinence change their behaviour, including restricting or limiting their activities in order to cope with the problems it presents. This frequently includes restriction of fluid intake but may also include restricting social activities such as visiting or shopping unless ease of access to toilet facilities is known to be available. Many older people will decline invitations to stay with family or friends or go on holiday as they are afraid they may 'have an accident' in the bed. Social and physical activities may be curtailed to avoid the embarrassment of being incontinent in public. This may have the effect of the person being thought of by others as being miserable and not wanting to 'join in'. Restricting or limiting behaviour may include poor compliance with drug treatments, especially diuretics, and cancelling or not attending clinic appointments.

Many people who are incontinent are very creative in their improvisations in order to prevent accidents, void more easily or cope with leakage. For those who have mobility problems this may involve methods of transferring on to the toilet or balancing in order to use a urinal. Some people are

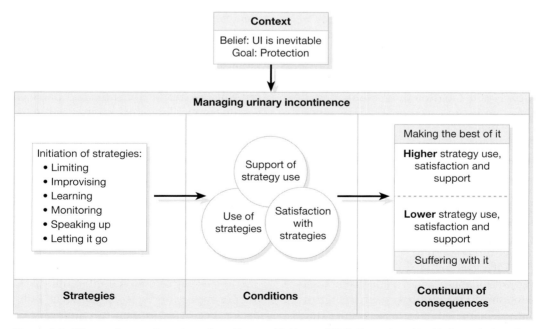

Figure 6.1 Theory of managing urinary incontinence (Robinson 2000). Reproduced by kind permission of Blackwell Science Ltd. UI, urinary incontinence.

very inventive like the old gentleman who devised a tubing system that drained into a bucket by the side of his chair. If commercial products or protective underwear are not being used, alternative innovative ways of containing leakage are often employed such as using old towels, kitchen roll or sanitary protection. Unfortunately many individuals, perhaps having sought help once but without success, will assume they 'have to get on with it' and will not ask for further assistance and continue with their improvisations. Whilst this may result in an acceptable outcome in some cases, there are other people who may be putting themselves at unnecessary risk – for example increased risk of falling and sustaining a limb fracture as a result of poor balance, where a raised toilet seat and other support or an appropriate urine collecting appliance could reduce such risks.

Some incontinent people attempt to learn more about their condition and increase their self-knowledge in order to manage their incontinence. This process of increasing self-knowledge can be used to help prevent or manage leakage through knowing how long it is safe to wait before leakage becomes inevitable or anticipating when to visit the toilet to prevent accidents. It may also include knowing where toilet facilities are available and their accessibility.

Coping with problems in isolation can be a significant source of anxiety. Many people with incontinence will monitor their bodily function and leakage, sometimes obsessively. This involves checking clothes for damp patches and comparing urinary or stool output with fluid and dietary input. This strategy may be as a result of the anxiety caused by the continence problem but can itself cause or increase distress.

An alternative approach concerns denial that there is a problem or underreporting the severity of the problem and this is very common indeed. It is frequently related to the fact that incontinence is still considered to be stigmatizing and a taboo subject for many older people who associate the meaning of incontinence with the Victorian definition of being out of control or lacking in restraint, with sexual implications. Robinson (2000) identified 'speaking up' as a coping strategy.

This relates to the communication, to doctors, nurses, carers, family and sometimes anyone who will listen, of needs, concerns, opinions and ideas in relation to the continence problem. It may concern specific treatment or management options in order to communicate the preferred methods. A key factor here seems to be the relief people often feel when they perceive that it is acceptable to discuss such issues and that they are not alone. It is sometimes surprising when at 'continence awareness sessions' people start talking, often quite publicly, about their problems. It is as if there is a need to be given permission to talk and this has been allowed because the professional leading the session is talking about continence problems in a natural way. When one person discusses their problem, this often leads to others joining in. This is important in terms of encouragement to individuals to acknowledge their continence difficulties and seek help but also in terms of ensuring that health professionals have up-to-date knowledge in order to respond to recognized needs.

Another aspect of continence behaviour is that some people will deliberately, accidentally or negotiate to void and 'let go'. Often, but not always, this involves the use of containment aids such as pads. It may be easier for the incontinent person than using the toilet especially when mobility or gross obesity is a problem. Health professionals and carers should always remember that to supply incontinence pads is giving permission to 'let it go' and may actually help to promote incontinence even if it is contained.

When strategies are used effectively, to the satisfaction of the individual and supported by others, Robinson identified a state of 'making the best of it' when quality of life was not significantly diminished. When strategies are used minimally, do not satisfy the individual and are not supported by others, the individual's quality of life is compromised, they may be depressed and withdrawn, and are 'suffering with it'.

The health professional must understand how people cope with their incontinence but that the experience of incontinence is unique to each person and must be considered when developing a management plan.

Research study 6.1 Managing urinary incontinence in the nursing home: residents' perspectives

Urinary incontinence affects a high proportion of residents in nursing home care. Despite there being evidence to show that behavioural programmes can significantly reduce or cure incontinence in this population these approaches often fail. Failure is often attributed to staffing issues such as apathy, ageism, ignorance, inflexibility, high workload, shortages and turnover but it is possibly also because the residents themselves lack motivation and initiative, preferring alternative, easier approaches to managing the problem.

This study by Robinson (2000) set out to explain the cognitive, psychosocial and behavioural aspects of living with urinary incontinence in American nursing homes. The study used a grounded theory approach. Data were obtained from interviews, participant observation and minutes from meetings of resident advisory councils. Analysis was by the constant comparative technique, a well-recognized qualitative research process which allows newly collected data to be continuously compared to earlier data. This process helps to refine the categories identified from the data which may then be used to develop theory to facilitate understanding.

Ten residents consented to be primary participants and gave an audiotaped formal interview, provided opportunities for observation and discussed their methods of bladder control and allowed access to their health records. A further 33 residents were secondary participants and agreed to provide opportunities for observation and gave informal interviews when their bladder control needs, issues or methods were visible to the investigator and appeared to be relevant to the evolving theory. The residents lived in one of three nursing homes in an American inner city area.

Data were collected over a period of 17 months. The emerging theory was that nursing home residents with actual or potential urinary incontinence engage in a process of managing their incontinence.

Managing urinary incontinence occurs in the context of the belief that incontinence is inevitable with ageing and the individual seeks to protect their physical, psychological and social integrity. Six specific strategies were identified as being used by residents to manage their continence problems. These were:

- *Limiting* – where individuals impose restrictions on their own activities and behaviour; this may include restriction of fluid, activities and outings.

- *Improvising* – individuals improvise by discovering or devising methods of preventing accidents, accomplishing voiding or dealing with their leakage.
- *Learning* – this refers to the acquisition of information or skills to deal with their incontinence.
- *Monitoring* – individuals monitor their bodily functions and in residential settings often observe their fellow residents.
- *Speaking up* – is when individuals communicate their needs, opinions and ideas about incontinence and its treatment/management.
- *Letting it go* – this refers to accidental, deliberate or negotiated voiding in other than the usually accepted location or receptacle.

Managing urinary incontinence is a dynamic process with consequences that are influenced by the degree to which the strategies identified are used with satisfaction by the resident and supported by the staff and others. The use of strategies, degree of satisfaction and the support of strategy use influenced outcomes and determined consequences on a continuum between making the best of it (the incontinence) or suffering with it.

This study provides important information of living with incontinence from the perspective of the nursing home resident but the application of the theory may be limited by methodological constraints, one being the sensitive nature of the topic and the risks of revealing intimate information to an outsider. This is borne out by the fact that seven eligible residents declined to participate and representation may have been inadequate by the exclusion of residents who were unable to discuss their problems.

Despite these limitations, important implications for practice come from this study and show clearly the need for education of residents and their families about incontinence and the many treatment options available. The way behavioural programmes are organized also needs to be examined to ensure an individualized approach with input from the resident at the planning stage rather than standardized protocols that do not consider the individual's needs. Staff resistance to change is often cited as an impediment to continence promotion but the findings from this study can help staff appreciate the reticence of residents and their apparent resistance to change may represent fear of being the cause of extra work for the staff. Collaboration of staff with residents in developing continence programmes should help encourage residents and staff to be proactive in their approach.

CAUSES OF INCONTINENCE IN OLDER PEOPLE

Urinary continence is dependent on effective function of the bladder, pelvic floor musculature, neural control centres in the cerebral cortex and pons and the integrity of neural connections that facilitate voluntary control (see Chapter 2). The bladder has two modes of operation: storage and voiding. Although disorders of voiding resulting in incomplete emptying may be associated with continence problems, disorders of storage are more likely to cause incontinence (de Groat et al 1999, RCP 1995).

Faecal continence depends on the integrity of bowel and sphincter anatomy, intact cerebral and spinal control and neuromuscular function. The rectum acts as a low pressure reservoir for formed stool but is not equipped to cope with liquid or irritant substances (Lamb et al 1991, RCP 1995) (see Chapter 7 for further details).

There are several normal physiological changes that occur as part of the ageing process that may have some impact on an older person's ability to maintain continence.

Renal function

Changes in kidney function are indicated by a reduction in glomerular filtration rate (GFR) from approximately 125 ml/min (at maturation, i.e. by 1 year of age) to about 60–70 ml/min by the age of 80 years, an effective decrease of 50% (Laker 1994, Mirpuri & Patel 1998). However, the renal changes have no great effect on the functioning of the kidney itself but they dramatically alter the ability of the body to compensate for external changes or stresses caused by disease states. For example, there is less efficient response to water depletion and older people tend to continue to produce more urine which is also less concentrated than that produced by a younger person (Addison 1999). The problem is caused by a reduced ability of the kidney to reabsorb sodium in the ascending loop of Henle. In turn this reduces the efficiency of the counter-current multiplier system that concentrates urine (Edwards 2001). There is evidence to show that levels of antidiuretic hormone (ADH) are diminished in some older people but also the kidney's response to ADH – i.e. water reabsorption by the kidney tubules – is less efficient with the effect of more urine being produced at night. The effects of dehydration and moving from lying to standing, which normally provoke an ADH response, also appear to be blunted in older people. A number of studies have demonstrated some success in reducing problems of nocturia by treatment with desmopressin, a synthetic analogue of vasopressin (ADH) (Asplund & Aberg 1993).

Bladder function

There are a number of ways in which ageing affects the lower urinary tract but Fonda et al (1999) argue that incontinence is not one of them. These changes are found in continent older people but age-related disease or illness will exacerbate these normal changes and impair an individual's ability to compensate for them.

Bladder capacity and urinary flow rate reduce with age in women but postvoid residual volume and uninhibited detrusor contractions increase in both sexes (Fonda et al 1999, Nazarko 1996). The bladder capacity of an elderly person may be reduced to half that of a young adult (600 ml to 250 ml) (Marieb 1992). Diokno et al (1988) found uninhibited detrusor contractions differed significantly between the sexes with 8% in women and up to 35% in men. They suggested that the presence of the prostate in men was the significant variable but there is evidence to show that older women have lower bladder capacities (Malone-Lee 2000) and show a tendency for the detrusor contraction to fail on initiation of voiding. These differences explain why the incidence of incontinence is higher in older women than in older men. In some frail elderly people detrusor hyperactivity is accompanied by impaired contractility of the bladder (Hogan 1997).

Reduction in the compliance of the bladder as a result of a 'stiff' bladder wall when there is continuous increase in intravesical pressure may be due to the replacement of muscle with collagen (Nazarko 1996, RCP 1995). Symptoms of a poorly compliant bladder are urgency, urge incontinence and frequency.

Afferent sensors in the bladder become less sensitive with age so the older person is not aware of the desire to void until their bladder is 90% full, giving them very little time to reach the toilet. A younger person, however, has warning much earlier when the bladder is about half full (Getliffe 1996a, Malone-Lee 2000). When this reduction in sensitivity is compounded by disability (e.g. poor mobility) incontinence is often inevitable.

In older men with benign enlargement of the prostate, the bladder enlarges and the bladder wall thickens to compensate for the outflow obstruction. The detrusor muscle becomes stretched and ineffective and the bladder becomes hypotonic or atonic (Mirpuri & Patel 1998).

Urethral changes

Compression of the urethral folds by the muscles of the pelvic floor is essential for the maintenance of continence. Strasser (1999) found there was reduction in striated muscle cells in the rhabdosphincter (external sphincter) in older subjects with an increased likelihood of incontinence. In some women reduced levels of oestrogen result in reduced urethral closing pressures due to changes in the muscles, ligaments and fascia (Kelleher & Versi 2000). It has been suggested that because the vagina and urethra are of the same embryologic origin, oestrogen therapy may be beneficial for some postmenopausal women but there is limited evidence to suggest oestrogen therapy is beneficial for patients with incontinence. Kelleher & Versi (2000) suggest that long treatment periods are necessary in order to produce significant effects and this may explain the poor results in some studies. Reduced vascularity of urethral tissues may also contribute to the reduction in urethral closing pressure.

In the older man, benign prostatic hyperplasia (BPH) can cause urethral obstruction displaying symptoms of frequency, nocturia, hesitancy, poor flow, residual urine and dribbling incontinence (Mirpuri & Patel 1998). Residual urine retention is not always entirely due to outflow obstruction caused by an enlarged prostate. The replacement of muscle fibres with fibrous tissue in the ageing bladder occurring at the same time prevents the detrusor from relaxing during filling. Consequently there is a rise in filling pressures and the reduction in compliance is responsible for the bladder symptoms. This was demonstrated by Holm et al (1995) who found no fibrosis in the bladders of young men but considerable replacement of muscle with fibrous tissue in the biopsies taken from older men.

After prostate surgery, incontinence is fairly common. It may only be temporary due to pelvic floor weakness or it may be more permanent caused by damage to the bladder neck, detrusor instability or residual obstruction (Jolleys 1993). In postprostatectomy incontinence, damage to the rhabdosphincter will cause stress incontinence.

There is greater risk of the incidence of urinary tract infection in older men who have urine retention due to BPH as there is less prostatic bactericide produced in older men (Nazarko 1996).

Lower gastrointestinal tract

In the healthy older adult, the effects of ageing should not significantly affect the normal digestion, absorption and elimination of waste products from the gastrointestinal (GI) tract. The main age-related changes are concerned with atrophy resulting in decreased motility and absorption, diminished sensation of rectal distension and reduced ability to distinguish between fluid and flatus in the anal canal (Getliffe 1996b, Watson 2001). There may also be a reduction in anal squeeze pressure (weak external sphincter), which is more common in women and may be an effect of childbirth (Getliffe 1996b). However, studies have found no reduction in the frequency of bowel movements in elderly people (Camilleri et al 2000) but that older people are more likely to increase laxative use (Wilson 1999). Some of the exaggerated concern of many older people about their bowel is the result of the upbringing of this generation. Despite older people being more likely to suffer from lower GI tract problems, these are unlikely to be due to ageing alone (Watson 2001).

Many older people are likely to develop diverticuli in the colon and this may be due to low fibre diets. When the diet is lacking in fibre, colonic residues are small, causing the colon to narrow. The powerful contraction of the muscles increases the pressure on the walls of the colon, resulting in diverticular pocket formation (Marieb 1992). Diverticuli do not normally cause problems but if the contents become infected, bleeding can occur which is seen in the stools. If the infected diverticuli rupture, the condition can be life threatening (Watson 2001).

Constipation is a common condition in older people but as constipation has many causes (see Chapter 7), it cannot be attributed solely to the ageing process. Irritable bowel syndrome in the older adult may be as a result of abnormal motility of the faecal mass, increased sensation and psychosocial disturbance but current research is being directed into neuroimmune dysfunction as a possible cause (Camilleri et al 2000).

Constipation and faecal impaction are common causes of faecal incontinence in the older person. Use of laxatives can also be part of the problem through contributing to soft stool, which is then difficult to pass effectively.

Neurological control

Neurological changes in the micturition centres in the cerebral cortex, pons and spinal cord will affect urinary function, often causing nocturia. Detrusor sphincter dyssynergia is a condition that occurs when there is poor coordination between detrusor contraction and relaxation of the bladder neck; the result is outflow obstruction. Neurological changes affecting continence in older people are often the result of disease or illness such as diabetes mellitus, hypertension, Parkinson's disease, Alzheimer's disease or stroke (Nakayama et al 1997). Loss of inhibitory nerve impulses from the brain causes detrusor instability and urge incontinence. Urge incontinence is reported to be the most common type of urinary incontinence in older people (Button et al 1998), especially in older women (Nasr & Ouslander 1998).

Incontinence following stroke is very common but only those people who have severe strokes should have ongoing problems. There are three main factors that will have an impact on continence status following stroke:

- Physiological changes affecting mobility, vision and visual fields and communication (dysphagia, dysarthria and receptive dysphagia) will restrict the individual's ability to move freely and communicate their needs.
- Damage to the higher micturition centres will affect continence and cause urgency, urge incontinence or detrusor sphincter dyssynergia (Nazarko 1998).
- Following a severe stroke where there has been considerable neurological damage, passive or reflex incontinence is likely.

The most likely problem with defecation as a result of neurological deficit in the central or peripheral nervous system such as stroke, Parkinson's disease or diabetic neuropathy is constipation. The main factors involved are the same as for urinary problems as already discussed above.

Damage to the peripheral nerves to the bladder or the lower spinal cord caused by pelvic lesions, diabetic neuropathy or lesions to the cauda equina makes the detrusor muscle underactive and unable to provide a sustained or adequate voiding contraction for micturition (Kirby 1994). Incomplete bladder emptying with residual urine may lead to dribbling/overflow incontinence.

Urinary incontinence is common in those who have impaired cognitive function or dementia, especially when their mobility is poor. However, it is not an inevitable consequence of dementia and in Alzheimer's disease often occurs late in the progression of the condition. Alternative explanations for incontinence, such as urinary tract infection, should therefore be sought when relatively mild disease is apparent (RCP 1995).

Cognitive impairment (including memory loss) may have the effect of the person forgetting they were on the way to the toilet or being confused as to where to go. For many people with dementia, each time they see a person or place, it is as if this is the first time. They have no memory of people or places (Jenkins 1999).

It has been a commonly held belief that incontinence in people with dementia is caused by detrusor instability but this opinion is now being challenged (Nazarko 1997). A study of 133 nursing home residents with continence problems found that despite 88% showing some cognitive impairment only 38% had detrusor instability, 16% had stress incontinence and 5% had dribbling/overflow incontinence. In 41% of the subjects, bladder function was established as being normal (Yu et al 1990). The authors of the study suggest that the high percentage of residents showing normal bladder function demonstrates that incontinence derives not necessarily from a primary bladder problem, i.e. nerve damage, but that mental and physical disabilities are more significant.

Cardiac function

The diurnal pattern of fluid excretion alters with increasing age due to reduced renal concentrating capacity, increased sodium excretion in the urine and loss of the daily rhythm of antidiuretic hormone secretion. The effect is larger quantities of fluid being excreted at night (Fonda et al 1999, Miller 2000). Cardiac dysfunction also leads to increased sodium excretion (Davis et al 1996) and when heart failure is present, fluid is retained in the extravascular spaces. At rest improved cardiac output improves venous return to the heart; the blood supply to the kidneys is thereby increased, resulting in an increase in urine production (Addison 1999). This nocturnal polyuria increases the likelihood of nocturnal enuresis.

Endocrine factors

The urethra and the trigone in the female develop embryologically from the same oestrogen-dependent tissue as the vagina. Following the menopause oestrogen levels are reduced and urethritis and trigonitis may occur in some women. The individual complains of symptoms similar to cystitis (i.e. urgency, dysuria and frequency) and these symptoms are associated with atrophic vaginitis (Swaffield 1996). The walls of the normal urethra are soft with many interdigitating folds. The oestrogen-deficient urethra is less soft and the folds are less pronounced, with resultant reduced efficiency of urethral closure. There is also a reduction in mucus production, which will lower surface tension making incontinence more likely.

Atrophic vaginitis is often a cause of urinary symptoms, including incontinence; other symptoms include urgency and scalding. It is important to identify atrophic vaginitis as it is very easy to treat with topical or low dose systemic oestrogen (Fonda et al 1999). Atrophic vaginitis is very common among older women with as many as 80% of women attending one clinic reported to have had evidence of its presence along with vaginal mucosal atrophy, friability, erosions and punctate haemorrhages (bleeding spots) (Fonda et al 1999). Harrington (2000) however cautions against always assuming that vulval and perianal itching is due to age-related dryness as there are several alternative conditions that could be responsible and oestrogen preparations will not improve symptoms. Because women often present for health care late, due to embarrassment, accurate assessment and diagnosis are very important.

Incontinence in an older person may be associated with undiagnosed recent onset of diabetes mellitus. Both diabetes mellitus and diabetes insipidus will cause polyuria and this may be a contributory factor in causing incontinence.

Impaired functional ability

Impaired functional status (especially immobility), impaired cognitive function and dementia strongly correlate with incontinence of urine, faeces and combined incontinence (Ouslander & Schnelle 1993). An environment that does not allow the individual to reach the toilet easily, lack of privacy or uncomfortable toilet facilities may also contribute to continence problems.

Reduced mobility may make it difficult for an older person to reach the toilet in time considering the age-related changes in the urinary tract already discussed. Moving may be painful as well as difficult or obesity may cause breathlessness on movement. Conditions such as osteoarthritis, vertebral disc disease or cervical scoliosis commonly cause painful movement in the older adult. Respiratory or cardiac conditions may dictate that mobilization is at a slow pace. Poor dexterity hinders the ability to remove clothing in order to void. Unsuitable clothing or footwear may increase the difficulties the older person experiences with dexterity or mobility. Poor eyesight may make finding the toilet a problem especially when the older person is not in a familiar environment.

Immobility and lack of exercise are common causes of constipation. Colonic activity is influenced by physical exercise which will also improve the appetite. Food also stimulates the movement of faeces into the rectum.

Drug clearance, toxicity and polypharmacy

In older people, drug treatment becomes more complex than in the younger adult due to the increased possibility of coexistent illness or disease. Medication is often prescribed indiscriminately, such as the administration of laxatives for constipation when diet change and increased fluid intake should be the first line in management.

Hogan (1997) defines polypharmacy as: ' ... *any drug regimen with at least one unnecessary medication*'. He considers the overuse of medication to be a serious, preventable public health problem that potentially increases the risk of illness, non-compliance and direct and indirect health-care costs.

One of the main problems with polypharmacy in older people is that the absorption, distribution, metabolism and elimination of drugs depend on processes that are affected by the ageing process. The most important consideration is drug elimination in the context of reduced renal function. The reduction in glomerular filtration rate reduces the excretion of renally excreted drugs such as digoxin, cimetidine, cephalosporins, oral hypoglycaemics and non-steroidal anti-inflammatory drugs (NSAIDs), resulting in drug toxicity unless dosage adjustments are made (Shepherd 1998). Other changes due to ageing, such as reduced hepatic function, have the result of drug tissue concentrations being increased by over 50%. The greater the number of drugs prescribed for an individual, the greater the risk of drug-to-drug interaction and toxicity. Prescribing a number of drugs can also contribute to non-compliance due to drug-to-drug interactions and adverse side-effects. Older adults with coronary heart disease or asthma/chronic obstructive pulmonary disease are slightly more at risk from adverse drug reactions (Veehof et al 1999). Renteln-Kruse (2000) found that elderly, frail adults were more likely to be prescribed numerous preparations and were more susceptible to adverse drug reactions.

Many acute hospital admissions are the result of adverse drug reactions in frail older people (Renteln-Kruse 2000) and it is common for drug treatments to be discontinued on admission. Therapeutic agents are then prescribed when necessary and only after careful monitoring.

Hogan (1997) suggests that some drugs prescribed for urinary incontinence can precipitate delirium or contribute to polypharmacy. It is important therefore to monitor the effects of any medication prescribed and titrate the dose to achieve the desired effect without unnecessary side-effects. Medication is discussed in more detail in Chapter 8, but some of the common drugs associated with urinary incontinence are mentioned here:

- Diuretics, especially the fast-acting loop diuretics, may cause urgency and frequency and cause or worsen incontinence. They may lead to severe dehydration and electrolyte imbalance.
- Anticholinergic agents including some antidepressants and antiparkinsonian drugs can cause urine retention.
- Sedatives and hypnotics reduce the level of awareness and ability to respond to bladder signals and may also cause disorientation and drowsiness during the day leading to secondary incontinence.
- Beta-blockers and antihistamines may reduce flow rates and cause voiding problems.
- Muscle relaxants may be prescribed following a stroke to reduce spasticity, but may cause incontinence by relaxing the muscles of the pelvic floor.
- Alcohol has sedative and diuretic properties.
- Caffeine has been found to have an excitatory effect on the detrusor muscle causing urgency and frequency, as well as having diuretic properties.
- Alpha-adrenergic antagonists may decrease tonicity in the proximal urethra causing stress incontinence in women.
- Alpha-agonists, found in many decongestants, may cause urinary retention in older men with prostate enlargement by increasing urethral muscle tone (Button et al 1998, Hogan 1997).

Drugs may also have an effect on bowel action. Analgesics, iron preparations, diuretics and anticholinergics (including some antidepressants) will cause constipation. Some antacid preparations will cause diarrhoea but antibiotics may cause either constipation or diarrhoea. Indiscriminate long-term use of aperients or laxatives causing soft stool can lead to faecal incontinence.

Transient incontinence

Older people frequently experience transient incontinence. This is incontinence of sudden onset, it is temporary or reversible and is usually related to a specific event, an illness or specific medical incident (Newman 1999). According to Fonda et al (1999), transient causes account for a third of cases of incontinence in older people living in the community, up to half of those with incontinence in acute hospital settings and a significant proportion of those with incontinence in residential care settings. The risk of transient incontinence is increased when physiological changes in the lower urinary tract are accompanied by illness or disease. A chest infection may exacerbate stress incontinence due to continual coughing or urinary tract infection may result in incontinence due to frequency of micturition.

Emotional distress such as a recent bereavement or change in environment can also cause transient incontinence. Very often older people experience incontinence following acute hospital admission, often due to the disorientation of an unfamiliar environment as well as the medical reason for admission. Continence should be restored when their health improves and they are no longer disorientated.

Fonda et al (1999), in a literature review, identifies eight main causes of transient incontinence. These are shown in Boxes 6.2 and 6.3 and can be recalled using the mnemonics DIAPPERS (Fonda et al 1999) or DRIP (Sander 1998). Delirium, a confusional state where inattentiveness and disorientation are observed, can be due to many illnesses, infections or drug reactions.

The incidence of transient incontinence emphasizes how continence is dependent on multiple factors: mental state, mobility, manual dexterity, health status and motivation as well as urinary function (Fonda et al 1999). 'Transient' incontinence may persist if left untreated so even when incontinence is of long duration it should not be dismissed as being untreatable or intractable. Assessment should seek the causes of incontinence with the aim of eliminating them to improve or cure the problem, thus improving the individual's overall function and quality of life.

Button et al (1998) list further risk factors that are strongly associated with incontinence, some of which may be applied to older people, such as smoking, body mass index, race, exercise and

---

Box 6.2 Transient incontinence (after Fonda et al 1999, Resnick 1990)	
D	Delirium or confusion
I	Infection (symptomatic urinary tract infection)
A	Atrophic urethritis/vaginitis
P	Psychological disorders (severe depression, neurosis)
P	Pharmacological factors (sedatives/hypnotics, anticholinergic agents, alpha-adrenoceptor agonists and antagonists)
E	Endocrine disorders (hypercalcaemia, hyperglycaemia), excess urinary output
R	Reduced/restricted mobility
S	Stool impaction

Box 6.3 Transient incontinence (after Sander 1998)	
D	Delirium
R	Reduced/restricted mobility, acute retention
I	Infection, inflammation, impaction of stool
P	Pharmaceuticals, polyuria, psychological disorders

previous surgery. However, statistically significant relationships have not been established in all cases.

CONSEQUENCES AND COMPLICATIONS OF INCONTINENCE IN THE OLDER ADULT

Incontinence can have adverse effects on physical health, psychological well-being and relationships. It may be associated with skin problems, pressure sores and urinary tract infection. An increased risk of falls associated with incontinence has been reported anecdotally but evidence is now emerging to substantiate this claim (Brown et al 2000).

Both urinary and faecal incontinence can affect every aspect of an older person's life. Chelvanayagam & Norton (2000) reported a range of emotional responses with the fear of public humiliation a recurrent theme.

Physical health

In a study by Roe et al (1996), people with incontinence were found to have a significantly lower health status than those who were continent. Problems with their feet, poor mobility and disturbed sleep with nocturia made more difficult by their poor mobility, were all more common. Other significant factors included gender, advanced age, increased body mass index and obesity. People who were incontinent were more likely to be living alone, without help from friends or relatives, than people who were continent. As a consequence, they needed more help with personal care and domestic activities and were more likely to have formal contacts and services such as community nurses, health visitors and other members of the community health and social care teams. In a further study, Johnson et al (1998) found that urinary incontinence was associated with self-rating one's health as poor despite the ability to perform specific activities of daily living (bathing, eating and dressing) without difficulties. As the incontinence became more severe, the odds of rating one's health as poor increased. However, when the ability to perform these specific activities of daily living was impaired, the association between incontinence and self-rated poor health became weaker, which suggests that the self-rating of health is related to the individual's perception of what they should be able to do.

Roe et al (1996) found that women who had incontinence tended to report better health status than men with incontinence, the reverse of gender differences in normative populations. An explanation for this finding may be a degree of acceptance by many women that incontinence is inevitably associated with childbirth and with increasing age.

Psychological well-being

Adults with incontinence are more likely to be depressed than those who are continent although depressive symptoms appear to be influenced by gender and physical health to a greater degree than incontinence. Adults with bladder control problems are likely to be more emotionally distressed than their continent counterparts. The likelihood of non-compliance to medical treatment is magnified by depression and it is probable that depressed individuals will not have the emotional strength to adhere to behavioural interventions such as pelvic floor exercises or bladder retraining programmes designed for them (Duggan et al 2000).

A recent study carried out in Australia found sufficient evidence to take seriously the possibility of depression being a risk factor for dementia and cognitive decline. The author suggests that further studies are needed to establish whether depression is a prodrome (predicting symptom) of vascular dementia and/or if depression is an early reaction to cognitive decline. The study poses the question: 'If depression is a risk factor for dementia, will treatment for depression help prevent the development of dementia?' (Jorm 2000). Treatment of depression in the older adult is recommended (Silverman et al 1997), especially as pharmacologic treatments are now safer and more effective.

The findings of the study by Jorm (2000), together with the overwhelming evidence of the correlation between depression and incontinence, reinforces the benefits of continence promotion, especially in the older population. With appropriate interventions, the disability associated with cognitive decline may be reduced (Jorm 2000).

Health-related quality of life is now accepted as an important patient outcome and is used to attempt to identify and quantify responses to disease or treatment (see also Chapter 1). The main aspects relating to quality of life reported by incontinent individuals focus on emotional disturbances and isolation. People with urge and mixed incontinence are reported to have more negative responses than those with stress incontinence. A likely explanation for these findings is the unpredictability of urge incontinence (DuBeau et al 1998, Grimby et al 1993, Harris 1999). More sleep disturbances are also reported by people with urge incontinence which can intensify depressive symptoms.

Incontinence is viewed by most individuals as loss of control. Schulz et al (1994) describe the disablement process in the elderly where loss of control accompanied by the failure to compensate by using control strategies will lead to negative emotional and psychological effects. Initially the response is heightened anxiety, with depressive effects becoming more dominant as the perception of the condition (incontinence) being a permanent state progresses.

Irritable bladder syndrome is a condition described by Hunt (1995) who suggests urgency and frequency may be due to infection or trauma or as a psychophysiological response to stress that affects the bladder and/or urethra. She suggests that in some patients physical factors and psychological processes interact where there is a chronic condition to maintain the dysfunctional state. This explanation appears feasible as it is common to experience frequency and urgency when in stressful situations such as attending for job interview or waiting to begin an examination. Although this phenomenon is not well understood, it is possible the stress involved with the fear of having an accident may compound the continence problem in some individuals and lead to incontinence or worsen an existing problem.

Relationships and sexuality

Incontinence may have a negative effect on relationships with family, friends or partners. Some drug treatments for existing medical conditions may affect continence status and may also be associated with male sexual dysfunction, such as antihypertensives, antidepressants, tranquillizers and phenothiazines. Gregoire (1999) suggests using strategies such as delayed dosing, reducing doses, substitution, withdrawal, 'drug holidays' or using adjunctive agents to manage side-effects.

The use of appliances, such as urethral catheters, to manage incontinence may be detrimental to body image and sense of masculinity or femininity and can contribute to the perception of being less attractive to the individual's partner (Milligan 2000). Sexual activity is commonly believed to be for the young and many older people may deny their need for sexual expression fearing derision (Grigg 1999, Heath 2000, RCN 2000b). Sexual behaviour is dependent on both physical and psychological factors but although there may be a decline in interest and capacity with advancing age (Box 6.4) it is not inevitable and should not be assumed by healthcare professionals and carers. A study reported by Gregoire (1999) found that in adults over the age of 80, 62% of the men and 30% of the women still enjoyed physical intercourse.

The ageing process is characterized by physiological, psychological, behavioural and sometimes

---

Box 6.4 Common age-related factors likely to lead to sexual dysfunction *(many potentially reversible)* (after Gregoire 1999)

- Physical disease – diabetic neuropathy, peripheral vascular disease
- Psychiatric disorders – dementia, depression
- Lack of willing partner, opportunity or privacy
- Lifestyle factors – smoking, alcohol consumption, lack of physical exercise, boredom, loneliness

---

Box 6.5 Age-related sexual changes (after Gregoire 1999, Grigg 1999)

- Decreased frequency of activity
- Reduced arousal in response to psychological stimuli (desire not necessarily less)
- Suppression of desire due to vaginal dryness causing dyspareunia
- Reduced tactile sensitivity of penis
- Reduction in vaginal contractions
- Shorter ejaculatory stage
- Increased rates of erectile dysfunction with age
- Decreased rates of premature ejaculation
- Shorter orgasm phase
- Increased refractory period after orgasm in men

---

pathological changes, all of which may affect sexual functioning (Box 6.5). Sexual expression includes behaviour that will enrich and enhance the relationship between a couple and Grigg (1999) suggests that older people need closeness, affection, intimacy, some romance and the need to feel feminine, or masculine. Sexual activity can also be considered from a therapeutic perspective in helping to reduce physical tension and psychological stress. Sexual intercourse may be beneficial for older women in helping to maintain muscular tone, reducing the risk of stress incontinence (Drench & Losee 1996, Heath 2000).

It is important for health professionals to acknowledge older people as sexual beings and be prepared to help them resolve difficulties if they exist. It is not possible or desirable for all health professionals to be practised in psychosexual counselling, but knowing what services are available and arranging referral when appropriate can go towards helping older people resolve their sexual concerns (see Chapter 12).

Skin problems

The ageing process affecting the skin is complex with changes to all skin structures and the subcutaneous fat. The epidermis will be reduced by 50% by the age of 80, collagen stiffens and elastic fibres thicken causing reduced elastic recoil and the formation of wrinkles. The sweat glands reduce in size producing less fluid and, in women, sebum secretion is reduced after the menopause. The effect of these changes is increased fluid loss from the epidermis, which is not adequately replaced by the normal processes, with the result that many older people complain of dry skin. Dry, fragile, puckered skin is more susceptible to damage from friction (Smoker 1999).

Children and older people are more at risk from incontinence dermatitis but it can occur at any age. Friction, chemical, enzymatic and microbial factors are all implicated in the causation of skin problems as a result of incontinence. Those people with faecal or double incontinence are at greater risk from incontinence dermatitis (LeLievre 2000, Smoker 1999). Incontinence dermatitis develops when permeability and pH of the skin increase, there is excessive hydration and microbials present can attack the skin. The increased pH occurs particularly when urine is mixed with faeces. Ammonia is produced from the breakdown of urinary and faecal urea as a result of faecal enzyme activity.

Excessive hydration of the skin can be caused by occlusive continence aids and the permeability will be increased causing a raised pH. The skin is more vulnerable to frictional damage when it is excessively hydrated and the permeability is increased (LeLievre 2000). Incontinence dermatitis can be superimposed with candidiasis or Staphylococcal infection (Smoker 1999).

Excessive cleansing, especially with soap and water, has been shown to be harmful for those with fragile skin and at risk from incontinence dermatitis. Soap is a detergent, designed to remove dirt and grease and will remove the natural skin oils, thus reducing the protective barrier properties of the skin. Alternative products specifically designed for skin cleansing following episodes of incontinence have been found to be clinically and cost-effective in cleansing gently and reducing the risk of damage to the skin. An added advantage is the ability of the skin cleansers to reduce odour more effectively than soap and water (LeLievre 2000, Whittingham 1998).

Talcum powder should also be avoided as the residue will cause encrustation in groin areas when dampened with urine or sweat adding to the possibility of frictional damage. Some talcs are believed to promote the development of candidiasis (LeLievre 2000, Smoker 1999).

Skin preparations such as barrier creams must be used with care as when used in conjunction with incontinence pads can render the pad ineffective by preventing urine being absorbed by the pad and increase hydration to the skin. Only a very thin layer of cream, such as zinc and caster oil, should be used.

Care must be taken when continence aids are needed. Incontinence pads containing superabsorbents are effective in reducing skin hydration and preserving skin integrity. Products must be chosen carefully to minimize their occlusive effects and they must be changed frequently enough to prevent excessive hydration. When appliances such as sheaths are being used, latex allergy should be considered when skin problems occur. Even though a patient has used the same aids for many years, latex allergy can suddenly occur. The need to change management methods can be distressing for an individual who is familiar with the aids they have used successfully for some time. LeLievre (2000) highlights the fact that patients can develop latex allergy when health professionals need to wear gloves during episodes of care, especially when dealing with body fluids.

Skin condition is also dependent on other factors such as nutritional status, hydration state and coexisting chronic conditions such as diabetes. These should be taken into account during assessment and in the planning of interventions.

Risk of falling

Falls are common in older people with approximately 30% of people over 65 and 50% over 80 years falling once a year. Almost half of Accident and Emergency department visits of people over

65 are as a result of falling. About 30% of falls result in an injury and hospital admission, with up to 9% sustaining fractures with a significant risk of mortality (Brown et al 2000, Close et al 1999, Oliver 2000, Stewart et al 1992).

Although incontinence has for a long time been associated with an increased risk of falling, evidence until recently has been mostly anecdotal. Brown et al (2000) found there was an association between incontinence and falling. Urinary frequency, nocturia and rushing to the toilet to avoid an episode of urge incontinence were most likely to increase the risk of falling and sustaining fractures. The study found that urge incontinence increased the risk of falling by 26% and the risk of fracture by 34% but stress incontinence was not significantly associated with falling. Getting up frequently at night to pass urine in a hurry can lead to trips and falls or incontinence can result in the person slipping in a puddle of urine. The fear of falling again or breaking a bone can lead to people curtailing their activities. Stewart et al (1992) identified an association between nocturia and the risk of falling in ambulant patients.

Nocturia is very common in older people and Fonda et al (1999) suggest there are many causes. The primary causes include bladder and sphincter abnormalities such as a small bladder capacity associated with ageing, low bladder compliance, detrusor instability and retention of urine with overflow. Secondary causes include a reduced ability to concentrate the urine and increased urine production at night after reabsorption of peripheral fluid.

Interventions designed to prevent and treat urge incontinence and nocturia should be implemented in an attempt to minimize the risk and prevent falls (Brown et al 2000, Stewart et al 1992). Environmental factors such as slippery or wet floors, poor lighting and clutter contribute to the risk of falling with many falls occurring in bathrooms (Rubenstein & Josephson 1993). Interestingly Sattin et al (1998) found one common associated hazard – throw rugs – was not linked with falling except in adults over 85. Their explanation for this was that people with throw rugs are aware of the hazards and are particularly careful.

There is more likelihood of a person being admitted to a nursing home with incontinence and following falls (Thom et al 1997, Tinetti & Williams 1997). Various preventative strategies could be used to reduce the number of falls and likelihood of nursing home admission such as modification to drug regimens. These include the use of commodes, rehabilitative interventions including strength and balance training and behavioural interventions designed to increase cerebral blood flow such as increased sitting and standing times (Brown et al 2000, Tinetti & Williams 1997, Wolf et al 2000). To facilitate these behavioural interventions, thorough assessment is essential to determine baseline ability and identify other problems such as anxiety about falling, neck stiffness or dizziness with neck movement in order to plan strategies to increase ability. Attention must be paid to posture, breathing and building up muscle strength which can often be done quite quickly. Strategies are taught to minimize problems such as dizziness by rising from lying to sitting or sitting to standing slowly and in stages. Standing still is discouraged and whilst standing movement should be maintained, such as rocking on heels or contraction and relaxation of calf muscles.

Urinary tract infection

Urinary tract infection (UTI) may be due to a variety of factors; it is not necessarily a consequence of incontinence but is often associated with continence problems and is a common problem in the older population. Old age is associated with a loss in immune competence and asymptomatic bacteriuria is more common in the elderly. In people aged 65–70, 20% of women and 3% of men, rising to 20–50% of women and 20% of men aged over 80 have bacteriuria (Malone-Lee 2000).

Although advancing age is a risk factor for both sexes, older women, as can be seen from the above percentages, are particularly at risk. The female anatomy is a significant factor. In combination with mobility or dexterity problems, a simple operation such as a woman cleaning herself after a bowel action may be a contributory factor. The majority of UTIs are due to normal bowel flora, with *Escherichia coli* being responsible for up to 80% (Stockert 1999), so if a woman wipes herself from back to front, the organisms will be swept towards the urethral orifice. Other organisms implicated in causing UTI are *Proteus mirabilis*, Klebsiella species, Pseudomonas, Enterococcus and Staphylococcus species (McCue 2000, Stockert 1999).

Raz et al (2000) compared 149 postmenopausal women with recurrent UTI with a control group of 53 age-matched women without a history of UTI and found 41% of the women with UTI were incontinent as opposed to 9% in the control group. In the study group 19% were found to have a cystocele and 28% were found to have postvoiding residual urine but in the control group none of the women had a cystocele and only 2% showed residual urine postvoid.

In postmenopausal women, the incidence of infection is possibly due to the reduction of oestrogen and the changes in the normal flora within the urethra (Raz et al 2000). In older women who are living in residential or nursing homes, catheterization, incontinence, antimicrobial exposure and poor functional status increase the risk of recurrent UTI (Stamm & Raz 1999).

UTI may be due to stasis of urine when there is residual urine caused by outflow obstruction or hypotonic bladder and as a result of trauma or the presence of fistulas (Stockert 1999).

In older people living in nursing homes, UTI occurs in up to 50% of residents but asymptomatic bacteriuria should not be treated with antimicrobial therapy as this can precipitate reinfection with resistant organisms (McCue 2000, Nicolle 1999). In older people in long-term care settings, complicated UTI is common and treatment differs from that for simple UTI in younger adults as initial treatments may not be effective. In complicated UTI other factors are present such as prolonged indwelling catheterization, urologic anatomic or functional abnormalities, immunosuppression, renal disease or diabetes.

Accurate assessment is essential as symptoms may be misleading, urinalysis can be undermined by the difficulty of obtaining uncontaminated specimens and treatments usually need to be long term (McCue 2000).

Rosser et al (1999) found that urosepsis was more likely to occur in patients over 60 years of age, in those with extended hospital stay and in patients who had been catheterized for a long time. Urinary tract infection is a major complication of urethral catheterization; 80% of all hospital-acquired UTIs are the result of urethral catheterization (Sedor & Mulholland 1999) (see also Chapter 9).

Methicillin-resistant *Staphylococcus aureus* (MRSA) has for several years been a considerable problem in hospitals and other settings such as nursing homes. A recent research project has demonstrated that MRSA readily adheres to silastic rubber surfaces (material used in some catheters) and the resultant biofilm grows rapidly. Neither vancomycin nor rifampicin was able to significantly reduce the biofilm thickness over 24 hours (Jones et al 2001).

Catheters should only be used when all other options have been explored. The research reported by Jones et al (2001) demonstrates how unacceptable catheterization is, especially in the older adult, unless all alternative options have been considered. Catheterization should only be considered after full comprehensive assessment that takes into account the associated risks.

ASSESSMENT

Assessment is the key to the effective treatment and management of incontinence for individuals of any age. The aim of assessment is to identify the underlying cause of which incontinence is a symptom. The process of continence assessment in older people is the same as for younger adults with more emphasis placed on certain aspects. Continence assessment is discussed fully in Chapter 2 (assessment for bowel disorders is discussed in Chapter 7) and only the aspects relevant to older people will be the focus of discussion here.

Continence assessment should have three main aims (Ouslander & Schnelle 1993) of identifying reversible factors, identifying those who need to be referred on for specialist evaluation and to determine management strategies (Table 6.2).

Table 6.2 The three main aims of continence assessment

Aim	Assessment
1	Identify reversible factors that may be causing or contributing to incontinence
2	Identify those individuals who need more specialist diagnostic evaluation such as urological or gynaecological examination and/or urodynamic investigations
3	Develop the most appropriate treatment or management plan

After Ouslander & Schnelle (1993).

The assessment process (Nazarko 1999) consists of:

- obtaining an accurate history
- performing simple investigations
- physical examination
- reaching a diagnosis
- determination of appropriate treatment/management strategies
- ongoing evaluation of treatment/management strategies.

The assessment process is ongoing and, especially in the older adult, all the relevant information may not be obtained at the first attempt. It is obtained gradually to enable a building up of the 'full picture'. A very important consideration that aids decisions about the treatment/management of incontinence is to establish the 'bothersomeness' of the symptoms being experienced by the incontinent person.

It is important to identify and exclude potentially reversible causes of incontinence (transient incontinence). This can be achieved using the mnemonic of DIAPPERS (Box 6.2) or DRIP (Box 6.3).

In older adults with cognitive disorders, an accurate history is difficult to obtain and the assessing professional will have to seek information from relatives and carers. The accuracy of the assessment is only as good as the information obtained and in reality, accurate information is often difficult to obtain even from cognitively intact individuals.

As an essential component of continence assessment, frequency/volume charts or bladder diaries (when intake is recorded as well as output) are robust methods of obtaining accurate information to aid diagnosis (Abrams & Klevmark 1996, Pfister 1999, Saito et al 1993). Some older people may find these extremely difficult to maintain and in these situations, attempts should be made to obtain frequency-only charts that exclude the measurement of urine.

Essential investigations include urinalysis, primarily to exclude urinary tract infection, and estimation of postvoid residual volume as significant degrees of urinary retention can occur without symptoms of outflow obstruction or hypotonicity of the detrusor (Fonda et al 1999, Nazarko 1995a, Ouslander & Schnelle 1995). Residual urine volume can be determined by an 'in out' catheterization, but a portable ultrasound bladder scan is preferable, since it is a non-invasive procedure. Urinalysis may also be the means of diagnosing covert diabetes.

Physical examination should not be restricted to the lower urinary tract but should aim to exclude undiagnosed cardiac conditions such as venous insufficiency or congestive cardiac failure and neurological conditions such as early signs of parkinsonism that might contribute to continence status (Ouslander & Schnelle 1995).

Rectal examination as well as assessing pelvic floor muscle strength should exclude faecal impaction and in men assess the prostate gland. An enlarged prostate, however, does not necessarily correlate with outflow obstruction. Pelvic examination should include assessment of perineal and vulval skin condition and exclude pelvic masses and prolapse. There should also be evaluation of the condition of the vaginal epithelium for inflammatory changes suggestive of atrophic vaginitis (Getliffe 1996a, Ouslander & Schnelle 1995). Before performing any invasive examination such as rectal or pelvic examination, it is essential to obtain consent from the patient. Performing such an examination on a frail elderly person who is unable to give real consent could be interpreted by relatives as abuse. Guidance should be sought and can be found in the literature (McKee 1999, Wallace 2000, Willis 2000) and from professional organizations. The Royal College of Nursing has published guidance for nurses in the UK on digital rectal examination and manual evacuation of faeces (RCN 2000a).

Functional assessment

Functional assessment is an essential component of continence assessment in the older person. The aim of functional assessment is to determine the type and amount of help or intervention required to resolve problems such as how to get to the bathroom, manipulate clothing and transfer to the toilet. The main goals of functional assessment in older people is to identify the problems, develop solutions, implement the solutions and evaluate progress. Although incontinence due to physiological factors (e.g. detrusor instability) is not specifically due to functional problems, functional deficit can have an impact on continence status (Williams & Gaylord 1990).

Functional assessment in continence includes assessment of both physical and cognitive function with consideration given to environmental and social factors. According to Williams & Gaylord (1990) functional assessment should include:

- *transfer ability* – from bed to chair, standing to sitting, i.e. onto a toilet, with or without help
- *mobility* – walking with or without aid or use of adjacent furniture
- *balance* – standing without help and ability to manipulate garments
- *arm strength and body flexibility* – ability to raise the toilet seat
- *manual dexterity* – ability to manipulate clothing, including buttons and zips
- *eyesight* – adequate vision to reach the toilet unaided
- *toileting ability* – able to wipe self or manage continence aids if used.

Cognitive function assessment

As has been discussed earlier in the chapter, poor mental function is associated with incontinence and greater numbers of incontinent to continent people demonstrate depressive symptoms. Cognitive assessment must establish if the person can interpret body signals of the need to void, if they can understand and obey instructions or attract assistance, and if they are motivated to overcome their continence problems.

Social function considerations

Social factors can have significant impact on continence status and the assessment should establish if the person lives alone or if there is someone available who is able to help. Other factors include relationship dynamics and the extent to which incontinence has reduced the person's social activity and involvement.

Environmental considerations

Environmental considerations can have a tremendous impact on continence status and assessment must establish problems being encountered due to unsuitable environmental factors such as:

- *bed* – height or furniture making access difficult
- *chairs* – height or ease of getting out of the chair
- *toilet access* – distance, ground floor or stairs to be negotiated, stairlift in place, height of toilet seat, wheelchair access, door to toilet or bathroom heavy and/or awkward
- *bedside commode* – availability, ease of use
- *lighting* – adequate, easy to turn on/off
- *supports* – rails and grab bars in suitable positions
- *clothing* – ease of adjustment and replacement, appropriate footwear to aid mobility and self-confidence.

Box 6.6 summarizes the psychological, environmental and social factors that may influence continence in older people, at home or in care facilities.

There are various tools advocated for functional assessment including the Barthel index and the Katz activities of daily living (ADL) scale that will give an overview of dependency status (Parker 1998, Williams & Gaylord 1990). Lewis (1999) has reported the General Health Questionnaire (GHQ) to be a useful tool to assess the psychological well-being of incontinent people. This questionnaire can be self-administered in suitable patients and consists of 60 questions to identify

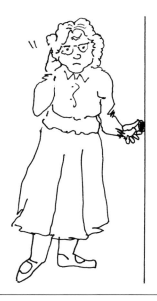 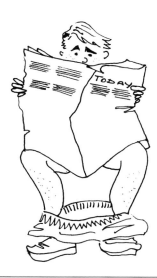

Box 6.6 Psychological, environmental and social factors that may influence continence in older people, at home or in care facilities

Unhelpful	Helpful
TOILETS	
Too far away	Close to bedrooms and living areas
Too few	Enough for 'peak demand' times
Too narrow for a wheelchair	Easy wheelchair access
Difficult to use	Raised toilet seat and rails available
Difficult to identify	Good signposting
Unpleasant to use – cold, smelly, dirty,	Easy to identify, e.g. doors colour coded
with lack of soft toilet paper	Warm and clean with spare toilet rolls in view
CLOTHING	
Difficult to adjust	Elasticated tracksuit bottoms
	Use of Velcro in place of zips and buttons
Unattractive and undignified clothing (e.g. no pants,	Attractive but practical
or dress open up the back) can reduce motivation	Special adaptations and gadgets may be
to be continent	available to help physically disabled people
CARERS AND OTHER PEOPLE	
Being rushed (e.g. by carers)	Sufficient time to make a leisurely and relaxed visit to the toilet
Lack of privacy (e.g. commode in a shared bedroom, door of toilet left open)	Neither overlooked, nor overheard
Lack of security (e.g. fear of being forgotten and left in the toilet)	Convenient means of summoning help
Carer's attitude is either: very critical of incontinence	Carer's attitude is one of support and encouragement to achieve continence
or continually gives permission for incontinence (e.g. 'it doesn't matter, we will clean it up')	
PATIENT PSYCHOLOGICAL PROBLEMS	
Depression amongst elderly people is not always recognized, but can be a major factor in impaired self-care. Alternatively, continence problems can cause anxiety and feelings of shame, making the individual feel that the problem is untreatable and therefore exacerbating feelings of low self-esteem.	

1.	**Physical function**					
1.1	Transfers	Independent	Independent with difficulty	Needs help		
		Needs help of two people	Usually stays in bed	Comments		
1.2	Mobility	Independent	Independent but slow	Mobile with aids		
		Mobile with 1 or 2 helpers	Stays in bed or chair	Comments		
1.3	Dressing	Independent	Independent but slow	Clothing adaptations		
		Needs help	Needs to be dressed	Comments		
1.4	Vision (with aids)	No problems	Able to read large print only	Partial vision		
		Registered blind	Needs helps	Comments		
1.5	Hearing (with aids)	No problems	Misses some conversation	Hears loud sounds only		
		Deaf (or almost), lip reads	Deaf, relies on others	Comments		
2.	**Cognitive function**					
2.1	Expression	Clear intelligent speech	Indistinct speech	Muddled speech		
		Makes gestures/signs only	Little or on communication	Comments		
2.2	Decision making	Can make own plans	Needs occasional prompting	Needs constant reminders		
		Frequently fails to respond	Unable to initiate any activity	Comments		
2.3	Comprehension	Mostly understands	Understands simple phrases	Understands signs only		
		Understands with help	No comprehension	Comments		
2.4	Orientation	Orientated to time and place	Occasional confusion	Uncertain about time and place		
		Wanders, needs supervision	Unaware of people and places	Comments		
2.5	Mood	Reasonably content and happy	Occasional anxiety/irritation	Anxious/depressed		
		Needs professional support	Often hysterical or suicidal	Comments		

3.	**Social function**				
3.1	General access	....	Indoors and outdoors	....	Indoors only	Downstairs only
		....	Upstairs only	....	One/two rooms only	Comments ....
3.2	Social activity	....	Active social life	....	Social activity reduced	Limited social life
		....	Social activity is rare	....	No social activities	Comments ....
3.3	Relationships	....	Relates well with others	....	Prefers own company	Lacks confidence, reserved
		....	Avoids social contact	....	Withdrawn or disruptive	Comments ....
3.4	Relatives/friends	....	Lives with family	....	Lives with spouse/partner	Lives alone, friends suppot
		....	Lives in sheltered housing	....	Lives in residential care	Comments ....
3.5	Food preparation	....	Independent	....	Independent with difficulty	Prepares food/drink with help
		....	Food/drink provided at home	....	Outside food provided	Comments ....
3.6	Shopping	....	Competent	....	Limited	By telephone (Internet)
		....	Needs help	....	Unable to manage	Comments ....
4.	**Environmental considerations**				
4.1	Access at home	....	Easy access	....	Access slow – stairs/furniture	Furniture impedes access
		....	Adapatations required	....	Access not appropriate	Comments ....
4.2	Bed access	....	No problems	....	Bed too high	Bed too low
		....	Furniture reduces access	....	Unable to access bed	Comments ....
4.3	Seating	....	No problems	....	Difficulty standing from chair	Independent with aids
		....	Needs help	....	Unable to transfer from chair	Comments ....

FURTHER COMMENTS _____

_____

_____

_____

_____

Figure 6.2 Functional assessment tool.

possible psychological disturbance. Positive answers to 12 or more indicates disturbance.

A comprehensive continence assessment should include all the elements of the functional assessment as discussed above as well as identifying lower urinary tract dysfunction. Figure 6.2 is an example of a functional assessment tool designed to include the components according to Williams & Gaylord (1990).

TREATMENT AND MANAGEMENT STRATEGIES

Ouslander & Schnelle (1993) make a distinction between 'treatment' and 'management' of incontinence. They describe the goals of treatment as being patient oriented and intended to change the functioning of the lower urinary tract. Treatment includes pelvic floor exercises, bladder retraining, drug therapy, biofeedback, electrical stimulation and surgery. Management strategies, however, are carer oriented and include approaches that will improve or even reverse incontinence but do not change urinary tract function (e.g. the implementation of toileting regimes and toileting assistance). Healthy older people with continence problems should respond to treatment strategies.

In one study of 128 adults over the age of 65 years, Silverman et al (1997) found that there was no evidence of treatment in 25 out of 55 patients with urinary incontinence, especially when cognitive impairment and depression were also present. The reasons given for no treatment interventions for incontinence were lack of motivation or acceptance, functional capacity limitations and lack of caregiver or caregiver support. However, it was significant that clinicians in this study did not perceive incontinence to be associated with substantial burden or risk and potential strategies for treatments were not familiar to most. The study identified the need for clinicians to be educated in the strategies appropriate for treating incontinence in the older adult.

Fonda (1990) classified nursing home patients according to their toileting capacity. This assists in the realistic planning of treatment or management and defines realistic outcomes (see Fig. 6.4). This classification of stages and levels of incontinence is a useful tool to assist with the planning of treatment or management for older people with urinary symptoms both in the community and in residential care. Independent continence is defined as not being wet and able to void independently without being reminded or assisted in any way during both day and night. Any person requiring a catheter or sheath system and any person not meeting the criteria of independent continence for a month is regarded as incontinent. Dependent continence is when continence is maintained in individuals with mental or physical disabilities when assistance is given to prevent incontinent episodes. When people are incontinent and the problem is well contained by the use of aids or appliances, social continence is achieved and personal dignity and carer morale should improve.

The treatment or management strategies used to promote or maintain continence in the older person are essentially the same as for younger people but treatment regimes may take longer to show significant results and a greater degree of support may be required to ensure compliance and sustain motivation.

Specific treatment and management methods are described in detail in other chapters in the book so only issues relating to the older person will be discussed here. The algorithm in Figure 6.3 shows the most usual methods used in the treatment or management of incontinence in the older adult.

Fluids

Older people with continence problems will often, as a coping mechanism, restrict their fluid intake hoping they will produce less urine. Although the reduction in fluid intake will reduce the amount of urine produced, the urine is highly concentrated and will irritate the bladder causing frequency and urgency. Reduced fluid intake can increase the risk of recurrent urinary tract infection and the incidence of constipation. Dehydration can lead to electrolyte imbalance and confusion (Anders 2000). Relatively minor fluid deprivation can, especially in the older adult, have serious consequences (Morrison 2000) but it

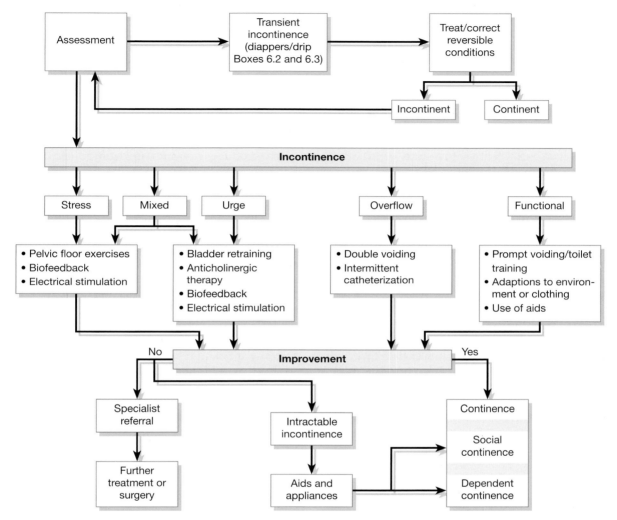

Figure 6.3 Management of incontinence in the older adult.

can be very difficult convincing older people of the need to drink more and for them to fully understand the benefits. Skin integrity is dependent on adequate hydration and it decreases susceptibility to pneumonia and urinary tract infection. Early diagnosis of dehydration is problematic in older adults due to many physical signs being less obvious in older people, possibly being overlooked as part of the 'ageing process' (Holben et al 1999).

Ageing has the effect of a decrease in total body water and older people are, as a consequence, at increased risk from dehydration (Fantl et al 1996).

A study in Aberdeen of 43 elderly people (of whom 24 lived in their own homes and 19 in institutional care) found that all the subjects were hypohydrated (Primrose 1999). This study showed that the people who were more frail and dependent had lower daily water turnover despite their total body water being similar to the healthy subjects.

A daily intake of 1.5 litres (eight cups or six mugs) of fluid a day is recommended to prevent dehydration (Fantl et al 1996, Madden 2000, Morrison 2000, Nazarko 2000a). However, there is limited evidence to suggest that encouraging a fluid intake above the level that is comfortable for an individual is beneficial (Lindeman et al 2000). Most of the 883 participants in their study, who had a mean age of 74 years, drank six or more glasses of fluid a day (71%) but for those that drank less, no adverse effects were found. Edwards (2001) suggests that the daily fluid intake of the average adult, taking into account food as well as fluid consumed and from oxidation of food during metabolism, is 2–2.5 litres. In a study of 121 adults aged 65–99 years old, living in a long-term care facility, symptoms of dehydration – see Box 6.7 – were noted in relation to documented fluid intake over 3 days. All meals and other foods as well as fluid given with medication were recorded. The findings showed that a minimum recommendation of 1500 ml of fluid per day was adequate to prevent symptoms of dehydration in older people who were not acutely ill (Holben 1999).

It has been suggested that thirst is reduced in older people (Bush 2000, Holben et al 1999, Nazarko 2000a) but the thirst mechanism is not a reliable indicator of dehydration as it is stimulated by increased blood sodium concentration. When there is sodium loss caused by sweating due to pyrexia or a hot environment, dehydration can occur without sensations of thirst (Madden 2000).

To ensure fluid intake is adequate, the best advice people can be given is to increase their intake of water. Many patients who are not drinking sufficient fluids are also consuming substantial quantities of drinks that can adversely affect the bladder such as coffee, carbonated drinks, citrus juices or alcohol. These fluids have diuretic properties and irritant effects on the bladder.

The most common sources of caffeine are to be found in the drinks most commonly consumed in our society such as coffee, tea and cola. Caffeinated products contain three compounds – caffeine, theophylline and theobromine – all part of the group of chemicals called methylxanthines. Methylxanthines are diuretics but caffeine is also a bladder irritant. Caffeine is found in coffee and cola, theophylline in tea and theobromine is in chocolate. Caffeine is also present in chocolate, over-the-counter medications, as a flavour enhancer in baked goods and in many processed foods (McKim & McKim 1993, Newman 1999). If caffeine consumption is abruptly stopped, withdrawal symptoms such as headache, fatigue and drowsiness may be experienced. This will persist for only a few days but reducing consumption gradually may be more acceptable. Decaffeinated substitutes are available but the methods used to remove caffeine involving the use of chemicals are associated with other health risks. It is preferable to select products where the caffeine has been extracted naturally with water or carbon dioxide (Addison 2000). To achieve compliance with advice it is not politic to demand that the patient eliminates the caffeine-containing drinks entirely but instead to suggest reducing consumption to acceptable levels. However, although tea contains caffeine in varying quantities, dependent on the plant variety, tea contains flavonoids that studies have shown can reduce blood pressure and cholesterol (Madden 2000). Although drinking coffee has been linked to cardiovascular disease, a recent study found that moderate coffee intake was not harmful to heart health (Kleemola et al 2000).

Other drinks such as alcohol, carbonated drinks and citrus juices have been found to cause urinary symptoms (Newman 1999) and should be consumed in moderate quantities. Alcohol has diuretic properties but drinks such as beer and lager quickly fill up the bladder causing

---

Box 6.7 Symptoms of dehydration requiring nursing or medical intervention (after Zembrzuski 1997)

- Dry, warm skin
- Dry mucous membranes
- Furrowed tongue
- Thirst (not a reliable indicator especially in older people)
- Reduced urinary output and concentrated urine
- Constipation
- Increasing lethargy and muscular weakness
- Reduction in skin elasticity and diminished skin turgor (bulk)
- Fever
- Daily weight loss
- Change in baseline mental function, increased confusional state (more than usual)
- Sunken eyes (severe dehydration)
- Tachycardia (severe dehydration)
- Hypotension (severe dehydration)

frequency. Carbonated drinks contain carbon dioxide, differing quantities of artificial sweeteners, flavourings, preservatives, colourings and some also contain caffeine. There is still considerable debate about the safety or otherwise of 'E numbers' and drinks (especially fruit juices) without additives are preferable (Madden 2000).

Cranberry juice has been found to be useful in the prevention of *E. coli* infections of the urinary tract by interfering with the bacterium's ability to adhere to the bladder mucosa (Avorn et al 1994, Howell et al 1998, Kuzminski 1996, Lavender 2000, Nazarko 1995b) although some scepticism about its effectiveness exists (Harkins 2000). Despite the many unanswered questions about the therapeutic use of cranberry juice, it offers a potential prophylactic which, if tolerated well, is preferable to antibiotic therapy with the inherent risks of resistance and side-effects. Cranberry juice has a distinctive taste which is not acceptable to all but it has no known side-effects in normal quantities (300–400 ml/day) and is a natural substance (Nazarko 1995b). Therefore, for older adults it is a potentially beneficial substance to reduce the risk of urinary tract infection and help in maintaining an adequate fluid intake.

In recent years the availability and number of herbal and fruit teas and infusions has increased significantly. In most cases the teas and infusions are harmless, caffeine free and useful substitutes for the less suitable drinks already mentioned. Although the substances these infusions contain are natural, care must be taken with some of the herbal teas as large quantities could be harmful (Madden 2000).

Rooibosch or red bush tea, an infusion made from a herb grown in South Africa, tastes similar to tea, is caffeine free, contains natural fluoride and can be substituted for tea. It can be drunk with milk if preferred, unlike most herbal or fruit teas. Fruit juices, preferably not citrus, may be enjoyed by an older person and can increase daily fruit and vegetable consumption as well as increasing fluid intake. Fruit juices may also help prevent constipation, with prune juice, in particular, having a laxative effect, probably because it contains magnesium salts (Newman 1999). Zembrzuski (1997) suggests experimenting with fruit juice combinations and cocktails to increase enjoyment of the flavours.

A survey of patients in hospital found that many older people were unable to drink adequately due to an inability to reach their drinks or that their cups were empty (Spencer et al 2000). Nazarko (2000a) and Zembrzuski (1997) suggest that when drinks are made attractive to the older person they will enjoy them and their fluid intake will increase. Alcoholic drinks such as weak spirit drinks, shandy or weak beer will not do any harm if consumed in moderation, will be enjoyable for the older person, increase their feelings of 'normality' especially when living in institutionalized environments as well as increasing their fluid intake.

The evidence that low fluid intake is implicated in the incidence of constipation is mixed, with some studies suggesting that increasing fluids does not necessarily increase stool output (Campbell et al 1993, Chung et al 1999). However, it does play an essential part in the prevention of simple constipation (Bush 2000, Madden 2000). A small study evaluated the effect of increasing fibre and fluid on bowel action and found that using natural means reduced the need for laxatives and faecal softeners (Rodrigues-Fisher et al 1993).

Older people may wish to restrict fluid at certain times of the day to enable them to maintain their social activities or to prevent excessive nocturia. This is acceptable providing they compensate at other times of the day to ensure their intake is at least 1.5 litres. If swallowing is difficult following stroke, more viscous or thickened fluids may be easier to manage than thin liquids (Nazarko 2000a). Cups or glasses may be too heavy for a frail older person to manage when full of liquid; filled only half full and kept topped up will encourage drinking. Plastic cups or glasses may be used to reduce weight, but unfortunately these often have an unpleasant taste that may discourage an individual from drinking sufficient fluid.

Ensuring an older person with incontinence has an adequate fluid intake of suitable quality should improve their continence status and may even cure their incontinence.

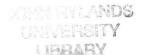

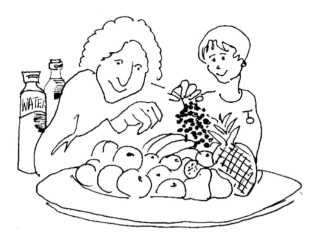

Diet

The fibre content of the diet has a significance for bowel function and many older people find it difficult to consume the recommended daily five portions of fruit and vegetables. However, certain foods may be implicated in bowel disorders such as diarrhoea and incontinence but this varies between different people. Certain foods may be found to cause symptoms in one person but not be a problem for another. It is worth keeping a food diary to identify any foods that may cause problems and to experiment with different foods and combinations whilst recording food intake (Norton & Kamm 1999).

Food intolerance has been implicated as being responsible for a wide spectrum of chronic illnesses such as irritable bowel syndrome amongst others but it is not regarded as a sound diagnosis by many doctors (Brostoff & Gamlin 1998, Graham & Varey 1999). Despite the recent trend for additive-free, so-called 'natural' foods, the greatest problems of intolerance come from naturally occurring foods and food ingredients (David 2000).

Foods most likely to contribute to looser stools are those foods high in fibre, spicy foods, dairy foods, chocolate and artificial sweeteners but certain foods such as arrowroot biscuits, marshmallows and ripe bananas are likely to make the stools more firm. Foods high in fat will reduce the food transit time (Norton & Kamm 1999).

It is possible that some foods may be implicated in causing urinary urgency and urge incontinence, such as citrus fruits and juices, tomatoes, highly spiced foods and artificial sweeteners (Newman 1999), but there is little information to substantiate this theory.

There is no doubt that nutritional status has an impact on physical health, psychological functioning and social well-being. Age-related changes that can affect nutritional status include sensory changes in taste, smell and vision, which may make food seem bland and tasteless. A reduction in the production of saliva and loss of natural teeth or wearing ill-fitting dentures can make chewing and swallowing more difficult. Depression may cause anorexia, and dementia can affect all aspects of nutrition from the ability to prepare food to its consumption and commonly, changes in food preferences (Clay 2001, Griep et al 2000, Harvey 2000).

The prevalence of malnutrition in older people living in the community is between 5 and 10% but in older people in residential care it is estimated to be between 30 and 60% (Griep et al 2000). Older people are prone to develop undetected malnutrition especially during illness and it is important to ensure that the diet is varied and contains all the necessary nutrients for health. Food can be made attractive to the older person in different ways and texture and flavour are important factors to be considered. For example, the person recovering from a stroke may require a soft diet but may prefer more flavour than the usual bland soft diets often provided in hospital or nursing homes. Interesting dishes in which the food is arranged attractively will make the meal more palatable. Help may be required with feeding or the provision of special utensils will aid independence. Ensuring the older person receives a well-balanced diet and adequate fluid intake will improve general health status and preserve skin integrity.

Behavioural interventions

Behavioural therapy is based on the theory of operant learning and the assumption that incontinent people have learned maladaptive voiding patterns or 'bad habits' (Newman 1999). Operant conditioning or learning is dependent on the individual and is essentially voluntary (Gross 1996). Continence is learned during childhood by toilet training, a behavioural modification process. The goal of behavioural treatments is for the person to relearn or regain continence learned in childhood (Newman 1999).

Pelvic floor exercises, biofeedback and electromuscular stimulation are described in Chapter 3 and bladder retraining in Chapters 3 and 11. These treatments are suitable for people of any age providing they are prepared to follow advice and are motivated to improve their continence status.

As behavioural interventions such as pelvic floor exercises, biofeedback and bladder retraining require active participation, comprehensive assessment that includes evaluation of cognitive ability and motivation is essential to determine if a particular treatment is appropriate. A knowledgeable and willing carer can help to ensure success (Fonda et al 1999). Although electromuscular stimulation is a passive exercise of the pelvic floor muscles it should only be used when the individual understands the procedure and is able to report comfort parameters during treatment (Fonda et al 1999, Laycock 1992). It is also necessary for the individual to 'join in' with the electrically induced contraction and learn to exercise the pelvic floor muscles (Laycock 1994). To maintain the improvement gained, motivation

and ability are required. Informed consent for biofeedback and electromuscular stimulation is essential and may preclude its use in cognitively impaired individuals (Fonda et al 1999).

Care must be taken when treating older women with biofeedback or electromuscular stimulation using vaginal probes as, especially with women who are not sexually active, they may complain of discomfort on insertion of the probes due to vaginal dryness. This can be sufficiently severe to preclude treatment but a course of topical oestrogen may render the treatment acceptable.

Pelvic floor exercises have been shown to be effective in improving continence status in stress and urge incontinence and following radical prostatectomy (Bo et al 1999, Boyington & Dougherty 2000, Burgio et al 1998, Burns et al 1990, Van Kampen et al 2000, Wyman et al 1998). Biofeedback enables individuals to identify their pelvic floor muscles, thus ensuring correct contraction during exercise. It also provides a record of progress during the initial treatment period. Burns et al (1990) found biofeedback significantly improved treatment outcomes in their study of 135 women with a mean age of 62 years. A formula using pretreatment and posttreatment incontinence was devised to calculate the percentage of improvement and although both exercise only and biofeedback groups showed similar self-reported improvement, electromyography (EMG) readings showed significantly increased EMG scores in the biofeedback group over the exercise only and control groups.

A more recent study examined outcomes in 104 women between the ages of 35 and 75, half of whom (52) had genuine stress incontinence with half of these having previously undergone gynaecological surgery. This group of women was compared with 52 women who had no urinary or prolapse symptoms and only 15% had had gynaecological surgery. The subjects underwent a 12 week programme of pelvic floor exercises and an increase in muscle strength as indicated by a validated intravaginal balloon device was found in both groups. The pelvic floor muscles were assessed for strength, endurance and contractility. There were no significant differences between each group but there was a tendency for the women without stress incontinence to demonstrate greater increase in pelvic floor muscle strength (Boyington & Dougherty 2000).

In their study comparing the treatment outcomes for behavioural treatment versus drug treatment, Burgio et al (1998) demonstrated that behavioural treatment which consisted of pelvic floor exercises and bladder retraining strategies was more effective in women with urge incontinence, than drug treatment. The study group consisted of 197 women between the ages of 55 and 92 years who were randomized into three groups to receive either behavioural therapy or drug treatment, the third group being the control who were given a placebo. Following treatment, the frequency of incontinence was lowest in the behavioural group, the highest being in the control group. The attrition rate was highest in the control group being only slightly lower in the drug treatment group. This rate of attrition in the drug group may be explained by the fact that oxybutynin was used in the study and compliance has been found to be a problem due to unpleasant side-effects. In a follow-up study, Burgio et al (2001) demonstrated that positive changes in psychological symptoms did not necessarily relate to changes in continence status and although a correlation was found between the improvement gained with behavioural or drug therapy there was improvement in all study participants. These findings suggest that reduction in distress was due to the interventions and support given by the healthcare professionals and that the expectations of benefit, encouragement and support given were the catalyst to positive outcomes and reduced distress.

Pelvic floor exercise can also be of value in men when incontinence occurs after prostatectomy. In a study of 102 men with a mean age of 65 years who had undergone radical retropubic prostatectomy, 50 men were allocated to a pelvic floor re-education programme. The remaining 52 were allocated to a placebo programme where they were given information about their incontinence and electromuscular stimulation to abdomen and thighs (that could not affect the pelvic floor muscles). Incontinence was rated using pad weight testing and only 10% of men in the treatment group were incontinent at 3 months and 4% at 1 year postoperatively in comparison to 44% and 17% in the placebo group (Van Kampen et al 2000).

Bladder retraining techniques can be effective in the treatment of urgency and urge incontinence (Abrams 1995, Anders 2000, McCreanor 1998, Sander 1998) but Kelleher et al (1997) found the medium-term improvement rate of behavioural and drug therapy disappointing at 54%, with a cure rate of only 5.5%. Interpretation of published studies can often be quite difficult since subjects may include different diagnoses (e.g. detrusor instability or low compliance bladder) and the treatments may be a combination of behavioural approaches and drug therapy. Where drug side-effects are not well tolerated compliance is likely to be poor and drop-out rates high. For example, in Kelleher et al's study 348 women with a diagnosis of detrusor instability ($n = 262$) or low compliance bladder ($n = 86$) were contacted by post 6–12 months after urodynamic investigations. Only 14 women were completely cured and 123 were significantly improved. A majority of the women had been prescribed oxybutynin but non-compliance was high with 82% discontinuing treatment mainly due to side-effects. Of 12 women who were instructed in bladder retraining, only eight were improved and four either the same or worse. The authors commented on these results being better than those from drug therapy and may have been the result of no side-effects or that the symptoms may have been less severe at the outset.

Swami & Abrams (1996) observe that individuals with sensory urgency (when lower urinary tract pathology is implicated, such as stones or infection) maintain improvement at better rates than individuals with motor urgency (neuropathic origin and possibly associated with bladder outlet obstruction). In reviewing the literature they found that initial improvement rates reported were in the region of 85% subjective and 50% objective but that many patients will relapse after initial improvement and after 6 months an improvement rate of 88% fell to 38%. An explanation for this may be the presence of comorbidity such as dementia or mobility problems.

Another issue of extreme importance, not always reported in the literature, is the long-term maintenance of improvement. In one study, 204 women with a mean age of 61 years were assigned to one of three groups and instructed in pelvic floor exercises with biofeedback, bladder retraining or both. The results showed the combination group initially had better results but that after 3 months there was no difference between the three groups. The authors suggest that the specific treatment modality may not be as important as having a structured intervention programme with education and patient support (Wyman et al 1998).

Burgio et al (2000) found that combining behavioural and drug therapy was of greater benefit than either treatment alone and in the study eight subjects crossed from behavioural treatment alone and 27 crossed from drug therapy alone to a combination of therapies. Both of these groups showed significant improvement and with the

---

Case study 6.1

Dorothy Sheffield, a 72-year-old grandmother of six, living in sheltered housing accommodation had had continence problems for the past 40 years since the birth of her last child. Her incontinence was relatively mild but in recent years had become more of a problem and she was buying large sanitary towels to wear, especially when she went out.

Mrs Sheffield saw a poster for the Continence Service in her local chemist's window and eventually plucked up the courage to telephone and ask for advice. An appointment was made for her at the local Continence Clinic. Initial assessment by the continence advisor identified mixed stress and urge incontinence. Dorothy said the most distressing part of her problem was the urgency and everyday events such as shopping had to be planned around available 'respectable' toilets. Outings that took her to unfamiliar territory caused such anxiety that it was easier not to go and this was making her feel 'rather low'.

The continence advisor assured Dorothy that there were several things she could do that would alleviate her symptoms. Dorothy's fluid intake was discussed with an explanation that by reducing her intake (which she had restricted to about 700–800 ml/day) she was possibly making the problems worse. She was advised about the effects of high caffeine drinks and encouraged to drink less tea and coffee and to try to drink more water. Targets were set to increase her daily intake slowly by just adding one extra cup or glass of drink a day until she felt she could add another one.

Dorothy was also taught how to strengthen the muscles of her pelvic floor and how to repress the urge to void when she experienced an urgent need to empty her bladder. She was instructed to sit down if possible and contract the pelvic floor muscles. Pressure on the perineum helps to repress the urge to void and it was explained that this was starting to retrain the bladder to hold more urine and empty less often. Dorothy had completed a frequency volume chart for a week before attending the clinic which showed that her bladder was capable of holding at least 300 ml of urine. This was the volume usually voided first thing in the morning but most of the remainder of the day she passed only 100–150 ml at a time and sometimes it was as low as 50 ml. As a consequence, she was constantly visiting the toilet, sometimes as much as 15 times a day. The advisor wrote the instructions down for her to take home to remind her and another appointment was made for her for 1 month later. A tick chart where she could record the times of voiding without also having to measure the urine was provided for completion before her next appointment to check on her progress.

At her second appointment Dorothy appeared much more cheerful. She felt much better after being able to discuss her problem and wasn't using the toilet quite so often. She was generally passing larger amounts although they were still small quantities at times.

The continence advisor checked that she was exercising her pelvic muscles correctly and instructed Dorothy to continue with these. She now suggested Dorothy started a bladder training programme. The times when Dorothy was to use the toilet were negotiated and identified as the times she would most likely need to empty her bladder. It is important to set realistic goals and the length of time between voids were no longer than she could achieve. The frequency volume and tick charts were valuable sources of information in setting Dorothy's goals. The continence advisor had not introduced a full bladder training programme on Dorothy's first appointment as she did not want to overload her with too much information.

Dorothy's condition had improved only slightly at her third appointment 1 month later and the continence advisor suggested that an anticholinergic agent to suppress her bladder irritability be included in her treatment. At the next clinic appointment Dorothy reported a great improvement and after 6 months' treatment, she was able to be discharged and felt she was now fully in control. Dorothy had reduced the number of times she was visiting the toilet to six or seven times a day and only once at night. She is now planning a trip to stay with her daughter who lives in New Zealand but prior to her treatment she had always been very nervous of travelling even relatively short distances!

This case study illustrates the difference relatively simple intervention strategies can make to improve the quality of life for a person with troublesome continence problems.

eight who added drug therapy to behavioural therapy the improvement rose from a mean 58% reduction in incontinence to 89%, and in the drug therapy group who added behavioural strategies the reduction in incontinence improved from 73% to 84%.

Abrams (1995) has recommended the use of bladder training techniques for the treatment of lower urinary tract symptoms in older men and endorses the continuance of conservative treatment for 3–6 months. He suggests that more active treatment can be implemented if improvement is poor or if symptoms deteriorate.

In older adults with cognitive impairment, the behavioural interventions already discussed will not be appropriate and toileting regimes or prompted voiding programmes are more suitable. When these are administered by motivated carers they can be very successful (Burgio et al 1994b, Chester 1998, Colling et al 1992, Ouslander & Schnelle 1995, Ouslander et al 1996, Schnelle 1990). For example, in a study of 165 nursing home residents with a mean age of 85 years (76% female) a 9–10 week prompted voiding programme was evaluated (Ouslander et al 1996). Of the subjects, 55% needed help with mobility and transfers. The main method of data collection in this study was physical checks for wetness. The checks were every hour during the daytime (08.00–18.00 h) with a total of 11 checks whenever possible. The researchers did not interrupt activities or meals and checks were not possible when subjects were away from the nursing home. Baseline data were collected over 3 days and the rate of incontinence was 34%. After 1 week of prompted voiding, 77 subjects showed an improvement, having an average of one or fewer episodes of urinary incontinence per day. After the 9–10 weeks of prompted voiding those who had responded well in respect of their urinary incontinence also showed less incontinence of stool.

Behavioural treatments can be effective for constipation and faecal incontinence. Muscle tone can be improved with pelvic floor exercises, biofeedback and electrotherapy to treat faecal incontinence (Getliffe 1996b, Kamm 1998, Norton 1996c) and biofeedback is now an established treatment for idiopathic constipation when laxatives,

increased dietary fibre and surgery have been found to be of limited value (Storrie 1997).

Successfully treating constipation and faecal impaction in older people will decrease the incidence of faecal incontinence but this can be difficult and Chassagne et al (2000) recommend a combination of laxative use and behavioural interventions.

Pharmacological treatment

Drug treatment that has been used successfully for treatment in younger adults is likely to prove effective for healthy older adults but care is necessary for the reasons already discussed earlier in this chapter. However, the use of pharmacological agents in frail older people is more likely to cause or contribute to incontinence rather than alleviate the problem (Fonda et al 1999).

For the pharmacological management of incontinence please refer to Chapter 8 where this is discussed in detail. This chapter will discuss only those issues pertinent to the older adult.

Although the use of drugs in older people requires care due to the increased likelihood of toxic effects, Malone-Lee (2000) suggests the increased sensitivity to pharmacological agents in older people can be used to advantage in the treatment of detrusor instability with successful treatment using lower doses.

Reported side-effects from oxybutynin used to treat detrusor instability are reversible confusional states in older people with Parkinson's disease, cognitive impairment, hallucinations, restlessness, disorientation and convulsions. Memory is mediated by acetylcholine (Drachman & Leavitt 1974, Drachman 1977) and short-term memory and cognitive function can be affected by taking oxybutynin (Katz et al 1998). Dimpfel et al (2000) found that oxybutynin had significant effects on the central nervous system measured by electroencephalogram but tolterodine and trospium chloride did not. It is important to be aware of the possibility of these effects. Anticholinergic agents can also be implicated in the development of glaucoma and those at risk and on long-term therapy should be monitored. Liver enzymes should be checked for those patients taking propiverine as reversible changes may occur but this is rare (Giles-Burness 2000).

Nocturia can be problematic for many older people causing sleep disturbance that may affect both health and well-being. The effect of nocturnal polyuria with age-related reduction in bladder capacity results in frequency, nocturia and sometimes incontinence (Miller 2000). Desmopressin, a synthetic analogue of vasopressin, the antidiuretic hormone, is effective in reducing nocturia and increasing diurnal diuresis (Asplund & Aberg 1993, Burgio et al 1996, Miller 2000). A study of 20 women with an average age of 71 years who passed at least 800 ml of urine at night found nocturnal diuresis reduced significantly with an associated increase in diurnal diuresis. Blood chemistry levels were monitored throughout the study and all values remained within normal parameters. Only two women had side-effects with one complaining of heaviness in the head in the morning and the other felt tired. Sleep improved in 11 of the subjects, deteriorated in one, remained the same in five and no data were available for the remaining three (Asplund & Aberg 1993).

Constipation is more common in the older population and laxatives and aperients are useful treatments but should not be the first option considered. Overuse of laxatives can produce large quantities of soft stools that are difficult to expel causing faecal loading and impaction with associated reduction in colonic motility (Norton 1996b, Winney 1998). Prolonged and excessive use of stimulant laxatives can cause nerve damage and resultant colonic inertia (Winney 1998).

Drugs for the treatment of diarrhoea such as loperamide and codeine phosphate should be used with caution as due to increased sensitivity to pharmacological agents in older people, constipation can easily be induced.

Catheterization

Indwelling catheterization should always be considered a last resort but intermittent self-catheterization may be a viable option when individuals have voiding difficulties or retain large quantities of urine (>150 ml) postvoid (Barton 2000). Age alone should not be considered a barrier to teaching this technique. Catharization and catheter care is discussed in detail in Chapter 9. When intermittent catheterization is unsatisfactory for women with voiding difficulties, a remote-controlled intraurethral insert may be a satisfactory option to produce artificial voiding. The insert is a short silicone catheter containing a valve and pump mechanism; it is produced in several sizes to fit individual urethras. It is inserted with a disposable inserter and is held in place by flexible silicone fins that open at the bladder neck. The insert is easily removed, the fins collapse on removal and the insert is changed monthly by the patient or a carer. An activator energizes the valve and pump mechanism that draws urine from the bladder at a rate of 10–12 ml per second (Madjar et al 1999). In a study of 92 women between the ages of 16 and 88 years, 47 were successfully treated with the intraurethral insert. The study concluded that this is a useful, safe method of managing voiding problems in women. Infection rates were reported as similar to those expected with clean intermittent catheterization (Madjar et al 1999).

Surgery

Surgery for incontinence is indicated only when conservative methods have been unsuccessful or the patient wants definitive treatment immediately. When detrusor instability and voiding dysfunction are present the patient must be warned that surgery may make the situation worse and treatment for these conditions should be established before surgery. The aims of surgery are to support the bladder neck or enhance urethral resistance or both (Chaliha & Stanton 2000).

Age itself is no barrier to surgery and older women should be considered for surgical treatment of stress incontinence when conservative interventions have been unsuccessful (Fonda et al 1999). A review of the literature has demonstrated good results following incontinence surgery in older women (Fonda et al 1999). Preoperative evaluation is essential for all age groups but it is especially important in the older patient to identify and stabilize comorbid conditions in order to minimize postoperative complications. However, frailty may preclude surgery in some women but recent developments of minimally invasive techniques will increase the population able to benefit from these procedures.

A very recent development, not yet reported in the literature but especially useful for treatment in older women, is the potential for repair surgery performed under local anaesthesia. To date over a hundred anterior and posterior repairs have been carried out as day cases. Success rates are similar (i.e. no better or worse) to those obtained when procedures are carried out under general anaesthetic but the risks of general anaesthesia are eliminated (Monga 2001).

Another useful surgical technique is the injection of bulking agents peri- or transurethrally. They act by bulking the tissue around the bladder neck and prevent the bladder neck opening prematurely. It is often necessary to administer several treatments to effect improvement or cure. The materials most commonly used include collagen and silicone. Most reports show subjective cure of 70–80% after 2 years with an objective cure of 50% and similar results have been reported in older women (Chaliha & Stanton 2000).

Chaliha & Stanton (2000) describe tension-free vaginal tape (TVT) as one of the most exciting and innovative procedures in the last 20 years. It is a sling technique but is placed without tension and is adjusted with cooperation from the patient who is conscious throughout the procedure. It can be done as a day case or at most an overnight stay in hospital and does not require a catheter. Voiding difficulties, urgency or frequency are not increased postoperatively.

For men with continence problems, surgical procedures should be considered only when conservative methods have failed. Preoperative evaluation is also important as has already been discussed with regard to female patients. The injection of bulking agents can also be used in men or the implantation of an artificial urethral sphincter to restore bladder control when incontinence is a complication of prostate surgery. With the artificial sphincter, a cuff is placed around the urethra, a pump in the scrotal sac and a balloon in the lower abdomen adjacent to the bladder.

The pump, cuff and balloon are all connected by tubing and the device is filled with fluid. The cuff keeps the urethra shut but when the pump in the scrotum is squeezed, the fluid is transferred from the cuff to the balloon releasing the urethra and allowing urine to be passed. After voiding the fluid returns to the cuff to close the urethra and prevent leakage (Newman 1999) (see also Chapter 4).

The artificial urethral sphincter can also be used for female patients, the only difference being that the pump is situated in either of the labium majus (Chaliha & Stanton 2000).

Surgical treatment for detrusor instability is limited and not without complications. Clam ileocystoplasty is the most reliable procedure but there are several potential complications including voiding dysfunction, stone formation, infection, mucus production and fluid and electrolyte disturbance (Venn & Mundy 2000) (see also Chapter 3).

Aids and appliances

When it is not possible for the older person to regain continence and/or sometimes during the time of ongoing treatment, it may be necessary for containment products to be used. There are more products on the market now for the containment of incontinence and the development of better products by manufacturers is a continuous process. The use of pads (and pants) and containment products should only be considered following comprehensive assessment as the inappropriate use of these aids may increase the number of incontinent episodes. The situations where the use of these products would be indicated and appropriate are shown in Box 6.8.

Box 6.8 Indications for the use of containment products (after Wang 2000)

- Whilst waiting for investigations
- When awaiting surgical treatment
- During treatment programme before treatment is effective
- Individuals who do not wish other more active treatment
- Individuals for whom active treatment/investigation is inappropriate

---

Absorbent products

When disposable absorbent products are used in continence care it is important to select the product that is most effective for each individual's needs. The majority of the disposable products available today contain superabsorbent polymers that enhance the performance of the product without increasing its bulk. There is often a tendency to supply products with more absorbency than required and an individual may be subjected to wearing a large bulky product unnecessarily. However, for residents living in nursing or residential care homes, carers often request the all-in-one diaper type of product. These products are not necessarily more absorbent than the body-worn pad and pants system but the perception is that they are more effective due to their all enclosing design. They are likely to be hot and uncomfortable for the user and may be implicated in the development of incontinence dermatitis by increasing skin permeability by overhydration of the skin.

Although containment of incontinence is required, absorbent products may not be the most effective option for an individual. In men a sheath system or, when this is not practicable, a body-worn collecting device may be more acceptable than wearing pads (see Chapter 4). For women, reusable absorbent products, when the incontinence is light, may feel more 'normal' and may help in the promotion of continence as there may be a more conscious effort not to wet the pants than when wearing pads.

Occlusive devices

There are now several occlusive devices available for women who have urinary incontinence. These are inserted into the vagina or urethra and prevent leakage by either applying pressure in the sagittal plane on the vesicourethral junction or occluding the urethra itself. The vaginal devices can be left in place all day but the urethral devices must be removed in order to pass urine. Use of these devices may not be acceptable to an older person but if they are tolerated and comfortable in use they should be available to them.

The anal plug, an occlusive device for anal incontinence, has recently become available on prescription in the UK. This is a very useful product for both men and women with faecal leakage, considerably improving their quality of life (see also Chapter 7).

Bed protection

Bed protection may be needed for some people with nocturnal incontinence and disposable and reusable bed pads are available. Disposable bed pads are not recommended for wide use as they represent a risk to the skin and the development of pressure sores, mainly through friction and becoming wrinkled and lumpy in use. They should only be used for faecal incontinence or for the very ill person who is unlikely to move much in bed except by the intervention of nursing staff and carers. Washable bed pads represent a more suitable option, they are comfortable in use, have considerable absorbency (at least 1 litre) and are easily washed. They are available in various sizes including complete bed size to fit the mattress and in double bed sizes.

Toilet access

When there is a problem reaching the toilet, urinals, commodes and aids to toileting may be used effectively. There are several hand-held urinals available for men and women, some of them so discreet they can be kept in a pocket or small bag. Some urinals are designed for use in bed or in a wheelchair and some are useful when travelling (see also Chapter 11).

Commodes can be useful for the person who is unable to reach the toilet due to poor mobility and/or manual dexterity. When used within an establishment such as a hospital, nursing or residential care home, privacy must be assured as most people will be inhibited if they are aware their bodily functions will be observed or heard by others in the vicinity. If a commode is provided for a person living in their own home, it is necessary to establish who will be able to empty the contents of the commode pan as this may be difficult for the user to manage. The use of a commode can also represent

---

Research study 6.2 Is there a risk of cross-infection from laundered reusable bedpads?

Reusable bedpads are used mainly for the management of urinary incontinence at night as an alternative to or instead of body-worn products. They are used in hospitals, residential and nursing homes and in the community. There are many different products available on the market but they are usually similar in construction, having three layers: a surface layer that is in contact with the skin, made of cotton or polyester fabric, a middle absorbent layer made of a rayon or polyester felt and a waterproof backing. Some products are available without the waterproof layer but used with a waterproof sheet to facilitate easy drying following laundering.

Bedding items have been considered by some authors as sources of infection as bacterial spores have been found to have an ability to adhere to fabrics when laudering practices have been inadequate (Croton 1990, Dixon 1990). This study by Cottenden et al (1999) evaluated the effects of laundering reusable bedpads following the standard foul wash procedure as specified by the NHS Executive (NHSE 1995). This specifies heat disinfection of bedpads and other fouled items of linen at 65°C for at least 10 minutes or at 71°C for at least 3 minutes. The study measured the microbial content of the bedpads after one night's use by incontinent adults and after laundering following the foul wash procedure as described above. Microbial content was measured on 145 bedpads from five different product designs.

Ten pads of the five pad types were used in random order on a long-stay elderly care ward. Nursing staff, laundry staff and the microbiologist were blinded to the brand names or the products being used. The used pads were placed in a clear plastic bag and delivered to the microbiologist within an hour of removal from the bed for sampling then sent to the laundry. Cultures were grown before and after laundering. On pads before laundry, growth was excessive and noted as more than 200 colony forming units (CFU) or were confluent. After laundering 90% of the bedpads tested had less than 20 CFUs and all colonies after laundering were very small numbers of commensal air contaminants and no anaerobic organisms were isolated.

This study concluded that all five products tested and laundered in accordance with the NHSE foul wash protocol were cleaned effectively and safe to reuse. It also suggested that ensuring individual bedpads are used for the same person each time is unnecessary, as the risk of cross-infection is minimized. The authors suggested that products without a waterproof backing (all products tested had an integral waterproof layer) would present an even lower risk of cross-infection.

The importance of close collaboration with laundry staff in the event of an organization considering the implementation of a reusable programme was stressed. The laundry must be able to cope with the soiled products and the recommended safe wash temperatures must be achieved, otherwise disposable products may be more appropriate.

---

a health and safety risk and safety for the user and carers must be assured by risk assessment.

Other aids to improve toilet accessibility may include raised toilet seats, rails and grab bars strategically placed to aid transfers and positioning. As part of the discharge planning process, the occupational therapist should carry out a home visit with the patient in order to arrange modifications to the home to ensure safe access for all activities including using the toilet.

INCONTINENCE IN RESIDENTIAL CARE SETTINGS

The number of people currently receiving care in an institution in the UK has increased considerably over the last 20 years with 157 500 older people living in nursing homes (of which 115 000 are public funded) and 288 750 living in residential care homes (of which 205 000 are public funded). Some older people are positive about the

transition to residential care but most commonly the move to living in an institution is viewed as rejection and of loss. Many admissions to long-term care facilities are as a result of breakdown in coping strategies of the older people themselves or their partners and carers (RCP et al 2000).

Many care home residents have complex medical needs that would have formerly been met in hospital settings and less than 40% of GPs, who are now responsible for their care, have had specialist education and training in the health and social care needs of older people. There are no statutory requirements for the nursing staff in nursing homes to obtain specialist knowledge, skills and expertise in the needs of older people in care homes and the capacity for specialist gerontological nurses is stifled by regulation (RCP et al 2000).

With high prevalence rates of urinary, faecal and combined incontinence in the residential and nursing home population the promotion of continence and management of incontinence is a

Case study 6.2

Derek Hancock, a 62-year-old man living in a residential care home, had recently suffered a stroke. He had made a good recovery but his mobility was slow and occasionally unsteady. Prior to his admission to the home, Mr Hancock had been homeless and he was clearly finding it difficult to adjust to living in the home.

He was referred to the District Nursing Service for symptoms of urge incontinence. A full continence assessment was carried out by a community nurse. Containment methods to achieve social continence were discussed and Derek agreed that a sheath system would be the most acceptable method of controlling his incontinence. The nurse requested the assistance of the local continence advisor to perform a bladder scan to exclude prostatic involvement. No residual urine was found and a sheath system was fitted.

Derek was happy for a member of staff to assist him with the sheath if he encountered problems due to his manual dexterity being slightly impaired and he understood he could stop using the sheath system at any time if he felt uncomfortable with it.

The continence advisor explained the method of application to both Derek and a member of staff from the home. Supplies for 7 days were left with Derek and the advisor promised to telephone the home within a week to enquire how Derek and the staff were coping. The continence advisor also offered to teach other members of staff the application of the sheath system if necessary.

However as the advisor was about to leave the home, the manager asked her to join him in his office with three female members of the staff who appeared distressed. The manager informed the advisor that he and his staff were not prepared to help Mr Hancock with fitting of the sheath system and that they considered it was not a suitable choice of management. The advisor was sympathetic and offered to instruct the staff about choosing sheath systems and when this was appropriate, the different types of sheath available and some tips on

overcoming embarrassment for the staff and resident. The staff remained adamant that they did not think the method chosen for this particular resident was appropriate and alternative methods of containment were discussed. It transpired that Derek was an alcoholic, had psychiatric problems and was often found masturbating when the staff entered the room early in the morning. He was not interacting well with other residents and was a disruptive influence in the home. The staff felt strongly that an indwelling urinary catheter was the most appropriate method of controlling his incontinence. The advisor explained why an indwelling catheter was not appropriate, including the potential risks of catheterization. She made counter-suggestions such as knocking at his door and waiting before entering and ensuring that only a male member of staff assisted him with the sheath.

It was clear that the staff in this residential care home had difficulty in dealing with this resident and his continence problem. They did not appear to consider the effect of Derek's health problems on his quality of life. It was agreed, in the interim, for continence pads to be provided to help Derek achieve social continence.

The issues raised by this incident showed the need for education about continence issues in the care home and the continence advisor arranged training sessions in liaison with the manager of the home. Assessment is only as good as the information gleaned and in this case the information was initially incomplete, demonstrating the need for effective communication. Following this unfortunate incident, the care home staff became more involved with all assessments of health needs to ensure all relevant information was included.

Derek was referred to his doctor for prostate assessment to confirm or eliminate prostatic involvement. He was also assessed by the community psychiatric team and was moved to an establishment more appropriate to his needs where the staff were experienced in dealing with people with behavioural problems such as those that Derek was exhibiting.

major issue. The effects of high prevalence rates can be low morale for both residents and carers and the possibility of complications of incontinence leading to illness. Incontinence increases workloads for care staff to unmanageable levels, can make staff feel inadequate and contributes to increasing staff turnover (Nazarko 1995a). The impact of increased turnover of staff is consistently low levels of knowledge in continence issues and requirement for education being a constant need of nursing and care staff.

As well as the physical and psychological costs of incontinence, the financial burden of

incontinence is considerable. In 1997 it was estimated that £1.4 billion per annum was spent on incontinence-related health care in the UK and that this would rise to at least £2 billion by 2020 without adjustment for inflation (Roy 1997, RCN 1997). These estimates do not take into account the hidden costs of the psychological consequences, informal care, inefficient delivery systems and inappropriate use of hospital beds (Roy 1997). The costs of incontinence were between 50 pence to £25 per day for people living at home to £120–200 for the most expensive hospital-based care. The incontinence-related costs within residential care settings was estimated to be approximately £300 per week (Roy 1997, RCN 1997) but Nazarko (1995b) estimated the nursing home costs of nurse time, laundry and incontinence products to be approximately £15 per day or £105 per week for each resident with incontinence. An average nursing home of 39 beds with a 60% level of incontinence was therefore costing £2457 each week or £127 764 per annum. These figures did not take into account indirect incontinence-related costs incurred due to the complications of incontinence such as incontinence dermatitis, pressure sores and infection.

It is possible to help older people regain continence and this will have positive effects on quality of life with residents enjoying greater confidence to participate in activities within the home and visiting their friends and relatives. Staff will feel motivated and encouraged by success and the achievement of continence or improvement in continence status. Continence promotion should initially be aimed at those residents most likely to respond in order to inspire and motivate the staff. The reduction in workload can be used to spend more time in social interaction with residents (Nazarko 1995a).

Both Chester (1998) and the RCP et al (2000) place an emphasis on staff education but Chester (1998) warns against assuming that staff with nursing or other health or social care qualifications are knowledgeable and have been adequately prepared during their professional training to be able to understand and deal appropriately with continence issues. Nurses' knowledge on continence promotion and management is often inadequate although they may not recognize this themselves. In their recent study of community nursing staff in one Trust, Bignell & Getliffe (2001) identified this lack of knowledge and awareness. They were able to demonstrate an association between an improvement in continence care, including heightened awareness, with the participation in a comprehensive education programme of the study group of nurses. This intervention group of nurses showed statistically significant changes in knowledge and awareness especially with regard to urge incontinence and an increased knowledge of potential

treatments. The authors also noted a decrease in the use of absorbent products being identified as a treatment for incontinence and speculated on whether this indicated a shift towards more proactive treatments being used rather than containment. In comparison, a control group of nurses, who had not participated in the programme, showed lower levels of knowledge and awareness even following the introduction of continence care guidelines.

Three main themes relating to the realistic provision of proactive continence care emerged from Bignell & Getliffe's (2001) study: assessment skills, patient capacity and role restrictions. Although assessment was recognized as being an important part of the nurses' role, the study identified the lack of confidence of many nurses in carrying out assessment and identifying the causes of incontinence and other contributing health, social and environmental factors. Many nurses considered themselves inadequately prepared for the more proactive role. Residents in residential care settings often have low capacity for improvement as they have low expectations and poor compliance to treatments, or frailty and complex problems may lead to the health professional recommending containment as the most appropriate option. Role restrictions identified in the study related to the lower priority that was given to continence care due to the multiple and complex problems of patients that nurses had to deal with in limited timescales.

In the nursing or residential care home staffing levels are often inadequate with low levels of qualified nursing staff who are able to give direction to care staff (Chester 1998). In residential care homes the care is provided mainly by care staff who do not usually hold professional qualifications and it is important for trainers to recognize that for some staff this subject may pose difficulties that need to be dealt with sensitively (Chester 1998). The necessity for assessment and ongoing evaluation must be understood by care staff who often appear to consider it a nuisance and waste of time. They may also feel threatened by regular evaluation/auditing in the belief that the aim of the assessor is to discontinue supply of continence aids. With educational intervention, care staff can learn the questions to ask when they are caring for residents who will often discuss their problems in more detail with them rather than the home manager or a visiting nurse. Box 6.9 contains questions suitable for care staff to use when caring for residents.

It is essential that the manager of the home recognizes and deals with low morale of staff due to feelings of hopelessness and acceptance of residents' incontinence by continually seeking positive actions and strategies. Continence should be easily and appropriately discussed between staff at handover times, when planning care and in staff meetings without causing undue embarrassment and disgust. It is important when these negative feelings are present in individuals or groups of staff that they are recognized and addressed (Chester 1998). Nazarko (1995b) observes that

nursing practice is often responsible for incontinence in nursing and residential care homes by encouraging dependency rather than rehabilitation, such as encouraging residents to use the pads they are wearing instead of using the toilet to void. Beds are often protected by plastic draw sheets routinely even when the person is not incontinent. This culture of dependency fosters a sense of powerlessness and residents can very soon become apathetic and disabled.

Many long-held beliefs about ageing are now being questioned and it is recognized that some changes previously attributed to the ageing process are largely a result of individual behaviour and environmental conditioning (RCN 2000c). Rehabilitation is not time limited but is continuous and may cover the lifespan of the individual. The role of the nurse or carer is a multifaceted one as re-enabler which is a positive role and involves identifying the things residents can do themselves and enabling them to do those things and increasing their ability where possible (RCN 2000c). The functions of the re-enablement role are shown in Box 6.10.

The central issue in the continence care of older adults in residential care settings is the need to treat each resident as an individual despite the temptation to treat all residents in the same way. For example, set times for toileting and providing

---

Box 6.9 Questions carers can use to ask residents about continence (after Sander 1998)

- What is the main problem?
- How long has it been a problem? When did it start?
- Did the problem start suddenly or gradually over several years?
- Do you ever leak if you cough or sneeze?
- Do you sometimes not quite make it to the toilet?
- Does the feeling of needing to pass urine come gradually or suddenly and urgently?
- Is there a particular time of day or night when this is more of a problem?
- When you leak, is it just a little or a sudden gush of urine?
- Do you constantly dribble urine? If so, are you aware of the dribbling?
- Tell me what you drink in an average day.
- What regular medicines or tablets do you take?
- How far is it to the nearest toilet? Can you reach it easily?
- Do you need help to get to the toilet? If so, do you get help when you need it?
- Is the toilet often occupied when you get there?
- Is the toilet comfortable, easy to use and in an acceptable condition?
- Can you get help easily when you need it?
- Do you have adequate privacy (including sound)?
- Have you noticed your urine is dark in colour or smells strong or 'fishy'?
- Is it a great effort to get to and use the toilet?
- Have you been feeling unwell recently?
- Have you been more thirsty than usual recently?
- Are you constipated?

Box 6.10 The functions of the re-enablement role (after RCN 2000c)

- Professional partnership with the individual aimed at maintaining or improving their quality of life.
- Recognize and respect the individuals' own needs, wishes and aspirations.
- Be a member of the multidisciplinary team, share activity with the individual, people close to them and the team. Recognize the value of each member's contribution.
- Be forward looking and positive.
- To search for things people can do for themselves and enabling them to continue to do them.
- Be a motivator and if necessary try to recapture motivation and hope for the future.
- Be creative and actively help the individual to make adaptations to changes in their life circumstances.
- Create the right atmosphere that is conducive to the rehabilitative process.

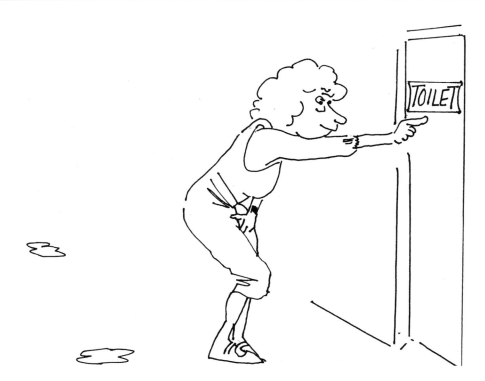

pads for everyone 'just in case' as happens in some of the less enlightened establishments is more likely to contribute to ongoing incontinence than improve it. Although helping residents to maintain continence has resource implications, time can be saved when assessment reveals the cause of the problems and appropriate management plans are established.

It is essential for staff to recognize the likelihood of transient incontinence in newly admitted residents as a result of the disorientation brought on by a change of environment and the need to help the older person become acclimatized to their new home.

Modifications within the home itself can aid the resident who is rather forgetful and vague by providing signed routes to the various essential facilities such as toilets and bathrooms. The door to toilets can be painted bright colours that are different from other doors so they stand out. A large picture of a toilet on the door will help some poorly sighted residents locate the correct place with clear indication whether for male or female

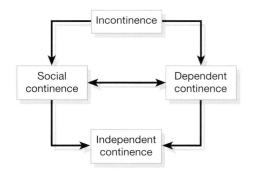

Figure 6.4 Stages and levels of incontinence (Fonda et al 1999). Reproduced by kind permission of Health Publication Ltd.

use. Many standard toilet signs are very small and a person with poor eyesight may make a mistake when using the toilet (meant for the other sex) and suffer considerable embarrassment.

Fonda (1990) suggests using the different stages and levels of incontinence (Fig. 6.4) in the institutionalized care setting to identify the dependency category. Management strategies should be

> **Box 6.11** Basic evaluation of the incontinent person living in residential care (after Fonda 1990)
>
> * Are staff sufficiently motivated and possess the skills to assess and manage incontinent residents?
> * What are the causes of the incontinence?
> * Can any of these causes be cured or modified?
> * What assistance (dependence) is needed, if any, for the resident to use the toilet?
> * Is the resident motivated to improve?
> * What dependency category does the resident fit into? (Table 6.3)

Table 6.3 Targeting management strategies and defining goals for continence

Nature of impairment	Management strategies	
	Goal	Strategies
Mental and physical	Social continence	Strict toileting and aids
Mental only	Dependent continence	Strict toileting programme
Physical only	Dependent continence (with or without social continence)	Bladder retraining programme
Neither mental or physical	Independent continence (with or without social continence)	Bladder retraining programme, pelvic floor exercises proactive strategies

After Fonda (1990).

targeted to achieve defined outcomes or goals within the stages/levels of incontinence (see Box 6.11 and Table 6.3). Using this approach should focus on each individual who is incontinent or has continence problems without making unrealistic demands on residents or staff.

It is important for the managers and staff of homes for older people to keep updated with current knowledge and information about treatments and facilities available for the older person with incontinence. A home can liaise with the local continence advisory service to ensure they have regular sources of the latest information as well as help with specific problems that staff have had particular difficulty in improving or resolving.

A study reported in 1998 found that many homes for older people were either not aware of

what help is available to them to promote continence or that they did not have the motivation to use services to help them (Chester 1998). Although most local continence services provide services into residential care homes, many do not provide services into nursing homes. When staff in a nursing home are enthusiastic about the promotion of continence, in the present climate of integrated working it is reasonable to expect more collaborative working with continence advisory staff providing advice, information and educational input.

The recently published National Service Framework (NSF) for Older People (DoH 2001) presents a 10-year programme of action linking services to support independence and promote good health for older people. It focuses on:

* rooting out age discrimination
* providing person-centred care
* promoting older people's health and independence
* fitting services around people's needs.

The NSF sets out a series of eight standards with key interventions to be achieved. These relate to: age discrimination; person-centred care; intermediate care; general hospital care; stroke; falls; mental health in older people; promotion of health and active life in old age. It is clear that continence is directly linked with all of these. The NSF also emphasizes the need to improve standards in care homes and presents a challenge to provide more integrated services regardless of professional and organizational boundaries. By April 2004, integrated continence services should be established in the UK, involving both health and social care systems.

There are more opportunities for staff working in nursing and residential care homes to further their education and gain recognizable qualifications by undertaking National Vocational Qualifications in Care programmes. Staff morale and retention can be enhanced by the achievement of awards by the home such as Investors in People (IiP). Nazarko (2000b) recognizes that the quality of care provided in a home is determined by the staff working there. She suggests the IiP standard enables homes to evaluate the skills of their

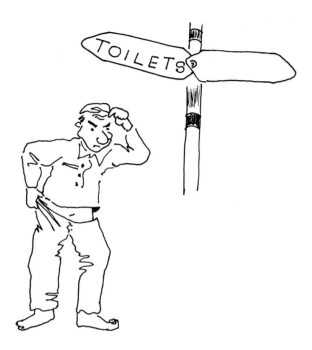

workforce and to plan and organize staff development. Staff who feel valued by the way the organization invests time in their further development will ultimately provide better quality care for their clients.

SERVICE PROVISION

Despite the high prevalence rates of incontinence, especially in the elderly population, and the overwhelming evidence that investment in continence services is clinically and cost-effective, service provision in the UK varies between different areas of the country. Some areas provide fully comprehensive services and others provide only continence aid supplies that are requested by community nursing staff.

The *Good Practice in Continence Services* guidance published by the Department of Health in March 2000 (DoH 2000) recommends more integration of services involved with continence-related issues to provide more cohesive and comprehensive services that include urinary and faecal incontinence, for people of all ages and people who live in their own homes and elsewhere. There are targets to be met that involve the participation of health authorities, primary care organizations, acute services and local authorities.

Continence clinics are usually provided by comprehensive services and these will include all aspects of continence-related problems and should be available for all client groups. Due to the embarrassment many incontinent people experience, continence clinics must be easily accessible, and open referral systems or 'drop in' facilities make this easier. GPs need to know how to refer appropriately to enable all the associated services to work well. Unfortunately there is some evidence to suggest that due to limited resources, some continence services do not attempt to market and publicize their services because they would not be able to cope with the resultant high demand (Anthony 1998).

User-friendly locations for health services are becoming more common and more unconventional non-healthcare settings are proving successful in persuading people to seek help. Examples include a leisure complex that includes a health suite and provides some classes specifically for older people. Local clinics in medical centres in the community are also more acceptable than at a hospital site, usually being nearer home for patients and often with better travel and parking facilities.

Many people with incontinence can be cured or improved, often with simple interventions or treatments and the emphasis of continence services is continence promotion. Services are able to give advice, information and support to anyone who is affected either directly or indirectly by incontinence including health or social care professionals, people with problems and their families and carers. They provide education to statutory and non-statutory groups and organizations and are usually involved locally with pre- and postregistration education and training of nursing and other healthcare staff.

Although continence services also provide continence aids to those people for whom they are indicated, it is essential that these are only supplied following comprehensive assessment. Requests for continence aids should be monitored to ensure inappropriate products are not being supplied and evaluation and assessment should be performed at least once a year as the situation may have changed or a more suitable product may be available (DoH 2000).

The absorbency capacity and quantity of aids supplied should be based on clinical need but most health organizations have rules and policies in place, some of which are restrictive. Anthony (1998) found that in 95% of areas out of 164, product supplies were subject to limits imposed by the organization.

Methods of providing continence aids vary between different continence services, with the most common method of acquisition of continence aids by the health organization being from a manufacturing company who will also supply computerized ordering and monitoring systems that include a client database of each individual's requirements. Other methods include using the NHS Supplies network or the subcontracting of a local delivery company to deliver products. With the two latter alternatives, more flexibility in the purchasing of continence aids by the health organization is possible as there is no obligation to purchase from only one source. In some areas

of the UK, supplies of continence aids are delivered direct to the user's place of residence but in other areas aids are delivered to health organization premises such as local health centres and require collection by the user or their representative. This can cause difficulties for some individuals, especially housebound older people but it should not be allowed to limit access to the service for these users (DoH 2000).

An essential role of the service includes the appropriate use of aids and appliances, other than disposable products, to enable individuals to obtain the optimum benefit. A display of products with advice and information available on their application, use and procurement is recommended (DoH 1991).

Continence services are expensive, and although continence services in the UK are available to residential care homes, nursing homes are often unable to access services for their residents. The Department of Health (2000) *Good Practice in Continence Services* guidance puts the responsibility of continence care on the homes themselves, suggesting each home should have staff trained in continence care but implies liaison with the local continence service. Where there is a good relationship with the primary healthcare team and the local continence services, an integrated approach is possible. Continence services will usually give advice and provide education opportunities to nursing home staff in response to interest and enthusiasm. The climate within healthcare is now towards integrated services and the breaking down of traditional boundaries should foster multidisciplinary and multiagency working.

PREVENTION OF INCONTINENCE IN THE OLDER ADULT

The prevention of incontinence in later life is, to a certain extent, dependent on proactive actions and strategies being used from a relatively early age. Hopefully, with a greater awareness of the risks of developing incontinence following certain events such as childbirth, and a greater emphasis on health education, the incidence of incontinence in older people will be reduced and reflect the culture of prevention rather than reaction. Continence promotion must be targeted at the general community, health services and the companies involved with the manufacture of continence products and drugs as well as those groups most at risk from developing incontinence. Continence promotion is taking place internationally through the work of the International Continence Society (ICS) working with national organizations to increase public awareness, provide education programmes, improve communication and introduce continence prevention strategies. The ICS website (see Chapter 12) conceived in 1995 is an important resource to achieve many of the continence promotion aims of the ICS (Fonda 1997, Lim & Fonda 1997).

There is very little information in the literature relating to the prevention of incontinence in older people. The principles of prevention for fit adults should apply to fit older adults but complications arise when frailty and disability are present (Fonda et al 1998). Prevention strategies can be divided into three categories: primary, secondary and tertiary (Fonda et al 1998, 1999) (Table 6.4).

Fonda et al (1999) found few data about successful use of prevention strategies but noted an increasing awareness of the risk factors implicated in continence problems in the older person (see Box 6.12). They suggested the prevalence and severity of continence problems can be reduced by concentrating on these risk factors to lessen their impact.

Primary prevention is no longer realistic in the frail older person due to the coexistence of lower urinary tract dysfunction, reduced mobility or impaired cognitive/mental status but it is often possible to use secondary preventative strategies effectively. The problem with secondary prevention of incontinence is that help is not usually requested by the incontinent person whilst they are asymptomatic. Empirical information is needed to determine the efficacy of specific preventative strategies that are appropriate for the older population to use when no symptoms are present (Fonda et al 1999).

The UK government has named the 'promotion of independence' as a national priority, with health and social services having a shared role. An objective has been set to prevent or delay the

Table 6.4 Prevention of incontinence

Prevention	Strategy
Primary	Intervention that prevents predisposing conditions from causing incontinence (childbirth trauma, pelvic muscle weakness, detrusor overactivity, impaired mobility, cognitive impairment)
Secondary	Intervention to reverse the predisposing condition(s) or prevent progression to incontinence
Tertiary	Management/treatment strategies to reduce the severity of consequences and complications of incontinence

After Fonda et al (1999).

Box 6.12 Risk factors associated with incontinence in older people (after Fonda et al 1999)

- Advancing age – especially female sex
- Cognitive impairment and decline
- Reduced or restricted mobility
- Functional disability, e.g. reduced dexterity, poor eyesight
- Constipation
- Chronic cough
- Diabetes mellitus
- Cerebrovascular disease
- Hypnotics and sedatives
- Diuretic therapy
- Previous genitourinary surgery
- Urinary tract infection, especially recurrent
- Lower urinary tract symptoms

loss of independence by the development of a range of preventative strategies that are targeted at those groups of adults who are most at risk (Continence Foundation 2000). The incidence of incontinence can erode independence and may precipitate premature admission to residential care so it is essential for proactive as well as reactive continence care to be provided to contribute towards the achievement of this objective.

SUMMARY

Incontinence is not inevitable in older adults and the reasons for its incidence are similar to those in the younger population. However, certain factors associated with ageing increase the risk of incontinence in older people, especially when there is the coexistence of illness or disease.

It is essential for education and training to be available for professionals and employed carers to displace the myth that incontinence is inevitable in old age and to raise awareness in those most at risk, their families and informal carers. It is essential for professionals to possess the skills of assessment in order to identify the cause of incontinence and determine the most appropriate methods of treatment or management. Older individuals are especially prone to transient incontinence that is reversible in most cases when effective treatment or management strategies are used.

The effects of incontinence are devastating for most individuals causing psychosocial and physical effects but in the older person can lead to isolation and may precipitate early admission to a residential care facility. Preventative strategies aimed at reducing the incidence or severity of incontinence should be used where possible to lessen the burden for the older person and enhance quality of life.

KEY POINTS FOR PRACTICE

- Incontinence is not an inevitable consequence of growing older. Professional and public attitudes to incontinence should understand and acknowledge this.
- Causes of incontinence in older adults are similar to those in younger people but older people are more susceptible to physiological, pharmacological and psychological risk factors that may affect their continence status.
- A thorough, individualized continence assessment and subsequent care plan is fundamental to good continence care. Use of a functional assessment tool can be a valuable component of the assessment process.

- Every person should be given the opportunity to achieve continence irrespective of frailty or disability. This can be:
  —independent continence
  —dependent continence (dry with assistance from a carer)
  —social continence (dry with use of continence aids or appliances; Fonda et al 1999).
- The philosophy and requirements of the National Service Framework for Older People (DoH 2001) must be incorporated within continence care.

Useful websites

AgeNet: http://www.agenet.com
Alzheimer's Association NSW (Australia): http://www.alznsw.asn.au
American Society of Consultant Pharmacists: http://www.ascp.com
British Geriatrics Society: http://www.bgs.org.uk

National Service Framework for Older People: http://www.doh.gov.uk/nsf/olderpeople.htm
Novartis Foundation for Gerontology: http://www.healthandage.com
On Health: http://onhealth.webmd.com

ACKNOWLEGEMENT

We are grateful to Christine Trimmings, Senior Territory Manager, Continence, Hollister Ltd. for her excellent illustrations in this chapter.

REFERENCES

Abrams P 1995 Managing lower urinary tract symptoms in older men. British Medical Journal 310: 1113–1117
Abrams P, Klevmark B 1996 Frequency volume charts: an indispensable part of lower urinary tract assessment. Scandinavian Journal of Urology and Nephrology Supplementum 179: 47–53
Addison R 1999 Nocturia, nocturnal polyuria and secondary nocturnal voiding. British Journal of Nursing 8(13): 877–880

Addison R 2000 Fluid intake: how coffee and caffeine affect continence. Nursing Times Plus 96(40): 7–8

Alessi C A, Henderson C, Linderborn K M 1993 A review of reseach on common bowel problems in the nursing home. In: Rubenstein L Z, Wieland D (eds) Improving care in the nursing home: comprehensive reviews of clinical research. Sage, Newbury Park, pp 160–194

Anders K 2000 Bladder retraining. In: Stanton S L, Monga A K (eds) Clinical urogynaecology. Churchill Livingstone, London, pp 575–581

Anthony B 1998 The provision of continence supplies by NHS trusts. Middlesex University, London

Ashford L 1998 Erectile dysfunction. Professional Nurse 13(9): 603–608

Asplund R, Aberg H 1993 Desmopressin in elderly women with increased nocturnal diuresis: a short-term study. British Journal of Urology 72: 42–45

Avorn J, Monane M, Gurwitz J H 1994 Reduction of bacteriuria and pyuria after ingestion of cranberry juice. Journal of the American Medical Association 271(10): 751–754

Barton R 2000 Intermittent self-catheterisation. Nursing Standard 15(9): 47–52

Bignell V, Getliffe K 2001 Clinical guidelines for promotion of continence in primary care: community nurses' knowledge, practice and perceptions of role. Primary Health Care Research and Development 2: 163–176

Bo K, Talseth T, Holme I 1999 Single blind, randomised controlled trial of pelvic floor exercises, electrical stimulation, vaginal cones and no treatment in management of genuine stress incontinence in women. British Medical Journal 318: 487–493

Boyington A R, Dougherty M C 2000 Pelvic muscle exercise effect on pelvic muscle performance in women. International Urogynaecology Journal 11: 212–218

Branch L G, Walker L A, Wetle T T, DuBeau C E, Resnick N M 1994 Urinary incontinence knowledge among community-dwelling people 65 years of age and older. Journal of the American Geriatrics Society 42(12): 1257–1262

Brostoff J, Gamlin L 1998 The complete guide to food allergy and intolerance. Bloomsbury, London

Brown J S, Vittinghoff E, Wyman J F et al 2000 Urinary incontinence: does it increase risk for falls and fractures? Journal of the American Geriatrics Society 48: 721–725

Burgio K L, Ives D G, Locher J L, Arena V C, Kuller L H 1994a Treatment seeking for urinary incontinence in older adults. Journal of the American Geriatrics Society 42(2): 208–212

Burgio L D, McCormick K A, Scheve A S et al 1994b The effects of changing prompted voiding schedules in the treatment of incontinence in nursing home residents. Journal of the American Geriatrics Society 42: 315–320

Burgio K L, Locher J L, Ives D G et al 1996 Nocturnal enuresis in community-dwelling older adults. Journal of the American Geriatrics Society 44(2): 139–143

Burgio K L, Locher J L, Goode P S et al 1998 Behavioural vs drug treatment for urge urinary incontinence in older women: a randomised controlled trial. Journal of the American Medical Association 280: 1995–2000

Burgio K L, Locher J L, Goode P S 2000 Combined behavioural and drug therapy for urge incontinence in older women. Journal of the American Geriatrics Society 48: 370–374

Burgio K L, Locher J L, Roth D L, Goode P S 2001 Psychological improvements associated with behavioural and drug treatment of urge incontinence in older women. Journals of Gerontology 56B(1): 46–51

Burns P A, Pranikoff K, Nochajski T, Desotelle P, Harwood M K 1990 Treatment of stress incontinence with pelvic floor exercises and biofeedback. Journal of the American Geriatrics Society 38: 341–344

Bush S 2000 Fluids, fibre and constipation. Nursing Times Plus 96(31): 11–12

Button D, Roe B, Webb C et al 1998 Consensus guidelines: Continence promotion and management by the primary health care team. London, Whurr

Camilleri M, Lee J S, Viramontes B et al 2000 Insights into the pathophysiology and mechanisms of constipation, irritable bowel syndrome and diverticulosis in older people. Journal of the American Geriatrics Society 48: 1142–1150

Campbell A J, Busby W J, Horwath C C 1993 Factors associated with constipation in a community based sample of people aged 70 years and over. Journal of Epidemiology and Community Health 47(1): 23–26

Chaliha C, Stanton S L 2000 Urethral sphincter incompetence. In: Stanton S L, Monga A K (eds) Clinical urogynaecology. Churchill Livingstone, London, pp 201–217

Chassagne P, Jego A, Gloc P et al 2000 Does treatment of constipation improve faecal incontinence in institutionalized elderly patients? Age and Ageing 29: 159–164

Chelvanayagam S, Norton C 2000 Quality of life with faecal continence problems. Nursing Times Plus 96(31): 15–17

Chester R 1998 Towards continence: a discussion document about approaches to continence in homes for older people. Counsel and Care for the Elderly, London

Chiang L, Ouslander J, Schnelle J, Reuben D B 2000 Dually incontinent nursing home residents: clinical characteristics and treatment differences. Journal of the American Geriatrics Society 48: 673–676

Chung B D, Parekh U, Sellin J H 1999 Effect of increased fluid intake on stool output in normal healthy volunteers. Journal of Clinical Gastroenterology 28(1): 29–32

Clay M 2001 Nutritious, enjoyable food in nursing homes. Nursing Standard 15(19): 47–53

Close J, Ellis M, Hooper R et al 1999 Prevention of falls in the elderly trial (PROFET): a randomized controlled trial. Lancet 353: 93–97

Colling J, Ouslander J, Hadley B J, Eisch J, Campbell E 1992 The effects of patterned urge-response toileting (PURT) on urinary incontinence among nursing home residents. Journal of the American Geriatrics Society 40: 135–141

Continence Foundation 2000 Making the case for investment in an integrated continence service. Continence Foundation, London

Cottenden A, Moore K N, Fader M, Cremer A W F 1999 Is there a risk of cross-infection from laundered reusable bedpads? British Journal of Nursing 8(17): 1161–1163

Croton C 1990 Duvets on trial. Nursing Times 86(26): 63–64

Darbyshire P 1986 When the face doesn't fit. Nursing Times September: 28–30

David T J 2000 Adverse reactions and intolerance to foods. British Medical Bulletin 56(1): 34–50

Davis K M, Fish L C, Minaker K L, Elahi D 1996 Atrial natriuretic peptide levels in the elderly: differentiating normal aging changes from disease. Journals of Gerontology 51A(3): M95–M101

de Groat W C, Downie J W, Levin R M et al 1999 Basic neurophysiology and neuropharmacology. In: Abrams P, Khoury S, Wein A (eds) Incontinence: 1st international consultation on incontinence. Health Publication Ltd, Plymouth, pp 105–154

Department of Health 1991 An agenda for action on continence services. DoH, London

Department of Health 2000 Good practice in continence services. DoH, London

Department of Health 2001 National Service Framework for older people. DoH, London

Dimpfel W, Todorova A, Vonderheid-Guth B 2000 Electrophysiological evaluation of potential adverse drug effects of tolterodine, oxybutynin and trospium chloride on the central nervous system. Journal of Urology Supplement 163(4): 226

Diokno A C, Brown M B, Brock B M et al 1988 Clinical and cystometric characteristics of continent and incontinent noninstitutionalized elderly. Journal of Urology 140: 567–571

Dixon B 1990 A real washday hazard. British Medical Journal 300: 528–529

Drachman D A 1977 Memory and cognitive function in man: does the cholinergic system have a specific role? Neurology 27: 783–790

Drachman D A, Leavitt J 1974 Human memory and the cholinergic system. A relationship to aging? Archives of Neurology 30: 113–121

Drench M E, Losee R H 1996 Sexuality and sexual capacities of elderly people. Rehabilitation Nursing 21(3): 118–123

DuBeau C E, Levy B, Mangione C M, Resnick N M 1998 The impact of urge urinary incontinence on quality of life: importance of patients' perspective and explanatory style. Journal of the American Geriatrics Society 46: 683–692

Duggan E, Cohen S J, Bland D R et al 2000 The association of depressive symptoms and urinary incontinence among older adults. Journal of the American Geriatrics Society 48: 413–416

Edwards S 2001 Regulation of water, sodium and potassium: implications for practice. Nursing Standard 15(22): 36–42

Fantl J A, Newman D K, Colling J et al 1996 Agency for Health Care Policy and Research (AHCPR). Clinical practice guideline for urinary incontinence in adults: acute and chronic management. US Department of Health and Human Services, Rockville

Fonda D 1990 Improving management of urinary incontinence in geriatric centres and nursing homes. Australian Clinical Review 10: 66–71

Fonda D 1997 Promoting continence as a health issue. European Urology 32(Suppl. 2): 28–32

Fonda D, Resnick N M, Kirschner-Hermanns R 1998 Prevention of urinary incontinence in older people. British Journal of Urology 82(Suppl. 1): 5–10

Fonda D, Benvenuti F, Castleden M et al 1999 Management of incontinence in older people. In: Abrams P, Khoury S, Wein A (eds) Incontinence: 1st international consultation on incontinence. Health Publication Ltd, Plymouth, pp 731–773

Getliffe K 1996a Urinary incontinence: assessing the problem. Primary Health Care 6(8): 31–38

Getliffe K 1996b Faecal incontinence in adults. Primary Health Care 6(10): 29–36

Giles-Burness D 2000 Drug treatment of urinary incontinence in adults. MeRec Bulletin 11(3): 9–12

Graham J, Varey M 1999 Food intolerance and chronic illnesses – a patient study. Positive Health March: 37–38

Gregoire A 1999 Male sexual problems. British Journal of Medicine 318: 245–247

Griep M I, Mets T F, Collys K et al 2000 Risk of malnutrition in retirement homes. Elderly persons measured by the 'mini-nutritional assessment'. Journals of Gerontology A55(2): M57–M63

Grigg E 1999 Sexuality and older people. Elderly Care 11(7): 12–15

Grimby A, Milsom I, Molander U, Wiklund I, Ekelund P 1993 The influence of urinary incontinence on the quality of life of elderly women. Age and Ageing 22: 82–89

Gross R D 1996 Psychology: the science of mind and behaviour. Hodder & Stoughton, London, pp 161–162

Harkins K J 2000 What's the use of cranberry juice? Age and Ageing 29: 9–12

Harrington C 2000 'I itch down below doctor': Managing vulval and perianal itch in older women. Geriatric Medicine June: 37–39

Harris A 1999 Impact of urinary incontinence on the quality of life of women. British Journal of Nursing 8(6): 375–380

Harvey R 2000 Food for thought: dementia, nutrition and the general practitioner. Geriatric Medicine July: 47–49

Heath H 2000 Sexuality and continence in older women. Elderly Care 12(3): 32–34

Hogan D B 1997 Revisiting the O complex: urinary incontinence, delirium and polypharmacy in elderly patients. Canadian Medical Association Journal 157: 1071–1077

Holben D H, Hassell J T, Williams J L, Helle B 1999 Fluid intake compared with established standards and symptoms of dehydration among elderly residents of a long-term care facility. Journal of the American Dietetic Association 99(11): 1447–1450

Holm N R, Horn T, Hald T 1995 Detrusor in ageing and obstruction. Scandinavian Journal of Urology and Nephrology 29(1): 45–49

Howell A B, Vorsa N, Marderosian A D, Foo L P 1998 Inhibition of the adherence of P-fimbriated Escherichia coli to uroepithelial-cell surfaces by proanthocyanidin extracts from cranberries. New England Journal of Medicine 339(15): 1085–1086

Hunskaar S, Arnold E P, Burgio K et al 1999 Epidemiology and natural history of urinary incontinence. In: Incontinence: 1st international consultation on incontinence. Health Publication Ltd, Plymouth, pp 197–226

Hunt J 1995 Irritable bladder syndrome: a void in the research? British Journal of Clinical Psychology 34: 435–446

Jenkins D A L 1999 Intimate caring skills. Urinary and faecal incontinence: a heightened problem when dementia is a factor. Dementia Services Development Centre, University of Stirling

Johnson T M, Kincade J E, Bernard S L et al 1998 The association of urinary incontinence with poor self-rated health. Journal of the American Geriatrics Society 46: 693–699

Jolleys J V 1993 Does detruser instability complicate BPH? Geriatric Medicine November: 56–58

Jones S M, Morgan M, Humphrey T J, Lappin-Scott H 2001 Effect of vancomycin and rifampicin on methicillin-resistant *Staphylococcus aureus* biofilms. Lancet 357: 40–41

Jorm A F 2000 Is depression a risk factor for dementia or cognitive decline? Gerontology 46: 219–227

Kamm M A 1998 Fortnightly review. Faecal incontinence. British Medical Journal 316: 528–531

Katz I R, Sands L P, Bilker W et al 1998 Identification of medications that cause cognitive impairment in older people: the case of oxybutynin chloride. Journal of the American Geriatrics Society 46(8): 8–13

Kelleher C J, Versi E 2000 Urogenital tract dysfunction and the menopause. In: Stanton S L, Monga A K (eds) Clinical urogynaecology. Churchill Livingstone, London, pp 373–385

Kelleher C J, Cardozo L D, Khullar V, Salvatore S 1997 A medium term analysis of the subjective efficacy of treatment for women with detruser instability and low bladder compliance. British Journal of Obstetrics and Gynaecology 104: 988–993

Kirby R S 1994 Non-traumatic neurogenic bladder dysfunction. In: Mundy A R, Stephenson T P, Wein A J (eds) Urodynamics: principles, practice and application. Churchill Livingstone, Edinburgh, pp 365–373

Kleemola P, Jousilahti P, Pietinen P et al 2000 Coffee consumption and the risk of coronary heart disease and death. Archives of Internal Medicine 160: 3383–3400

Kuzminski L N 1996 Cranberry juice and urinary tract infections: is there a beneficial relationship? Nutrition Reviews 54(11): S87–90

Lagro-Janssen T, Smits A, Van Weel C 1992 Urinary incontinence in women and the effects on their lives. Scandinavian Journal of Primary Health Care 10(3): 211–216

Laker C 1994 Anatomy and physiology of the urinary system. In: Laker C (ed) Urological nursing. Scutari, London, pp 1–35

Lamb J F, Ingram C G, Johnston I A, Pitman R M 1991 Essentials of physiology. Blackwell, London

Lavender R 2000 Cranberry juice: the facts. Nursing Times Plus 96(40): 11–12

Laycock J 1992 Pelvic floor re-education for the promotion of continence. In: Roe B (ed) Clinical nursing practice: the promotion and management of continence. Prentice Hall, New York, pp 95–126

Laycock J 1994 Electrotherapy. In: Laycock J, Wyndaele J J (eds) Understanding the pelvic floor. Neen Health Books, Dereham, Norfolk, pp 101–113

LeLievre S 2000 Care of the incontinent client's skin. Journal of Community Nursing 14(2): 26–32

Lewis G 1999 Assessing psychological well being of incontinent patients. Journal of Community Nursing 13(9): 40–43

Lim P H C, Fonda D 1997 The ContiNet of the International Continence Society. Neurourology and Urodynamics 16: 609–616

Lindeman R D, Romero L J, Liang H C et al 2000 Do elderly persons need to be encouraged to drink more fluids? Journals of Gerontology 55A(7): M361–M365

Madden V 2000 Nutritional benefits of drinks. Nursing Standard 15(13–15): 47–52

Madjar S, Sabo E, Halachmi S et al 1999 A remote controlled intraurethral insert for artificial voiding: a new concept for treating women with voiding dysfunction. Journal of Urology 161(3): 895–898

Malone-Lee J 2000 The elderly. In: Stanton S L, Monga A K (eds) Clinical urogynaecology. Churchill Livingstone, London, pp 387–399

Marieb E N 1992 Human anatomy and physiology. Benjamin/Cummings, Menlo Park, California

McCreanor J 1998 Comparing therapies for incontinence. Professional Nurse 13(4): 215–219

McCue J D 2000 Complicated UTI: effective treatment in the long-term care setting. Geriatrics 55(9): 48–61

McKee D 1999 The legal framework for informed consent. Professional Nurse 14(10): 688–690

McKim E M, McKim W A 1993 Caffeine: how much is too much? The Canadian Nurse 89(11): 19–22

McNeil S 1995 Expected and accepted. Community Outlook January: 19–20

Miller M 2000 Nocturnal polyuria in older people: pathophysiology and clinical implications. Journal of the American Geriatrics Society 48(10): 1321–1329

Milligan F 2000 Urethral catheterisation in older men. Elderly Care 12(2): 35–38

Mirpuri N, Patel P 1998 Crash course: renal and urinary systems. Mosby, London

Mitteness L S 1990 Knowledge and beliefs about urinary incontinence in adulthood and old age. Journal of the American Geriatrics Society 38(3): 374–378

Monga A K 2001 Anterior and posterior repair under local anaesthetic. Personal communication

Morison M J 1998 Family attitudes to bed-wetting and their influence on treatment. Professional Nurse 13(5): 321–325

Morrison C 2000 Helping patients to maintain a healthy fluid balance. Nursing Times Plus 96(31): 3–4

Nakanishi N, Tatara K, Naramura H et al 1997 Urinary and fecal incontinence in a community-residing older population in Japan. Journal of the American Geriatrics Society 45(2): 215–219

Nakayama H, Jorgensen H S, Pedersen P M et al 1997 Prevalence and risk factors of incontinence after stroke: the Copenhagen Stroke Study. Stroke 28(1): 58–62

Nasr S Z, Ouslander J G 1998 Urinary incontinence in the elderly: causes and treatment options. Drugs and Aging 12: 349–360

Nazarko L 1995a Nursing in nursing homes. Blackwell Science, Oxford

Nazarko L 1995b The therapeutic uses of cranberry juice. Nursing Standard 9(34): 33–35

Nazarko L 1996 A matter of urgency. Nursing Times 92(32): 62–67

Nazarko L 1997 The whole story. Nursing Times 93(43): 63–68

Nazarko L 1998 A passing phase. Nursing Times 94(32): 83–87

Nazarko L 1999 Assess all areas. Nursing Times 95(6): 68–72

Nazarko L 2000a How age affects fluid intake. Nursing Times Plus 96(31): 8

Nazarko L 2000b Good investments. Nursing Management 7(7): 8–11

Nelson R, Norton N, Cautley E, Furner S 1995 Community-based prevalence of anal incontinence. Journal of the American Medical Association 274: 559–561

Newman D K 1999 The urinary incontinence sourcebook. Lowell House, Los Angeles

NHS Executive 1995 Hospital laundry arrangements for used and infected linen. HMSO, London

Nicolle L E 1999 Urinary infections in the elderly: symptomatic or asymptomatic? International Journal of Antimicrobial Agents 11(3–4): 265–268

Norton C 1996a Faecal incontinence in adults 1: prevalence and causes. British Journal of Nursing 5(22): 1366–1374

Norton C 1996b The causes and nursing management of constipation. British Journal of Nursing 5(20): 1252–1258

Norton C 1996c Faecal incontinence in adults 2: treatment and management. British Journal of Nursing 6(1): 23–26

Norton C, Kamm M A 1999 Bowel control: information and practical advice. Beaconsfield Publishers, Beaconsfield, Bucks

Oliver D 2000 Falls in the elderly: the role of the GP and the hospital. Geriatric Medicine December: 9–11

Ouslander J G, Schnelle J F 1993 Assessment, treatment and management of urinary incontinence in the nursing home. In: Rubenstein L Z, Wieland D (eds) Improving care in the nursing home: comprehensive reviews of clinical research. Sage, Newbury Park, pp 131–159

Ouslander J G, Schnelle J F 1995 Incontinence in the nursing home. Annals of Internal Medicine 122(6): 438–449

Ouslander J G, Simmons S, Schnelle J, Uman G, Fingold S 1996 Effects of prompted voiding on fecal continence among nursing home residents. Journal of the American Geriatrics Society 44(4): 424–428

Parker A 1998 Using the Barthel index in care homes. Elderly Care 10(3): 12–14

Perry S, Shaw C, Assassa P et al 2000 An epidemiological study to establish the prevalence of urinary symptoms and felt need in the community: the Leicestershire MRC Incontinence Study. Journal of Public Health Medicine 22(3): 427–434

Pfister S M 1999 Bladder diaries and voiding patterns in older adults. Journal of Gerontological Nursing 25(3): 36–41

Primrose W R 1999 Indices of dehydration in elderly people. Age and Ageing 28: 411

Raz R, Gennesin Y, Wasser J et al 2000 Recurrent urinary tract infection in postmenopausal women. Clinical Infectious Diseases 30(1): 152–156

Renteln-Kruse W 2000 Does frailty predipose to adverse drug reactions in older patients? Age and Ageing 29(5): 461–462

Resnick N M 1990 Initial evaluation of the incontinent patient. Journal of the American Geriatrics Society 38: 311–316

Roberts R O, Jacobsen S J, Reilly W T et al 1999 Prevalence of combined fecal and urinary incontinence: a community-based study. Journal of the American Geriatrics Society 47(7): 837–841

Robinson J P 2000 Managing urinary incontinence in the nursing home: residents' perspectives. Journal of Advanced Nursing 31(1): 68–77

Rockwood K, Stadnyk K, MacKnight C et al 1999 A brief clinical instrument to classify frailty in elderly people. Lancet 353: 205–206

Rodrigues-Fisher L, Bourguignon C, Good B V 1993 Dietary fiber nursing intervention: prevention of constipation in older adults. Clinical Nursing Research 2(4): 464–477

Roe B, Wilson K, Doll H, Brooks P 1996 An evaluation of health interventions by primary health care teams and continence advisory services on patient outcomes related to incontinence. Health Services Research Unit, University of Oxford

Rosser C J, Bare R L, Meredith J W 1999 Urinary tract infections in the critically ill patient with a urinary catheter. American Journal of Surgery 177: 287–290

Roy S 1997 The cost of continence. In: The cost of continence. Royal College of Nursing, London, pp 3–4

Royal College of Nursing (RCN) 1997 A briefing paper on the cost of continence (publication code 000 809). Royal College of Nursing, London

Royal College of Nursing (RCN) 2000a Digital rectal examination and manual removal of faeces: guidance for nurses (publication code 000 934). Royal College of Nursing, London

Royal College of Nursing (RCN) 2000b Sexuality and sexual health in nursing practice (publication code 000 965). Royal College of Nursing, London

Royal College of Nursing (RCN) 2000c Rehabilitating older people (publication code 000 058). Royal College of Nursing, London

Royal College of Physicians 1995 Incontinence: causes, management and provision of services. Royal College of Physicians, London

Royal College of Physicians (RCP), Royal College of Nursing (RCN) and British Geriatrics Society 2000 The health and care of older people in care homes: A comprehensive interdisciplinary approach. Royal College of Physicians, London

Rubenstein L Z, Josephson K R 1993 Clinical research on falls in the nursing home. In: Rubenstein L Z, Wieland D (eds) Improving care in the nursing home: comprehensive reviews of clinical research. Sage, Newbury Park, pp 216–240

Saito M, Kondo A, Kato T, Yamada Y 1993 Frequency-volume charts: comparison of frequency between elderly and adult patients. British Journal of Urology 72: 38–41

Sander R 1998 Promoting urinary continence in residential care. Elderly Care 10(3): 28–35

Sattin R W, Rodriguez J G, DeVito C A, Wingo P A 1998 Home environmental hazards and the risk of fall injury events among community-dwelling older persons. Study to Assess Falls Among the Elderly (SAFE) Group. Journal of the American Geriatrics Society 46: 669–676

Schnelle J F 1990 Treatment of urinary incontinence in nursing home patients by prompted voiding. Journal of the American Geriatrics Society 38: 356–360

Schulz R, Heckhausen J, O'Brien A T 1994 Control and the disablement process in the elderly. Journal of Social Behaviour and Personality 9(5): 139–152

Sedor J, Mulholland S G 1999 Hospital-acquired urinary tract infections associated with the indwelling catheter. Urologic Clinics of North America 26(4): 821–828

Shepherd M 1998 The risks of polypharmacy. Nursing Times 94(32): 60–62

Silverman M, McDowell B J, Musa D, Rodriguez E, Martin D 1997 To treat or not to treat: issues in decisions not to treat older persons with cognitive impairment, depression and incontinence. Journal of the American Geriatric Association 45: 1094–1101

Simons J 1985 Does incontinence affect your client's self-concept? Journal of Gerontological Nursing 11(6): 37–40

Smoker A 1999 Skin care in old age. Nursing Standard 13(48): 47–53

Spencer B, Pritchard-Howarth M, Lee T, Jack C 2000 Won't drink? Can't drink? Age and Ageing 29(2): 185

Stamm W E, Raz R 1999 Factors contributing to susceptibility of postmenopausal women to recurrent urinary tract infections. Clinical Infectious Diseases 28(4): 723–725

Stewart R B, Moore M T, May F E, Marks R G, Hale W E 1992 Nocturia: a risk factor for falls in the elderly. Journal of the American Geriatrics Society 40: 1217–1220

Stockert P A 1999 Getting UTI patients back on track. Registered Nurse 62(3): 49–52

Storrie J B 1997 Biofeedback: a first-line treatment for idiopathic constipation. British Journal of Nursing 6(3): 152–158

Strasser H 1999 Urinary incontinence in the elderly and age-dependent apoptosis of rhabdosphincter cells. Lancet 354: 918–919

Swaffield J 1996 Continence in older people. In: Norton C (ed) Nursing for continence, 2nd edn. Beaconsfield Publishers, Beaconsfield, Bucks, pp 258–282

Swami S K, Abrams P 1996 Urge incontinence. Urologic Clinics of North America 23(3): 417–425

Thom D H, Haan M N, Van den Eeden S K 1997 Medically recognised urinary incontinence and risks of hospitalisation, nursing home admission and mortality. Age and Ageing 26(5): 367–374

Tinetti M E, Williams C S 1997 Falls, injuries due to falls, and the risk of admission to a nursing home. New England Journal of Medicine 337(18): 1279–1284

Van Kampen M, De Weerdt W, Van Poppel H et al 2000 Effect of pelvic floor re-education on duration and degree of incontinence after radical prostatectomy: a randomised controlled trial. Lancet 355: 98–102

Veehof L J G, Stewart R E, Meyboom-de-Jong B, Haaijer-Ruskamp F M 1999 Adverse drug reactions and polypharmacy in the elderly in general practice. European Journal of Clinical Pharmacology 55(7): 533–536

Venn S, Mundy T 2000 Detruser instability. In: Stanton S L, Monga A K (eds) Clinical urogynaecology. Churchill Livingstone, London, pp 219–226

Wallace B 2000 Nurses and consent. Professional Nurse 15(11): 727–730

Watson R 2001 Assessing the gastrointestinal (GI) tract in older people: 2 The lower GI tract. Nursing Older People 13(1): 27–28

Whittingham K 1998 Cleansing regimens for continence care. Professional Nurse 14(3): 167–172

Williams M E, Gaylord S A 1990 Role of functional assessment in the evaluation of urinary incontinence. Journal of the American Geriatrics Society 38: 296–299

Willis J 2000 Bowel management and consent. Nursing Times Plus 96(6): 7–8

Wilson J A P 1999 Constipation in the elderly. Clinics in Geriatric Medicine 15(3): 499–510

Winney J 1998 Constipation. Nursing Standard 13(11): 49–53

Wolf S L, Riolo L, Ouslander J G 2000 Urge incontinence and the risk of falling in older women. Journal of the American Geriatrics Society 48: 847–848

Wyman J F, Harkins S W, Fantl J A 1990 Psychosocial impact of urinary incontinence in the community-dwelling population. Journal of the American Geriatrics Society 38(3): 282–288

Wyman J F, Fantl J A, McClish D K, Bump R C and the Continence Program for Women Research Group 1998 Comparative efficacy of behavioral interventions in the management of female urinary incontinence. American Journal of Obstetrics and Gynecology 179: 999–1007

Yu L C, Rohner T J, Kaltreider D L et al 1990 Profile of urinary incontinent elderly in long-term care institutions. Journal of the American Geriatrics Society 38: 433–439

Zembrzuski C D 1997 A three-dimensional approach to hydration of elders: administration, clinical staff and in-service education. Geriatric Nursing 18: 20–26

7

Down, down and away! An overview of adult constipation and faecal incontinence

Claire Edwards
Mary Dolman
Nicky Horton

'Quietly he read, restraining himself, the first column, and yielding but resisting, began the second midway, his last resistance yielding, he allowed his bowels to ease themselves quietly as he read, reading still patiently, that slight constipation of yesterday quite gone. Hope it's not too big, bring on piles again. No, just right. So. Ah!'

James Joyce, Ulysses

INTRODUCTION

James Joyce's description of one day in the life of Mr Bloom would not have been complete without including his 'daily bowel motion', whilst, of course, reading the newspaper. Although *Ulysses* was written almost a century ago, for some people the emphasis on the daily bowel motion is as strong today as it seemed to be then.

This preoccupation with bowel habit sends 1 in 100 people to their general practitioner (GP) each year, i.e. 400 000 consultations annually (Royal College of Physicians, 1995). As with urinary incontinence, the number visiting their GP is only a small proportion of those suspected of actually suffering from problems of constipation. Population surveys demonstrate that as many as 10–20% suffer from constipation and/or straining at stool. As age increases, so does the incidence of constipation, and it is the elderly who most commonly present with symptoms (see Chapter 6). Fewer than 10% of the general population do not have at least one bowel action daily, and 1% have a bowel action less than three times a week.

During childhood, constipation is more common in boys than in girls. Later, constipation presents more commonly in women. As age increases the sexes are equally affected (Devroede 1992). Constipation is a costly business, not only in terms of the health and comfort of the individual but also financially. Each year, millions of pounds are spent on laxatives, more than 50% of such sales being made to the elderly population with doctors writing approximately a quarter of a million prescriptions for laxatives. A National Audit (Phase I) for chronic constipation took place in 2001 in 20 different audit centres, when it was established that over 121 different combinations of laxatives were being prescribed. From this guidelines are being devised to form a standard 'essence of care' to reduce the number of laxatives being used. Regular audits will take place and plans are being made for the 2002 audit. At present laxative use is costing £61 million in the UK. Many other approaches to treating constipation can be found in this chapter before resorting to laxatives.

Difficulties with regular bowel motions can have a considerable effect, not only on the sufferer, but also indirectly on family and friends. Whether or not a sufferer is successful on the toilet can influence the entire household on a day-to-day basis; on the other hand there are people who seem to accept constipation as being one of those everyday ailments, not important enough to trouble the nurse or doctor with.

Left untreated, constipation may cause such miseries as haemorrhoids, rectal bleeding, abdominal and anal pain, reduced appetite, headache, urinary retention and/or urinary and faecal incontinence. The aim of this chapter is to highlight the problem of constipation and to help alleviate any possible misconceptions regarding its treatment. Research-based knowledge is combined with concise practical advice.

Constipation leading to faecal impaction with overflow diarrhoea is by far the most common cause of faecal incontinence, particularly in the elderly, but other possible causes are presented in

---

Box 7.1 Causes of faecal incontinence

Severe diarrhoea
This may result from:

- infection
- medication
- radiation therapy
- colorectal disease
  —ulcerative colitis
  —diverticular disease
  —carcinoma.

Anorectal muscle weakness
The main abnormality is weakness of the anal sphincter and pelvic floor muscles, which may result from:

- surgical or traumatic division of the anal sphincters
- denervation atrophy of the external anal sphincter and/or puborectalis muscles
- pudendal nerve neuropathy occurring during childbirth or due to chronic straining at stool (Swash 1988)
- reduced strength of contraction of external sphincter occurring with age (Laurenberg & Swash 1989).

Pelvic floor muscle exercises may help in many cases. In severe cases, surgery may be indicated (e.g. postanal repair, rectopexy for rectal prolapse).

Bowel surgery
Faecal incontinence can be a temporary or a longer-term consequence of surgical procedures performed on the bowel (Ness 1994), when one or more of the complex factors, which control continence, are disturbed. The anal sphincter is commonly divided or stretched during the operation (see previous heading). Colonic absorption is significantly reduced in patients who have had part or all of their colon removed, and this leads to the production of a more liquid stool which may be difficult to control.

Neuropathic disorders
Any neuropathic disorder (e.g. multiple sclerosis, stroke, dementia, spinal injury) can affect faecal continence. Very careful individual assessment and management are required, but it is often possible to plan a regime of bowel evacuation that maintains continence (see also Chapter 11).

Faecal impaction
This is by far the most common cause of faecal incontinence, particularly in the elderly, and is dealt with in depth in the main body of this chapter.

Box 7.1. Refer also to Chelvanayagam and Norton (1999) who have focused on the causes and assessment of faecal incontinence. Further classification, or grading, of faecal incontinence (Box 7.2) may be made based on such criteria.

Box 7.2   Classification or grading of faecal incontinence

A number of different classification systems exist, making comparisons between research studies difficult. In addition, there is a need for a common definition of the terms used to describe factors such as stool consistency. One example of a simple classification system is provided below (Karanjia et al 1992).

1. Bowel frequency
2. Ability to distinguish flatus from faeces
3. Ability to defer defecation
4. Frequency of soiling

Further factors that should not be ignored are the social and psychological effects of faecal incontinence on the patient's lifestyle.
    See also Bristol Stool Scale (p. 205).

WHAT IS CONSTIPATION?

The word 'constipation' comes from the Latin word *constipare*, meaning to 'crowd together'. This perhaps implies that stools are hard and large. However, in modern medicine the word 'constipated' is normally used to describe a symptom that is identified either by the infrequent passage of stools – i.e. less than every 3 days – or excessive straining when having the bowel open (Storrie 1997). It is generally accepted that the passing of at least three stools per week, without straining, may be considered as normal.

Nagengast et al (1988) identified possible reasons why elderly patients who complained of constipation were passing soft stools. Contrary to common belief and practice, assessing stool consistency alone is not a reliable measure of constipation. Donald et al (1985) recognized that digital examination of the rectum in elderly patients was also an unreliable measure of the degree of constipation.

In clinical practice patients sometimes express concern about 'normal' bowel habits. Since childhood training may well have conditioned them to expect at least a daily bowel motion, it is often difficult to reassure patients that, medically speaking, their habits are considered normal. These patients often needlessly take laxatives on a daily basis (see Chapter 6).

As well as identifying normality concerning the regularity of bowel movement, *what* happens and *how* it happens are also important. This will be discussed next.

PHYSIOLOGY OF THE LARGE BOWEL

This section reviews the physiology of the large bowel or colon, which comprises the last 1.5 metres of the gastrointestinal (GI) tract. Understanding the function of the large bowel is elementary. Originating from the Latin word *botulus*, meaning 'sausage', the large bowel is part of the GI tract 'team'. As with all teams, each member has a specific job to perform in order to ensure that the ultimate goal is achieved. In this case, the goal is that the body should receive a constant supply of nutrients and fluids and that material not considered necessary is conveniently disposed of.

The GI tract is also rather like a factory production line. Various functions are performed at various sites in order that the article in question, in this case food and fluid, is processed effectively to produce an end result – the faeces. If, at any time, the conveyor belt breaks down, the result may be devastating to production and severely threaten an individual's state of health.

The large bowel has several important roles:

- *Absorption of water, salts and some medication.* In a 24-hour period, approximately 500 ml of fluid enters the colon, from which about 400 ml of water is reabsorbed.
- *A habitat for micro-organisms.* A range of micro-organisms commonly inhabit the large bowel. Some such as *Escherichia coli* and *Streptococcus faecilis*, although harmful in other areas of the body, perform a valuable function in the bowel by synthesizing vitamin K which is important for the production of the blood clotting agent, prothrombin. They also play a role in the synthesis of folic acid, important for red blood cell development.
- *Defecation.* The large bowel is responsible for removing faeces (the end result of the digestive process), mucus, micro-organisms and epithelial

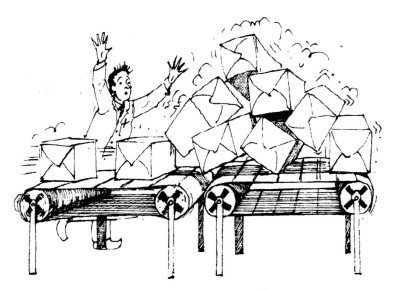

'The GI tract is rather like a factory production line.'

cells. Faeces are made up mainly of water and cellulose (the walls of plant materials that cannot be digested). It is usually brown in colour owing to the bilirubin content, derived from the breakdown of haemoglobin.

Parts of the large bowel

The large bowel begins after the ileum, that is the last part of the small intestine. It starts at the caecum and finishes at the anus, with the colon, rectum and anal canal in between (Fig. 7.1).

The caecum

This is the shortest part of the large bowel. It has a blind end to which the vermiform appendix is attached. Where the caecum and ileum join is the ileocaecal junction which acts as a 'one-way' valve, forcing the contents to travel in the direction of the caecum only and preventing their return. Passing upwards from the caecum is the ascending colon.

The ascending colon

The ascending colon is the first part of the colon. It continues upwards until it reaches the liver.

It then bends sharply. This bend is known as the right colic or hepatic flexure.

The transverse colon

The transverse colon continues from the hepatic flexure, across the abdomen, passing in front of the stomach and duodenum. It bends sharply at the left colic or splenic flexure.

The descending colon

The descending colon passes downwards from the splenic flexure, through the pelvis. At approximately the level of the left iliac crest, it forms an S-shaped curve known as the sigmoid colon.

The rectum and anal canal

The rectum makes up the last 15–17 cm of the large bowel. At the level of the pelvic floor, the last 2–3 cm of the rectum becomes the anal canal, collectively known as the anorectum.

Above the anal canal, the rectum has a slightly larger diameter than the rest of the colon. The anal canal begins at the anorectal junction, passes through the *levator ani* muscle, and ends at the

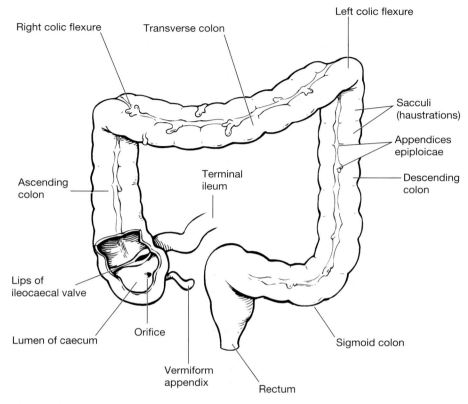

Figure 7.1   The colon. Reproduced with permission of Hodder/Arnold Limited from Barrett (1993).

anal orifice. One of the muscles of the pelvic floor, the *puborectalis* muscle, forms a sling around the anorectal junction. When this muscle contracts the anorectal junction is pulled upwards and forwards, decreasing its angle, thus preventing faeces from passing into the anal canal.

The internal anal sphincter

The internal anal sphincter is formed by a thickening of smooth circular muscle. It surrounds the anal canal. It is not under voluntary control.

The external anal sphincter

The external anal sphincter is formed by a sheet of striated muscle. It surrounds the bottom of the internal anal sphincter, overhanging it slightly. It is under voluntary control.

Tissues of the large bowel

There are four main layers of tissue which form the large bowel: the outer, muscle, submucous and mucous layers.

The outer layer

Also known as the adventitia or serosa, this layer is made up of connective tissue and epithelium and forms part of the peritoneum – the largest serous membrane in the body. This part of the peritoneum anchors the large bowel to the back of the abdominal wall, preventing excessive movement and friction.

The muscle layer

This layer is mostly made up of two sheets of smooth, involuntary muscle. The inner sheet comprises circular muscle fibres, and the outer sheet longitudinal muscle fibres. These longitudinal fibres are divided to form flat strips called taeniae coli, which run the length of almost all the large bowel. It is the muscular tone of these strips that gives the colon its familiar pleated appearance, gathering it up into pouches called 'haustra'.

The submucous layer

This layer comprises loose connective tissue, within which are a large number of blood vessels and lymphoid tissue.

The mucous layer

The types of cell found within the mucous layer are related to the degree of wear and tear to which each particular area of the large bowel is subject. Columnar epithelial cells and mucus-producing goblet cells are found in the colon and upper part of the rectum. The anal canal, which may be subject to a larger degree of wear and tear, has a mucous layer consisting of non-keratinized stratified squamous epithelium.

Nervous control

The nervous control of the colon, anorectum and pelvic floor is not fully understood. The hypothalamus and medulla oblongata are the main areas of the brain which coordinate the passage of faeces through the colon. Amongst other functions, the hypothalamus is involved in controlling the autonomic nervous system. The medulla oblongata, continuous with the spinal cord, is involved in autonomic reflex activity.

Most of the activities which take place in the colon are not under voluntary control. Generally, the colon is insensitive, so that the person does not have conscious awareness of physiological activity within the colon. The rectum and pelvic floor, however, do contain sensory nerve endings which are stimulated by stretch. It has also been shown that sensory nerve endings in the anal canal are stimulated by pain, touch and temperature; they can distinguish between stool and flatus.

Different nerves supply different parts of the large bowel. Because the colon is made up of smooth involuntary muscle fibres, it is supplied by the autonomic nervous system, which is part of the peripheral nervous system. The autonomic nervous system is divided into the sympathetic and the parasympathetic systems. Generally, sympathetic nerves prepare the body for excitement or danger, whereas parasympathetic nerves 'calm things down'. Working together, these nerves maintain the body's nervous harmony.

Parasympathetic motor innervation of the ascending colon and approximately half of the transverse colon occurs via the vagus nerve (the 10th cranial nerve). This nerve arises from sacral nerve roots S2, S3 and S4. Parasympathetic motor innervation of the rest of the transverse colon, the descending colon, the sigmoid colon, the rectum and the anal canal mainly occurs via the sacral nerves, arising from the sacral nerve roots S2, S3 and S4. It is mostly involved in contracting the colon.

Sympathetic motor innervation of the colon and rectum mainly occurs via the lumbar colonic and hypogastric nerves. Both of these nerves are principally involved in reducing muscle contractions. Parasympathetic motor control of the internal anal sphincter is thought to occur mostly via sacral nerve segments S2, S3 and S4. Sympathetic motor control occurs via the hypogastric network of nerves.

Motor and sensory somatic innervation of the external anal sphincter is thought to occur via the pudendal nerve, arising from sacral nerve roots S2, S3 and S4.

Blood supply to the large bowel

The main sources of oxygenated blood to the large bowel are the superior and inferior mesenteric arteries. The superior and inferior mesenteric veins carry deoxygenated blood from the large bowel, eventually joining the portal vein.

Musculature of the pelvic floor

The pelvic floor plays an important role in the maintenance of faecal continence and successful defecation (Fig. 7.2).

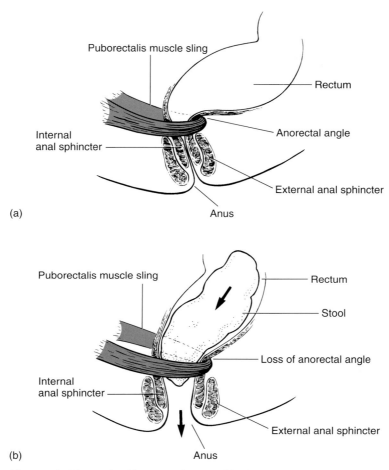

Figure 7.2 The anal sphincter mechanism: (a) with the rectum empty, and (b) during defecation.

The pelvic floor consists of three main layers. For the purposes of faecal continence and defecation, the levator ani muscle – which makes up one layer of the pelvic floor – is of primary importance. In fact, to be more specific it is the puborectalis muscle that plays the major role. This muscle is one part of the levator ani muscle and stretches from the pubic bone to the rectum. This thick band of muscle is responsible for creating an angle, ranging from approximately 60–110° between the rectum and the upper anal canal. This angle is known as the 'anorectal' angle and is formed as a result of the rectum being pulled towards the pubic bone. As long as the angle remains below 110°, faeces in the rectum cannot pass into the anal canal; this is achieved by contraction of the puborectalis muscle. Relaxation of the muscle results in an increase in the anorectal angle, thereby allowing the easy passage of faecal contents from the rectum into the anal canal. If the angle did not increase, the person would experience great difficulty when attempting to defecate, particularly with larger, harder stools. There are individuals with specific problems of this nature, and these will be discussed later.

DEFECATION
Awareness of the need

In order to control the opening of the bowel, it is necessary to be aware of the need. This conscious awareness occurs via sensory pathways, when faeces move from the sigmoid colon into the rectum, thus expanding it. Lack of awareness as a result of impaired feeling in the rectum, however, does not necessarily mean that an individual will suffer from faecal incontinence.

Early awareness is a very individual factor since the rectum of one person may expand more than that of another before there is awareness of the need to defecate.

As the rectum expands, the internal anal sphincter relaxes, thus reducing anal pressure. This is known as the *inhibitory reflex*. It is at this point that the individual becomes aware that something is in the rectum. Finely tuned nerve endings inform the cortical centre whether the stool is solid or liquid, or whether it is just flatus. As the rectum becomes accustomed to its new size, it no longer inhibits the contraction of the internal sphincter, and the sphincter is able to return to its contracted state, thus restoring anal pressure. When this happens the external anal sphincter contracts, thus closing the anus. The puborectalis muscle also contracts, decreasing the anorectal angle. This is known as the *inflation reflex* (Fig. 7.3).

How to 'go' at a convenient time

Successful defecation relies on several mechanisms. As long as the anal sphincters maintain a higher pressure within the rectum than within the anal canal, it is possible to defecate effectively. It is the internal sphincter that is mainly responsible for exerting this pressure. When it is convenient to defecate, and the individual is sitting comfortably, the pressure within the rectum rises. This rise in pressure is brought about by a rise in abdominal pressure which occurs due to muscular contraction of the diaphragm and abdominal wall. The pressures exerted by the internal and external sphincters decrease. This mechanism is important, as rectal pressure must be higher than anal pressure for defecation to be effective. The pelvic floor descends as a result of the relaxation of the puborectalis muscle. Relaxation of this muscle increases the anorectal angle and allows faeces to pass more easily into the anal canal (Fig. 7.4).

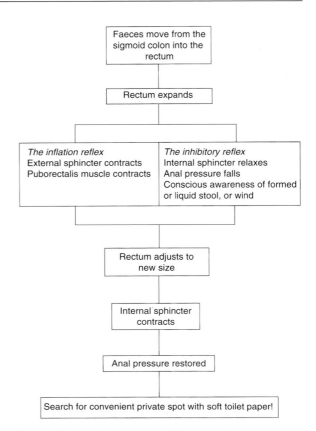

Figure 7.3   How to know when it is time to 'go'.

Throughout the procedure the body's posture is extremely important as the downward force exerted by the abdominal muscles helps expel the faeces, by pushing the walls of the rectum and sigmoid colon inwards (known as the Valsalva manoeuvre). Posture will be discussed again later.

How not to 'go' at an inconvenient time

No doubt most people have been in this situation at some time. The pain, nausea, sweating and general feelings of anxiety that can sometimes accompany the 'unwanted call to stool' may be an experience that would rather be forgotten. Of course, there are occasions when it may be absolutely necessary to ignore the urge to defecate and the rectum and anal canal cope very well with such occasions. The external anal sphincter,

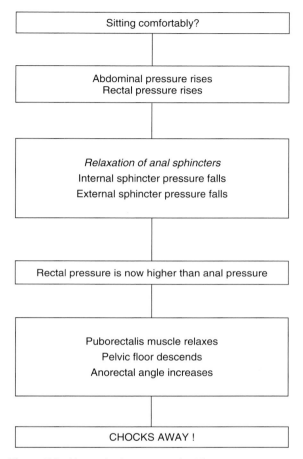

Figure 7.4 How to 'go' at a convenient time.

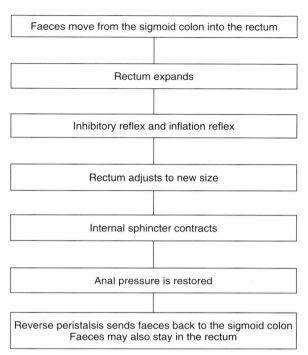

Figure 7.5 How not to 'go' at an inconvenient time.

normally relaxed during defecation, contracts and the anal pressure rises. Rectal pressure falls and the puborectalis muscle contracts, pulling the rectum back towards the pubic bone, thus reducing the anorectal angle (Fig. 7.5). Over a prolonged period of time, if the call to stool is ignored too frequently, constipation may result. This will be discussed later.

Flatus

Before the advent of modern medical models, Ayurvedi medicine – an ancient Indian theory related to disease – recognized health as a balance between phlegm, bile and flatulence. One may argue that, far from being healthy, the flatulent fellow is often uncomfortable and unpopular.

Excessive flatus or wind may accompany some bowel disorders. Even under normal circumstances flatus can be a very embarrassing problem, but if the sufferer has no control over flatus they may become completely socially isolated. There are no hard and fast rules concerning the amount of wind passed – it varies between 200 ml and 2400 ml daily, with between 25 and 100 ml being passed on each occasion.

Flatus mainly occurs owing to the activity of the bacteria which help to speed up the chemical changes required to produce faeces. This fermentation process generates gaseous substances, namely carbon dioxide, nitrogen, hydrogen and methane. Flatus also occurs as a result of swallowing air whilst eating. Some sufferers of irritable bowel syndrome have been found to eat their food very quickly, and gulp air as they eat.

The type of food eaten can also affect the 'wind status'. Eating small, regular meals and avoiding such foods as onions, dairy products and carbonated drinks can help. Some herbal remedies may be helpful (see below).

A herbal remedy for excessive flatus
One herbal remedy consists of an equal mixture of fennel seeds, anise seeds and caraway seeds, crushed and put into boiling water. The mixture should be left for 10 minutes and then taken before a meal. Peppermint and ginger teas may also be helpful (Gosling 1985).

CAUSES OF CONSTIPATION

Constipation is a symptom, not a disease. As with any symptom, constipation should be thoroughly investigated. It may cause a great deal of physical and psychological distress to individuals and their families.

Some of the causes of constipation are easily identified by reassessing certain aspects of the individual's lifestyle, while other causes are more complex. At times it may be difficult to discern whether the *apparent* causes of constipation are *actual* causes, or whether they are the *consequences* of constipation. One thing is certain, however: everyone, regardless of age or lifestyle, is potentially vulnerable to constipation and the misery it can bring.

There are situations when it can be anticipated that constipation will occur. Most people know how their own 'body clock' ticks and how, sometimes, even subtle changes in a routine may disrupt the bowel habit (e.g. going abroad for a holiday). Dietary and time changes which accompany foreign travel, together with the general change of routine can often affect people's normal bowel habits.

The part played by the environment, and the facilities available to assist healthy defecation, cannot be underestimated. There are few people who can say that they feel comfortable defecating in a public toilet, or even at a friend's house. Not only is there the worry of making noises when defecation takes place, there is also the worry of odour. The amount of time spent in the toilet, and the odours left behind, clearly point the finger. Of course, different people deal with these problems in their own way, but it is hardly surprising that nature's call can often be ignored until a

---

Box 7.3 Causes of constipation

- Bowel blues — Depression and constipation
- Coming when you are called — Ignoring the 'call to stool'
- Dietary disasters — Lack of dietary fibre
- Hormonal happenings — Pregnancy, childbirth and the puerperium
  Hypothyroidism
  Hyperparathyroidism
  Addison's disease
  Diabetes mellitus
- Motionless motions — Mobility and constipation
- Pharmacological facts — Medication and constipation
- Suitable surroundings — The environment and constipation
- Surgical side-effects — The effects of surgery of the bowel
- The bothersome bowel — Tumours
  Diverticular disease
  Irritable bowel syndrome
  Haemorrhoids
  Megacolon and megarectum
  Slow-transit constipation
  Normal-transit constipation
  Rectal prolapse
  Rectocele
- The neurological niche — Parkinson's disease
  Multiple sclerosis
  Cerebrovascular accident
  Senile dementia
  Spinal injury
- The retired rectum — Constipation in old age

---

pleasantly private toilet with a lockable door is found, with no other human beings in close proximity. Soft toilet paper may also be an important part of the equation!

Because the causes of constipation are many and varied, for ease of reference they will be discussed in alphabetical order. Box 7.3 can be used as an index.

Bowel blues: depression and constipation

One of the difficulties with constipation in association with a psychiatric disorder is in identifying whether the disorder causes constipation, or whether the bowel problem is a consequence of the disorder. People suffering from depression feel varying degrees of hopelessness and despair. Many are unable to concentrate and lose interest in life. They may lose their appetite and take little interest in exercise or looking after themselves. The call to stool may be neglected. Such changes may cause a constipation problem or exacerbate an existing one. Tricyclic and monoamine oxidase inhibiting antidepressants may increase the problem, owing to the anticholinergic effect reducing tone and peristalsis within the large colon.

Coming when you are called: ignoring the 'call to stool'

There may be times when it is necessary to ignore the fact that the bowel needs to be 'opened'. This is done by voluntarily contracting the external anal sphincter. In turn, this creates a fall in intrarectal pressure and reverse peristalsis may push faeces back into the sigmoid colon. Faeces may also stay in the rectum. As water continues to be reabsorbed, faeces dry out and thus become more difficult to pass. Longer, more difficult and possibly painful defecation follows. Because of this the individual may be reluctant to defecate and the situation worsens. Expansion of the rectum continues, and as the rectum becomes accustomed to the accommodation of larger quantities of faeces, the feeling of wanting to defecate becomes less frequent. Therefore, the individual goes to the toilet less frequently and constipation may follow.

Dietary disasters: lack of dietary fibre

During eating or after eating a meal the peristaltic action within the colon increases. Lack of fibre in the diet can cause constipation. Since the 16th century bran has been used to treat constipation. However, the benefits of fibre on bowel health were positively identified through studies demonstrating that bowel diseases such as carcinoma and symptoms such as constipation are rare in Africa. Africans enjoy foods such as maize and root crops, all of which provide a diet rich in fibre. Initially, dietary fibre was referred to as 'the skeletal remains of plant tissues'. This definition was then changed to 'dietary fibre' and describes the collective name given to the constituents of plant cell walls in food (Southgate 1992).

More recently fibre has been redefined as 'non-starch polysaccharides' (NSPs). (See Chapter 8 for details.)

Dietary fibre can be divided into *soluble* fibre (e.g. fruit, oats and barley), and *insoluble* fibre (e.g. wheat, vegetables and grains). This grouping has been derived from the fact that different sources of fibre dissolve in water at different rates. In the large colon, insoluble fibre tends to be more effective than soluble fibre.

How does fibre work?

Fibre has been shown to increase the weight and bulkiness of stools, thereby aiding defecation. Fibre made up of larger particles produces more bulky stools than an identical source of fibre made of smaller particles (Heller et al 1980).

It has also been recorded that pieces of plastic will do the same job as fibre in that they will also bulk the stool. In countries where fibre intake is high, daily stools can average in excess of 450 g, with an average transit time of 35 hours. However, in the United Kingdom, stools weigh an average of 153 g with transit times of between 18 and 144 hours (Burkitt et al 1972).

Some forms of fibre are broken down into simpler substances more readily than others. Fibres, such as starch, are digested in the small intestine. This is an enzymatic action. Other forms of fibre, such as cellulose, are partially digested in the large intestine. This is a bacterial action. The bacteria produce gas which becomes trapped in the stool, thereby adding bulkiness to the stool. Products such as wheat bran resist such breakdown and, therefore, due to their undigested state, add to the bulk of the stool. Bulky stools increase colonic movement, resulting in shorter transit times, and are consequently wetter, softer and easier to pass than harder stools.

However, other factors, such as mobility, also influence transit time. This is considered later in the chapter.

Who will benefit from taking more fibre?

The fibre story can be a difficult one to follow, and great care must be taken when advising patients to increase their fibre intake. Patients can easily be subjected to a complicated array of different advice. By contrast, simply being advised to 'up the fibre intake' by sprinkling bran on breakfast cereal and eating 'lots of fresh fruit and vegetables' may be too limited if little advice is given on how much fibre to take and what side-effects are likely to be experienced. It is perhaps for this reason that some people say that increasing the fibre in their diet either makes no difference or gives them unacceptable wind and abdominal pain.

There are circumstances where an increase in dietary fibre is not helpful. Donald et al (1985) demonstrated that high dietary fibre intake by elderly immobile patients led to faecal loading, a term used to describe a colon loaded with either soft or hard stool (Barrett 1993). Other studies have shown that increasing fibre in the diets of elderly immobile patients leads to an increase in faecal incontinence (Ardron & Main 1990), as softer faeces are more likely to leak than harder faeces (Barrett 1988).

Increasing dietary fibre in patients suffering from idiopathic slow-transit constipation may cause increased abdominal pain and bloating. The cause is thought to be the fact that faeces remain in the colon for longer periods. Therefore, owing to continued bacterial action, there is a large build-up of gas in the colon.

How much fibre is needed?

The recommended daily intake of fibre in Britain is 30 g (just over 1 oz). This does not sound much. However, considering that a slice of white bread contains only 0.8 g and that a person would need about 37 slices in order to meet the recommended daily intake, the task of achieving the recommended intake is, perhaps, a little more daunting. Figure 7.6 shows the fibre content of some foods commonly consumed.

It is estimated that in Britain daily fibre consumption is in the region of 24 g for men and 18 g for women, compared with over 100 g reportedly consumed daily in rural African populations (Southgate 1992). Younger women take less fibre than older women. There are also regional variations; for example the Scottish population takes

less fibre than people living in the North of England. In the 20th century there was a decline in fibre intake, mainly due to the amount of dairy products consumed, with less priority placed on foods such as potatoes.

As previously discussed, some forms of fibre are broken down into simpler substances more readily than others. For this reason, it is important to take a variety of different foods such as wholemeal bread, high-fibre cereals, potatoes and vegetables, as opposed to increasing bran intake alone. This will help ensure that individuals benefit not only from more satisfying defecation, but good general health as well.

Hormonal happenings

Pregnancy, childbirth and the puerperium

Hormonal changes take place during pregnancy. Oestrogen and progesterone levels rise in order to prepare the uterus for the foetus. It is thought that hormonal changes, particularly the rise in the level of progesterone, reduce smooth muscle tone in the large colon (Davis & Platz 1965). This may lead to slower transit times and faeces remaining in the large colon for a longer period.

Pregnancy may impose restrictions on normal exercise regimes, and in turn this may influence the movement of faeces into the rectum. Another contributory factor to constipation in pregnancy may be that in the later stages the colon is rather compressed by the weight and size of the gravid uterus, and the passage of faeces through the colon is hindered. Trauma caused during childbirth can sometimes result in problems with defecation. It is certainly recognized that trauma such as anal sphincter muscle damage and pudendal nerve damage can lead to the underreported symptom of faecal incontinence (Sultan et al 1993).

Hypothyroidism

Hypothyroidism, or myxoedema as it is commonly known, occurs due to a lack of the hormone thyroxine. The thyroid hormones T3 and T4 produced from the thyroid gland in the neck stimulate cellular oxygen consumption and metabolism.

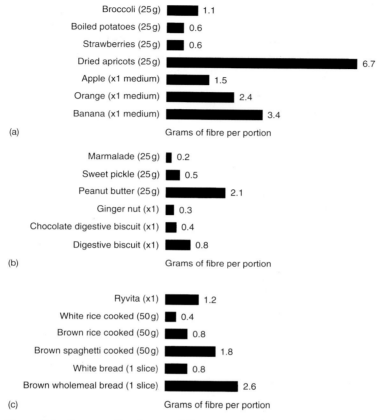

Figure 7.6 Focus on fibre (grams of fibre per portion): (a) fruit and vegetables, (b) biscuits and preserves, (c) bread, crispbread and pasta.

Any reduction in circulating levels of these hormones will result in reduced metabolism, including impairment in colonic movement.

Hyperparathyroidism

Hyperparathyroidism is due to an excess of parathormone, a hormone secreted by the parathyroid glands which are attached to the thyroid gland. The main function of parathormone is to regulate calcium and phosphorous levels in the blood. Normal calcium concentrations are essential in maintaining nerve and muscle responses. High levels of circulating calcium depress such responses, thereby diminishing muscular tone of the large colon.

Addison's disease

Addison's disease is caused by a deficiency in the hormonal steroid, cortisol. Because cortisol is important in the maintenance of blood sugar level, deficiency may cause lack of energy, electrolyte imbalance and a general slowing down of the metabolism.

Diabetes mellitus

Diabetes mellitus is caused by a deficiency or total absence of the hormone insulin. Insulin is synthesized in the pancreas and is essential for effective transport of glucose from the blood to the body cells. Long-standing high levels of circulating blood glucose damage nerves and blood vessels.

It is not uncommon for diabetic patients to suffer from neuropathy relating to the gastrointestinal tract. Such side-effects as constipation, diarrhoea and faecal incontinence may occur. It is thought that diabetic patients presenting with faecal incontinence suffer from impaired rectal sensation reflex, where the external anal sphincter fails to contract in response to rectal distension. Either the inflation reflex is not present at all, or gross rectal distension is required before the reflex occurs (Wald & Tunuguntla 1984).

Motionless motions: mobility and constipation

The onward movement of faeces into the rectum has been shown to be influenced by physical activity (Holdstock et al 1970). Immobility is one of the most common causes of constipation in the elderly, and in those individuals affected by diseases which threaten mobility such as strokes, multiple sclerosis or spinal injuries.

Exercise produces change in abdominal pressure by relaxing and contracting the abdominal muscles and diaphragm. Exercise also improves the appetite and the consumption of food, and is recognized as influencing the movement of faeces into the rectum. It is not understood how much exercise is needed before significant improvements occur. One study identified that an hour's worth of exercise such as jogging produced significantly shorter gut transit times (Oettle 1991). Unfortunately, such an exercise regime is not practical for many individuals. Because of mobility problems, many rely on others to take them to the toilet and when they need to 'go' may or may not coincide with when they are taken. Lack of exercise and the inability to respond each time to the call to stool may result in constipation.

Pharmacological facts: medication and constipation

'I do not want two diseases – one nature made, one doctor made.'

Napoleon Bonaparte, 1820

The therapeutic action of certain prescribed medications may cause constipation. This can cause great distress for patients who, on the one hand, are benefiting positively from their treatment and yet, on the other, are struggling with such a troublesome side-effect. It is important to have a basic knowledge of the commonly used drugs likely to cause constipation in order that the most appropriate advice can be given. An overview of these drugs is given below. However, for further information please refer also to Chapter 8.

Anticholinergics

Anticholinergic drugs reduce muscular spasm by blocking the nerve transmitter acetylcholine. Patients presenting with an unstable bladder often benefit from the controlled use of an anticholinergic; but as well as reducing the troublesome urinary symptoms of frequency and urgency, this also reduces tone and peristalsis within the large colon. As a result of this smooth muscle relaxation, transit time is prolonged. For this reason these drugs may be useful in the treatment of colitis, but may also cause constipation. In addition there is a possibility of worsening any urinary symptoms, by adding pressure on the bladder from a loaded rectum.

Opiates

Opiate analgesics such as morphine, and derivatives such as codeine and pethidine, are widely used for pain control. Opiates cause contraction of the smooth muscle of the large colon, and curtail peristaltic action. This is because the colon is in a state of continuous muscular contraction, as opposed to intermittent contraction. Transit time is therefore reduced, and constipation may follow.

Antidepressants

Antidepressant drugs help relieve the symptoms of depression, and may be divided into two main groups: tricyclic antidepressants, such as imipramine and amitriptyline, and monoamine oxidase inhibitors (MAOIs). Antidepressants in the tricyclic group are more commonly used than those in the MAOI group, but both groups may cause constipation owing to their anticholinergic effect, resulting in a relaxation of smooth muscle and a reduction in transit time.

Diuretics

Diuretics promote increased loss of salt and water from the body. They increase urine production, primarily by preventing the reabsorption of sodium and, therefore, water (the osmotic principle). Despite the fact that large amounts of water are reabsorbed from faeces as they pass through the large colon, 60–70% of the total weight of faeces still consists of water. When individuals are taking diuretics the general 'drying' effect and possible electrolyte imbalance may cause the stool to become drier, harder and more difficult to pass.

Iron supplements

The specific effects of iron on the intestine are still not certain. A slight overdose, and sometimes even an ordinary dose, can cause constipation or diarrhoea, accompanied by nausea and abdominal pain. A change in the iron compound prescribed may sometimes relieve these side-effects.

Antacids

Magnesium compounds used as antacids tend to cause diarrhoea. They are therefore also used as laxatives. Other compounds used in antacids, such as calcium carbonate and aluminium hydroxide, tend to constipate. They have an osmotic effect, drawing water out of the stool making it smaller, harder and more difficult to pass.

Suitable surroundings: the environment and constipation

Despite the many anecdotes about toilet facilities and their effect on the bowels, is it safe to assume that the environment is a definite contributing factor to bowel problems? There is evidence to suggest that overcrowding and access to toilets are related to the degree of urinary and faecal incontinence experienced by the elderly and people with a learning disability. Indeed some studies have indicated that if improvements to living conditions are made, continence can improve (Shrubsole & Smith 1984).

Surgical side-effects

Unfortunately, undergoing surgery of any kind may disrupt the bowel routine. Food and fluid intake are often restricted, as well as mobility. The environment may change and patients may find themselves without the private facilities to which they are accustomed. The anaesthetic not only sends patients to sleep, but sends their colon to sleep as well! Anaesthetics relax the muscular walls of the colon, thereby reducing the muscular contractions which move faeces along the colon. Following abdominal surgery, scar tissue formation and adhesions can result, causing pain and obstruction. Local parasympathetic nerve damage can occur when women undergo operations such as hysterectomy. This may result in severe difficulty when trying to empty the bowel. Pre- and postoperative analgesic medication may also constipate patients.

The bothersome bowel

Because the large colon is responsible for transporting faeces from the inside to the outside, any disorder which interferes with this process will produce symptoms. Some problems are idiopathic in origin (that is, of unknown cause), others are the consequences of recognizable disease processes.

Tumours

The second most common carcinoma in the UK is that of the colon. Whether benign or malignant, any tumour has the potential to hinder the passage of faeces along the colon, or to obstruct it completely. Generally, the longer faeces remain in the colon, the harder they become and the more difficult they are to pass. Intermittent constipation with diarrhoea may occur.

Diverticular disease

Diverticular disease occurs as a result of weakness within the mucosal wall of the large colon.

This weakness results in small pouches developing within the walls. The muscular contractions of the colon create a rise in pressure, which is useful when bulky faeces need to be propelled along the length of the colon. However, without such bulk this pressure exerts a force against the wall of the colon, pushing it outwards. Constipation may occur as a result of muscular spasm interfering with the normal muscular contractions of the colon, and therefore affecting the movement of faeces. Diarrhoea and pain are also common.

Irritable bowel syndrome

It has been estimated that 50–70% of referrals to gastroenterological outpatient departments in Britain are for people suffering from irritable bowel syndrome, and 500 new referrals are made each week (Digestive Disorders 2002). Irritable bowel syndrome (IBS) affects a third of the population at some time or other and about one in ten people suffer from symptoms bad enough to go to the doctor (IBS Network 1991). The cause is still not fully understood, but symptoms may include the following:

• Abdominal pain and spasm
• Diarrhoea
• Constipation
• Feeling bloated; rumbling noises; flatus
• Urgency to defaecate
• A feeling of incomplete bowel evacuation
• Faecal incontinence
• Pain in lower rectum
• Nausea
• Belching and vomiting.

The prevalence of IBS is about the same in both males and females; however, more females tend to seek medical help. It commonly starts between 15 and 40 years of age, but may occur at any time. Symptoms differ between patients and may vary from time to time but the above mentioned symptoms will be present in most cases.

IBS is linked to stress and diet. Attacks of this condition are often triggered by an event such as a bereavement, or feeling overworked and undervalued, arguments, a car accident, etc. Some people seem to react to these incidents with their bowels! Psychological factors which might have occurred in the past influence this condition (e.g. unhappy childhood) and ongoing emotional tension is the commonest reason for bowel sensitivity. When the gut is sensitive, anything passing through will give rise to symptoms, hence the symptoms seem to be caused by so many different foods. It is difficult to identify which particular food is causing the problem as it is not so much the food but the sensitive gut that is simply at fault. Often this can relate to an emotional state that has happened but IBS is *not* psychological, it is real. Excellent patient leaflets and information on all digestive disorders can be found on the Web at http://www.digestivedisorders.org.uk.

There is ongoing research into the cause of IBS but meanwhile the treatments available include: relief of anxiety states; support for coping mechanisms; dietary changes and lifestyles; understanding of IBS; elimination of other bowel dysfunctions (e.g. cancer). Some patients respond to drug therapy as in control of constipation and diarrhoea but this should not be the long-term goal. Emotional support is paramount.

Irritable bowel syndrome is *not*:

• hereditary, but other members of the family may have similar symptoms
• 'all in the mind' when tests results are normal
• a food allergy even though some patients may have certain food intolerance
• an infection
• bowel inflammation as in ulcerative colitis or Crohn's disease
• caused by cancer, ulcers, gallstones or other serious digestive diseases but sometimes these conditions have symptoms similar to IBS.

Haemorrhoids

A haemorrhoid is the term used to describe a swelling formed by the haemorrhoidal veins within the anal canal. The haemorrhoid may or may not be visible; it may cause pain, particularly on defecation, when it sometimes bleeds. There is evidence to suggest that constipation causes haemorrhoids (Gibbons et al 1988), possibly owing to the destruction of venous drainage by hard stools.

Unfortunately a vicious circle may develop, whereby pain on defecation encourages the sufferer to ignore the call to stool because defecation is associated with pain and best avoided. This may then cause constipation.

Megacolon and megarectum

Megacolon and megarectum are terms used to describe gross enlargement of the colon, the cause of which is not fully understood. Constipation, pain and bloating are characteristic symptoms, as faeces continue to build up in the dilated portion of colon. Colonic dilation is also characteristic of the condition Hirschsprung's disease which can affect both children and adults. In this condition, a characteristic narrowing of the colon occurs above the dilated portion.

Slow-transit constipation

Slow-transit constipation is the name given to a condition characterized by the abnormally slow movement of faeces through the colon, particularly the transverse, descending and sigmoid colon. It presents mainly as a problem in young women. Depending on the severity of the problem, sufferers may have their bowels open between only once weekly and once every 4 weeks. The cause of this problem is not yet fully understood, but it is thought that colonic nerve damage or a condition known as *anismus* may be significant. The latter is characterized by inappropriate pelvic floor contractions during defecation. Defecation is difficult and sufferers will often strain considerably. It is believed that there may also be a strong psychological link to the cause of slow-transit constipation (Gattuso & Kamm 1993).

Normal-transit constipation

It is not only people with 'slow' colons who suffer from constipation; those with 'normal' transit times may also experience difficulties. As with slow-transit constipation, sufferers of normal-transit constipation are mainly female. They experience difficulty in emptying the bowel completely and will often strain considerably.

The cause is thought to be associated with nerve damage.

Interestingly, Gattuso & Kamm (1993) identified that up to half of sufferers with constipation of unknown origin may have suffered some kind of bereavement, or sexual, physical or emotional abuse in childhood.

Rectal prolapse

Rectal prolapse is the term used to describe descent of the rectum. When the prolapse is complete the lower part of the rectum may not distend as it does not fill with faeces. This is due to intussusception, whereby one part of the bowel descends into another part below. The sufferer may experience difficulty in completely emptying the bowel, often straining at stool.

Rectocele

Rectocele is the term used to describe the protrusion of the anterior rectal and posterior vaginal wall into the vagina. This protrusion forms a pouch in which faeces become trapped. The sufferer may experience difficulty in completely emptying the bowel, often straining at stool.

The neurological niche

Neurological disorders such as Parkinson's disease, multiple sclerosis, cerebrovascular accident and spinal injury may cause constipation (see also Chapter 11).

Parkinson's disease

Parkinson's disease is thought to occur as a result of degeneration of the corpus striatum of the brain. The corpus striatum is a basal ganglia, which is a mass of grey matter located in each cerebral hemisphere of the brain and it controls skeletal muscle contractions. Degeneration of the corpus striatum is believed to reduce levels of dopamine, a chemical essential in the transmission of some nerve impulses. The disease manifests itself in many ways, but the main contributory factors to constipation are mobility problems, treatment with anticholinergic drugs such as levodopa and trihexyphenidyl (benzhexol hydrochloride), difficulties in chewing and swallowing, and general neurological deterioration.

Multiple sclerosis

Multiple sclerosis (MS) occurs as a result of degeneration of the myelin sheath, although the precise cause is unknown. This sheath covers the larger axons, i.e. those nerve processes which convey impulses away from a cell. The sheath increases the speed at which an impulse may travel and protects the axon.

Constipation is a grossly underreported symptom in patients with MS: 39–68% of sufferers experience constipation or faecal incontinence (Carvana et al 1991). Pressure tests have identified decreased resting anal tone, decreased external anal sphincter pressures and abnormal rectal sensation (Anderson & Bradley 1976). Hinds et al (1990) suggested that constipation could possibly be an early presenting symptom of MS in non-diagnosed patients. They also reported that constipation was still more common in mobile and active patients with MS whose use of constipating medication was no more common than in the non-constipated controls. They concluded that factors other than immobility and medication may be responsible for causing constipation problems (see Chapter 11).

Cerebrovascular accident (CVA or stroke)

A stroke may result from an interruption in the blood supply of the brain. Brain cells starved of vital oxygenated blood are damaged. There are, of course, a host of problems caused by a stroke which can contribute to constipation. Many stroke sufferers present with mobility problems, swallowing difficulties upset their normal eating and drinking habits, and communication problems prevent them from responding to the call to stool because they are unable to say when they want to 'go'. The main problem is that of faecal loading.

Dementia

Dementia mainly affects the elderly population, and its cause is still not fully understood.

Abnormal proteins, known as senile plaques, have been found within the cell bodies of neurones and excessive amounts of aluminium have also been identified as a possible contributory factor. The side-effects of the disease are crippling: patients may suffer varying degrees of memory loss, confusion and irritability, failing to recognize themselves or those around them.

The main bowel-related problem for patients with dementia is that of faecal loading. It seems that many sufferers are treated with laxatives for a faecal impaction problem when in fact they may be loaded with soft stool as opposed to hard stool. Demented patients are often not aware of the call to stool and huge amounts of soft or hard stool may build up in the rectum. Remembering that the definition of constipation is excessive straining at stool, or the infrequent passage of stools, sufferers loaded with soft stool may still be constipated.

Spinal injuries

The symptoms experienced by the individual with spinal injuries will depend on where the spinal injury has occurred. Symptoms may range from impaired rectal sensation and external anal sphincter activity, to complete inhibition of the inflation and inhibitory reflexes, particularly if the sacral nerve roots S2, S3 and S4 have been damaged. Immobility and impaired squeeze pressure contribute to the constipation problem.

The retired rectum: constipation in old age

Constipation is a major cause of faecal incontinence in elderly people. It can affect the efficiency of the anorectal angle and rectal sensation. The main contributing factor to constipation in elderly people seems to be that of mobility (Donald et al 1985). Immobility at any age may contribute to a constipation problem, but elderly people are particularly at risk because of many of the other age-related disorders that threaten mobility (see Chapter 6).

Some studies have compared transit times of immobile elderly people in long-stay care against

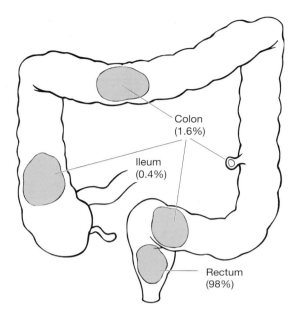

Colon
(1.6%)

Ileum
(0.4%)

Rectum
(98%)

Figure 7.7 Sites and frequency of faecal impactions.
Reproduced with permission from Dresden & Kratzer
(1959); © American Medical Association.

those of active independent elderly people
(Brocklehurst & Kahn 1969, Brocklehurst et al
1983). The main difference in transit times
appears to occur in the sigmoid colon and rectum, where the passage of faeces is shown to be
much slower in the immobile group. If the elderly person is forced to rely on someone else to
take them to the toilet, the call to stool may often
be neglected and faeces build up in the rectum.
Poor food and fluid intake may contribute to constipation in elderly people. Those struggling with
the effects of disorders such as Parkinson's disease and stroke may have difficulty in maintaining an adequate food and fluid intake, as well as
suffering the effects of immobility.

The main manifestation of constipation is that
of faecal loading. The rectum may be filled with a
large quantity of soft or hard stool. Leakage of
soft faeces may be mistaken for spurious diarrhoea. This is the leakage of liquid faeces around
hard impacted faeces, and occurs because hard
faeces irritate the lining of the colon causing it
to produce mucus which dissolves and liquefies
the bowel contents. Barrett (1988) has shown that

faecal incontinence is more likely to occur with
soft stool than with hard stool; hence great care
should be taken if laxatives are prescribed,
because softening the stool may cause faecal
incontinence. Figure 7.7 shows sites and frequency of faecal impactions.

BOWEL INVESTIGATIONS

It has been established that there are many causes
of constipation, some more complex than others.
For this reason, it is extremely important that the
actual cause be identified. A treatment plan may
then be implemented, based on what is known,
not on what is assumed to be known. Many
patients find the thought of any kind of bowel
investigation overwhelming and frightening.
Clear accurate information given in a supportive
manner can enhance confidence about undergoing such intimate procedures. Patients can then
see such investigations as being an important part
of their overall care, contributing to their welfare
as opposed to hindering it.

There are a number of tests available to help
diagnose the various causes of constipation.
Investigatory techniques are continually updated
as more is known about the physiology of defecation. Some patients may only require a careful history to be taken, followed by a general physical
examination of the back passage, both digitally
and with a sigmoidoscope, and an examination of
the abdomen.

Taking a history

Time is the key to history taking. This may sound
idealistic, but a great deal of information can be
learned by giving the patient time to talk about
what he or she perceives as the problem. It takes
time to allow someone to gain confidence in talking openly about such a basic human function – a
function that takes place behind closed doors and
is rarely talked about. Time also gives the individual the opportunity to establish his or her
own vocabulary with reference to colonic function and the act of defecation.

Most primary and secondary care Trusts have
a bowel policy which will aim to promote bowel

continence and improve the quality of life for persons suffering bowel dysfunction (Chelvanayagam & Norton 2000). The main objective is to ensure that all persons with bowel problems have a full assessment and an accepted plan of action and that the outcomes of treatment are measurable. This provides an audit tool to demonstrate how effective treatment is and the ways in which quality of life has been improved. It will also highlight the prevalence of bowel disorders in any one Trust (Norton & Chelvanayagam 2000).

The history should include the following:

- Normal defecation habits: what happens when the patient wants to defecate? What happens when the patient does defecate? Is there any flatus, abdominal bloating or anorectal pain?
- Date of onset: has the patient always been constipated?
- Description of stools passed using the Bristol Stool Form Scale (see below).
- Description of daily food and fluid intake.
- Description of sensation on defecation: pain, urgency, straining?
- Recent changes in environment/lifestyle.
- History of past surgery: obstetric and general.
- Any childhood bereavement? Any sexual or physical abuse? Although these require extremely delicate handling, the psychological history related to constipation is as important as the physical one.
- Medications taken: including any over-the-counter preparations, and homeopathic or herbal remedies.

Bowel care pathways

In a similar way to urinary care pathways (Chapter 2), care pathways for the bowel have been developed (Bayliss 2000). It is the same format as for urinary care where a basic first level assessment must be completed by nurses who have been trained to use the pathway. In the community this training programme has been widely available and many Trusts use it alongside their own policies and guidelines. The first level assessment is basic knowledge of what should be happening and patients need to complete a

bowel diary for at least 1 week (longer if necessary). Many patients find it difficult to explain the type and consistency of their stools and so the Bristol Stool Form Scale (Heaton et al 1992) assists by grading the type of stool as seen in Figure 7.8.

It is essential that the first level assessment includes a bowel habit diary (Fig. 7.9) and a 1-week recording of dietary intake. These two records form the basis of making a diagnosis and along with the above 'history taking' completes the verbal assessment.

Examination

Many people consider a rectal examination to be one of the most uncomfortable and undignified experiences they will ever have to endure. However, they should be informed that an abdominal and rectal examination may be necessary. Distension, pain and tenderness on abdominal examination may indicate the presence of gas, fluid or an obstruction of some kind. Rectal examination may reveal such problems as faecal impaction, a tumour, perineal descent or a rectocele. For practical guidelines on how to perform a digital rectal examination (DRE) refer to Addison (1999). There are also guidelines from the Royal College of Nursing on *Digital Rectal Examination and Manual Removal of Faeces* (1999).

It is often not possible to 'reveal all' by abdominal palpation and digital rectal examination alone. An individual may have to undergo an endoscopic examination – a sigmoidoscopy or proctoscopy. For any investigation of this nature the colon needs to be clear of faeces. Because a sigmoidoscopy is an examination of the anal canal, rectum and sigmoid colon only, a local enema is usually all that is required. Patients may be asked to restrict fibre intake beforehand.

During the procedure the person is asked either to kneel on all fours, which can be rather undignified, or to lie on their left side with knees bent upwards. Sigmoidoscopy examination involves the passing of a rigid, hollow tube into the anorectum. This tube has a light on the end, and if necessary air may be pumped through it to distend the colon. This is an uncomfortable procedure, but it can be very helpful in assessing rectal stability and

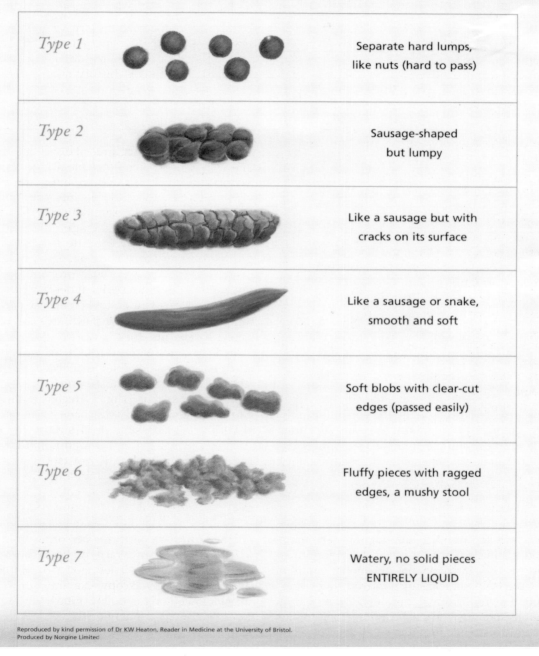

THE BRISTOL STOOL FORM SCALE

Type 1		Separate hard lumps, like nuts (hard to pass)
Type 2		Sausage-shaped but lumpy
Type 3		Like a sausage but with cracks on its surface
Type 4		Like a sausage or snake, smooth and soft
Type 5		Soft blobs with clear-cut edges (passed easily)
Type 6		Fluffy pieces with ragged edges, a mushy stool
Type 7		Watery, no solid pieces ENTIRELY LIQUID

Reproduced by kind permission of Dr KW Heaton, Reader in Medicine at the University of Bristol.
Produced by Norgine Limited

Figure 7.8   The Bristol Stool Form Scale. Reproduced by kind permission of Norgine Ltd from Heaton et al (1992).

BOWEL HABIT DIARY

Record accurately for 7 days

Name:

Date/Time	Bristol stool type	Did you feel the urge to go?		Accident or soiling	Comments e.g. laxative/fluids
		YES	NO		

Figure 7.9 The bowel habit diary.

the nature of any reported anorectal pain. More severe problems of sudden onset may require further investigations.

Radiography

X-rays are useful in assessing the general 'health' of the colon and in identifying any disorder that may affect colonic function, such as intestinal obstruction, megacolon or inflammatory bowel disease. A barium enema and plain abdominal films of the colon are the main X-rays undertaken.

The patient is required to take a stimulant laxative such as sodium picosulfate the day before a barium enema in order to clear the colon completely. This laxative increases colonic motility and decreases water absorption from the colon. Its action is rapid and severe and it can cause abdominal cramps and dehydration. Food intake is usually restricted but fluids should be consumed freely. In the X-ray department, the patient will be given an enema of barium, and asked to

turn in differing positions in order to coat the colon. X-rays are then taken as the patient is turned on a moving couch. After expelling as much barium as possible, further X-rays may be required. As with a sigmoidoscopy, the procedure is uncomfortable, particularly when air is inserted into the colon. Because of the constipating effects of barium and possible dehydration due to the sodium picosulfate, it is important to remind patients to drink extra fluid in order to avoid such side-effects.

Colonic transit-time studies

These studies are performed in order to identify whether or not there is a prolonged colonic transit time. Three days prior to the procedure, all laxatives are stopped. Three radiopaque markers are swallowed on each of the 3 days leading up to the procedure. Each set of markers is a different shape, and traces the 'journey' made from the mouth to anus, giving an indication of the time taken (Barrett et al 1990).

Manometry

As well as investigating the structure of the colon, its function may also need to be assessed. Manometric tests measure the effectiveness and strength of the anal sphincters, together with the degree of sensation felt within the rectum. The test usually takes approximately 30 minutes and involves passing a soft plastic tube, which resembles a latex Foley catheter, into the rectum. When the balloon is distended, it will demonstrate the effectiveness of rectal contraction and expansion, relaxation of the internal anal sphincter and contraction of the external anal sphincter (the inhibitory and inflation reflexes). The individual will then be asked to pass the balloon out as if it were a stool, and the catheter is gradually pulled out as the pressures are measured.

Balloon capacity and compliance

This test evaluates how well the rectum expands and contracts in response to the entry of faeces. It usually takes approximately 45 minutes and involves the passing of a deflated balloon into the rectum, which is then inflated with air or water. The patient is asked to indicate when he or she first feels the balloon in the rectum, when the urge to defecate is felt, and when further rectal distension can no longer be tolerated.

Balloon expulsion

This test evaluates the degree of puborectalis muscle relaxation during defecation. Relaxation of this muscle results in an increase in the anorectal angle, thereby allowing the easy passage of faecal contents from the rectum into the anal canal.

Electromyography

An electromyogram (EMG) records electrical activity within muscles. This test is used to identify and measure any pelvic floor muscle damage. Surface needle electrodes or an intra-anal plug are placed in selected areas of the external anal sphincter and puborectalis muscle. When the muscle contracts, electrical activity is measured. It can be an extremely uncomfortable test, but gives a good indication of whether or not pelvic floor damage is causing or contributing to a constipation problem. Alternative ways of measuring the electrical activity which are less uncomfortable are by using surface adhesive electrodes or an anal probe (see also Chapter 3).

Some centres measure electrical activity continuously over a 24-hour period, which gives an extremely reliable and detailed picture.

BIOFEEDBACK FOR FUNCTIONAL BOWEL DISORDERS

Constipation is a common problem that may affect up to 20% of the adult population at one time or another (Drossman et al 1993a). Men and women of all ages are affected, and as many as one in ten women will experience constipation (Heaton & Cripps 1993).

Idiopathic constipation can be described as an infrequent or incomplete evacuation not caused by disease or medication. Constipation has many possible predisposing factors such as psychological issues, pregnancy and childbirth, change in routine, abdominal surgery and old age.

Using the Rome II criteria (Thompson et al 1999) to diagnose constipation, two or more of the following must be present for at least 12 weeks, which need not be consecutive, in the preceding 12 months:

- Straining for >25% of defecations
- Lumpy and/or hard stools in >25% of defecations
- A sensation of incomplete evacuation in >25% of defecations
- Sensation of anorectal obstruction/blockage in >25% of defecations
- Manual maneouvres to facilitate >25% of defecations (e.g. digital evacuation, support of the pelvic floor)
- Fewer than three defecations/week.

Biofeedback therapy is useful where patients are resistant to laxatives and require increasingly larger doses.

The results of surgery for bowel disorders are variable. Kamm et al (1988) looked at 44 patients following colectomy: 22 patients had a normal bowel frequency, 17 had diarrhoea and five had persistent or recurrent constipation. Two-thirds of patients still experienced abdominal pain, and some still required laxatives. As a result, biofeedback has become a first-line treatment for constiaption (Storrie 1997). About two-thirds of patients benefit from biofeedback therapy, and this is maintained on long-term follow-up (Chiotakakou-Faliakou et al 1998).

Functional abnormalities

Biofeedback therapy can be used to treat a variety of evacuation disorders. The functional group includes:

- idiopathic constipation
- constipation in irritable bowel syndrome.

Idiopathic constipation

Patients with constipation may experience a number of symptoms such as a decrease in bowel actions, incomplete evacuation, straining at stool, bloating and pain.

Constipation in irritable bowel syndrome

Irritable bowel syndrome can cause alternating constipation and diarrhoea which can cause unpredictable and unwanted symptoms. It is very difficult to find a cause for IBS but factors such as stress and/or tension, certain food and drink, psychological problems, or an erratic lifestyle can influence the way the gut functions. Symptoms include abdominal pain and spasms, bloating and increased wind, diarrhoea and/or constipation. One or all of the above may be experienced. It is important for patients to know they don't have a disease, but a collection of symptoms as indicated earlier.

Physical or structural abnormalities

Other disorders can be classed as physical or structural abnormalities:

- solitary rectal ulcer syndrome
- rectal prolapse
- rectocele

- ileoanal pouch
- megarectum/megacolon.

Solitary rectal ulcer syndrome

Solitary rectal ulcer syndrome is a condition where there is a benign ulceration of the rectum. It is a relatively uncommon condition. The cause is unknown but these patients seem to have a behavioural disorder (Vaizey et al 1997). Excessive straining, prolonged periods of time spent in the toilet, digitating per rectum to extract stool and constipation may be contributory factors.

Commonly patients experience a frequent urge to defecate and make repeated attempts to open their bowels. Often the evacuation feels incomplete so they strain excessively and digitate to aid evacuation. The more attempts that are made to defecate, the more the ulcer is aggravated. Blood and mucus are often passed with stool, or on their own with excessive straining. The ulcer gives a 'false' urge and a sensation of incomplete evacuation. Biofeedback therapy can reduce the attempts of defecation and improve symptoms (Vaizey et al 1997).

Rectal prolapse

Rectal prolapses are usually caused by excessive straining. A rectal prolapse can either refer to the prolapse of the rectal lining (intussusception) or a complete prolapse of the rectum. This can be attributed to muscle weakness, childbirth and chronic straining during defecation. This condition can result in symptoms such as difficult evacuation, perineal heaviness and incomplete evacuation. This can lead to patients straining more which in turn can worsen the prolapse. Blood and mucus may be passed, and patients may experience incontinence. The prolapse may occur only when defecating or at other times.

Rectocele

Rectoceles may be caused by excessive or chronic straining, childbirth and/or ageing. Common symptoms include difficult defecation, incomplete evacuation and vaginal discomfort.

Such symptoms can lead to numerous attempts at trying to defecate. This increased straining can weaken the muscles further. The sensation of incomplete evacuation means increased straining which can exacerbate the rectocele and therefore worsen the problem. Often these women have to digitate vaginally or rectally or both to aid evacuation. Biofeedback therapy can help reduce the severity of these symptoms in some women (Mimura et al 2000).

Surgery may be required to repair a rectocele. Biofeedback therapy is a good way of re-educating the patient on how to use their defecatory muscles properly which will help them postoperatively.

Ileoanal pouch

Pouch emptying problems may be due to inability to utilize the correct defecatory muscles. This can lead to incomplete evacuation, pain in the pouch and abdomen, and trapped wind in the pouch.

Megarectum

Megarectum is where the rectum is grossly dilated. The colon, however, is usually of normal size. The condition often begins in childhood or adolescence. Symptoms of a megarectum include a delay in feeling rectal contents which can lead to faecal impaction, loss of normal reflexes causing soiling and diarrhoea due to the liquid stool passing around the hard stool in the rectum. Patients can achieve spontaneous and satisfactory bowel actions without laxatives following biofeedback therapy.

Megacolon

Megacolon is where the colon has been overstretched, and is wider and longer than a normal colon. The passage of waste through the megacolon will be slower than through a normal colon. The condition often begins in adulthood. Symptoms of a megacolon include abdominal pain and bloating, heartburn and no 'urge' to open the bowels.

Patterns of presentation

A diverse group of patients present to the biofeedback clinic. Some patients have been raped or sexually abused in the past which may

have caused their bowel disorder (Drossman 1993b). These people disassociate themselves from the pelvic area; they mentally cut themselves off from the waist down and therefore have problems with opening their bowels. Some people are very tense and find it hard to relax to open their bowels, others are too busy to go to the toilet and put off the urge so often they 'lose' this urge. There is a group of patients that have a dislike of the toilet. This may be from a childhood experience or because it's always a struggle to go. Some people are very obsessional about their bowels, spend far too much time in the toilet and think about their bowel habit continuously. Some patients are 'normal'.

Aims of treatment

The aims of biofeedback therapy are to improve coordination of the defecatory muscles and improve defecatory control without the use of laxatives, suppositories and enemas. Patients should feel that their bowel symptoms have improved. The frequency of bowel actions is not the most important factor, but rather how the patient feels. It is important to feel comfortable after each bowel action and to stay comfortable until the next bowel action. Patients must take responsibility for their treatment. The therapist can give advice and information but it is up to the patient to go home and change what they are doing.

Prior to biofeedback therapy commencing most patients will have a transit study (Evans et al 1992). Two capsules are taken for 3 consecutive days. These capsules contain 60 radiopaque shapes in total. On day 6 a plain abdominal X-ray is taken. Slow or normal colonic transit is determined by counting the number of shapes left. All laxatives, suppositories and enemas are stopped during this test. Biofeedback therapy can be successful for treating slow and normal transit constipation (Emmanuel & Kamm 2000).

Biofeedback therapy

A course of biofeedback therapy normally consists of a total of five appointments, at 4-weekly intervals. The patient sees the same therapist for the course. The components of a biofeedback therapy session include taking a detailed bowel assessment, health education, defecatory muscle exercises, behavioural therapy and psycho/social support.

Detailed bowel assessment

When patients first attend the biofeedback clinic they are asked a series of bowel-specific questions so that a detailed assessment can be made. It is also important to ask about life in general (e.g. work, home, etc.) and whether bowel symptoms restrict daily activities.

Patients are asked about stress and links are made with the possible broader psychological issues that may be at the root of the problem.

Health education

Patients are asked how they sit on the toilet when defecating. They are taught to lean forwards with their shoulders relaxed. Some patients find it helpful to raise their feet on a block or stool (Fig. 7.10).

The basic function of the digestive tract is explained using a simple diagram. Few patients actually understand what happens to food when it enters the body, and how stools are formed. Test results can be explained at this point. If a patient has slow transit it is important to stress they have 'slow' transit, not 'no' transit. The colon still functions, but just more slowly. Patients should understand that 'normal' bowel frequency differs from one individual to another.

Defecatory muscle exercises

During examination the patient will lie on a couch, facing the therapist, and covered with a sheet to maintain dignity. A balloon (see Fig. 7.11) is inserted into the rectum and inflated with 50 ml of air. This simulates the urge to defecate, so the patient has something to work with. The therapist can manually assess what the patient can and can't do with their muscles, by holding onto the end of the balloon. Initially the patient is asked to contract their external anal sphincter as if they are 'holding on'. This demonstrates to the patient and the therapist that the patient can control these

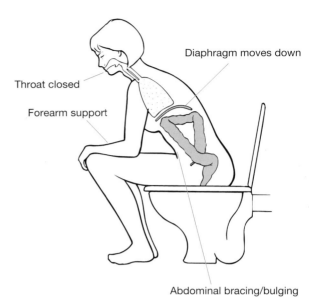

Figure 7.10 The right way to open the bowels. Reproduced from Chiarelli & Markwell (1992).

muscles. The patient is then asked to push the balloon out. The majority of patients demonstrate incoordination of their defecatory muscles. Specifically they may demonstrate the following:

- *Poor propulsion:* The patient holds their breath and strains, often tensing head, neck and shoulders. This straining may result in a bowel action but the patient is unlikely to evacuate completely, and straining can lead to other anorectal problems such as haemorrhoids.
- *Paradoxical contraction:* The patient contracts the external anal sphincter when trying to expel the balloon, instead of relaxing it. This makes it more difficult to evacuate stools on the toilet, and may lead to retrograde peristalsis and slower transit (Klauser et al 1990).

The patient may demonstrate one or both of these problems. At this point in the initial assessment the patient may ask why they are demonstrating incoordination of their defecatory muscles. It is difficult to explain why some people demonstrate this but the following possible reasons should be explored with the patient.

- Following abdominal or perineal/anal surgery (gynaecological/colorectal) patients may

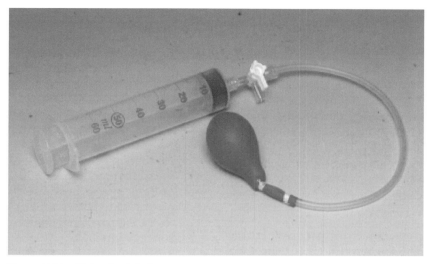

Figure 7.11 Biofeedback balloon.

develop bad habits during defecation. Initially it may be painful to have a bowel action, and patients may tense their external sphincter instead of relaxing it. Some may compromise the way in which they push in order to protect the surgical incision. This incoordination may continue once the patient has recovered.

- Many women experience difficulties following childbirth. They may feel pain in the abdominal and/or perineal area irrespective of the mode of delivery. This pain may cause incoordination, which may continue after the pain has eased.
- Patients who have been raped, or have a history of physical or sexual abuse, have difficulty thinking about their pelvic region in any way, and as a result may demonstrate incoordination of their defecatory muscles. They are no longer able to associate themselves with these muscles. These patients tend to demonstrate paradoxical contraction.

Teaching the exercises

The exercises are taught with the patient lying on the couch as before. At home, the patient is advised to sit correctly on the toilet and relax their shoulders, arms and legs. They should breath normally, and not hold their breath. The following two exercises can be taught.

The 'Brace'. An effective way for the patient to locate the abdominal oblique muscles needed to brace with, is to place their hands on either side of their waist and cough. Their waist should widen and become barrel shaped. The following steps should then be followed:

- Slowly brace outwards (widen the waist, without coughing). When fully braced, push/propel from the waist back and downwards into the back passage.
- Relax for 1 second, very slightly (i.e. maintain the level of pressure with the brace muscles, do not push with them).
- Brace outwards and push downwards again. This should be repeated.

The 'Lift'. Initially the patient is asked to contract their external anal sphincter as if they are 'holding on'. This is a good way of demonstrating to the patient which muscle to focus on. This exercise is explained using a lift analogy. When relaxed, the external anal sphincter is the equivalent of a lift resting on the first floor. In tightening the external sphincter, this is the equivalent of the lift moving upwards. The patient is advised that during defecation they should use their anal sphincter muscles in the opposite way, i.e. relax. Once the patient understands which muscle to use, they need to focus on relaxing this muscle by following the procedure outlined below:

- Imagine your back passage is a lift, resting on the first floor.
- Slowly push the lift down to ground floor, down to basement, down to cellar.
- Take the lift down as far as it will go.
- If you relax for a second do not allow the lift to rise.
- When the lift has come down as far as possible, push your waist out wide and channel the strength from your waist down to your back passage.

It is important to emphasize that the exercise teaches the patient to correctly coordinate their defecatory muscles. This enables them to achieve an effective bowel action and therefore relieve any symptoms.

Behavioural therapy

Stop medication

All patients must stop laxatives on day 1 of treatment. The aim is for the patient to achieve a satisfactory bowel action without the use of any medication. This is a slow process and patients should understand this will take hard work and willpower. Patients may feel worse before any benefit is felt, and should be aware of this.

Diet

Many patients will have been told to increase their fibre intake as a way of improving their bowel condition. This may work in some cases, but rarely for those with chronic constipation. If a patient has slow transit, fibres merely add bulk. Decreasing dietary fibre may help relieve symptoms of bloating and abdominal pain. Bloating may be reduced by avoiding the following:

- Wholemeals/wholegrains
- Dried fruit and nuts
- Muesli, bran, porridge
- Sprouts, broccoli, cabbage.

To maintain a balance, fibres can be found from other sources, i.e. fresh fruits and other vegetables. Patients should be advised to eat regularly, even if bloating is a problem. Although dietary advice is helpful it is a small component of this therapy.

At home

The aim of this routine is to teach the patient to:

- make time to go to the toilet every day
- sit correctly on the toilet
- relax before opening bowels
- 'brace' or widen waist for effective propulsion
- relax the external anal sphincter instead of squeezing it.

An individual routine is devised which will be followed until the next appointment. The exercise is given in written form to reinforce what is learnt at the first session.

Routine for patients with constipation and irritable bowel syndrome. The focus is to increase the frequency of bowel actions, improve evacuation and establish a good bowel routine:

- Patients must practise their exercises each day at a similar time. This will help establish a routine. Many patients with constipation will only attempt to open their bowels after taking laxatives or when they get the urge so this may mean that attempts are infrequent.
- The patient should sit on the toilet about 30 minutes after breakfast, or evening meal. Eating will stimulate peristalsis which may give the patient an urge to go. Regardless of an urge being present, or whether anything is passed, it is important for patients to do this. This time allows the patient to focus and establish a routine.
- Regular practising should also stimulate the bowel to work more effectively. This enables the patient to improve the coordination of their defecatory muscles, which will help them evacuate more effectively.

Routine for patients with solitary rectal ulcer syndrome, rectocele, rectal prolapse and frequency. The main focus is to reduce the number of attempts to defecate, reduce pressure exerted on the pelvic floor through excessive straining and establish a better bowel routine:

- Patients must not strain when opening their bowels.
- Patients are advised not to digitate per rectum to aid evacuation. This can exacerbate solitary rectal ulcers.
- Patients are advised to only attempt defecation a maximum of three times daily. This should be after mealtimes. This reduction of attempts should lessen the pressure in the rectum and vagina. Ultimately the aim is for patients to have a bowel action once or twice daily.
- Patients may need to find distractions to prevent more frequent attempts in the toilet (e.g. go for a walk).
- Time spent at each attempt in the toilet should be a maximum of 10 minutes.
- To reduce the feeling of pressure in the rectum and/or vagina the patient should pull the muscles of the rectum and vagina inwards and upwards and hold for 10 seconds then relax. This can be repeated. This is particularly useful before lifting an object, or coughing and sneezing.
- Some women find it helpful to support their perineum during defecation. It may also help to digitate per vagina; this will assist evacuation of a rectocele. Patients should be informed that further damage will not be caused by doing this.

Solitary rectal ulcers can take a long time to heal so patients are usually reviewed in the outpatient department so that the ulcer can be monitored. Some patients can relapse with time and revert back to disordered defecation. All patients with solitary rectal ulcers may benefit from having a 'refresher session' to maintain benefit (Malouf et al 2001).

Further appointments

It is important that the patient attends regularly so that the therapist can monitor the progress made. At each appointment the same questions are asked to monitor symptom improvement, and the coordination of the defecatory muscles

is assessed by using balloon expulsion. Patients can contact the therapist by telephone between scheduled appointments should they have any concerns. Symptoms may become worse and patients need encouragement to persevere with the therapy.

Psychological issues

If patients have experienced any type of abuse they may cite this as the cause of their problem. It is essential that psychological referrals can be made should the need arise. If patients disclose for the first time that they have been raped or abused it is important to be able to offer professional help should it be required. If referrals can not be made it is perhaps not prudent to offer biofeedback therapy. This is a vital component of the care package.

If psychological support is required then this can sometimes run concurrently with the biofeedback therapy. Patients can have the practical treatment for their physical problem, and also take active steps to tackle their psychological problems.

Discharge

When patients are discharged it is important that they continue with the biofeedback programme. It can take up to 12 months for patients to gain

---

Case study 7.1

Mrs P., a 40-year-old married woman, had a 20-year history of constipation which started when she was sexually abused by her first husband. The bowel habit diary revealed bowels open once a week after large daily doses of a laxative. She was Type 1 Bristol Stool and also passed some blood and mucus. There was abdominal bloating and anal pain which at times were so severe she could hardly sit down. She had been advised by her GP that she might need to have a colostomy. However, after only five sessions of biofeedback training which included psychological support and encouragement, she started passing soft, formed stools (Type 4) daily without the use of laxatives. There was no blood or mucus. The abdominal bloating and anal pain improved and she was able to sit more comfortably.

maximum benefit from this treatment. Some patients may need a 'refresher session' to remind them what to do.

If the biofeedback therapy fails, patients can be offered an appointment for review in the outpatient department. These patients usually need conservative management of their residual symptoms. What they have learnt with biofeedback therapy is insight into their condition, and a better ability to cope with their symptoms.

OTHER TREATMENTS FOR CONSTIPATION

Because there are many causes of constipation, it is understandable that there are also many ways of treating it successfully. Once the cause is identified treatment can commence. Accurate diagnosis is important since the resultant treatment prescribed is more likely to control symptoms and rectify the problem effectively, causing minimum discomfort to the individual. It is also more likely to ensure that treatment will be cost-effective and prompt. As the treatment of constipation depends on the cause, recommended treatments will be discussed under some of the causes which have already been described.

Treating bowel blues

The main aspect of treating constipation related to depression is re-education. Individuals may need advice on the importance of exercise, eating regularly and responding to the call to stool. Such advice will need to be given hand-in-hand with effective medical treatment of the depression. If medication is used to treat the depression problem, advice should be given on any associated side-effects, such as constipation. Biofeedback therapy is often the first line of treatment (see above).

Treating hormone imbalance

Once the underlying hormone imbalance has been identified and treated, the problem of constipation may be resolved. However, opportunities to discuss the effectiveness of fibre in the diet, adequate fluid intake and exercise should not be missed.

Because the constipation is related to muscular weakness within the walls of the colon, brought about by hormonal changes, the colon may become impacted. It is important to ensure that the bowel is clear before embarking on any dietary changes, or introducing a bulk-forming laxative. The rectum should be cleared from below with stimulant suppositories such as glycerin or bisacodyl. Further details on managing an impacted bowel are given under 'Treating the retired rectum'.

Treating the effects of immobility

It is often difficult to counter the effects of immobility if it is the result of underlying disease. However, this is an important consideration and should be given high priority, particularly when planning care for elderly people.

In addition, the importance of posture during defecation should not be underestimated (Fig. 7.10). Correct posture can help to make defecation easier and more comfortable. Those who have had to suffer the discomfort of sitting on a bedpan will understand the influence of posture. In their book *Let's Get Things Moving: Overcoming Constipation*, Pauline Chiarelli and Sue Markwell describe how to do it in eight simple steps (Box 7.4). Have a practice yourself.

Treating the bothersome bowel

Tumours

The treatment offered will depend on the individual and the type and site of any intestinal tumour. The usual choice of treatment for malignant tumours is a surgical resection of the colon with an anastomosis, resulting in either a temporary or permanent stoma.

Diverticular disease

To help relieve the symptoms and prevent further constipation in individuals with diverticular disease, an increase in dietary fibre is usually recommended. It is also important to ensure an adequate fluid intake, particularly if wheat bran is being taken.

Box 7.4   Let's get things moving: overcoming constipation (after Chiarelli & Markwell, 1992)

1. Sit on a chair with both hands over the front of your stomach.
2. Draw up the sling (pelvic floor muscles).
3. Relax the sling, noting what happens to the abdominal wall. It should bulge.
4. Keeping your hands in place, imagine you are opening your anal muscles – *make the anus wide*. You should feel a greater swelling/tension/bulge underneath your hands as you do this.
5. Now move one hand to your waist. This time, when you open your anal muscles, feel the bulge under your front hand and the widening as you widen your waist. This is the normal pattern – you should resemble a pear. This is what should happen when you go to the toilet successfully. It is known as *brace and open out*.
6. Keep your lips slightly open and your teeth apart. This will help your anal muscles relax and release faeces. A relaxed jaw means an open pelvic floor. Breathe out. (So *brace and open out* is followed by *grunt*!)
7. Pull up the anorectal muscles as you finish emptying. This will improve the closing reflex and *turn off the switch*.
8. Remember those three simple instructions – *brace, open out, grunt*!

Irritable bowel syndrome

The type of symptoms suffered will determine the treatment offered. Constipation problems may occur intermittently with diarrhoea. Bloating and pain may also be present. An increase in dietary fibre and bulk-adding laxatives may be helpful, although too much wheat bran may make bloating worse. It may be worth avoiding such foods as dairy products, spicy hot dishes, and fried dishes, and beverages such as alcohol and coffee in order to help relieve the troublesome symptoms of pain and bloating (see Biofeedback above).

Haemorrhoids

The most important aspect of treatment for constipation related to haemorrhoids is to prevent the individual from straining at stool. An increase in dietary fibre will make stools large, wetter and easier to pass. Stools may initially need to be softened with a faecal softener, and a bulk-adding laxative may be required. General advice should

be given on the importance of responding to the call to stool. Depending on the severity of the problem, the haemorrhoids themselves may require treatment. This usually takes the form of injection therapy or a haemorrhoidectomy.

Megacolon and megarectum

Because of the huge build-up of faeces in the dilated portion of colon, the aim of treatment initially is to empty the rectum completely and maintain stools of a manageable consistency, i.e. not too hard and not too soft. Depending on the severity of impaction, emptying the rectum may need to be performed under anaesthetic. This is very invasive and expensive so biofeedback (as above) may now be the first line of treatment.

Daily micro-enemas or suppositories may be given, and may need to be continued for between 7 and 14 days. Maintaining a soft, manageable stool requires further treatment with osmotic laxatives or enemas. Such treatment must continue on a regular basis in order to prevent the recurrence of faecal impaction.

Surgery may also have a place in managing this condition. Depending on the extent of the problem, surgical treatment usually consists of a colectomy and ileorectal anastomosis, a coloanal anastomosis, a colostomy or ileostomy. This would be a last resort only.

Slow-transit constipation and normal-transit constipation

These problems are best managed using stimulant suppositories or osmotic rectal laxatives to empty the rectum regularly. Biofeedback may be helpful. The use of wheat bran should be avoided.

Rectal prolapse and rectocele

Biofeedback is again the first line of treatment but if this fails then the regular administration of suppositories may help sufferers to empty the rectum more easily. It is important that the stool remains soft, bulky and manageable, as harder small stools will not only be uncomfortable but also more difficult to pass. It may be helpful for those suffering from a rectocele to insert a finger into the vagina and support the vaginal wall as this will often help to empty the rectum more successfully.

Treating the retired rectum

Faecal loading with hard or soft faeces is often the problem for individuals suffering from constipation of a neurological nature or associated with old age (Fig. 7.12).

As with a megacolon, the initial aim of treatment is to empty the rectum completely. It is important to establish whether the bowel is loaded with hard or soft stool, as the appropriate long-term management differs. If the stool is hard and is causing discomfort, daily micro-enemas or suppositories should be administered until the rectum is empty. It may take between 7 and 14 days to achieve this. A study conducted by Abd-el-Maeboud et al (1991) showed that suppositories are more likely to be successfully retained if they are inserted blunt end first. If this treatment does not solve the problem, an osmotic laxative such as lactulose should be introduced. If impaction continues to be a problem, a stimulant laxative, such as dantron or senna, may then be given. A combination of osmotic and stimulant laxatives may be helpful.

If the stool is soft and causing discomfort, the rectum must be emptied with daily micro-enemas or suppositories. If additional treatment is required, a stimulant laxative may be introduced together with further micro-enemas if necessary.

Once the rectum is empty, the aim of treatment is to maintain a soft but manageable stool, preferably without the use of laxatives. Depending on the individual's general state of health, an increase in dietary fibre may be appropriate. This measure should be closely supervised, particularly if mobility and/or fluid intake is severely impaired.

Since the movement of faeces along the colon into the rectum is encouraged by the ingestion of food, a good time to go to the toilet is after a meal, particularly after breakfast which is when the urge to defecate most commonly occurs. Do not forget to consider the issues of good posture and the suitability and privacy of facilities. Patients should be encouraged to sit on the toilet for 10-minute intervals after each meal. This is known as 'prompted toilet-sitting' or 'stimulus control'. There is evidence to suggest that behavioural training programmes are successful in reducing the incidence of faecal incontinence amongst elderly people with dementia. Rewarding successful trips to the toilet is thought to be helpful, provided that rewards and punishments are given immediately after the event (Smith & Smith 1993). There is debate concerning the rewarding of 'dry pants' as it is thought that individuals suffering from constipation may become more constipated in an attempt not to soil. There is, however, no specific evidence to support this.

Smith & Smith (1993) concluded from available evidence that organized, well-supported behavioural training programmes do work well. However, in cases of chronic constipation and faecal impaction it may be impossible to verify a pattern of defecation. Houts et al (1988) recognized that a regular pattern of defecation is achievable by increasing dietary fibre whilst a prompted toilet-sitting regime is in progress (see also Chapter 6).

Spinal injury

Many individuals with a spinal injury are able to control bowel movements by stimulating the anus with a finger. This causes a reflex emptying of the rectum. Where such control is not possible suppositories or micro-enemas should be administered to ensure that the rectum is regularly emptied (see Chapter 11).

Nerve stimulators are now being used for carefully selected individuals with damage to the sacral nerve roots S2, S3 and S4. The stimulator is implanted at the roots of these sacral nerves and receives electrical impulses from a receiver which is implanted in the chest wall. When it is necessary to empty the rectum a signal is transmitted to the receiver via a hand-held control. This is a little like having a radio-controlled bottom!

MORE ABOUT LAXATIVES

Four different classes of laxative can be identified: bulk-forming, stimulant, osmotics and stool

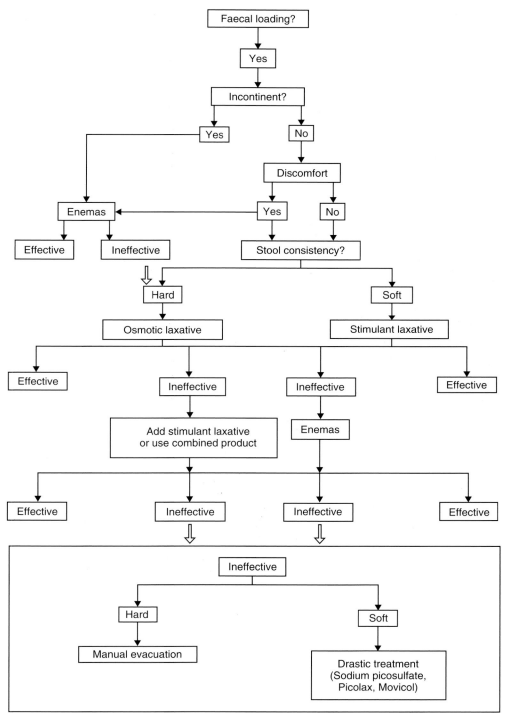

Figure 7.12 A simplified scheme for the management of faecal loading in elderly and disabled patients.

Case study 7.2

Fiona, aged 38 years, had always managed to lead a full and active life despite the fact that she had been suffering from multiple sclerosis for some 15 years. As a result of the disease her eyesight was poor and she dragged her left leg slightly, particularly when she was tired. She also suffered from urgency of micturition due to an unstable bladder, but she always managed to reach the toilet on time and had never felt that this problem had affected her quality of life.

However, her condition began to deteriorate and her mobility became so poor that she was unable to walk more than a few metres. Consequently, the urgency of micturition had become a significant problem, with sporadic episodes of urge incontinence. Oxybutynin hydrochloride, 5 mg twice daily, was considered suitable for controlling the symptoms of the unstable bladder as there was no significant residual urine identified.

Previously, the subject of bowel management had never really been raised with Fiona. Unfortunately, she was now faced with three major factors contributing towards constipation: an underlying diagnosis of multiple sclerosis, immobility and anticholinergic drug therapy. Her bowel movements soon became infrequent and stools were hard and difficult to pass. Owing to her inactivity and her loss of independence regarding toileting, she had reduced her food and fluid intake. In turn this increased the constipation problem and worsened the urinary incontinence. To try to soften the stool Fiona had decided to take lactulose, as straining at stool not only required a great deal of energy but had now become extremely painful. Although the lactulose did help soften the stool, evacuating the rectum completely still remained a problem. She also found the softened faeces difficult to control on occasions and sometimes leaked. Fiona started to wear large incontinence pads to contain any faecal leakage. She became very depressed and began to lose interest in many of the pastimes she had previously enjoyed. It was only when she had reached her lowest ebb that she confided in a friend who suggested she seek further help.

After reassessment, a bowel programme was planned for Fiona as follows:

- The lactulose was stopped.
- The rectum was emptied daily using micro-enemas. Fiona found these easier than suppositories to administer herself, as suppositories would slip out of her hands.
- As well as micro-enemas, Senokot was given in order to help propel the soft faeces through the colon. This treatment continued for 8 days until the rectum was clear. Once the rectum was clear, the aim of treatment was to maintain a soft but manageable stool. This was achieved by:
  —giving advice with reference to the association of bowel movements and the intake of food and fluid
  —deciding on the best time for Fiona to empty her bowels. It was agreed that in the morning after her breakfast and a warm drink would be the most suitable time
  —planning a 'walking' regime, which observed the importance of exercise and its association with bowel movement. Fiona had previously lost all interest in exercise mainly due to the fact that her incontinence pad was bulky and insecure!
  —adding bulk to the diet in order to moisten and enlarge the stool. Fiona was not keen on 'fibre-rich' foods but this was mainly because she associated fibre with foods such as bran and prunes. An appointment with the dietician clarified the meaning of 'high-fibre', and Fiona's food and fluid intake improved dramatically following this. At this point, the introduction of a bulk-adding laxative was discussed. Fiona found that daily Fybogel helped achieve a bulky stool which was easier to pass.

Although the bowel programme took time to implement and evaluate, it was clear that this time had been well spent. It had addressed many issues relating to Fiona's lifestyle, independence and self-esteem, and positively improved her general state of health.

---

softeners. The successful treatment of constipation should be possible with a single laxative or combination of laxatives, although discovering the cause of the constipation is the main priority. The main laxatives which are commonly used are considered here but a more in-depth discussion is provided in Chapter 8.

Bulk-forming laxatives

Bran

Bran's laxative properties have been generally accepted for centuries. Bran absorbs water, thus expanding and softening the stool. The increased bulk also promotes peristaltic action. Bran passes through the intestine undigested. This leads to a decrease in transit time, which in turn reduces the amount of water absorbed by the colon.

Bran should produce results within a few days and is quite safe for long-term treatment although fluid intake should be maintained. Bran is available in tablet form but the easiest way to administer it is by changing diet, or it may also be taken mixed with a drink such as fruit juice. Wheat bran should be avoided in conditions such as coeliac disease, and all brans should be avoided in cases of intestinal obstruction, colonic atony or faecal impaction.

Ispaghula

Ispaghula husk is derived from the seeds of the psyllium plant (*Plantago psyllium*). Ispaghula absorbs water in the gastrointestinal tract and expands. As with bran, this expansion stimulates peristalsis and leads to wetter, bulkier stools. Ispaghula is available in several forms, the most common of which are Fybogel, Isogel, Konsyl and Regulan. All of these come in either granular or powdered form and should be taken with water. It is important that fluid intake be maintained. Fybogel and Regulan are gluten-free; Konsyl is available in gluten-free and sugar-free formulations.

As with all bulking agents, ispaghula may cause flatulence and/or abdominal distension and should not be used in cases of intestinal obstruction, colonic atony or faecal impaction.

Methylcellulose

Methylcellulose is made from indigestible vegetable fibre. It absorbs water to form a colloid, increasing its volume by up to 25 times. As with bran, this water absorption and swelling stimulates peristalsis and leads to bulkier, moister stools.

Methylcellulose is available in tablet form (Celevac) or as diluent water ('methylcellulose mixture'). As with other bulking agents, methylcellulose may cause abdominal distension and/or flatulence and should not be used in cases of intestinal obstruction or colonic atony. Methylcellulose may be used in cases of faecal impaction as it is also a faecal softener.

Sterculia

Sterculia is derived from the seeds of the kola plant and acts in much the same way as other bulk-forming laxatives. Normacol and Normacol Plus are examples of sterculia-based laxatives and come in granular form. As with bran they should be taken with water, maintaining fluid intake, and

should not be used in cases of intestinal obstruction, colonic atony or faecal impaction.

Stimulant laxatives

Bisacodyl

Bisacodyl is a synthetic polyphenolic diphenylmethane derivative. It is generally believed that stimulant laxatives act by nerve stimulation to induce peristalsis, but they also decrease water reabsorption from the colon by inhibiting sodium–potassium–ATPase, leading to large, more moist stools.

Bisacodyl comes in both tablet and suppository forms. Tablets (Dulco-lax) act in about 10–12 hours and suppositories in about 20 minutes to 1 hour. Bisacodyl and other stimulant laxatives can cause abdominal cramps as they increase intestinal motility. Bisacodyl should not be administered in cases of intestinal obstruction, or over any long period as it can lead to colonic atony and hypokalaemia. Ideally, it should be avoided in the treatment of children.

Senna

Senna is a member of the anthraquinone group and is derived from the leaves and seed pods of the Arabian shrub *Cassia angustifolia*. Soluble anthraquinone derivatives are absorbed in the small intestine and excreted into the colon. It is believed that they then stimulate the Auerbach's plexus in the large intestine to give physiological purgation. Senna comes in tablet, granular, liquid and syrup forms (e.g. Manevac and Senokot) and acts in about 6–10 hours. Senna pods can also be infused in water and drunk somewhat like tea, although this makes dose control difficult. As with the other stimulant laxatives, senna may cause cramps and should not be used in cases of intestinal obstuction or for long-term treatment. It also causes the urine to be coloured brown or red.

Cascara

Cascara is another member of the anthraquinone group and comes from the bark of the Californian Buckthorn *Coscara sagrada*. Cascara acts in the same way as senna but is not as effective. It generally comes in tablet form and the same precautions should be taken as with senna. Cascara should be avoided by breast-feeding women.

Dantron

Dantron is a polyphenolic derivative which is usually combined with a stool-softener poloxamer (co-danthramer) or with another stimulant, docusate sodium (co-danthrusate). Dantron comes in capsule form (co-danthrussate – Normax) and as a suspension (co-danthramer – Codalax and Codalax Forte). It acts in about 6–12 hours. Dantron's use should be limited to elderly patients, to those with cardiac conditions where straining should be avoided, and for analgesic-induced constipation in terminal cases. It should be avoided by pregnant and breast-feeding women.

Sodium picosulfate

Sodium picosulfate is a polyphenolic laxative which increases intestinal motility and decreases water absorption. It is most often used in powdered form with magnesium citrate (Picolax) and is taken for bowel evacuation. Sodium picosulfate should not be prescribed in cases of intestinal obstruction or on a long-term basis. Its possible side-effects are cramps, nausea and vomiting.

Glycerol

Glycerol (glycerin) suppositories are fairly widely used. Not only do they lubricate the anorectum but they also stimulate defecation by a mild irritation effect. No significant contraindications or side-effects have been reported.

Osmotic laxatives

Lactulose

Lactulose is a semi-synthetic disaccharide which is made up of fructose and lactose. It is broken down to form lactic and acetic acids in the colon. These stimulate peristalsis and the osmotic effect leads to softer stools. Lactulose comes in liquid form and can often take up to 3 days to be effective. Lactulose should not be used in cases of abdominal obstruction or galactosaemia, and may cause flatulence and abdominal cramps.

Movicol

Movicol contains polyethylene glycol and various electrolytes but there is limited evidence that it is an advantage over lactulose (Attar et al 1999). Further comparable studies are required to show its efficacy as it does remain expensive. It is used for impacted faeces and chronic cases where other interventions have failed (MeReC Bulletin 1999).

Magnesium salts

Magnesium salts such as magnesium hydroxide, magnesium sulphate or magnesium citrate are osmotic agents which attract water into the bowel, having passed through the intestine relatively unabsorbed. This increases the volume of the stool, keeping it moist, and also stimulates peristalsis. Magnesium compounds are extremely effective and can act in as little as 2 hours when taken orally. These laxatives should be used only in the short term for rapid evacuation of the bowel. They should not be used in cases of intestinal obstruction, and because of their osmotic properties care must be taken to avoid dehydration.

Rectal phosphates

Rectal phosphates such as sodium acid phosphate (Carbalax) are administered as suppositories. They have a direct osmotic and stimulant effect and produce evacuation in about 30 minutes. As with magnesium compounds, phosphates should be used only in the short-term to produce rapid bowel evacuation. They should not be used in cases of abdominal obstruction or acute gastro-intestinal conditions and are not recommended for treatment of children.

Rectal sodium citrate

Rectal sodium citrate is administered as an enema (Micolette Micro-enema, Micralax Micro-enema,

Relaxit Micro-enema) and acts in much the same way as rectal phosphates. In addition to the cautions already mentioned, care should be taken in cases where sodium salts could be contraindicated (e.g. cardiac failure).

Stool softeners

Docusate sodium

Docusate sodium (dioctyl sodium sulphosuccinate) has detergent and emulsifying properties which soften the stool. It also acts as a stimulant. It is available in tablet and syrup forms (Dioctyl) and as an enema (Fletchers' Enemette). By mouth, docusate sodium usually acts within 24–48 hours. As with other laxatives, docusate sodium should not be used in case of intestinal obstruction or over any long period, and it may cause abdominal cramps.

Arachis oil

Arachis oil is derived from peanuts. Used as an enema (Fletchers' Arachis Oil Retention Enema) it is effective in softening the stool in cases of impaction. It also helps promote bowel motion.

A ROLE FOR COMPLEMENTARY THERAPIES?

The World Health Organization estimates that only 15% of the world's population has access to the kind of Westernized health services to which Britain is accustomed. It is hardly surprising, therefore, that ancient forms of treatment such as herbalism, acupuncture and reflexology continue to play important roles in the treatment of disease and in the maintenance of health for individuals worldwide. Interest in these and other complementary therapies is increasing in Britain, and some services, such as acupuncture, are now available through the National Health Service.

A brief review of therapies which offer potential benefits in relation to problems of constipation is provided here. However, it must be emphasized that none of these therapies should be practised without guidance from a qualified practitioner.

Colonic massage

Since 3000 BC the Chinese have been practising massage. It was also widely used by the Greeks and Romans. Julius Caesar himself would be massaged daily. There are many forms of massage, of which manual colonic massage is one. Slow massage relieves muscle tension, thereby improving blood circulation and lymphatic drainage. Different degrees of pressure may be used and each person has their own preference. Oils such as baby oil or lavender may be used to avoid friction on the skin, but aromatherapy oils must only be used by an experienced practitioner. In her book *The Magic of Massage*, Ouida West explains the technique:

> Sit at the receiver's side. Gently lay both hands on the abdomen with extreme tenderness, for this part of the body is especially vulnerable. Unless you proceed with the utmost caution, the receiver will jump with a start. Once your hands are gently resting on the receiver's abdomen, you are ready to begin the technique. Keeping your hands on the abdomen, begin a clockwise circular motion. Move from the lower right side of the abdomen up, across and down the left side of the abdomen. Use two hands, one after the other following the direction of faeces (sic).

This procedure should be repeated three to five times per treatment session. Ouida West suggests that some improvement may be noted within 2 weeks, but for significant improvements to become apparent it may take months of numerous daily treatments.

Acupuncture

Acupuncture is an ancient Chinese healing art developed some four to six thousand years ago. It is based on the principle that health is maintained by a 'balance of energy'. Fine adjustments may be made to the energy potential of bodily organs in order to improve and maintain the body's equilibrium.

Acupuncture treatment consists of inserting a small sterile needle into a certain point, located along identified meridians or energy pathways. The needle acts as a centre point through which energy may enter and leave the body, resulting in a subtle adjustment to the energy potential of such a point. Acupuncture of points both close to the organ requiring treatment, and of points further away, form the basis of treatment. Points located in the hand and arm are used to treat conditions of the large intestine.

Shiatsu

Shiatsu developed from ancient Chinese massage techniques and is similar to acupuncture, but pressure is applied to the points with the fingertips, rather than inserting needles. Pressure is firm and may be held for seconds or up to 1 minute, depending on how much treatment is required. Each pressure point relates to a certain part of the body; shiatsu uses acupuncture pressure points, encouraging healing through stimulation.

Herbalism

Herbalism is an ancient form of treatment which seems to be returning to popularity in the Western world's desire to favour 'green' and 'ecofriendly' ideals. The use of plant-derived drugs or plant extracts is only one step away from the pharmacist, but herbal medicine has a different approach.

Herbal medicine uses remedies that do not directly attack a disease. They support the body and stimulate its own natural defences, and help in the recovery process. A tablespoon of linseeds, soaked overnight, may be sprinkled over food and added to soups and stews, adding bulk to the diet. Liquorice root and chickweed also relieve constipation, and may be taken as an infusion. This can be made using 25 g (1 ounce) of the desired herb to 600 ml (1 pint) of water and bringing gently to the boil. *Successful Herbal Remedies* by Nalda Gosling and *The Herb Book* by John Lust are just two of the many books available which discuss herbs and their medicinal uses.

Reflexology

Reflexology has been practised for thousands of years by the Indians, Chinese and Egyptians, and was introduced into the West early in the 20th century. In reflexology the body is divided vertically into ten different sectors or zones which extend into the feet and hands. Pressure applied to these zones on the feet or hands is said to stimulate the vital organs in the appropriate sector, by improving the blood and nerve supply and removing uric acid and calcium deposits from nerve endings.

Although pressure zones differ in individuals, it is generally agreed that pressure applied to the outer, fleshy area at the very base of the thumb corresponds to the large colon in hand reflexology. In foot reflexology the arch of the foot corresponds to the large colon, and pressure applied to the heel of the foot is known to treat haemorrhoids (Figure 7.13 shows a much simplified side view). Two or three treatments daily are usually required.

Homeopathy

Homeopathy is an ancient Greek method of treatment which basically treats like with like. In homeopathy the symptoms of an ailment are considered to be the body's reaction to that ailment. Therefore if a substance which produces the same symptoms is administered this reaction will be stimulated, thus helping the body to overcome the ailment. Homeopathy is a natural healing process which stimulates the body's natural forces of recovery. It is difficult to give any specific treatment regimens because remedies are prescribed on an individual basis according to the patient's personal traits. *Homeopathy for the Family*, published by the Homeopathic Development Foundation (1985), is a useful introductory guide.

Aromatherapy

One of the most popular of the complementary therapies, aromatherapy, has been practised for many thousands of years. In 3000 BC the Egyptians used aromatic treatments for many different ailments.

The therapy uses the essential oils of aromatic flowers, herbs, spices and trees. The oils may be applied either topically in the form of a skin

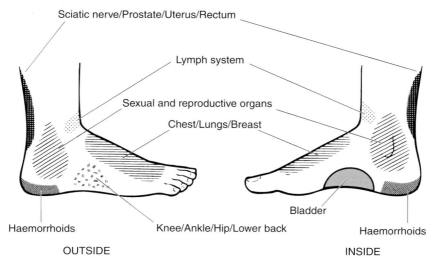

Sciatic nerve/Prostate/Uterus/Rectum

Lymph system

Sexual and reproductive organs

Chest/Lungs/Breast

Bladder

Haemorrhoids

Knee/Ankle/Hip/Lower back

Haemorrhoids

OUTSIDE

INSIDE

Figure 7.13 A simplified illustration of foot reflexology (side views).

massage, bath oil, cream, lotion or compress, or as an inhalation. The application may be hot or cold, depending upon the condition requiring treatment. Marjoram, rosemary and juniper are often used to treat constipation. They are massaged into the abdomen, using the same technique as for colonic massage. When the oils come into contact with the skin they stimulate the nerve endings, muscles and tissues, and increase circulation and lymphatic drainage around the affected area. An example of a blend of oils which may be used to promote peristalsis is provided in Chapter 8. Because aromatherapy uses a holistic approach, the therapy prescribed will not only treat the physical aspects of the disease but also any underlying psychological and emotional ones as well.

All of these complementary methods consider constipation fairly seriously, in that the retention of faeces leads to the reabsorption of toxins or waste products which upset the body's 'balance'. They all have treatments for constipation, the largest selection being herbalism. This is logical, considering that the majority of proprietary laxatives are derived from plants. The fruits and vegetables which have laxative properties are fairly well known, and include examples such as asparagus, aloe, figs, prunes, psyllium, rhubarb, chicory, linseed, castor bean and walnuts.

Finally, it must be re-emphasized that none of these therapies should be practised without guidance from a qualified practitioner.

FAECAL FINALE

'Estrie finis aut initium finis, aut finis initii, aut initium…?'

Beard (1993)

'Is it the end, or the beginning of the end, or the end of the beginning, or the beginning…? This may be the end of the chapter, but really it is just the beginning. The responsibility of health professionals lies in the restoration and preservation of healthy independent living for all individuals. In order to be effective, health professionals need to be able to offer sound, sensitive advice and dispel some of the myths surrounding bowel habits and 'the high-fibre diet'.

Although constipation is not considered a life-threatening problem, effective management may be life-saving in that it can relieve psychological distress, social indignity and physiological pain.

KEY POINTS FOR PRACTICE

The old aviators' expression 'chocks away!' refers to the removal of small wooden wedges from the wheels of an aeroplane so that it is able to take off. Using this as a basis, here is a final reminder of some of the points made in the chapter.

- **C**onstipation is a symptom identified as the passing of fewer than three stools per week, or excessive straining when having the bowel open.
- **H**ormonal changes may cause constipation.
- **O**ther causes of constipation may be related to diet, mobility, environment, medication and neurological conditions.
- **C**onstipation in the elderly may be controlled by diet, exercise, toileting after meals, and the administration of suppositories or microenemas if necessary.
- **K**eep a record of dietary fibre intake as care should be taken when recommending such

diets for the elderly and/or the immobile patient.
- **S**uccessful treatment depends on accurate diagnosis, as constipation is a symptom not a disease.
- **A**re you sitting comfortably? Correct posture can help to make defecation less strenuous.
- **W**hen administering a laxative, consider the diagnosis and ensure the laxative is appropriate.
- **A**lternatives? Complementary therapies such as acupuncture, herbalism, homeopathy and reflexology have been with us for centuries.
- **Y**es! You can help your patient as 'The size of a deed is measured not so much by its effort, as by its impact' (Lenzkes 1987).

The call of the old aviator to remove a simple obstacle may well be all that is required to set the wheels (or bowels!) in motion.

REFERENCES

Abd-El-Maeboud K H, El-Nagger T, El-Hawi E M M, Mahmoud S A R, Abd-el-Hay S 1991 Rectal suppository: common sense mode of insertion. Lancet 338: 798–800

Addison R 1999 Digital rectal examination. Nursing Times 95(40): Supplement

Anderson J T, Bradley W E 1976 Abnormalities of detrusor and sphincter function in multiple sclerosis. British Journal of Urology 48: 193–198

Ardron M E, Main A N H 1990 Management of constipation. British Medical Journal 300: 1400

Attar A, Leman M, Ferguson A et al 1999 Comparison of a low dose polyethylene glycol electrolyte solution with lactulose for treatment of chronic constipation. Gut 44: 226–230

Barrett J A 1988 Effect of wheat bran on stool size. British Medical Journal 296: 1127–1128

Barrett J A 1993 Faecal incontinence and related problems in the older adult. Edward Arnold, Sevenoaks

Barrett J A, Brocklehurst J C, Kiff E F, Ferguson G, Faragher E B 1990 Rectal motility studies in geriatric patients with faecal incontinence. Age and Ageing 19: 311–317

Bayliss V 2000 North Hampshire bowel care pathway. Norgine Ltd, Uxbridge, Middlesex

Beard H 1993 Latin for all occasions. HarperCollins, London

Brocklehurst J C, Kahn M Y 1969 A study of faecal stasis in old age and the use of Dorbanex in its prevention. Gerontologia Clinica 11: 293–300

Brocklehurst J C, Kirkland J L, Martin J, Ashford J 1983 Constipation in long-stay elderly patients: its treatment and prevention by lactulose, poloxalkoldihydroxy anthroquinolone and phosphate enemas. Gerontology 29: 181–184

Burkitt D P, Walker A R P, Painter N S 1972 Effect of dietary fibre on stools and transit times, and its role in the causation of disease. Lancet ii, 1408–1411

Carvana B J, Wald A, Hinds J P, Eidelman B H 1991 Anorectal sensory and motor function in neurogenic faecal incontinence: comparison between multiple sclerosis and diabetes mellitus. Gastroenterology 100: 465–470

Chelvanayagam S, Norton C 1999 Focus on continence: causes and assessment of faecal incontinence. British Journal of Community Nursing 4(1): 28–35

Chelvanayagam S, Norton C 2000 Quality of life with faecal continence problems. Nursing Times 96(31): 15–17

Chiarelli P, Markwell S 1992 Let's get things moving: overcoming constipation. Gore & Osmet, Rush Cutters Bay, Australia

Chiotakakou-Faliakou E, Kamm M A, Roy A J, Storrie J B, Turner I C 1998 Biofeedback provides long term benefit for patients with intractable, slow and normal transit constipation. Gut 42: 517–521

Davis M E, Platz E F 1965 Obstetrics, 13th edn. Saunders, Philadelphia

Devroede G 1992 Editorial. Constipation: a sign of disease to be treated surgically or a symptom to be deciphered as non-verbal communication? Journal of Clinical Gastroenterology 15(3): 189–191

Digestive Disorders 2002 www.digestivedisordersorg.uk/leaflets/ibs.html

Donald I P, Smith R G, Cruikshank J G, Elton R A, Stoddart M E 1985 A study of constipation in the elderly living at home. Gerontology 31: 112–118

Dresden K A, Kratzer G L 1959 Sites and frequency of faecal impactions. Journal of the American Medical Association 170: 644–647

Drossman D A, Li Z, Andruzzi E et al 1993a U.S. householder survey of functional gastrointestinal disorders. Digestive Diseases and Sciences 38: 1569–1580

Drossman D A, Leserman J, Nachman G et al 1993b Sexual and physical abuse in women with functional disorders of the lower gastrointestinal tract. International Journal of Colorectal Diseases 113: 828–833

Emmanuel A V, Kamm M A 2000 Laser doppler flowmetry as a measure of extrinsic colonic innervation in functional bowel disease. Gut 46: 212–217

Evans R C, Kamm M A, Hinton J M, Lennard-Jones J E 1992 The normal range and a simple diagram for recording whole gut transit time. International Journal of Colorectal Diseases 7: 15–17

Gattuso J M, Kamm M A 1993 Review article: the management of constipation in adults. Alimentary Pharmacology and Therapeutics 7: 487–500

Gibbons C P, Bannister J J, Read N W 1988 Role of constipation and anal hypertonia in the pathogenesis of haemorrhoids. British Journal of Surgery 75: 656–660

Gosling N 1985 Successful herbal remedies for treating common ailments. Thorsons, London

Heaton K W, Cripps H 1993 Straining at stool and laxative taking in an English population. Digestive Diseases and Sciences 38: 1004–1008

Heaton K W, Radvan J, Cripps H et al 1992 Defecation frequency and timing and stool form in the general population: a prospective study. Gut 33: 818–824

Heller S N, Hadder L R, Rivers J M et al 1980 Dietary fibre: the effect of particle size of wheatbran on colonic function in young adult men. American Journal of Clinical Nutrition 33: 1784

Hinds J P, Eidelman B H, Wald A 1990 Prevalence of bowel dysfunction in multiple sclerosis: a population survey. Gastroenterology 98: 1538–1542

Holdstock D J, Misiewicz J J, Smith T, Rowlands E N 1970 Propulsion (mass movements) in the human colon and its relationship to meals and somatic activity. Gut 11: 91–99

Homeopathic Development Foundation 1985 Homeopathy for the family, 5th edn. Homeopathic Development Foundation Ltd, London

Houts A C, Mellon M W, Whelan J P 1988 Use of dietary fibre and stimulus control to treat retentive encopresis: a multiple baseline investigation. Journal of Pediatric Psychology 13: 435–445

IBS Network 1991 www.ibsnetwork.org.uk

Joyce J 1969 Ulysses, 9th impression, revised edn. Bodley Head, London

Kamm M A, Hawley P R, Lennard-Jones J E 1988 The outcome of colectomy for severe idiopathic constipation. Gut 29: 969–973

Karanjia N D, Schache D J, Heald R J 1992 Function of the distal rectum after low anterior resection for carcinoma. British Journal of Surgery 79: 114–116

Klauser A G, Voderholzer W A, Heinrich C A, Schindlebech N E, Muller-Lissner S A 1990 Behavioural modification of colonic function. Digestive Diseases and Sciences 35: 1271–1276

Laurenberg S, Swash M 1989 Effects of ageing on the anorectal sphincters and their innervation. Diseases of the Colon and Rectum 32: 737–742

Lenzkes S L 1987 A silver pen for cloudy days. Zondervan Publishing, Michigan

Lust J 1986 The herb book. Transworld Publishing, London

Malouf A J, Vaizey C J, Kamm M A 2001 Results of behavioural treatment (biofeedback) for solitary rectal ulcer syndrome. Diseases of the Colon and Rectum 44: 72–76

MeReC Bulletin 1999 National Prescribing Centre: the management of constipation. MeReC 10(9): 33–36

Mimura T, Roy A J, Storrie J B, Kamm M A 2000 Treatment of impaired defecation associated with rectocele by behavioural retraining (biofeedback). Diseases of the Colon and Rectum 43: 1267–1272

Nagengast F M, van der Werf S D J, Lamers H L M et al 1988 Influence of age, intestinal transit time, and dietary composition on faecal bile and profiles in healthy subjects. Digestive Diseases and Sciences 33: 673–678

Ness W 1994 Silent problem: faecal incontinence. Nursing Times 90(36): continence suppl.

Norton C, Chelvanayagam S 2000 A nursing assessment tool for adults with fecal incontinence. Journal of WOCN 27(5): 279–291

Oettle G J 1991 Effects of moderate exercise on bowel habit. Gut 32: 941–946

Royal College of Nursing 1999 Digital rectal examination and manual removal of faeces. RCN, London

Royal College of Physicians 1995 Report of a working party: Incontinence – causes, management and provision of services. RCP, London

Shrubsole L, Smith P S 1984 The effect of change in environment on incontinence in profoundly mentally handicapped adults. British Journal of Mental Subnormality 30: 44–53

Smith L, Smith P S 1993 Psychological aspects of faecal incontinence in the elderly. Faecal Incontinence and Related Problems in the Older Adult 23: 182–185

Southgate D A T 1992 Starch and dietary fibre. Briefing Paper. Health Education Authority 29

Storrie J B 1997 Biofeedback: a first-line treatment for idiopathic constipation. British Journal of Nursing 6(3): 152–158

Swash M 1988 Childbirth and incontinence. Midwifery 4: 13–18

Sultan A H, Kamm M A, Hudson C N, Thomas J M, Bartram C I 1993 Anal sphincter disruption during vaginal delivery. New England Journal of Medicine 329: 1905–1911

Thompson W G, Heaton K W 1980 Functional bowel disorders in apparently healthy people. Gastroenterology 79: 27–30

Vaizey C J, Roy A J, Kamm M A 1997 Prospective evaluation of the treatment of solitary rectal ulcer syndrome with biofeedback. Gut 41: 817–820

Wald A, Tunuguntla A 1984 Anorectal sensorimotor dysfunction in faecal incontinence and diabetes mellitus: modification with biofeedback therapy. New England Journal of Medicine 310: 1282–1287

West O 1984 The magic of massage. A new and holistic approach. Century, London

8

Medication and continence

Mel Smith

'Principiis obsta; sero medicina paratur cum mala per longas convaluere moras.'
(Stop it at the start, it's late for medicine to be prepared when disease has grown strong through delays.)

Ovid, 43BC–AD17

INTRODUCTION

This chapter (for which the author has copyright) discusses the drugs that can be used to treat incontinence. The treatment of constipation complements information in Chapter 7 and is covered in detail because this is the area where, with the introduction of nurse prescribing and the availability of over-the-counter medicines, healthcare professionals other than the general practitioner will have more control in the future.

This chapter attempts to review some drugs and classes of drugs that may adversely affect patients in their ability to be continent. Questions that need to be asked when setting guidelines in treatment are suggested, and a sample of a set of guidelines currently in use is included. It is hoped that the information in this chapter will aid healthcare workers in treating patients, remembering always that drugs are not the only answer and that it is a person who is being treated.

THE TEAM APPROACH

In industry, the age of hierarchical management has given way to a flatter structure. This has been found to be more productive and more efficient.

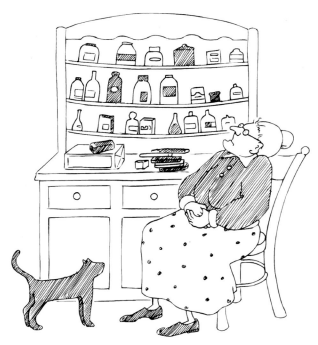

'A pill for every ill?'

Medicine needs to take its lead from industry. In patient care the team approach is the way forward. To improve the outcome in any treatment regime it is necessary to involve all the healthcare professionals who are treating the patient, as well as the carers, relatives and the patient in the plan for care (Sandars 1995).

The major part of this chapter looks at the effects of drugs *on the continent patient*. It is important that there is an holistic approach to patient care. This requires information from all the above people. The information must be coordinated and used to form a complete picture of the patient's needs. Only when the total needs have been identified should the possible treatments and outcomes be considered. There is rarely only one solution to a medical problem, which is why it is necessary to consult with all involved. Finally, with agreement of all parties, the protocol for treatment should be started. It is then important that the treatment is monitored. This is necessary as the patient's state may alter. The patient will get older, their physical and mental

condition may alter. The disease state may alter: it may be self-limiting, the underlying cause may be removed, or the treatment may be effective. If the condition alters then the treatment should be reviewed. While the monitoring and review of treatment may be carried out by the team, the patient if possible should be consulted, informed and agree to all aspects of the treatment by discussion with a single member of the team. The patient should not be confused by receiving different information from different members of the team.

There are more drugs available now than ever before. Many of these drugs are extremely potent and no drug is without side-effects. Some drugs are contraindicated in certain conditions. Some drugs interact with other drugs or with certain foodstuffs. Treatment for one condition may aggravate or even cause another condition. It is essential that these facts be borne in mind when drug therapy is being chosen. It is also useful to discuss this with the patient before treatment starts, if certain side-effects are likely to occur.

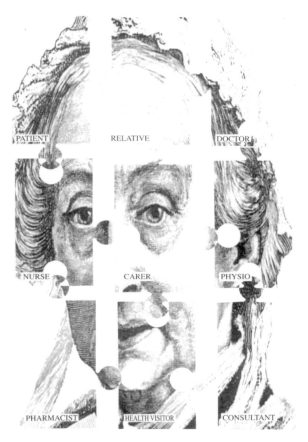

Information from all professionals involved in the patient's care must be obtained to create the whole picture.

Patients receiving cytotoxic treatment will not avoid going bald by being told that hair loss is a side-effect of the treatment; they may, however, be less traumatized if they know what is likely to happen, and this may help them to cope with the treatment. Side-effects themselves may be so serious as to require treatment in their own right. This can lead to a vicious circle of treatment, side-effect, and treatment of side-effect.

While patients with self-limiting acute conditions may only require symptomatic relief, patients with chronic conditions may require continuous medication. Side-effects may not occur with short-term treatment, but will almost certainly occur during continuous long-term treatment.

The above information may appear to have little to do with the treatment of the patients that you see. This is a general introduction to the treatment of any patient with a long-term illness. In the past, unless the patient was hospitalized the doctor dictated the treatment after making a diagnosis, the pharmacist dispensed the medications according to the prescription written, and the nurse in hospital or the community carried out the wishes of the medical staff with respect to the medication or other materials dispensed. More recently this situation has changed. The introduction of primary care groups and primary care trusts is leading to a review of existing prescribing habits and drug management systems. The increase in administration of the GP's practice is making the devolvement of some duties to other staff essential. This, together with the introduction of prescribing by other healthcare professionals, is set to change the way that patients will be treated in future. Already pharmacists are aiding medical staff to review patient medication and to introduce practice formularies and protocols. These will form the basis of medical audit, which will almost certainly lead to peer review of treatment. When all this is in place, the team approach to treatment will be functional.

With a team approach, communication between members of the team is essential. Although Blanchard (1993) says that the leader of the team can vary, this may be too radical for the healthcare team to accept at present. Those who see the patient most frequently will be able to brief the rest of the team on the patient's progress. Liaison between all members of the team is important, although regular meetings of the whole team may not be possible. It is therefore important for all members to keep each other up-to-date with the patient's progress.

This continual monitoring and reporting serves several important functions. The most obvious is to ensure that changes in the patient's condition are monitored and subsequently reviewed. The patient's compliance with medication regimens can be checked. This is especially important with patients taking several medicines concurrently (see Case study 8.1) where confusion may be a problem. If the patient is not taking the medication prescribed, is taking it incorrectly or is adding in another 'favourite' treatment, then the condition may not improve or other symptoms may present. This can be seen when the patient misuses laxatives and presents with diarrhoea. The treatment of the diarrhoea may not be effective if the patient continues to take laxatives. The review and modification of treatment, without knowing that the patient is complying with the present treatment, is not desired. The addition of stronger medication to the regimen – because medication already prescribed, but not taken, appears not to work – can be avoided. The hoarding of unused medicaments can be stopped. This will not only ensure that the patient is getting the best treatment, but also saves the medical practice money on medicines that are prescribed but not used. Finally, the patient's progress is checked against the treatment used and not against the treatment prescribed.

KEY POINTS: CARE FOR CHRONICALLY ILL PATIENTS

- All professionals and carers plus relatives and patient if possible should be involved in reviewing the patient's case.
- An holistic approach to the patient must be taken.
- A coordinated plan of treatment should be agreed by all.
- The plan must be monitored and reviewed regularly.
- The patient and/or carers should be kept informed of what treatment the patient is receiving and how it may affect them.
- Finally the patient's progress is checked against the treatment used and not against the treatment prescribed.

DRUG THERAPY

Drugs can affect continence in various ways:

- They can *treat* constipation or urinary retention.
- They can *cause* constipation or urinary retention.
- They can *treat* diarrhoea or urinary incontinence.
- They can *cause* diarrhoea or urinary incontinence.
- Some drugs may fit into more than one category.

For convenience this chapter looks at each group separately, and there is a final section on how combinations of drugs may lead to continence problems even though the treatment was for some other disease. This is known as the 'iatrogenic effect'.

TREATMENT OF CONSTIPATION: GENERAL PRINCIPLES

Chapter 7 discusses the causes of constipation and introduces the main drugs. To recap, the main causes of simple constipation are: a poor diet (i.e. inadequate fluid and dietary fibre); ignoring the call to stool; lack of exercise.

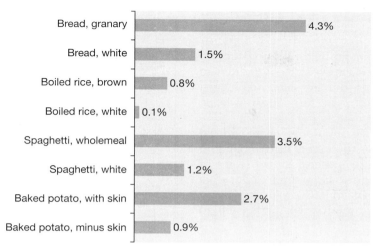

Figure 8.1 The fibre content of selected foodstuffs, determined by the Englyst method.

The term 'dietary fibre' was considered too imprecise by the Committee on Medical Aspects of Food Policy (COMA) (Whitehead 1991). The committee supported the proposition that the term 'dietary fibre' should become obsolete and be replaced by the more precise term 'non-starch polysaccharides' (NSPs). NSPs can be measured by the Englyst–Cummings technique (Englyst & Cummings 1984, Englyst et al 1982). It has been recommended that an NSP figure be used when labelling food in the United Kingdom. Figure 8.1 shows some examples.

The COMA recommendation was that the diet should include 18 g of NSPs per day (Whitehead 1991). It is estimated that adults in the UK consume only 12–13 g per day (calculated as NSP). At least 2 litres (4.5 pints) of fluid should be drunk. This should not include alcohol, which acts as a diuretic. Tea and coffee that contain caffeine, which also has a mild diuretic effect, should be limited.

It is possible to increase the intake of NSPs by substituting foods higher in NSPs for those that are lower. However, increasing the intake by this method may be unacceptable: the patient may not be able to tolerate the increase in food volume or may find the food unpalatable. It is then necessary to look at the use of bulking agents. These are often referred to as 'bulk-forming laxatives'

(*British National Formulary*), but the majority are natural products, standardized and formulated for convenient use. These will be discussed with the laxatives.

Fluid should not be restricted in the mistaken belief that it increases the risk of urinary incontinence.

Education of a patient who has continually ignored the call to stool may require the use of laxatives (Abrahams 1964, Haward & Hughes-Roberts 1962) to help restore natural bowel function.

Gentle exercise is all that is required to help the process of peristalsis. In patients who are physically handicapped the use of colonic massage may alleviate the problem without the need for drug intervention (Emly 1993). If drugs are required then the doses may be reduced if massage is used. The use of massage may also increase the patient's general well-being and some guidelines for this method are given later in this chapter and in Chapter 7.

KEY POINTS: CAUSES OF SIMPLE CONSTIPATION

- Poor diet: too little fibre (NSPs) and/or fluids.
- Ignoring the call to stool.
- Lack of exercise.

LAXATIVES: DRUGS THAT TREAT CONSTIPATION

These fall into four main groups: bulk-forming laxatives, stimulant laxatives, faecal softeners and osmotic laxatives. Box 8.1 shows the drugs included in each group by the *British National Formulary*.

The use of laxatives should be related to the patient's regimen as discussed in the opening part of this chapter. It is useful to have a set of guidelines as to when each type of laxative should be used and The Medical Resource Centre (MeReC) have issued the following information (MeReC 1999):

- Initial assessment should involve investigation of possible causes of constipation, such as drugs or poor diet. However, it is not always possible to identify an obvious underlying cause.
- Colorectal cancer should be suspected in any adult aged over 45 who presents with alarm symptoms or altered bowel habit without an obvious cause. Such patients should be referred for further investigation.

Box 8.1 Laxatives

- **Bulk-forming laxatives**
  Bran
  Ispaghula husk
  Methylcellulose
  Sterculia

- **Stimulant laxatives**
  Bisacodyl
  Dantron
  Docusate sodium
  Glycerol
  Senna
  Sodium picosulfate

- **Faecal softeners**
  Arachis oil
  Liquid paraffin

- **Osmotic laxatives**
  Lactitol
  Lactulose
  Macrogols
  Magnesium salts
  Phosphates
  Sodium citrate

- Along with removal of possible causes, dietary advice is the first step in the management of uncomplicated constipation. Laxatives should be reserved for cases where dietary intervention has failed, unless rapid relief of symptoms is required.
- Where appropriate, patients should be encouraged to gradually increase their NSP intake. They should aim to eat at least one fibre-rich food at every meal, as well as drinking two litres of fluid a day. However, a high fibre intake should be avoided in certain patients, such as immobile, elderly patients and those with faecal impaction.
- In pregnancy, if dietary and lifestyle measures fail, bulk-forming laxatives or stimulant laxatives such as senna may be used.

Bulk-forming laxatives

These can be thought of as a method of supplementing the fibre content of the diet. The Department of Health recommends a daily intake of NSPs of 18 g per day, while the suggested range is 12–24 g (Whitehead 1991). This range is low, because the report states that intakes of NSPs up to 32 g/d have been shown to increase stool weight.

All bulk-forming laxatives have the following in common:

- they must be taken with fluid – they absorb liquid and this causes them to swell to produce a soft mass
- the increase in bulk increases peristalsis, thus decreasing the transit time through the colon.

The reduction in time that the faecal mass is in contact with the colon has two effects. Firstly it reduces the amount of fluid absorbed from the faeces. Secondly it decreases the amount of time that noxious chemicals in the faeces are in contact with the colon. Many of the bulk-forming agents are fermented by bacteria in the colon. The products of this fermentation include gaseous substances. The production of these may initially lead to flatulence and abdominal distension, but they also stimulate peristalsis. These side-effects subside with continuation of the treatment as the bacteria in the bowel change. An adult evacuates up to 1.5 litres of gas per day as part of normal digestion (Tomlin et al 1991) (see Chapter 7). Although it is believed that bulk-forming laxatives are slow acting, it has been shown that they usually work within 24–36 hours in the majority of patients.

Bran

Wheat bran is what most people think of as fibre, or roughage. It is available as coarse unprocessed flake or is incorporated in breakfast cereals, snack bars, etc.

While wheat bran is a good source of fibre (36.4%; McCance & Widdowson 1991), it is high in insoluble fibre and low in soluble fibre (80:20). It also contains phytic acid, which chelates metal ions. This may lead to malabsorption, especially of iron and calcium. The amount of phytic acid may be reduced by processing the wheat bran.

The problems with bran as a source of fibre are mainly due to the quantity required (about 80 g/d) and palatability. It is worth noting that while All-Bran, with 29% fibre, is nearly pure bran, other high-fibre cereals contain only a small percentage of bran and therefore quite low levels of dietary fibre – for example, Kellogg's Fruit'n Fibre contains 9% fibre, Kellogg's Bran Flakes 15%, Rice Krispies 1.5%, Shredded Wheat Bitesize 11.6%, and Hot Oat Cereal 7.3%. Figure 8.2 shows the amount of bran-based cereal that would have

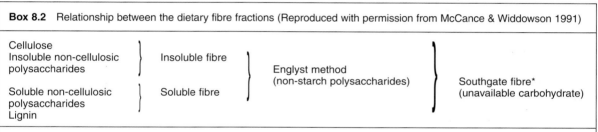

Box 8.2 Relationship between the dietary fibre fractions (Reproduced with permission from McCance & Widdowson 1991)

Cellulose
Insoluble non-cellulosic polysaccharides } Insoluble fibre }
Soluble non-cellulosic polysaccharides
Lignin } Soluble fibre } Englyst method (non-starch polysaccharides) } Southgate fibre* (unavailable carbohydrate)

* The Southgate values (this is the value obtained by using the Southgate method of analysis) are generally higher than NSP values because they include substances measuring as lignin, and also because the enzymatic preparation used leaves some enzymatically resistant starch in the dietary fibre residue. A 'resistant starch' value can be obtained from the NSP procedures, but because this uses different conditions and enzymes this may or may not be the same as the enzymatically resistant starch in the Southgate method.

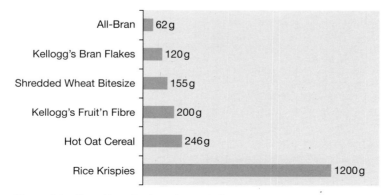

Figure 8.2 Quantities of selected cereals (in grams) needed to supply 18 g of NSP.

to be eaten if the total daily requirement of NSPs were to be taken as breakfast cereal. However, bran is available as the pharmaceutical preparation Trifyba.

Trifyba. Available as sachets containing 80% wheat fibre.

Adult: 1 sachet two to three times a day.

Child: ½–1 sachet once or twice daily, depending on age and size.

It should be mixed with food. For maximum effect adequate fluids should be taken. This product contains gluten and should be avoided in patients suffering from coeliac disease.

Ispaghula husk

This is the husk of the plant *Plantago Ovata Forsk*, which is native to the Canary Islands and the Mediterranean regions of southern Europe (Fig. 8.3). It is grown as a cash crop in India in the states of Gujarat and Rajasthan. The husk is separated from the seed by a process of milling

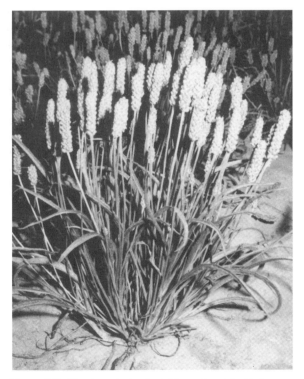

Figure 8.3 The ispaghula plant. Reproduced by kind permission of Reckitt Benckiser Healthcare (UK) Ltd.

and sieving. The husk is an extremely rich source of fibre containing between 80 and 85% dietary fibre. It is very low in phytic acid and has a high level of soluble fibre – the ratio of soluble to insoluble being approximately 80:20. Therefore, compared with wheat and oat bran, the total level of fibre and the level of soluble fibre in ispaghula husk is very high (Fig. 8.4).

The husk itself is an off-white flake, which needs processing to make it palatable. A fine balance has to be struck between texture, taste and gelling time to produce a product that is acceptable to most people. Ispaghula, like all bulk-forming laxatives, must be taken with liquid to avoid intestinal or oesophageal obstruction. It is therefore preferable to give ispaghula as a drink. If the patient cannot tolerate ingesting ispaghula in this way, refer to the recipes at the end of the chapter. In all cases a good supply of water should be taken throughout the day. As stated earlier, a lack of fluid intake is a possible cause of constipation, so educating the patient to drink more should always be part of treatment.

Fybogel. Available in plain, orange- or lemon-flavoured granules which are gluten-free and sugar-free, packed in sachets containing 3.5 g of ispaghula husk.

Adults: The contents of 1 sachet dissolved in 150 ml of water and taken twice a day.

Child over 6 years: ½ to 1 level 5 ml spoonful mixed as above and given twice daily.

Child below 6 years: On medical advice only.

Isogel. Bulk granules containing 90% ispaghula husk.

Adult: 2 teaspoonsful in water once or twice a day, preferably at mealtimes.

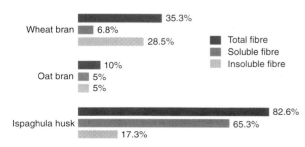

Figure 8.4 The fibre compositions of wheat bran, oat bran and ispaghula husk.

Child: 1 teaspoonful as above.

Konsyl Orange. 3.5 g ispaghula husk as orange-flavoured sugar-free powder per sachet.

Adult: 1–3 sachets per day in liquid.

Child 6–12 years: half the adult dose.

Regulan. Effervescent powder, gluten-free and sugar-free, packed in sachets containing 3.4 g ispaghula.

Adult: 1 sachet dissolved in 150 ml of water one to three times a day.

Child 6–12 years: 2.5–5 ml spoonful as above.

Methylcellulose

This is a synthetic bulking agent produced by modifying cellulose. The degree of modification affects the properties. The main property of methylcellulose is its ability to produce a viscous solution in cold water. There are many grades of methylcellulose: to identify each grade, the thickness or viscosity of a standard 2% solution is measured at 20°C (*British Pharmacopoeia* 2000, *United States Pharmocopeia* 2000). The higher the value obtained, the thicker or more viscous the solution. The value obtained from measuring this standard solution is appended to the description of the methylcellulose, for example Celevac contains methylcellulose '450'.

The medium- or high-viscosity grades are used as laxatives and work by taking up moisture to increase the bulk of the stools and hence increase peristalsis.

The side-effects of methylcellulose are similar to those of other bulk-forming laxatives. It should be avoided in gastrointestinal obstruction or threatened bowel obstruction. It must be taken with plenty of fluid (300 ml) (British National Formulary (BNF) 2002). Methylcellulose should not be used in the first trimester of pregnancy unless the expected benefit is thought to outweigh any possible risk to the foetus.

Celevac. Pink chewable tablets containing 500 mg methylcellulose '450' BP.

Dose: 3–6 tablets twice daily, to be taken with at least 300 ml of liquid. The tablets should be chewed before swallowing. The dose may be reduced as normal bowel function is restored.

Sterculia

This is a gum obtained from the plant *Sterculia urens* and other species of sterculia. Its action is similar to that of ispaghula. It should not be taken if intestinal obstruction, faecal impaction or total atony of the colon is suspected. It should not be taken immediately before going to bed.

Normacol. White-coated granules containing sterculia BP 62%, available in sachets containing 7 g of granules or bulk packs of 500 g.

Adults: 7–14 g taken once or twice daily after meals. The granules should be placed dry on the tongue and, without chewing or crushing, swallowed immediately with plenty of water.

Children 6–12 years: Half of the above dosage taken as described above.

Recommendations for bulk-forming laxatives

The aim of this group of laxatives is to add to the daily intake of NSPs. While bran is the cheapest source of dietary fibre, its lack of palatability and levels of phytic acid make it a questionable first choice. In some patients with irritable bowel syndrome, bran makes their symptoms worse (Francis & Whorwell 1994). These products are best taken mixed with fluid to avoid them causing obstruction. This may occur if they are taken dry and swell on contact with saliva. Owing to the high bulking capability of ispaghula husk, this is recommended as first-line treatment, but it is important to remember that not all patients are the same and if possible the patient's preference should be used. Clinical guidance on the use of bulk-forming laxatives is given in Box 8.3.

Box 8.3 Bulk-forming laxatives: the facts

- First-line treatment for simple constipation, after education on diet and lifestyle.
- Must be taken with plenty of fluids.
- Preferable to use a ready-hydrated product because there is less chance of causing obstruction.
- May cause flatulence and abdominal distension, which will subside within the first few days of treatment.
- Can be used long-term if necessary and during pregnancy.

Stimulant laxatives

All these drugs work by stimulating the nerve endings in the muscular wall of the colon. This stimulation causes an increase in peristalsis and secretion of fluid into the colon. The increased intestinal motility reduces colonic transit time, thus reducing the time for the absorption of fluid from the stools. This, along with the lubricating and softening effect of the secretions, aids evacuation of soft stools. These drugs usually act within 6–12 hours. They should only be used short term, when dietary advice or bulk-forming laxatives have proved ineffective. The continual use of stimulant laxatives can reduce muscle tone in the colon and can lead to colonic atony. They can be used when bulk-forming laxatives are contraindicated. Because of their action in stimulating secretion of fluid into the colon, chronic long-term use of this class of laxatives may lead to potassium depletion and dehydration.

KEY POINTS: CHRONIC LONG-TERM USE CAN CAUSE

- colonic atony
- potassium depletion and dehydration.

Bisacodyl

This is a synthetic diphenylmethane stimulant laxative. Although little of the active compound is absorbed, it exerts its stimulant effect throughout the gastrointestinal tract. This is the cause of its main side-effect – abdominal discomfort such as colic or cramps. In an attempt to limit this effect the tablets are enteric-coated, which stops the tablet releasing the bisacodyl in the upper gastrointestinal tract as the coating does not dissolve in the low pH of the stomach. To protect this coating, the tablets must be swallowed whole. They should not be taken with or soon after an antacid. Bisacodyl is available as a suppository for rectal use, but prolonged use rectally may cause irritation, proctitis or sloughing of the skin.

Dulco-lax. Available as enteric-coated tablets containing 5 mg bisacodyl; also as suppositories containing either 5 mg or 10 mg bisacodyl.

Adults and children over 10 years: 2 tablets at night or one 10 mg suppository in the morning. *Children under 10 years*: 1 tablet at night or one 5 mg suppository in the morning.

Because the tablets are enteric-coated they should not be crushed or chewed.

In cases of overdose, gastric lavage should be performed where appropriate. Adequate hydration must be maintained and the serum potassium levels should be measured. Particular care about fluid and electrolyte balances should be taken in the elderly and the young. Antispasmodics may be of some value in reducing the colicky lower abdominal pain.

Dantron

This is a synthetic stimulant anthraquinone laxative. It is normally given in combination with a surfactant poloxamer '188' (co-danthramer – Codalax) or docusate sodium (co-danthrusate – Normax). The action of dantron is similar to that of senna. It is, however, partly absorbed from the small intestine and it is excreted in the faeces and urine, and to some extent in other secretions including breast milk.

Dantron has been shown in some animal studies to cause the development of tumours in the liver and intestines. These studies were in rats and mice, and the administration of dantron was chronically at very high doses. For this reason dantron is limited in use to the treatment of constipation in the terminally ill (MCA 2000).

Dantron colours stools, urine and the perianal skin pink. This may interfere with urine tests, which rely on colour change. If the skin is left in contact with dantron then superficial sloughing of the discoloured skin may occur. This is seen in incontinent patients or young children in nappies; dantron should be avoided in these patients.

Normax. Dark brown capsules containing dantron 50 mg and docusate sodium 60 mg (co-danthrusate capsules). Docusate sodium is an anionic surfactant, which works by stimulating the secretion of electrolytes and water into the intestines. Owing to its surfactant properties it aids the penetration of the faecal mass by these secretions. It does have some laxative effect in its own right.

Adults (including elderly patients): 1–3 capsules taken at bedtime.

Children 6–12 years: 1 capsule at bedtime.

Prolonged use is not recommended.

Normax should not be used when intestinal obstruction is suspected. Normax is contraindicated in pregnancy or lactation. Where there is overdose, the patient should be encouraged to drink fluids to avoid dehydration and anticholinergic preparations may be used to reduce excessive intestinal motility.

Codalax and Codalax Forte suspension. An orange-coloured, peach-flavoured suspension. Each 5 ml dose contains either poloxamer '188' 200 mg and dantron BP 25 mg (Codalax, co-danthramer 25/200) or poloxamer '188' 1000 mg and dantron BP 75 mg (Codalax Forte, co-danthramer 75/1000).

Poloxamer '188' is a non-ionic surfactant, which is used as a wetting agent in the treatment of constipation. It increases the penetration of water into the faecal mass and helps to prevent it from drying and hardening excessively. It may also act as a lubricant. It may increase the absorption of fat-soluble substances such as liquid paraffin.

Dosage co-danthramer suspension:

Adult: One to two 5 ml spoonfuls at bedtime.

Child: Half to one 5 ml spoonful at bedtime.

Dosage co-danthramer forte suspension

Adult: Half to one 5 ml spoonful at bedtime or as directed.

Child: Not recommended for children under 12 years.

Docusate sodium

Dioctyl, Docusol. This agent probably acts as both stimulant and softening agent. It is included in the stimulant laxatives section of the BNF, but is classified as a faecal softener in the *Monthly Index of Medical Specialities* (MIMS).

Yellow capsules containing 100 mg docusate sodium (Dioctyl) or a solution containing 50 mg docusate sodium in 5 ml (Docusol). A paediatric solution is available containing 12.5 mg in 5 ml.

The tablets and solutions should be swallowed whole with a glass* of water. Due to the enteric coating these tablets should be swallowed whole.

Adults: Up to 500 mg daily in divided doses.

Children 2–12 years: 12.5–25 mg three times a day.

Infants over 6 months: 12.5 mg three times a day.

Because of its surfactant properties, docusate sodium will increase the absorption of mineral oil, so concurrent administration of mineral oil is contraindicated. As docusate sodium increases the absorption of anthraquinone derivatives, the dose of anthraquinone derivatives (senna and dantron) should be reduced when administered with docusate sodium.

Fletchers' Enemette. A ready-to-use self-contained single-dose enema containing 90 mg docusate sodium BP and 3780 mg glycerol PhEur.

Adults: The contents of one 5 ml enema as required.

Children under 3 years: Not recommended.

Glycerol

This is an osmotic dehydrating agent with hygroscopic and lubricating properties. Its action when administered rectally in the form of suppositories is localized. It is thought to have a local stimulating effect. It is also classified as a hyperosmotic laxative and is thought to draw water into the lower colon. It will also lubricate the faeces. These three actions are probably responsible for the fast action of glycerin suppositories. They normally work within 15–30 minutes of administration.

Adult: 4 g.

Child: 2 g.

Infant: 1 g.

To aid insertion the suppositories should be dipped in water before administration.

Senna

This is a natural anthraquinone stimulant laxative, obtained from the pods of the senna plant.

---

*Throughout this chapter a glass of liquid is estimated to measure 250 ml.

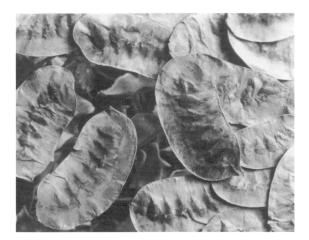

Figure 8.5 A close up view of natural senna pods. Reproduced by kind permission of Reckitt Benckiser Healthcare (UK) Ltd.

There are two types: *Cassia acutifolia* known as Alexandrian senna, and *Cassia angustifolia* known as Tinnevelly senna (Fig. 8.5).

In the past, an infusion of between four and twelve pods steeped in a cupful of water for 12 hours and taken at bedtime was used for the treatment of constipation. This produced variable results, and in 1950 the School of Pharmacy at the University of London, in collaboration with Westminster Laboratories (now part of Reckitt Benckiser), produced a chemical method for standardizing senna. This led to an entirely new manufacturing process to separate the senna seeds from the pods. The deseeded material is stabilized and assayed before being used to yield a product with a standard amount of the active ingredients, known as sennosides A and B. Tablets, syrup and granules contain a standard amount of these sennosides which have predictable results.

When senna is taken it is inactive. It is hydrolysed in the colon by the colonic bacteria, so releasing active free anthraquinones. It is these anthraquinones that produce a laxative effect. It has been suggested (Leng-Penschlow 1993) that senna does not damage epithelial cells, unlike bisacodyl, phenolphthalein, ricinoleic acid, docusate sodium and magnesium sulphate. Senna is the mildest of the stimulant laxatives (MIMS).

Senokot. Small brown tablets, each containing standardized senna equivalent to 7.5 mg total sennosides. It is also available as brown chocolate-flavoured granules (one 5 ml level spoonful (2.73 g) contains standardized senna equivalent to 15 mg total sennosides) and as a brown fruit-flavoured syrup (one 5 ml spoonful contains senna equivalent to 7.5 mg total sennosides). In all cases the total sennosides are calculated as sennoside B.

Adults: 2–4 tablets or one to two 5 ml spoonsful of granules or 10–20 ml of syrup at bedtime. On medical advice the dose may be up to twice that stated.

Children over 6 years: Half the adult dose taken in the morning.

Children 2–6 years: Use Senokot syrup, half to one 5 ml spoonful in the morning. Temporary mild griping may occur during adjustment of dosage. In cases of overdose, conservative measures are usually sufficient. Give generous amounts of fluids.

Sodium picosulfate

Sodium picosulfate is available as Dulco-lax Liquid, Laxoberal, and Picolax. Picolax is used for bowel cleansing prior to examination by radiography, endoscopy or surgery.

Dulco-lax Liquid, Laxoberal. Each contains 5 mg/5 ml sodium picosulfate.

Adults: 5–10 ml at night.

Children: under 4 years: 0.25 ml/kg
4–10 years: 2.5–5 ml at night
10 years and above: adult dose.

NB Dulco-lax is an example of 'umbrella branding': Dulco-lax tablets and suppositories contain bisacodyl, while Dulco-lax Liquid contains sodium picosulfate.

Picolax. Sachets containing sodium picosulfate 10 mg and magnesium citrate 13.1 g.

Adults: First dose before 8 a.m. of the day prior to examination. The contents of the sachet are dissolved in approximately 150 ml of water and swallowed. Second dose between 2 p.m. and 4 p.m. on the day prior to examination. The second dose should be made up in the same way.

Children: Timings as above.

1–2 years: Quarter sachet in morning, quarter sachet in afternoon.

2–4 years: Half sachet in morning, half sachet in afternoon.

4–9 years: One sachet in morning, half sachet in afternoon.

9 years and above: Adult dose.

A low-residue diet is recommended for 2 days prior to the examination. Plenty of fluids should be taken. This product is only used in specialized units. It is important that you are aware of the side-effects and the effects on the patient of this treatment if you should be asked to use it. It is, however, not usually used for treatment of constipation.

The patient should be warned to expect frequent loose stools within 3 hours of the first dose. The patient must drink large quantities of fluids during the treatment – this aids the passage of the stools and helps to avoid dehydration. It is usually advised that the patient has no food during the 24 hours before the procedure.

Recommendations for stimulant laxatives

These drugs work by stimulating the nerve endings in the colon wall to decrease the transit time of faecal matter through the colon. They also cause fluid to be secreted into the colonic lumen, which softens the stools. For oral use either senna or bisacodyl can be recommended. However, because senna is only active in the colon, where it is broken down by colonic bacteria and there is some evidence that it is less harmful to the epithelial layer of the colon wall (Leng-Peschlow 1993), senna has the gentlest action of the stimulant laxative group (MIMS). If a combination product is required then dantron in combination with a surfactant as co-danthramer or co-danthrusate is recommended. These products are now only licensed for use in the terminally ill.

For rectal use glycerin suppositories are safe and effective. It should be remembered that if possible the patient's preference should be taken into account, with regard to type, presentation and ingredient(s).

For simple constipation stimulant laxatives should only be used in the short term. If no effect

---

Box 8.4 Stimulant laxatives: the facts

- Can be used for acute simple constipation, particularly if dietary advice and bulk-forming laxatives are not effective.
- Short-term use only.
- Long-term chronic use may cause colonic atony and electrolyte disturbances.
- Dantron now only recommended for use in terminally ill patients.
- Senna has the gentlest action of the group.

---

is seen within 3 days then medical advice should be sought. In patients on long-term treatment with drugs that may cause constipation, it may be better to give prophylactic treatment to save the patient from more severe treatment when constipation does occur. Box 8.4 provides clinical guidance on the use of stimulant laxatives.

Faecal softeners

Docusate sodium and poloxamer '188', mentioned above, could fit into this section as they help water to penetrate and soften the faeces. They also have a stimulant action and have therefore been covered in the previous section. The *British National Formulary* (2002) includes just two products in the faecal softeners section: arachis oil and liquid paraffin.

These work by coating the faecal mass and the lower bowel with a hydrophobic layer. The stools retain water, which keeps them soft. The stools and colon are coated in oil, which acts as a lubricant to help easy passage of hard stools.

When given orally, liquid paraffin mist may be inhaled and can lead to lipoid pneumonia. Long-term use of liquid paraffin can affect fat-soluble vitamin absorption. The use of liquid paraffin can cause soiling of undergarments by anal seepage of the oil and stools. For these reasons the use of liquid paraffin in the treatment of constipation is now not routinely recommended.

Arachis oil

This is a refined oil from the seeds of *Arachis hypogaea*. It is normally given as an enema to soften and aid evacuation of impacted faeces.

Fletchers' Arachis Oil Retention Enema. Supplied as a ready-to-use single-dose enema containing 130 ml of arachis oil BP.

Adults and elderly patients: The contents of one enema as required.

Children over 3 years: Reduce the dose in relation to the child's bodyweight.

Children under 3 years: Not recommended.

The enema should be warmed to body temperature prior to use by placing it in warm water. As with all enemas, care should be taken not to use undue force during administration. This is particularly important in elderly or debilitated patients or those with neurological disorders.

Recommendations for faecal softeners

Nowadays oral administration of faecal softening laxatives with the exception of docusate sodium (see Stimulant laxatives) is not recommended. The use of arachis oil enemas may be helpful in aiding the passage of hard or impacted stools. Box 8.5 provides clinical guidance on the use of faecal softeners.

Osmotic laxatives

These work by keeping fluid in the faeces by osmotic pressure, or by drawing fluid into the faeces from the surrounding area. While they may have special uses, the continual use of these products can lead to dehydration and electrolyte disturbances. It is important that these laxatives are taken with large quantities of water. They normally produce semifluid evacuation.

Box 8.5 Faecal softeners: the facts

- Useful when straining is a problem.
- Only docusate sodium (classified as a stimulant in the BNF) is recommended for oral use.
- Arachis oil as an enema may be useful in aiding the passage of hard or impacted stools.
- Liquid paraffin may cause lipoid pneumonia and should not be routinely used in the treatment of constipation.

Lactitol and lactulose

These are semi-synthetic sugars, which are not absorbed when taken orally. They produce their actions by holding or drawing water in the food mass during passage through the colon. They are broken down by bacteria in the colon. The breakdown products include lactic acid, which exerts a local stimulant effect. The lactic acid also lowers the colonic pH – this action is used in hepatic encephalopathy. The low pH selectively promotes the growth of colonic bacteria. This and the lower pH reduce the production and absorption of ammonium ions and other toxic nitrogenous products. The side-effects of these products are flatulence, cramps and general abdominal discomfort. Although lactitol is tasteless, the sweet syrupy taste and volume required make lactulose unpalatable for some patients. These products may take up to 48 hours to work. The full dose must be taken regularly during the treatment course for them to be effective. It is now recommended that these are not used as first-line treatment for simple constipation (MeReC 1999).

Lactitol. Sachet containing 10 g fine white powder.

Adults: Initially 20 g taken morning or evening with a meal; adjust the dose to produce one stool daily, usually 10 g daily. The powder should be mixed with food or liquid and one or two glasses of liquid should be drunk with the meal.

Children 6–12 years: Between 5 g and 10 g daily.

Children 1–6 years: Between 2.5 g and 5 g daily.

Lactulose solution BP. A clear colourless or brownish-yellow solution containing lactulose (with some lactose and galactose). Also as branded products Duphalac and Lactugal. Each dose may be taken with water or fruit juice.

Adults: 15 ml twice a day.

Children 5–10 years: 10 ml twice a day.

Children 1–5 years: 5 ml twice a day.

Children under 1 year: 2.5 ml twice a day.

Magnesium salts

The most common magnesium salt used for constipation is magnesium sulphate (Epsom salts).

Because magnesium salts are poorly absorbed they hold water in the food mass. Care must be taken in using magnesium salts in patients with impaired renal function as the increased absorption of magnesium may produce toxic effects.

Adults: 5–10 g dissolved in a tumblerful of water will produce bowel evacuation in 2–4 hours.

Other salts are used for preparation of patients before radiological or surgical procedures, for example magnesium citrate (Citramag).

Phosphates

These preparations are administered rectally. They should only be used when other treatments have proved ineffective or before radiological or surgical procedures. As they are administered locally their action is usually rapid.

Fletchers' Phosphate Enema. A ready-to-use disposable 128 ml enema containing sodium acid phosphate 12.8 g and sodium phosphate 10.24 g.

Adults: The contents of one enema to be administered when required.

Child: In proportion according to age and bodyweight.

This product should be used with caution in patients on a reduced sodium intake or with a disease that alters the absorptive capacity of the colon. If used chronically, electrolytes must be checked and a balance maintained.

Sodium citrate

This is administered rectally in combination with surfactants and other osmotic laxatives. Prolonged use of these enemas may lead to local irritation.

Micolette Micro-enema. A ready-to-use 5 ml disposable enema containing sodium citrate 450 mg, sodium lauryl sulphoacetate (a surfactant) 45 mg, glycerol 625 mg, together with citric acid, potassium sorbate and sorbitol.

Adults and children over 3 years: The contents of one or two enemas as required.

Micralax Micro-enema. A ready-to-use 5 ml disposable enema containing sodium citrate 450 mg, sodium alkylsulphoacetate (a surfactant) 45 mg, sorbic acid 5 mg, together with glycerol and sorbitol.

Adults and children over 3 years: The contents of one enema as required.

Relaxit Micro-enema. A ready-to-use 5 ml disposable enema containing sodium citrate 450 mg, sodium lauryl sulphoacetate (a surfactant) 75 mg, sorbic acid 5 mg, together with glycerol and sorbitol.

Adults and children over 3 years: The contents of one enema as required.

Recommendations for osmotic laxatives

The osmotic group of laxatives covers drugs with a variety of actions, side-effects and costs. Magnesium sulphate acts within 2–4 hours, can cause hypermagnesaemia and is very cheap. Lactulose can take up to 72 hours to work. The taste, possibility of dehydration and quantity required should restrict the use of lactulose to second-line treatment. This is reflected in the recommendations of the National Prescribing Centre (MeReC 1999). Enemas may be useful in treating impacted faeces, but their use as routine treatment for elderly patients should be deplored. Box 8.6 provides clinical guidance on the use of osmotic laxatives.

Prescribing treatments

Under the nurse prescribing regulations suitably qualified nurses will be allowed to initiate treatment for constipation. This section of the

---

Box 8.6 Osmotic laxatives: the facts

- Essential that plenty of fluid be taken with these products to avoid dehydration.
- Can have a variable speed of action.
- Can produce watery stools and osmotic diarrhoea.
- Not recommended as first-line treatment (MeReC 1999) but use when other laxatives have failed to produce an effect.
- Enemas may be useful for removal of impacted faeces.
- May cause electrolyte imbalance (electrolytes need to be monitored, particularly in elderly patients on chronic treatment).

chapter has included details on products and dosages to help with that responsibility. Many hospitals and general practice surgeries have guidelines on what to prescribe for constipation. It can be helpful to develop a set of guidelines locally in consultation with colleagues, or adopt an existing set (Fig. 8.6). Box 8.7 shows a proforma for writing new guidelines (see Chapter 7).

DRUGS THAT CAUSE DIARRHOEA

In the previous section details of products and dosages have been given. In this section groups of drugs will be considered which may have the ability to cause diarrhoea as a side-effect. Proprietary names are given only where it is felt necessary for clarity and doses will not be mentioned unless the side-effect is dose related.

Many of the groups of drugs used to treat constipation can themselves cause diarrhoea. The exception to this is the bulk-forming laxatives. Overuse of stimulant laxatives in the short term may cause diarrhoea. Chronic use leads to colon atony and the lack of colonic motility causes constipation. While liquid paraffin does not cause watery diarrhoea, it does lead to anal seepage. The osmotic laxatives by their action produce watery stools. Chronic use or high doses can cause osmotic diarrhoea.

> Many of the groups of drugs used to treat constipation can themselves cause diarrhoea.

Antacids

Some antacids such as magnesium salts cause diarrhoea, while others like calcium and aluminium cause constipation. Sometimes in branded antacids a combination of agents is administered to try to neutralize the effect (e.g. magaldrate and hydrotalcite). Magaldrate is a combination of aluminium and magnesium hydroxides. Hydrotalcite is aluminium magnesium carbonate hydroxide hydrate. Another combination is calcium carbonate and light magnesium carbonate.

Box 8.7 Proforma for writing guidelines for the treatment of constipation

- **Identify causes**   Take a detailed patient history
  Inform patient of lifestyle changes (dietary measures)
- **Define condition**
- **Define treatment**   What it will achieve
  What the end point is
- **Discuss treatment with patient**   Education
- **Review patient and treatment**   Set time scale
- **Adjust treatment as necessary**

A co-dried gel is made from aluminium hydroxide and magnesium carbonate.

Magnesium salts (i.e. magnesium carbonate, magnesium hydroxide, magnesium oxide and magnesium trisilicate) are all used as antacids.

Antibiotics

These may cause diarrhoea by altering the bacterial content of the gastrointestinal tract. This is seen only with orally administered antibiotics. It is common with penicillin antibiotics, fluoroquinolones, macrolides and tetracyclines although less so with the cephalosporins. Giving yoghurt which contains live lactobacillus can help in the treatment of patients who have been on long courses of antibiotic therapy or who develop diarrhoea.

Antidepressants

Selective serotonin reuptake inhibitors (e.g. fluoxetine hydrochloride and fluvoxamine maleate) can cause diarrhoea. Lithium products can cause either diarrhoea or constipation.

Beta-adrenoceptor blocking agents

These can cause gastrointestinal (GI) upsets leading to diarrhoea or constipation. In one study, GI disturbances accounted for 11.2% of all adverse reactions (Kock-Weser 1974). It appears that diarrhoea is more common than constipation.

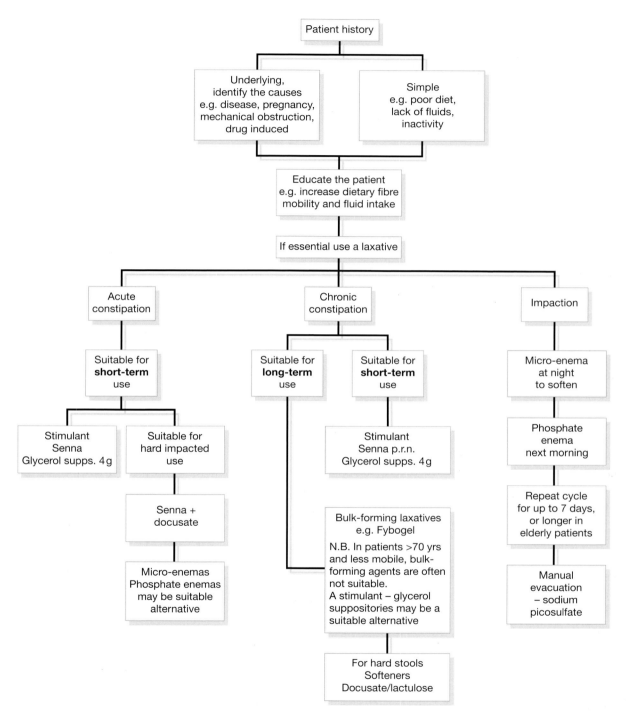

Figure 8.6   Suggested guidelines for the treatment of constipation in adults.

Oral hypoglycaemic agents

These may cause diarrhoea. Some, especially glibenclamide and glipizide, have a mild diuretic effect.

Antineoplastic agents

Many of these agents cause inflammation of the gastric mucosa. This may lead to diarrhoea. Combination with radiotherapy may increase the toxicity of some of these agents to the GI tract.

Dantrolene sodium

The skeletal muscle relaxant dantrolene sodium, used in the relief of spasticity, may cause diarrhoea severe enough to necessitate withdrawal of treatment.

Diuretics

Because of their ability to alter electrolyte balances, diuretics may cause either constipation or diarrhoea. Spironolactone can cause diarrhoea, while amiloride and the thiazides can cause either constipation or diarrhoea. Furosemide (frusemide) rarely causes GI disturbances.

Iron preparations

These can cause GI disturbances leading to either constipation or diarrhoea. In cases of overdose, diarrhoea predominates.

Lipid regulating drugs

The fibric acid derivatives cause diarrhoea, while colestyramine and the resins cause constipation.

Xanthines

Theophylline, aminophylline and caffeine can all cause diarrhoea.

Foods

Foods, including non-absorbed sugars such as sorbitol and lactose, may cause diarrhoea. Sorbitol is found in diabetic and sugar-free foods. Lactose is found in many nasogastric feeds, as well as milk products.

Box 8.8 Drugs that may cause diarrhoea

- Antacids
- Antibiotics
- Antidepressants
- Antineoplastic agents
- Beta-adrenoceptor blocking agents
- Dantrolene sodium
- Diuretics
- Iron preparations
- Lipid regulating drugs
- Oral hypoglycaemic agents
- Xanthines
- Foods containing non-absorbed sugars, sorbitol and lactose.

When treating a patient it is important to review the existing regimen. It is undesirable to add further medication to counteract the side-effects of existing treatment.

ANTIDIARRHOEAL DRUGS

The *British National Formulary* divides these into two categories: adsorbents and bulk-forming laxatives, and antimotility drugs. A third type can be added – oral rehydration therapy – in this chapter referred to as 'electrolytes'.

The most important part of treatment is the correct diagnosis. Paradoxically, diarrhoea can be as the result of faecal impaction. Two types of constipation have been identified as causing this type of diarrhoea. The colon may become full of faecal material, which because of increased transit time loses too much water and becomes hard round pellets. Alternatively transit time may be normal but, owing to delay in transit through the sigmoid colon to the rectum, the colon fills with a large mass of putty-like faecal material. In the final stages the flow of faeces around this large mass causes the passage of offensive smelling watery stools which can be mistaken for diarrhoea. In elderly patients 98% of faecal impaction is rectal (Smith 1983). It may be caused by the effects, side-effects or interactions of other drugs – the 'iatrogenic effect'.

Diarrhoea may be due to infection, food poisoning or a disease state which alters the GI tract, such as cancer or an inflammatory bowel condition like Crohn's disease or diverticulitis. It can also be due to changes in neurological state (see also Chapter 11).

The treatment regime will depend on the diagnosis. In cases of acute diarrhoea, usually caused by infection, it is important to maintain the body's fluid and electrolyte balances. In cases of faecal stasis it is important to remove the impacted faecal mass prior to re-educating the bowel. In cases of chronic diarrhoea, as well as ensuring that the patient is well hydrated, drug intervention may be required.

Oral rehydration salt (ORS) therapy

The World Health Organization (WHO) recommends a formula suitable for the treatment of acute diarrhoea (Box 8.9). This mixture should be dissolved in sufficient water to produce 1 litre of solution. Anhydrous glucose dissolves more quickly than either sucrose or glucose monohydrate.

The solution should be administered after each loose stool in the volume of 200–400 ml. In severe cases up to 4 litres can be administered in a 4-hour period. The solution should *not* be diluted, as this is the optimal for the absorption of the electrolytes in patients who are severely dehydrated. In these people the body's normal homeostatic mechanism is not working, so if more liquid is required then extra drinks of water should be administered *between* the doses of rehydration solution. It is important that uncontaminated water be used to make up the solution.

The *British Pharmacopoeia* gives three formulae for ORS (Table 8.1). For patients in the UK, where severe dehydration is less of a problem, formula A is recommended as this is lower in sodium and higher in glucose. This solution is more beneficial in mild to moderate diarrhoea where the body's homeostatic mechanisms are still working. Note that formula B corresponds to the WHO bicarbonate formulation and formula C to the WHO citrate formulation. All of these solutions should be used within 24 hours of preparation and if possible they should be kept in a refrigerator.

In cases of severe dehydration the body tries to preserve fluid by modifying its normal functions. This leads to the alteration of absorption of electrolytes and carbohydrates. To help the absorption, cereal flour and rice starch have been used

---

Box 8.9 The WHO recommended formula for acute diarrhoea

• Sodium chloride	3.5 g	
• Potassium chloride	1.5 g	
• Sodium citrate	2.9 g	or
sodium bicarbonate	2.5 g	
• Anhydrous glucose	20 g	or
glucose monohydrate	22 g	or
sucrose	40 g	

Table 8.1 The British Pharmacopoeia formulae for ORS

	Formula A	Formula B	Formula C
Sodium chloride	1 g	3.5 g	3.5 g
Potassium chloride	1.5 g	1.5 g	1.5 g
Sodium bicarbonate	1.5 g	2.5 g	–
Anhydrous glucose	36.4 g	20 g	20 g
OR			
Glucose monohydrate	40 g	22 g	–
Sodium citrate	–	–	2.9 g
Water to	1000 ml	1000 ml	1000 ml

---

in place of some or all of the glucose. These solutions may be more effective. The need to prepare the solution by boiling and the increased risk of bacterial growth mean that they are not generally recommended.

> All solutions must be made up in clean water, preferably boiled and cooled. ORS must be kept in a refrigerator and used within 24 hours of reconstitution.

Adsorbents and bulk-forming laxatives

The bulk-forming laxatives mentioned in the earlier section on constipation can be effective in diarrhoea. They could effectively be reclassified as drugs for regulating colonic transit, or 'drugs for regularity'. In India, one of the main uses for ispaghula husk is in the treatment of diarrhoea. Those bulk-forming agents containing soluble fibre have a twofold action:

- They hold water in the colon, by their gelling action. In constipation this bulking action stimulates peristalsis.

- In diarrhoea the viscosity of the gel slows the passage of the watery mass, allowing more time for absorption of water by the colon.

Details of the bulk-forming laxatives are to be found in the section on constipation. One study on chronic diarrhoea showed that the administration of calcium and ispaghula was as effective as loperamide, had fewer side-effects and was cheaper (Qvitzau et al 1988).

Adsorbents

These are now *not* recommended for acute diarrhoea, which is usually due to bacterial infection. Adsorbents could hold the bacteria in the gut and so prolong the infection. In the past they were widely used to treat faecal incontinence. A letter to *The Lancet* in 1960 outlined five cases where alternate treatment with kaolin and Senokot was used to successfully treat patients with neurogenic incompetence (Jarrett & Exton-Smith 1960). Adsorbents work by absorbing water and thickening the faecal mass. Kaolin, attapulgite and chalk work in this manner. Adsorbents are usually combined with antimotility drugs, as in the mixture of kaolin plus morphine.

Kaolin mixture BP. Each 10 ml dose contains light kaolin 2 g, light magnesium carbonate 500 mg, sodium bicarbonate 500 mg, with peppermint flavouring and chloroform water as a preservative.
Adults: 10–20 ml every 4 hours.

Kaolin and morphine mixture BP. Each 10 ml dose contains light kaolin 2 g, sodium bicarbonate 500 mg, tincture of chloroform, and morphine 0.4 ml. It may be found that giving the dose in warm water has a soothing effect.
Adults: 10 ml every 4 hours.

Kaopectate (OTC). An off-white suspension containing 1.03 g of kaolin per 5 ml dose.
Adult: 10–30 ml every 4 hours.
Children 1–5 years: 10 ml every 4 hours.
Children up to 1 year: 5 ml every 4 hours.

Antimotility drugs

These drugs work by reducing the motility of the intestinal tract. The increase in transit time allows the absorption of more water from the faecal mass and reduces the frequency and fluidity of the stools.

Modern theory has little place for these drugs. For acute diarrhoea, oral rehydration solution (ORS) therapy is the treatment of choice. In chronic diarrhoea, treatment of the cause of the diarrhoea if possible, plus ORS therapy and if necessary bulk-forming laxatives, would be most appropriate. If antimotility drugs *are* used, the patient still needs to be given oral rehydration therapy. Treatment with antimotility drugs should normally be in the short term.

Codeine phosphate

Like all the opioid analgesics, codeine reduces intestinal motility. It is less constipating than morphine, but is used in the treatment of diarrhoea as it has less of a sedative effect. It produces less euphoria than morphine and is less likely to produce addiction. Morphine-type dependence is seen in some users, especially those on long-term high doses. It can also be found in some cough mixtures, where it is used as a cough suppressant, and overuse of these products may be the cause of constipation in some patients.

Codeine phosphate tablets. In the treatment of diarrhoea.
Adults: 30 mg three to four times a day.
Children: Not recommended.

Diphenoxylate hydrochloride

This is a derivative of pethidine. It is metabolized in the liver to produce diphenoxylic acid, which is the major active metabolite. As it is a derivative of a narcotic it may produce morphine-like dependence in chronic use or at high dosage. To try to prevent abuse and deliberate overdose, a subtherapeutic amount of atropine sulphate is added. This preparation has the generic name of co-phenotrope.

Treatment with co-phenotrope should be in the short term. In acute diarrhoea, if no improvement is seen within 48 hours, then treatment with this drug should be discontinued. In cases of chronic diarrhoea, if no improvement is seen after 10 days with a dose of 20 mg, then treatment should be discontinued.

Lomotil. Available as white tablets containing diphenoxylate hydrochloride 2.5 mg with atropine sulfate PhEur 25 μg.

Adults: Starting dose of four tablets, followed by two tablets every 4 hours.

Children 13–16 years: Two tablets three times a day.

Children 9–12 years: One tablet four times a day.

Children 4–8 years: One tablet three times a day.

Before using this in elderly patients, consideration should be given to the diagnosis of constipation. Is there any underlying disease or iatrogenic effect of other treatment?

Loperamide hydrochloride

As well as inhibiting intestinal motility, loperamide inhibits gastrointestinal secretions. It should be used with caution in patients with liver disease as it is metabolized in the liver. Use in these patients may lead to toxic effects at normal therapeutic doses. It may cause toxic megacolon if given to patients with inflammatory bowel disease or pseudomembranous colitis. It should not be used alone in acute dysentery. It should not be used if constipation has to be avoided.

Treatment should be short term only in the case of acute diarrhoea, for no more than 5 days. Constipation has been observed in patients after treatment with lopermide.

Imodium. Available as a grey and green capsule containing 2 mg loperamide or as a red fruit-flavoured syrup containing 1 mg of loperamide per 5 ml dose. Capsules and syrups are also available to the public (Arret, Diocalm Ultra).

Adults: For acute diarrhoea, 2 capsules at the start followed by 1 capsule after every loose stool for up to 5 days. The usual dosage is 3–4 capsules per day. The maximum dose should not exceed 8 capsules per day. For chronic diarrhoea, the normal dose required is between 2 and 4 capsules daily in divided doses. When the correct dose has been titrated, the patient should be given the maintenance dose in a twice-daily regimen.

Children 9–12 years: 10 ml spoonful of the syrup or 1 capsule four times a day.

Children 4–8 years: 5 ml spoonful four times a day.

TREATMENTS FOR SPECIFIC DISEASES WHERE DIARRHOEA IS A PROBLEM

The following six diseases have diarrhoea as a symptom: irritable bowel syndrome (IBS), malabsorption syndrome, ulcerative colitis, Crohn's disease, pseudomembranous colitis and diverticular disease.

While all patients need fluid and electrolyte replacement, some patients will require diet modification. The treatment for these diseases tends to be symptomatic although in some cases some specific drugs may be effective. These drugs are discussed below. In many of these conditions the use of antimotility drugs is contraindicated because they may precipitate paralytic ileus or megacolon.

Irritable bowel syndrome (IBS)

Diagnosis should be made using the Rome II criteria (Jones et al 2000). The treatment should be related to the symptoms as shown in Figure 8.7.

The use of bulk-forming laxatives such as ispaghula may be beneficial, although bran may make the condition worse (Francis & Whorwell 1994). Combination of ispaghula with the antispasmodic mebeverine (Fybogel Mebeverine) has been shown to be effective in cases of IBS where spasm together with bowel irregularity is a problem.

Refer to Chapter 7 where the use of biofeedback to treat IBS is described.

Malabsorption syndrome

In this condition, identifying the condition or the food group that gives rise to the symptoms is important. Coeliac disease requires the avoidance of gluten-containing foods such as wheat starch products. Pancreatic deficiency such as cystic fibrosis and pancreatitis requires supplements of pancreatin.

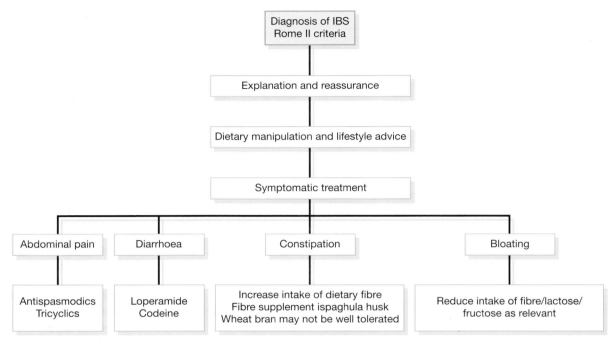

Figure 8.7 Outline of protocol for managing the symptoms of IBS.

Ulcerative colitis and Crohn's disease

Ulcerative colitis requires treatment with steroids in the acute phase. Balsalazide, mesalazine, olsalazine and sulfasalazine can be used for treatment and to prevent relapse. Infliximab, a monoclonal antibody that inhibits the proinflammatory cytokine, has recently been introduced for use in the treatment of severe acute Crohn's disease refractory to corticosteroid or immunosuppressant therapy.

The drugs used in ulcerative colitis can also be used for the treatment of Crohn's disease. Metronidazole may be of benefit if bacterial overgrowth in the bowel occurs.

Pseudomembranous colitis

This is due to colonization of the colon with *Clostridium difficile*. This usually follows antibiotic therapy, especially with clindamycin, and can be successfully treated with vancomycin and metronidazole.

Diverticular disease

This can be treated conservatively with bulk-forming laxatives such as ispaghula husk. Antispasmodics such as mebeverine are useful when colic is a problem. In diverticulitis, antibiotics may be needed to fight infection.

A summary of clinical guidance on treatment for diarrhoea is given in Box 8.10.

DRUGS CAUSING CONSTIPATION

As stated in the sections on diarrhoea, with the exception of the bulk-forming laxatives, the products used in the treatment of diarrhoea can cause constipation. This can occur in overdose or in chronic use. Other drugs which cause constipation are discussed below and are summarized in Box 8.11.

Some drugs have the side-effect of gastrointestinal disturbance. This may be either constipation or diarrhoea, depending on the patient

---

Box 8.10 Treatments for diarrhoea

Acute diarrhoea
- Maintain electrolyte and fluid balances using oral rehydration salt (ORS) therapy.
- Bulk-forming laxatives may be added.
- A *short course* of antimotility drugs can be used.
- Should be self-limiting within 3–5 days.

Chronic diarrhoea
- Examine for underlying cause: may be faecal impaction with overflow, laxative overuse or drug side-effects.
- Remove or treat cause.
- Keep patient hydrated.
- In all cases, review.

---

and the condition being treated. These drugs have already been covered in the section on drugs causing diarrhoea.

Opioid analgesics

This is a class of drugs commonly associated with causing constipation. The action on smooth muscle is to reduce motility. It is usual to prescribe a stimulant laxative to counteract the reduction of gastromotility caused by these drugs. While morphine and diamorphine are well known, others in this class are dextropropoxyphene, an ingredient of co-proxamol, and dihydrocodeine, and an ingredient of co-dydramol (DF118). Some proprietary cough suppressant medicines contain codeine.

This is a major problem in patients in terminal illness, when strong painkillers are often required. For mild-to-moderate pain the use of analgesics which do not contain opioid derivatives is advised. Aspirin, paracetamol, ibuprofen or one of the other non-steroidal anti-inflammatories may provide a suitable alternative.

Antacids

While magnesium-based antacids can cause diarrhoea, aluminium- and calcium-based antacids can cause constipation. To try to neutralize the effects, combinations have been developed (see Drugs that cause diarrhoea). Aluminium hydroxide and calcium carbonate are both used as antacids.

Antidepressants

Amitriptyline and imipramine, along with other tricyclic antidepressants, may cause constipation. This is due to their antimuscarinic side-effects. Monoamine oxidase inhibitors (MAOIs) like phenelzine sulfate can also cause constipation.

Antihypertensive agents

Clonidine, which in low doses is also used for the prophylaxis of migraine, causes constipation in about 10% of patients.

Antimuscarinic agents

Atropine, dicycloverine (dicyclomine), hyoscine and propantheline are used in the treatment of smooth muscle spasm. Trihexyphenidyl (benzhexol) and procyclidine are used in the treatment of Parkinson's disease. Oxybutynin is used for the management of urgency and incontinence in neurogenic bladder disorders. All these antimuscarinic agents can cause constipation by reducing muscle tone of the colon and thus inhibiting peristalsis.

Anxiolytics, sedatives, hypnotics and neuroleptics

Phenothiazides such as chlorpromazine, thioridazine and clozapine have antimuscarinic properties. These can cause constipation and difficulty in micturition. Other drugs within this category can cause confusion, which, while not affecting bowel habit directly, may cause forgetfulness. This can cause incontinence of all types.

Barium sulfate

This is used as a contrast medium in radiological examinations. While such an examination is unlikely to take place in a patient in the community, if the patient has been to hospital recently they should be asked whether a radiological examination was performed.

Box 8.11 Drugs that may cause constipation

- Analgesics
- Antacids
- Antidepressants
- Antihypertensive drugs
- Antimuscarinic drugs
- Anxiolytics, sedatives, hypnotics, neuroleptics
- Barium sulphate
- Diuretics
- Iron and resins

Box 8.12 Drugs that may be used to treat urinary retention

Alpha-adrenoceptor blockers
- Alfuzosin
- Doxazosin
- Indoramin
- Prazosin
- Tamsulosin
- Terazosin

Parasympathomimetics
- Bethanechol
- Carbachol

Diuretics

All diuretics can cause dehydration, which may cause constipation. Amiloride and hydrochlorthiazide may cause either constipation or diarrhoea.

Iron supplements and resins

Iron can cause gastrointestinal upset, which may present as either diarrhoea or constipation and seems to be patient and/or iron salt related.

Colestyramine and colestipol are used to lower lipids. These resins are used to bind cholesterol and remove it from circulation. Constipation is a common side-effect and they may even cause faecal impaction. A summary of drugs that may cause constipation is provided in Box 8.11.

URINARY CONTINENCE

This section looks at drugs used in urinary retention and urinary incontinence. It reviews the drugs that may contribute to these conditions.

The basis of treatment should be as stated previously. The team approach combined with the identification of a desired outcome should enable treatment to be tailored to the individual's need. Drug therapy should be only a part of patient management. The patient's condition should be reviewed regularly. This will ensure that the treatment is still relevant and that side-effects are not developing.

Urinary retention

In acute urinary retention there is great pain as well as the desire to urinate. The treatment is normally by catheterization (see Chapter 9). In chronic conditions there may be no need to catheterize the patient. Depending on the cause of the retention various drug treatments can be tried. Urethral stricture may be due to benign prostatic hyperplasia (see Chapter 4).

Drugs that may be used to treat urinary retention are summarized in Box 8.12.

Alpha-adrenoceptor blockers

The obstruction caused by benign prostatic hyperplasia may be increased by the stimulation of the prostatic alpha-adrenoceptors. Stimulation of these receptors will increase prostatic muscular tension. For this condition, prazosin (Hypovase), alfuzosin (Xatral), indoramin (Doralese), doxazosin (Cardura), tamsulosin (Flomax MR) or terazosin (Hytrin BPH) can be used. These drugs work by selectively blocking the alpha$_1$-adrenoceptors, which decreases smooth muscle tone.

In low doses these products have been shown to improve the urinary pressure profile in patients with urinary obstruction (Lepor 1989). They are indicated in the treatment of patients in whom surgical treatment is unsuitable or in patients awaiting prostatic surgery. These drugs also decrease peripheral vascular resistance. They are used in the treatment of hypertension, so it is important that patients taking these drugs have their blood pressure carefully monitored. The possibility of postural hypotension, dizziness and the loss of consciousness must be borne in mind. Urinary incontinence and frequency have also been seen in patients on this treatment.

Parasympathomimetics

Carbachol and bethanechol (Myotonine) are the two agents usually used in the treatment of urinary retention. They act at the muscarinic sites on smooth muscle in a similar way to acetylcholine (Goodman & Gilman 1985). As they are not inactivated by cholinesterases their action is more prolonged. Their action is not specific to the smooth muscle of the bladder (detrusor); they affect the smooth muscle in the stomach and the gastrointestinal tract. Bethanechol has been used for the treatment of congenital megacolon and oesophageal reflux.

The side-effects of these drugs include frequency of micturition, lower abdominal cramps and blurred vision. Nausea and vomiting may occur if they are taken immediately after food. As they are administered orally and are poorly absorbed, untoward effects relating to the cardiovascular system are rare.

Urinary incontinence

Urinary tract infection

Infection of the urinary tract may be detected by testing the urine. The presence of protein or an unpleasant fishy odour together with frequency could be an indication of infection. A midstream urine (MSU) specimen should be sent for testing and treatment with a suitable antibiotic should be started. The use of a broad-spectrum penicillin such as ampicillin (e.g. Penbritin), a cephalosporin such as cefalexin (Ceporex, Keflex) or the antibacterial agent trimethoprim (Monotrim, Trimopan) is effective in most cases.

Genuine stress incontinence

Drug treatment using sympathomimetics has been tried for patients with genuine stress incontinence, identified by urodynamic investigation, although a definite place for these drugs has yet to be established (Andersson 1988). Some benefit has been shown in the treatment of mild cases (Wise & Cardoso 1992). The alpha-adrenoceptor agonists, ephinedrine and phenylpropanolamine, cause contraction of the smooth muscle of the neck of the bladder, while relaxing the detrusor muscle of the bladder wall. Due to adverse reports of phenylpropanolamine in the United States by the Food and Drug Administration (FDA), it is unlikely that it will be used in the future. These drugs should be used with caution in patients with hyperthyroidism or severe heart disease, or in patients who have been on monoamine oxidase inhibitors in the past 14 days.

Detrusor instability

While surgery is the treatment of choice in genuine stress incontinence or urinary retention, most cases of detrusor instability can be improved by drug treatment and/or combined with electrical stimulation (see Chapter 3). The contraction of the detrusor muscle is instigated by acetylcholine. Drugs which competitively inhibit the action of acetylcholine at the muscarinic receptors are called antimuscarinic drugs. Antimuscarinic drugs are not specific in their action; treatment with this group of drugs may cause dry mouth, blurred vision, tachycardia, constipation and relaxation of the oesophagus leading to oesophageal reflux. Propantheline (Pro-Banthine) has been widely used for incontinence due to detrusor instability, but owing to the high incidence of side-effects it is now used only in adult enuresis.

Flavoxate hydrochloride (Urispas) and emepronium bromide (Cetiprin) have been used to treat detrusor instability, but the effectiveness of both has been questioned (Meyhoff et al 1983). These drugs have now been replaced by oxybutynin hydrochloride (Ditropan) – as well as its anticholinergic action it is reported to have direct effects on smooth muscle and some local anaesthetic properties. Clinical studies show that there is symptomatic improvement in patients taking oxybutynin over those on placebo (Moisey et al 1980). The side-effects of oxybutynin mean that it is unsuitable for patients with intestinal atony, severe ulcerative colitis or toxic megacolon, myasthenia gravis or glaucoma, and it is contraindicated during pregnancy. Research study 8.1 highlights the intravesical use of oxybutynin for patients with neurogenic bladder dysfunction. Tolterodine tartrate (Detrusitol), trospium (Regurin) and Propiverine (detrunorm) are also antimuscarinic drugs, which have recently been introduced as treatment for detrusor instability, Detrusitol has been shown to have greater selectivity for the bladder than the salivary glands in animal tests; however the clinical significance of this has not been established.

Research study 8.1   Intravesical use of oxybutynin

One of the key advantages of locally introduced instillations of therapeutic reagents is that lower doses can be used so that systemic side-effects are commonly reduced or absent. In the managment of patients with neurogenic bladder dysfunction resulting in detrusor hyperreflexia, anticholinergic agents can be effective. However, oral anticholinergic drugs can produce pronounced and distressing side-effects which include dry mouth, constipation and visual disturbances in more than 60% of patients (Thuroff et al 1991).

Some reports have demonstrated a positive effect on urodynamic parameters and reduced symptomatic side-effects in patients after intravesicular instillation of oxybutynin hydrochloride (Mizunaga et al 1994, O'Flynn & Thomas 1993, Prasad & Vaidyanathan 1993). In these studies 5 mg of oxybutynin hydrochloride were dissolved in water and instilled into the bladder either twice or three times daily and retained for up to 3 hours. Patient follow-up ranged from 6 hours to 16 months. These studies centred on patients practising clean intermittent self-catheterization, but such therapy could also be of potential benefit to patients with an indwelling catheter who suffer from frequent bypassing of urine or expulsion of their catheters. See also Chapters 9 and 11. Imipramine is useful when the patient needs to keep dry for a short period, such as a holiday (Haycock 1985).

Nocturnal enuresis

Drugs are not the first-line treatment for this condition and should be reserved for use when other methods have been unsuccessful.

The drugs used for the treatment of nocturnal enuresis are normally the tricyclic antidepressants imipramine (Tofranil) and amitriptyline. Imipramine is the one used most often. It has lower sedative properties than amitriptyline.

Tricyclics act by inhibiting the reuptake of noradrenaline and 5-hydroxytryptamine (5HT) into the presynaptic membrane. This potentiates the action of noradrenaline and 5HT and results in relaxation of the detrusor and an increase in outlet resistance. It is also believed that the tricyclics may alter the level of sleep, allowing increased awareness of bed-wetting.

Although imipramine is particularly successful in the treatment of enuresis, the relapse rate on withdrawal is high (Kales et al 1987). It is doubtful whether the dryness persists beyond the period of drug administration.

The side-effects of the tricyclic drugs would make their use in patients under the age of 6 years inadvisable, and Tofranil is not licensed for use under this age.

Desmopressin (DDAVP), a synthetic analogue of vasopressin, is regarded as useful in the short-term control of enuresis. It has prolonged anti-diuretic activity with little or no pressor activity. It has been suggested that enuretic children may lack the normal nocturnal rise in plasma vasopressin (George et al 1975, Norgaard et al 1985), and the use of desmopressin may correct this deficiency (see Chapter 5 for desmopressin treatment in children). As with the tricyclics the relapse rate after treatment is high, but the drug should be withdrawn for at least 1 week in every 3 months to reassess the situation. The patient should also be regularly monitored for fluid overload. The introduction of a tablet form of desmopressin makes treatment with this drug more acceptable than the previous intranasal product.

Urinary incontinence as a result of constipation

The pressure of a full bowel on the bladder may cause urinary incontinence. This form of incontinence will usually resolve when normal bowel function has been re-established (see the section on constipation). A summary of other drugs, which may be used to treat urinary incontinence, is given in Box 8.13.

Drugs that cause urinary retention

It is important to be aware that the drugs mentioned in this section are capable of affecting the bladder and urinary flow, although not all patients taking these drugs may experience side-effects.

The following drugs relax smooth muscle and can result in voiding difficulties and urinary

---

Box 8.13 Drugs that may be used to treat urinary incontinence

- **Urinary infection**
  Antibiotics

  Broad-spectrum penicillin (ampicillin)
  Cephalosporin (cefalexin)
  Trimethoprim

- **Genuine stress incontinence**
  Sympathomimetics Ephedrine

- **Detrusor instability**
  Antimuscarinics

  Flavoxate hydrochloride
  Oxybutynin
  Propantheline
  Propiverine
  Tolterodine tartrate
  Trospium

- **Nocturnal enuresis**
  Tricyclic antidepressants

  Amitriptyline
  Imipramine

  Synthetic analogue of vasopressin Desmopressin

Box 8.14 Drugs that can cause urinary retention

- **Drugs that relax smooth muscle**
  Phenothiazides

  Chlorpromazine
  Thioridazine

  Antiparkinsonism drugs Levodopa
  Antihypertensives Hydralazine
  Minoxidil

- **Drugs that increase smooth muscle tone**
  Sympathomimetics

  Phenylpropanolamine
  Salbutamol (taken orally or intravenously)

  Antihypertensives Propranolol
  Antimigraine Ergotamine

Box 8.15 Drugs that may cause urinary incontinence

Antihypertensive
- Methyldopa

Cardiac glycosides
- Digoxin

Indirect effect
- *Diuretics* increase the amount of urine produced and the frequency of micturition.
- *Sedatives* and *hypnotics* may cause the individual to be less responsive to body signals (call to stool, bladder signals).
- *Alcohol* acts as both a sedative and a diuretic.

---

retention: phenothiazides such as chlorpromazine (Largactil), which are used as neuroleptics and antiemetics; the antiparkinsonism drug levodopa; and the antihypertensive drugs hydralazine (Apresoline) and minoxidil (Loniten) which act by peripheral vasodilatation.

The following drugs increase smooth muscle tone in the outflow tract: salbutamol (Ventolin), a sympathomimetic used in the treatment of asthma; phenylpropanolamine, found in various over-the-counter cold products as a nasal decongestant (for reasons stated earlier this drug is likely to be removed from sale); the antihypertensive propranolol (Inderal); and the ergot alkaloid ergotamine which is used to treat migraine (Migril). They may cause voiding difficulties, but they may also relieve stress incontinence.

Drugs that can cause urinary retention are summarized in Box 8.14.

Drugs that cause urinary incontinence

The antihypertensive methyldopa (Aldomet) may cause stress incontinence by decreasing the smooth muscle tone in the outflow tract. The cardiac glycoside digoxin (Lanoxin) can increase smooth muscle tone, causing increase in bladder pressure and decrease in capacity (see Box 8.15).

INDIRECT EFFECTS OF DRUGS

While drugs may not have a direct effect on a patient's continence, many may affect the patient in such a way as to cause bowel or bladder problems (Box 8.15). For example, a bed-bound patient administered a powerful diuretic such as furosemide (frusemide) (Lasix) may suffer from urinary incontinence owing to the inability to get to a toilet. Similarly, lack of exercise due to infirmity will predispose the patient to constipation. Drugs that can cause confusion or stupor may lead to poor toilet habits and thus constipation. In these cases the drugs may not be the direct cause but the result is a problem of continence.

It is important to take the physical and social conditions of the patient into account when prescribing treatment, which may have such effects. The use of diuretics in elderly patients with reduced mobility may cause the patient to suffer from urinary urge incontinence. The patient may choose to reduce fluid intake in the belief that it will reduce the risk of urinary incontinence. This may lead to fluid and electrolyte imbalances. The reduction of fluid combined with the lack of mobility may lead to constipation.

MASSAGE IN THE TREATMENT OF CONSTIPATION

In cases where exercise is not practicable, such as with a hemiplegic or paraplegic patient, or when mobility is restricted for any reason, colonic massage may be used successfully to aid peristalsis and promote faecal evacuation (see Table 8.2). It is also possible to improve the patient's sense of well-being by the close contact established with the masseur (Emly 1993). The patient will not be subjected to the indignity of enemas and manual evacuation. This technique is described in Chapter 7 together with further discussion of other complementary therapies.

Aromatherapy has also shown to be beneficial in treating constipation in some people. The following essential oil mixture is suggested (courtesy Mrs Lynne Ward): 10 drops of marjoram, 10 drops of rosemary, 2 drops of black pepper, 2 drops of peppermint, 2 drops of sweet fennel – mixed to 100 ml with sweet almond oil.

Colonic massage is contraindicated in some people. It should not be used:

- during pregnancy
- premenstrually or during menstruation
- for clients with any medical condition unless permission has been given by the client's doctor.

ISPHAGULA RECIPES

Fybogel has been used in testing these recipes; however other brands of isphagula should

Table 8.2 Aromatherapy for colonic massage

Action	Rationale
1. Apply some mixture (size of £2 coin) to palms and smooth hands together gently	To even out the amount of oil to be applied, to reduce the possibility of overloading any area
2. Apply oil to abdomen effluage (30 seconds)	To provide even distribution of oil
3. Follow bowel pattern – start in right iliac fossa: use flat hand stroke five times	To increase abdominal pressure to aid peristaltic action
4. Use fingertips five times	To stimulate peristalsis
5. Repeat (3)	
6. Use daily	To maintain peristaltic action

produce similar results. Fybogel is formulated as a pleasant-tasting orange or lemon drink, but in some patients the consumption of a glassful of fluid in one go may be difficult. On standing, Fybogel forms a gel that can be resuspended by stirring, but for patients who cannot consume Fybogel as a drink the following recipes may prove useful. It is important to note that the patient should consume plenty of fluids throughout the day and that Fybogel should not be taken dry as it could cause a blockage. The use of Fybogel Plain is recommended in the recipes.

Heating ispaghula to 70°C alters the fibre content, so to avoid this food should be cooled to 60°C before Fybogel is added.

All the recipes are for a single portion, except where stated. The quantities can be increased in these recipes and Fybogel added to a single portion at the end.

Instant soup
1 packet soup in a cup (e.g. tomato, chicken)
300 ml (½ pint) boiling water
1 sachet Fybogel

Method
1. Place soup powder in a bowl.
2. Pour on boiling water and mix well.
3. Leave for 10 min to cool below 60°C.
4. Stirring briskly with a fork, pour in Fybogel.
5. Serve immediately.

Jelly

¼ packet of jelly cubes
200 ml (⅓ pint) boiling water
1 sachet of Fybogel

Method

1. Break the jelly into cubes and put into jug.
2. Pour on boiling water and stir until jelly is dissolved.
3. Leave until cool (below 60°C).
4. Sprinkle on Fybogel and mix with a fork or whisk.
5. Put in a dish, in the fridge to set.
6. Eat within 24 hours.

Instant Whip

½ packet instant whip
150 ml (¼ pint) milk
1 sachet of Fybogel

Method

1. Add the Fybogel to the instant whip powder and mix.
2. Pour the milk into a bowl or jug.
3. Add the instant whip/Fybogel mixture.
4. Mix well until thick and creamy.
5. Put into a dish and leave to set.
6. Eat within 24 hours.

Fruit purée

75 g (⅛ pint) cooled stewed fruit (e.g. apple, rhubarb, plums)
or 50 g (2 oz) soft fruit (e.g. raspberries, strawberries)
or half a 450 g (15 oz) tin of fruit minus juice
12–25 g (½–1 oz) sugar or sweetener (to desired sweetness)
1 sachet of Fybogel

Method

1. Mash fruit or mix in a blender.
2. Add the Fybogel and mix briskly or blend until smooth.
3. Add sugar or sweetener.
4. Consume within 24 hours with custard or ice cream.

Fruit fool

¼ of 450 g (15 oz) tin of fruit including juice
12–25 g (½–1 oz) sugar or sweetener (to desired sweetness)

75 g (⅛ pint) custard: use ready-made carton or make thick custard and allow to cool
Half small pot of whipping cream (optional)
1 sachet of Fybogel

Method

1. Mash fruit or mix in a blender.
2. Mix the Fybogel with 25 ml (1 fl oz) of the fruit juice and allow to set.
3. Add the Fybogel/juice mixture to the fruit.
4. Beat vigorously or mix in the blender.
5. Add custard and beat/blend again.
6. Pour into serving dish.
7. Can be topped with whipped cream.
8. Chill well and eat within 24 hours.

This recipe works best if made in a blender.

Milkshake

200 ml (⅓ pint) milk
1 sachet of Fybogel
1 tablespoon vanilla ice-cream
4 tablespoons milkshake syrup

Method

1. Place all the ingredients in a blender in the order stated.
2. Blend until well mixed.
3. Pour into a glass or cup and drink at once.

Soup soubise

300 ml (½ pint) chicken stock
1 medium onion cut into 5–6 pieces
¼ leek sliced
1–2 whole black peppercorns
Salt to taste
1 sachet of Fybogel

Method

1. Put all ingredients except Fybogel into a saucepan.
2. Bring to boil.
3. Turn down heat and cook until vegetables are soft.
4. Put into a soup bowl and allow to cool for 10 min (below 60°C).
5. Sprinkle on Fybogel and mix well.

Parsnip soup

200 ml (⅓ pint) water
½ chicken stock cube
125 g (¼ lb) parsnips peeled and chopped into
  small pieces
½ small carrot sliced
1–2 whole black peppercorns
¼ teaspoon curry powder (optional)
Salt to taste
1 sachet of Fybogel

Method

1. Put all the ingredients except Fybogel into a
   saucepan.
2. Bring to boil.
3. Turn down the heat and cook until vegetables
   are soft.
4. Put through a sieve or blend until smooth.
5. Leave for 10 min to cool below 60°C.
6. Sprinkle on Fybogel and mix well.

*This can be made in larger quantities and the Fybogel
just added to a single portion.*

Chicken korma

Sufficient for 2 servings
2 chicken breasts, boned and diced
50 g (2 oz) butter or margarine
2 cloves of garlic, peeled and chopped
1 onion peeled and chopped
½ teaspoonful powdered ginger
50 g (2 oz) desiccated coconut
Small tin chopped tomatoes
150 ml (¼ pint) chicken stock
150 ml (¼ pint) natural yoghurt
1 teaspoonful ground coriander
½ teaspoonful turmeric
½ teaspoonful paprika
Salt and pepper to taste
1 sachet of Fybogel (per portion)

Method

1. Melt the butter in a large saucepan.
2. Fry onion, garlic, ginger, coriander, turmeric
   and paprika until onions are soft.
3. Add chicken and cook for another 10 min.
4. Stir in the coconut, chopped tomatoes and
   yoghurt.
5. Add chicken stock, cover the pan and cook
   for another 30 min.
6. Divide between two dishes and leave to
   stand for 10 min to cool below 60°C.
7. Sprinkle on Fybogel and mix into a
   portion.
8. Serve with boiled rice.

Case study 8.1

The complexity of polypharmacy prescribed for some patients is illustrated by this case study. The prescription below was presented by a male patient:

Atenolol 50 mg	60 tablets	One in the morning
Slow-K 600 mg	240 tablets	Two twice a day
Diltiazem 60 mg	180 tablets	One three times a day
Furosemide (frusemide) 40 mg	120 tablets	Two in the morning
Chlorpromazine 25 mg	180 tablets	One three times a day
Warfarin 3 mg	60 tablets	One at night
Warfarin 1 mg	60 tablets	No instructions!
Co-proxamol	200 tablets	One to two when required
Allopurinol 300 mg	60 tablets	One daily
Epanutin 100 mg	240 tablets	Two twice a day

The following possible interactions should be considered:

Warfarin plus
• allopurinol   may increase the effect of warfarin
• co-proxamol   may increase the effect of warfarin

• epanutin   increases the risk of bleeding (rare case of epanutin intoxication reported)

Atenolol plus
• chlorpromazine   frequently causes postural hypotension
• diltiazem   rarely, unpredictably produces bradycardia/hypotension

Epanutin plus
• chlorpromazine   occasionally and unpredictably affects epanutin action
• furosemide (frusemide)   reduces or abolishes the effect of furosemide (frusemide)
• allopurinol   increases the effect of epanutin.

This patient may be stabilized on this regimen, but it does illustrate the complex interactions between different drugs a patient may be given. A review of this patient by the team is suggested, with the aim of simplifying the treatment.

REFERENCES

Abrahams A 1964 A re-educative regimen for chronic (functional) constipation. British Journal of Clinical Practice January: 181–185

Andersson K E 1988 Current concepts in the treatment of disorders of micturation. Drugs 35: 477–494

Blanchard K 1993 The one minute manager builds high performing teams. Fontana, London

British National Formulary 2002 BNF43. British Medical Association and Royal Pharmaceutical Society of Great Britain, London

British Pharmacopoeia 2000 The Stationery Office, London, p 1027

Emly M 1993 Abdominal massage. Nursing Times 89(3): 34–36

Englyst H N, Cummings J H 1984 Simplified method for the measurement of total non-starch polysaccharides by gas–liquid chromatography of constituent sugars as alditol acetates. Analyst 109: 937–942

Englyst H, Wiggens H S, Cummings J H 1982 Determination of the non-starch polysaccharides in plant foods by gas–liquid chromatography of constituent sugars as alditol acetates. Analyst 107: 307–318

Francis C Y, Whorwell P J 1994 Bran and irritable bowel syndrome: time for reappraisal. Lancet 334: 39–40

George C P L, Messerli F H, Genest J et al 1975 Diurnal variation of plasma vasopressin in man. Journal of Clinical Endocrinology and Metabolism 41(2): 332–338

Goodman L S, Gilman A et al (eds) 1985 Goodman and Gilman's The pharmacological basis of therapeutics, 7th edn. Macmillan, New York

Haward L R C, Hughes-Roberts H E 1962 The treatment of constipation in mental hospitals. Gut 3: 385–390

Haycock G 1985 Monthly Index of Medical Specialities November: 1541–1546

Jarrett A S, Exton-Smith A N 1960 Letter to the Editor. Lancet 23 April: 925

Jones J, Boorman J, Cann P et al 2000 British Society of Gastroenterology guidelines for the management of the irritable bowel syndrome. Gut 47(Suppl. 2): ii1–ii19

Kales A, Soldatos C R, Kales J D 1987 Sleep disorders: insomnia, sleepwalking, night terrors, nightmares, and enuresis. Annals of Internal Medicine 106: 582–592

Kock-Weser J 1974 Adverse reactions to beta-adrenergic receptor blocking drugs: a report from the Boston Collaborative Drug Surveillance program. Drugs 7: 118–129

Leng-Peschlow E 1993 Sennoside-induced secretion is not caused by changes in mucosal permeability or Na, K-ATPase activity. Journal of Pharmacy and Pharmacology 45: 951–954

Lepor H 1989 Nonoperative management of benign prostatic hyperplasia. Journal of Urology 141: 1283–1289

MCA 2000 Current problems in pharmacovigilance. May: 26

McCance R A, Widdowson E M 1991 In: Holland B et al (eds) McCance and Widdowson's the composition of foods, 5th edn. Royal Society of Chemistry/MAFF, Cambridge

MeReC 1999 The management of constipation. Medical Resources Centre Bulletin 9(10): 33–36

Meyhoff H H, Gerstenberg T C, Nordling J 1983 Placebo – the drug of choice in female motor urge incontinence? British Journal of Urology 55: 34–37

Mizunaga M, Miyata M, Kaneko S, Yachiku S, Chiba K 1994 Intravesical instillation of oxybutynin hydrochloride therapy for patients with a neurogenic bladder. Paraplegia 32: 25–29

Moisey C U, Stephenson T P, Brendler C P 1980 The urodynamic and subjective results of treatment of detrusor instability with oxybutynin chloride. British Journal of Urology 52: 472–475

Norgaard J P, Pedersen E B, Djurhuus J C 1985 Diurnal antidiuretic hormone levels in enuretics. Journal of Urology 134: 1029–1031

O'Flynn K J, Thomas D G 1993 Intravesical instillation of oxybutynin hydrochloride for detrusor hyper-reflexia. British Journal of Urology 72: 566–570

Prasad K V R, Vaidyanathan S 1993 Intravesical oxybutynin chloride and clean intermittent catheterisation in patients with neurogenic vesical dysfunction and decreased bladder capacity. British Journal of Urology 72: 719–722

Qvitzau S, Matzen P, Madsen P 1988 Treatment of chronic diarrhoea: loperamide versus ispaghula husk and calcium. Scandinavian Journal of Gastroenterology 23: 1237–1240

Sandars J 1995 The team is dead: long live the team. Update 50: 737

Smith R G 1983 Long-term care in faecal incontinence. Journal of the American Geriatrics Society 3(11): 694–697

Thuroff J W, Bunke B, Ebner A et al 1991 Randomised double blind, multicentre trial on treatment of frequency, urgency and incontinence related to detrusor hyperactivity: oxybutynin versus propantheline versus placebo. Journal of Urology 145: 813–817

Tomlin J, Lowis C, Read N W 1991 Investigation of normal flatus production in healthy volunteers. Gut 32(6): 665–669

United States Pharmacopoeia National Formulary 2000 Note 911, p 1079. Rockville, Maryland

Whitehead R G (chair) 1991 Report on Health and Social Subjects 41: Dietary reference values for food energy and nutrients for the United Kingdom. HMSO, London

Wise B, Cardozo L 1992 Urinary incontinence, retention and enuresis. Prescriber 579–593

9

Catheters and catheterization

Kathryn Getliffe

'The operation of introducing the catheter, if it do not require intrepidity and courage, requires at least peculiar delicacy, a perfect knowledge of the parts, and above all, a humane and steady temper ...'

John Bell, 1810

INTRODUCTION

Urinary catheterization is not a pleasant experience, but then neither is urinary incontinence. For some patients faced with long-term urinary dysfunction, catheterization may be viewed depressingly as the 'beginning of the end', marked by the need for an invasive device to control what should be a normal bodily function. But for others a catheter can provide a sense of freedom and independence in the knowledge that their urine loss is contained. However, long-term catheterization is rarely completely free of complications and can, in extreme cases, be a contributory factor in life-threatening bacteraemia resulting from urinary tract infection. Therefore, the decision to catheterize should only be considered where other options are inappropriate or unsuccessful, and should never be based solely on convenience.

The aim of this chapter is to examine the appropriate use of catheters in the promotion of continence; to discuss the choice of catheter and drainage equipment for individual patients; and to consider catheter management and minimization of problems. The major research evidence underpinning care is presented throughout. Figure 9.1 provides an overview of the complexity

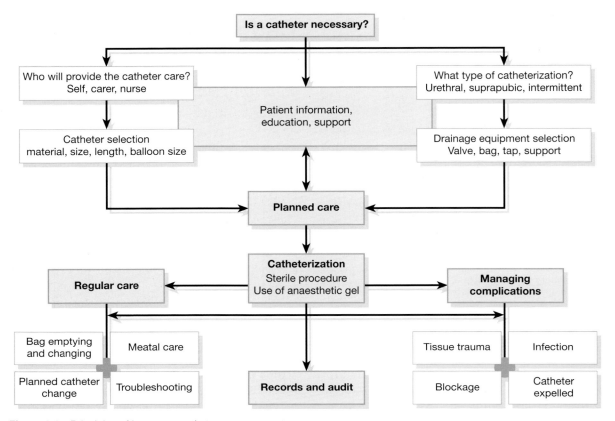

Figure 9.1 Principles of long-term catheter management.

of issues concerned in long-term catheter management. These are discussed in detail throughout the chapter.

PATIENT PERSPECTIVES

Advances in the understanding of urodynamics and alternative treatments for urinary dysfunction have meant that the use of long-term catheters is commonly considered to be a last resort. Careful planning and thought can often allow effective management of incontinence without catheters. Since catheterization is associated with a number of potential complications, non-invasive approaches to management and care should be considered in the first instance and reviewed on a regular basis. Nevertheless there are some patients for whom catheterization can be the most appropriate form

of care. These include:

- patients with difficulty in complete emptying of the bladder, often as a result of neurological disease or injury
- patients with bladder outlet obstruction who may be unfit for surgical repair
- patients who are chronically incontinent, often with associated debility or confusion, for whom alternative methods are inappropriate or unsuccessful.

An indwelling catheter may be inserted into the bladder via the urethra or a suprapubic cystotomy but is contraindicated in confused patients where there is a risk of the catheter being forcibly removed. Intermittent catheterization, in which the catheter is removed as soon as drainage has ceased, may be appropriate for some patients and may be performed by patients themselves or a carer. The principles supporting the use and management of different forms of catheterization are discussed later in the chapter but it should be recognized that urinary catheterization and catheter care remain primarily a nursing responsibility. Promoting 'best practice' based on a sound knowledge base is critical to providing effective and supportive patient care and nurses need to ensure that the care they provide is supported by evidence.

Some 10–12% of all patients admitted to hospital will have an indwelling catheter at some time during their stay (Crow et al 1988). The most common indications are drainage of urine postoperatively, accurate monitoring of urine output in acute illness and management of urinary retention. In most cases the catheter will be for short- or mid-term use, up to 28 days (Crow et al 1988). Figures on the prevalence of long-term catheterization, for patients in institutionalized settings or in the community, are variable and more difficult to obtain but the procedure has been employed in around 4% of patients nursed in the community (Getliffe 1994a). A further group of catheterized patients – commonly younger people with neurological injuries – may be largely unknown to the nursing services because they are self-caring.

Whilst it is not the purpose of this chapter to consider in detail the psychological and social implications of incontinence these effects are considerable and cannot be ignored (see Chapter 1). Similarly the psychological and social effects of long-term catheterization are of concern and patients may require a great deal of educational help and support, particularly in the early days following catheterization. For this reason it is important that wherever possible the decision to catheterize should be a joint one between the patient, carer (if at home) and the health professional, and should never be made solely for the convenience of the latter. Whilst some patients consider the catheter as a sign of declining independence and a cause for embarrassment, others may be grateful for improved control of their urinary dysfunction and the opportunity for social activity without fear of incontinence (Getliffe 1995). For some, a catheter can make the difference between coping at home and the alternative of institutional care.

Careful assessments are clearly important in the selection of long-term catheterization as the most appropriate form of care for individual patients, but it should be remembered that assessment is an ongoing process and healthcare professionals need to reassess regularly and to ask the question: 'Is a urinary catheter still the most appropriate form of care for this patient?'.

URINARY CATHETERS
Historical perspectives

Urinary catheters have been used since ancient times to relieve the pain of overfilled, obstructed bladders. Urinary retention is mentioned in most of the earliest recorded histories of civilization (Bloom et al 1994, Herman 1973) and early catheterizations were accomplished with reeds, straws and curled-up palm leaves. The thin, hollow leaves of the Allium (onion) family were used effectively by the Chinese, but breakage and difficulties in pushing the dried leaves past obstructions limited their value (Bloom et al 1994). Metal catheters were more robust, and tubes of gold or bronze were used by the Egyptians and Greeks to relieve obstruction. Similar metal catheters were recovered during the excavations of Pompeii (Fig. 9.2). Silver catheters, although expensive, remained popular until the advent of modern latex and plastics. The antibacterial properties of silver are still employed in some modern silver-alloy-coated catheters (Liedberg & Lundeberg 1990).

Early records suggest that catheterization was a painful procedure since it was often difficult to obtain the patient's consent! (Murphy 1972). To reduce patients' suffering, catheters made of cloth or animal skin were designed. These materials were impregnated with wax and moulded on a metal former. The catheter was introduced with

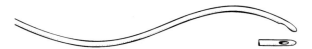

Figure 9.2 Representation of an early metal catheter recovered during excavations at Pompeii.

the help of a metal or bone stylet, but rapid softening and collapse often occurred following removal of the stylet.

At the end of the 17th century, the Dutch surgeon Van Solingen constructed a catheter of flat silver wire, wound spirally, and designed to accommodate itself to the irregularities of the urethra. To avoid damage to the mucosa by the metal grooves, it was covered with parchment held in place with a silk thread and impregnated with wax to fill in any crevices. One patient is known to have used such a catheter for 2 years, leaving it in place for 4 or 5 days at a time (Murphy 1972). The use of silk, woven catheters, soaked in linseed oil and then dried was described by Louis Mercier in the early 19th century, but like previously used materials, these catheters could not be sterilized effectively and were subject to breaking during use, with resultant tissue damage and retention of fragments. As a consequence, catheterization was still generally a rather desperate measure (John Bell 1810: cited by Bloom et al 1994).

Although early attempts were made to incorporate rubber into loosely woven material, dramatic advances in catheter manufacture became possible after a method of forming and shaping rubber, known as vulcanization, was developed by Goodyear in 1844 and patented in 1851. In less than a decade, Auguste Nelaton of Paris, physician to Napoleon III, was using this method to produce a flexible rubber catheter. Modern plastic catheters of this design with a solid tip and a single eye, are still known as the Nelaton catheter, and are used extensively for collection of bladder urine samples and by patients practising intermittent self-catheterization.

When retention of the catheter within the bladder was required, most early designs were tied or taped to the penis in males and sometimes sewn to the urethral orifice in females. Clearly this was unsatisfactory! – a catheter which could be retained through its own configuration was needed. In 1892, Malecot demonstrated his four-winged catheter and this was followed shortly by the de Pezzer 'mushroom' (Fig. 9.3). There was, however, considerable risk of tissue trauma during removal of these catheters.

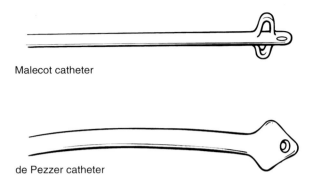

Malecot catheter

de Pezzer catheter

Figure 9.3 Early self-retaining catheters, Malecot and de Pezzer.

Many attempts were made to produce a catheter with an attached bag (balloon) which could be inflated within the bladder. In some cases the design aimed to relieve strictures by inflation of the bag and, in others, to apply pressure to control haemorrhage, rather than to facilitate continuous urinary drainage. Some early designs incorporated bags made of 'goldbeater's skin', a submucosal layer of the intestines of oxen, tied to the catheter and inflated through a separate channel. In the mid-19th century, Reybard designed two self-retaining catheters, one held in place by a moveable flange and the other fitted with a small inflatable balloon. However, most early designs did not prove satisfactory in practice. Finally during the 1930s, when latex rubber became available, the forerunner of the modern indwelling catheter was developed by Frederick Foley of St Paul, Minnesota. By dipping and coagulating latex on metal formers it became possible to manufacture a one-piece catheter and balloon. The first production model was demonstrated at an annual meeting of the American Urology Association in 1935.

Modern catheters

The Foley catheter is now the most commonly used of all urethral catheters. In its usual form it has a double lumen shaft (one lumen for urine drainage, the other for inflation and deflation of the retention balloon), a rounded tip and two drainage eyes proximal to the balloon (Fig. 9.4). A variety of alternative tip designs is available, with either opposed or staggered eyes proximal

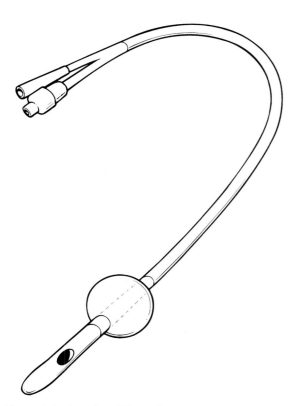

Figure 9.4 A modern Foley catheter.

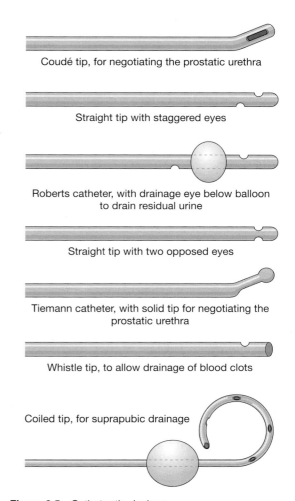

Coudé tip, for negotiating the prostatic urethra

Straight tip with staggered eyes

Roberts catheter, with drainage eye below balloon to drain residual urine

Straight tip with two opposed eyes

Tiemann catheter, with solid tip for negotiating the prostatic urethra

Whistle tip, to allow drainage of blood clots

Coiled tip, for suprapubic drainage

Figure 9.5 Catheter tip designs.

to the balloon; an additional eye distal to the balloon to facilitate drainage of residual urine (Roberts catheter); or a terminal opening for maximal drainage of blood clots postoperatively (Fig. 9.5). Some catheters have a third channel for irrigation or instillation purposes.

The French were the foremost manufacturers of catheters during the 19th century and their terminology is still used to describe certain catheter features, for example coudé and bicoudé (curved or 'elbow' tips). The invention by Mercier of the coudé catheter, designed to help negotiate strictures, was of immense value in the treatment of bladder neck obstruction and urethral strictures.

Catheter size or gauge is measured as the external diameter of the catheter shaft, and is defined in either Charrière units (Ch) (after Joseph Charrière, a 19th century Parisian instrument maker), or French gauge (Fg). Both scales are identical with one unit equivalent to a third of

a millimetre (e.g. an 18 Ch or 18 Fg catheter has an external diameter of 6 mm, Fig. 9.6). The inflation valve on the catheter is colour coded according to Ch size and most also have the balloon infill volume printed on them (Table 9.1). The diameter of the internal lumen may vary, however, depending on the catheter material and the manufacturing process. For example, catheters formed by the extrusion of a single material, such as silicone, usually have relatively thin walls and large lumens compared to catheters of the same gauge produced by building up layers through dipping and coating on a former. The shape of the lumen also varies and where this is 'crescent-shaped'

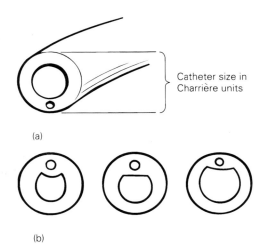

(a)

(b)

Figure 9.6 (a) Catheter size is measured by the external diameter of the catheter; (b) the size of the internal lumen depends on the manufacturing process.

Table 9.1 Charrière size and colour coding of inflation valves

Charrière size	Colour of inflation valve
10	Black
12	White
14	Green
16	Orange
18	Red

Larger catheters of Charrière sizes 20–24 may be required following urological intervention but further guidance should be sought on continued use of these catheters.

rather than round there is potential for accumulation of mineral deposits in the 'corners'. Problems of recurrent catheter blockage associated with mineral precipitation and encrustation are considered later in the chapter.

The standard male length catheter (41–45 cm) is available to men and women, but a shorter female length of approximately 25 cm may be more comfortable and discreet for some patients (Fig. 9.7). Whilst the female length should never be used for males as inflation of the balloon within the urethra could result in severe trauma, the longer male length catheter may be more practical for some women, particularly obese women, as it provides easier access to the catheter/drainage bag junction. Paediatric catheters are usually approximately 30 cm long.

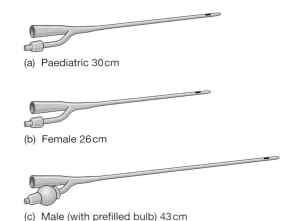

(a) Paediatric 30 cm

(b) Female 26 cm

(c) Male (with prefilled bulb) 43 cm

Figure 9.7 Catheter lengths.

Table 9.2 Selection of appropriate catheter material

Duration of catheterization	Catheter material
Short term (up to 14 days) (up to 28 days)	Latex or plastic Teflon-coated latex
Long term (more than 14 days)	All silicone Silicone–elastomer-coated latex Hydrogel-coated latex

Catheter materials

An ideal catheter should be soft for comfort and yet sufficiently firm for easy insertion and maintenance of lumen patency *in situ* (Table 9.2). For efficient drainage, the largest possible lumen is required for the smallest possible external diameter. The material used needs to have elastic recoil, so that an inflated balloon can be deflated again to almost its original size, thus minimizing discomfort during catheter removal. The aim of current research in catheter design and manufacture is to develop a biocompatible material which, whilst meeting the previous criteria, also:

- is comfortable and causes minimal tissue reaction
- inhibits colonization by micro-organisms
- resists encrustation by mineral deposits.

These catheter-associated problems will be discussed in detail later in this chapter.

Many people experience discomfort and cramps when they are first catheterized. This usually subsides within 24 hours and can be minimized by careful choice of appropriate catheter type and size. Modern catheters are usually composed of polyvinyl-chloride (PVC or plastic), latex with or without a coating, silicone or metal. Plastic catheters are relatively cheap to manufacture, and are commonly chosen for short-term use, up to 14 days. Because they have a thin wall they provide the largest lumen, and since water absorption by plastic is low, overall diameters remain unchanged *in situ*. Although plastic is relatively soft at body temperature, it can be uncomfortable to sit on, and is not designed for long-term use. Plastic catheters without a balloon are used for intermittent self-catheterization (ISC).

Latex catheters are soft and flexible but their high surface friction may result in discomfort during insertion or removal. Latex may also cause urethral tissue inflammation and these catheters are subject to rapid encrustation (Bruce et al 1974, Cox et al 1989). Furthermore, the absorption of water and body fluids by latex may lead to an increase in overall diameter, or a reduction in lumen size, thus limiting the catheter's effectiveness. Latex allergies have also been implicated in the development of urethritis and urethral strictures and may result from both catheter material and/or use of latex gloves during catheterization procedures. There is some evidence that the coating on a latex catheter does not necessarily provide protection and patients at risk of latex allergy need to be identified prior to catheterization (Woodward 1997). For these reasons latex catheters are restricted to short-term use, and have become less common as newer materials are developed.

Long-term catheters

Attempts to minimize friction during catheterization and to reduce tissue reactions led to the coating of latex catheters with a tightly bonded layer of material designed to provide a smoother, less irritant surface which also minimizes the absorption of water. Teflon-coated catheters are still in use (for medium-term use, up to 28 days) but

silicone–elastomer or hydrogel-coated catheters are recommended for long-term use (Roberts et al 1993, Talja et al 1990).

Hydrogels are hydrophilic polymers that absorb aqueous fluids to produce a soft slippery surface that reduces trauma on insertion or withdrawal of the catheter. They are highly biocompatible, relatively inert and are extensively used in other medical applications such as contact lenses, synthetic cartilage and drug delivery systems (Nacey & Delahunt 1991). Hydrogel-coated catheters are also available prefilled with a bulb on the inflation arm which contains the correct quantity of sterile water (Fig. 9.8). After inserting the catheter the balloon can be inflated by removing a clip and squeezing the bulb, thus avoiding the need for syringes and ampoules of sterile water, and the possibility of over- or underinflating the balloon.

Catheters made of 100% silicone also minimize tissue irritation (Nacey et al 1986, Talja et al 1990) and are latex free. These catheters are manufactured by an extrusion process and provide a larger drainage lumen than coated catheters. However, silicone allows the slow diffusion of water, which in time may occasionally lead to deflation of the balloon and the catheter falling out.

Catheter and balloon size

The key message here is: use the smallest size of catheter that allows good drainage. Urinary flow rate is proportional to the internal diameter of the catheter, and this in turn depends on the manufacturing process. However, the smallest Charrière size (usually 12 for adults) can easily drain normal quantities of urine, including the large volumes produced during diuresis (Ebner et al 1985). Size 12–14 Ch is usually suitable for females and 12–16 Ch for males. If blood clots, debris or rapid encrustation are apparent, a larger size may be appropriate, but larger catheters are usually reserved for use following urological procedures. Smaller sizes (6–10 Ch) are available for children.

Large catheters and balloons are believed to increase bladder irritability, causing spasms and leakage of urine, and may occlude the paraurethral glands which produce the mucus lining

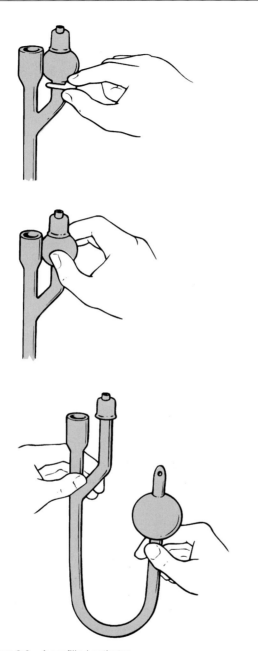

Figure 9.8 A prefilled catheter.

of the urethra, protecting against ascending infection (Blandy & Moors 1989, Kennedy et al 1983). Larger catheters may also exert greater pressure against the urethral or bladder wall, giving rise to ulceration and possible stricture formation.

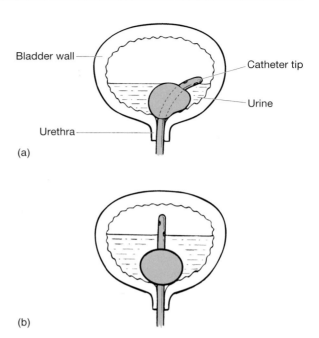

(a)

(b)

Figure 9.9 (a) Catheter balloon inflation. Underinflation of the balloon causes the catheter tip to be angled to one side. (b) A fully inflated balloon allows the tip to be located symmetrically.

Small balloons are recommended for all patients, 10 ml balloons for adults and 2.5–5 ml balloons for children. Larger balloon sizes of 30 ml (originally designed to provide pressure to reduce postoperative bleeding) should be avoided. Not only is there an increased risk of urethral damage if large balloons are expelled (e.g. by patients who are prone to bladder spasm), but they also tend to sit higher in the bladder allowing a greater volume of residual urine to collect below them. This may result in urinary leakage and also provide a reservoir for infection. The greater height of the catheter tip can also irritate the trigone area of the bladder causing spasm. The weight of water in the balloon will also exert pressure at the base of the bladder and since 1 ml of water weighs 1 g a balloon filled with 30 ml of water will weigh over 30 g (Robinson 2000).

It is important that balloons are inflated with the correct amount of sterile water, as stated on the catheter. Both over- and underinflation can result in balloon distortion so that the tip is angled to one side (Fig. 9.9) which could result in pressure ulceration of the bladder wall. If the balloon is underinflated there is a possibility that the catheter may become dislodged causing trauma to the prostatic urethra in males and urethra in females. Risks of overinflation are similar to those associated with use of large balloons but also include the possibility of balloon rupture, leaving fragments inside the bladder. It is important that sterile water is used, as filling with air allows the balloon to float on top of the urine, thereby reducing efficient drainage and potentiating risks of pressure necrosis caused by contact of the tip with the bladder mucosa. Filling with saline or tap water could lead to blockage of the deflation channel by small particles or crystals.

Catheter information and storage

Manufacturers are required to ensure that their products conform to the strict specifications laid down in the British Standards, BS 1695 (1990). However the correct use of equipment, together with ensuring that it is in a satisfactory state, is the responsibility of the individual practitioner. It is important, therefore, that the manufacturer's recommendations are followed during catheter management. Information is provided on both the catheter and its outer packaging, which includes the size and name of the catheter, the name of the manufacturer and a code number (which should be recorded on the patient's notes to allow faulty equipment to be traced). The outer packaging also carries the sterilization and expiry dates (Fig. 9.10). Out-of-date catheters should be discarded. Catheters should be stored flat in the boxes in which they are supplied, away from sources of heat and direct sunlight. This practice will reduce risks of damage to the packaging with resultant loss of sterility.

Drainage equipment

The choice of drainage equipment is particularly important for the promotion of patient independence and self-care, and it is a nursing responsibility to match choice with the individual patient. A wide range of products is available in

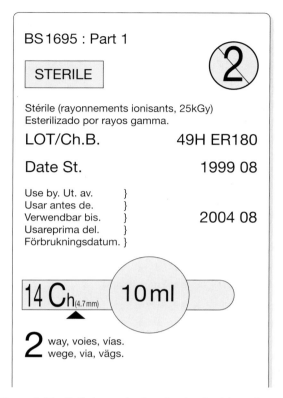

Figure 9.10 Catheter packaging showing the lot number.

the community on prescription (Figs 9.11–9.15), but availability in hospital may be subject to local purchasing agreements. Nevertheless, for patients catheterized in hospital, it is preferable for them to go home with the system that they will continue to use. Whenever possible patients should have the opportunity to try out:

- different bags, to decide for themselves which type of tap they find easiest to open and close
- different support systems for body-worn bags, to find the most practical and comfortable, e.g. a drainage bag supported by a holster suspended from a belt around the waist, or a leg bag supported by straps around the thigh or calf, etc.

Drainage bags, which are connected directly to an indwelling catheter, must be sterile, but non-sterile bags can be used for attachment to externally applied urinary drainage sheaths where there is no direct open pathway to the bladder.

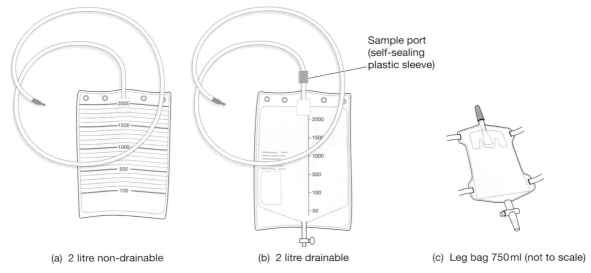

Sample port
(self-sealing
plastic sleeve)

(a) 2 litre non-drainable

(b) 2 litre drainable

(c) Leg bag 750 ml (not to scale)

Figure 9.11 Drainage bag designs.

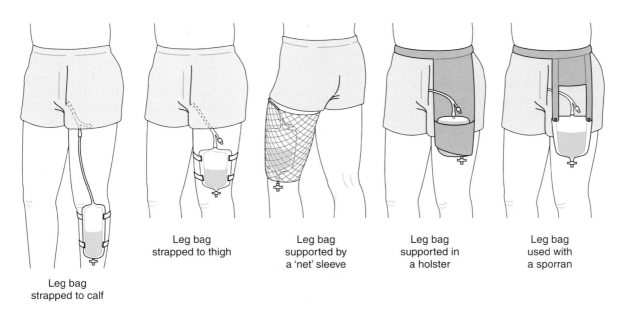

Leg bag
strapped to thigh

Leg bag
supported by
a 'net' sleeve

Leg bag
supported in
a holster

Leg bag
used with
a sporran

Leg bag
strapped to calf

Figure 9.12 Drainage bag suspensory systems.

Body-worn bags are preferable for most patients since their attachment to the leg, or suspension from the waist, allows maximum freedom combined with concealment beneath clothing. However, it is extremely important that the bag is emptied frequently to avoid it becoming too heavy and that it is adequately supported so that it cannot suddenly slip, pulling on the catheter and causing urethral trauma. Leg bags are available in a range of capacities (e.g. 350 ml, 500 ml and 750 ml), with choice being dependent on how frequently the bag is likely to be emptied and the desire for effective concealment.

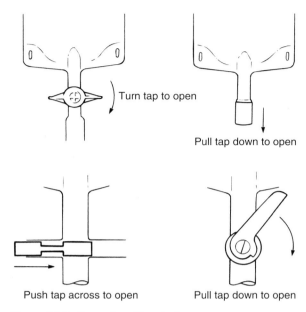

Turn tap to open

Pull tap down to open

Push tap across to open

Pull tap down to open

Figure 9.13 Examples of tap designs.

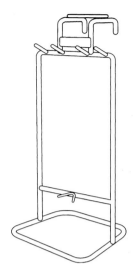

Figure 9.15 Support for a night bag.

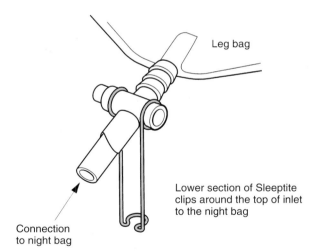

Leg bag

Lower section of Sleeptite clips around the top of inlet to the night bag

Connection to night bag

Figure 9.14 The Sleeptite device (Simpla).

A further feature, which influences the ease with which the bag can be accessed for emptying, is the length of the inlet tube. Tube lengths vary from around 5–40 cm, but on some bags the length of tubing can be adjusted by adding an extension piece or by cutting off a portion and reapplying the connecting piece. To reduce the

problem of bulkiness as the bag fills and embarrassing sounds caused by movements of urine, some manufacturers have designed bags which are divided into vertically arranged subcompartments which promote even distribution of urine and greater conformity to the shape of the leg.

Choice of drainage bag outlet tap is subject to individual preference. All taps are designed to be opened with one hand but patients commonly find one style more satisfactory than another. This is often related to ease of opening, particularly for those with limited manual strength or dexterity, or to confidence that the tap is securely closed after emptying.

Plastic surfaces can cause discomfort when worn next to the skin and some drainage bags have a woven 'coverstock' backing for greater comfort, although this backing can deteriorate with bathing. One solution is to insert the bag into a 'coverstock' sleeve during normal wear, which can be removed for bathing.

At night a larger, freestanding, night drainage bag (capacity 2–4 litres) may replace the smaller leg bag, or be 'linked' to it via an extension to the outlet tap. A simple restraining device is available to minimize the risk of separation of the linked bags during the night since the leg bag tap is left open to allow free drainage. The night drainage bag should be supported on a cardboard or plastic-coated metal stand, which can be obtained on prescription. Failure to use a stand could result in a heavy bag falling with resultant damage to the urethra and the risk of separation of the link system. At home, where risks of cross-infection are low, bags may be reused for up to 1 week if they are rinsed with water and allowed to dry between uses. In hospital and other institutionalized settings patients should have a new, non-drainable bag each night which is disposed of the following morning. Bags should not be reused once removed from the patient because of potential cross-infection. Catheter-associated infection is discussed in further detail later in the chapter.

Aspiration of urine samples

All drainage bags provide a sample port for the aspiration of urine for analysis. Commonly this is a self-sealing plastic sleeve located on the inlet tubing, through which a syringe needle can be inserted (Fig. 9.11). To prevent the risk of needle-stick injury by pushing the needle right through both sides of the tubing some manufacturers have provided a hard plastic backing section to the sampling area. It is important that samples are taken from the port and not from the bag, via the tap, since the urine in the bag is likely to contain greater numbers of micro-organisms which have had the opportunity to multiply within the reservoir of urine collecting in the bag.

Catheter valves

The urine drainage system may be dispensed with altogether if a catheter valve is inserted into the end of the catheter, allowing bladder filling and intermittent drainage (Fig. 9.16). However, catheter valves are inappropriate for patients with poor bladder capacity, detrusor overactivity, ureteric reflux or renal impairment. Patients must be able to manipulate the valve and empty the bladder regularly to avoid overfilling, with the accompanying risk of backpressure on the

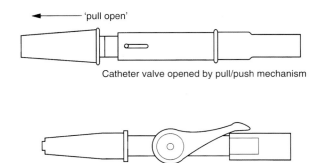

Figure 9.16 Catheter valves.

upper urinary tract. At night a drainage bag may be appropriate, in which case a valve designed for the attachment of a bag should be chosen.

A spigot is not a suitable alternative to a catheter valve since it must be removed from the catheter to allow drainage, thereby breaking what is essentially a closed system and increasing the risk of infection. Valves are available in several different designs ranging from simple, inexpensive types to more complex, longer lasting forms which patients may have to purchase for themselves. At home valves can be reused after cleaning under running water, soaking in an antiseptic solution overnight and then storing in a sealed, airtight, plastic box. Patients normally have two valves, one in use and one being stored. In hospitals or other institutions valves should not be reused and a sterile valve should be connected whenever the catheter/valve junction is broken. Much of the evidence supporting beneficial effects of catheter valves (in terms of reduced problems with encrustation and blocking) is anecdotal, but the flushing effect which results from bladder filling and emptying seems likely to contribute. There is stronger evidence of benefits in terms of patient comfort and independence (Fader et al 1997, German et al 1997). Fader et al evaluated a range of catheter valves from the user's perspective and identified certain key criteria. Valves must be easy to manipulate, leak free, comfortable, inconspicuous and an integral part of the closed system. In this study the Flip-flo valve (Bard Ltd, Crawley) was preferred by over 80% of users.

PRINCIPLES OF CATHETER MANAGEMENT

The main aims of catheter management are:

- to relieve and manage urinary dysfunction
- to recognize and minimize risks of secondary complications
- to promote patient dignity and comfort
- to assist patients to reach their own potential in terms of self-care and independence through appropriate education and support
- to provide a cost-effective service.

The skills and knowledge necessary to achieve these aims are complex (Fig. 9.1) and include ongoing assessment of patients and evaluation of both care products and procedures. Nurses are accountable and clinical governance requires them to be proactive in their clinical practice to prevent the risk of complications (Scally & Donaldson 1998). Catheterization can be an effective means of managing urinary dysfunction for appropriate patients and the issues concerned with selection of patients and equipment have been discussed above. However, risks of catheter-associated complications are high, with up to 75% of all patients experiencing one or more recurrent problems (Getliffe 1994a).

Catheterization is always an aseptic procedure (with the exception of clean intermittent self-catheterization which will be discussed later). Local policies for aseptic technique, hand washing and catheterization procedure should be referred to, but should include use of anaesthetic gel for both males and females.

There are three main categories of complications, which can arise during long-term catheterization:

- tissue damage
- urinary tract infection
- catheter encrustation leading to blockage.

They are discussed in detail in the following sections, together with the scientific bases for approaches to their management.

TISSUE DAMAGE

Tissue damage associated with long-term catheterization occurs as an inflammatory reaction in response to the presence of the catheter and/or as a result of trauma to urethral and bladder tissues.

Inflammatory response

As a 'foreign body' the catheter initiates an inflammatory response ranging in severity from mild oedema to haemorrhage and damage to mucosal epithelium (Nacey & Delahunt 1991). The choice of a material, which minimizes tissue reaction, is therefore extremely important, particularly during long-term use. In the past leaching of toxic substances from certain materials has been implicated in subsequent formation of urethral strictures (Blacklock 1986, Talja et al 1985), and recognition of this problem led to the enforcement of stricter controls on catheter materials and catheter manufacture (BS1695 part I, 1990).

The materials most commonly chosen for long-term catheterization are:

- all silicone
- silicone–elastomer-coated latex
- hydrogel-coated latex.

There is little research evidence to suggest that any of these materials produces significantly less tissue inflammation than the others, although the hydrogel coating is claimed to cause minimal friction on insertion.

Pressure necrosis

In addition to the problems of urethral irritation, tissue damage can also occur as a result of pressure necrosis. In the bladder there is potential for this to occur if continued pressure is exerted by the catheter tip in one location. Regular changing of the catheter and hence the position of the tip will reduce this risk. The urethra is also vulnerable to pressure necrosis, particularly in the male (Fig. 9.17) if continued tension is applied to the catheter, for example from the weight of a heavy drainage bag hanging unsupported or by tubing becoming caught in a wheelchair (Blandy & Moors 1989). Long-term pressure of this type can result in erosion of the tissue of the urethral meatus. Effective support should be provided for

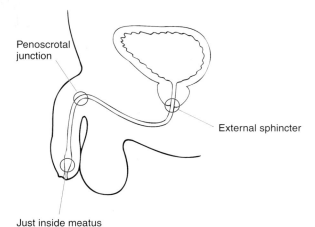

Figure 9.17 Diagram of penoscrotal flexure and potential pressure points.

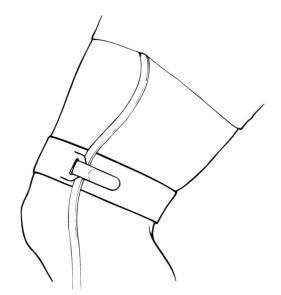

Figure 9.18 Catheter support strap.

the drainage bag, together with frequent emptying (e.g. when no more than two-thirds full), and also for the catheter itself. Traditionally this has been achieved by securing the catheter or tubing to the patient's thigh with adhesive tape whilst ensuring there is sufficient slack to allow free movement, and in males to allow for penile erection. However, adhesive tape can sometimes cause local irritation, especially when the skin is moist from sweat, and furthermore may not stick well to catheter materials chosen for their smoothness. If insufficient slack is allowed, this can result in 'shunting' of the catheter backwards and forwards within the urethra and bladder as the patient moves, with increased risk of tissue damage and infection. A number of alternative catheter supports have been designed to provide a secure support whilst preventing pulling, some of which are available on prescription (Fig. 9.18). If a catheter support is used, it is important that it is not allowed to constrict the catheter or tubing causing a restriction in the urine flow.

Correct positioning of the drainage bag is also important to minimize risks of hydrostatic suction causing the bladder mucosa to be sucked into the catheter eyes. The catheterized bladder is shrunken in comparison to a normally functioning bladder and a vacuum effect can be produced as the urine drains. Positioning the bag no more than 30 cm below the bladder should minimize this risk.

Tissue trauma on catheter insertion or removal

It is clear that the urethral catheterization procedure must be performed carefully to minimize risks of trauma. Removal of the catheter usually presents less difficulty but may be painful if urethral secretions have formed hard crusts around the meatus, or encrustations have formed on the external surface of the catheter and balloon within the bladder. Meatal secretions can be removed by gentle washing with soap and water, but catheters should also be observed for signs of encrustation immediately following removal. Measures to deal with recurrent encrustation are discussed later in this chapter.

CATHETER-ASSOCIATED INFECTION

At the outset of this section it is important to recognize that there is a distinction to be made between 'clinical infection' involving tissue invasion by micro-organisms with resultant systemic symptoms, and 'colonization' by micro-organisms which is indicated by the occurrence of bacteriuria, in the absence of clinical symptoms. It is not

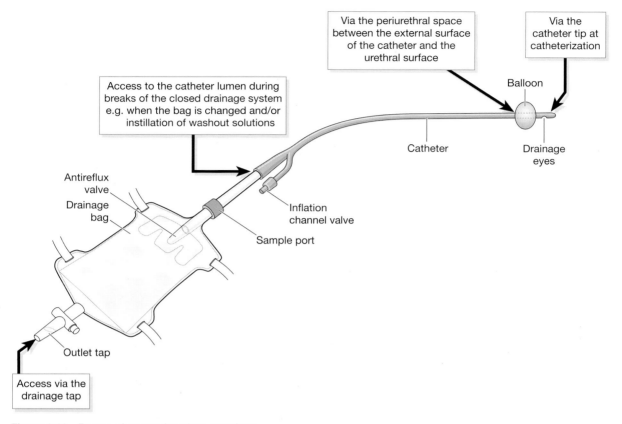

Figure 9.19 Routes of access for micro-organisms.

uncommon to find the generic term 'infection' being used in the literature to refer to both situations. In the absence of clinical symptoms it is generally accepted that bacteriuria should not be treated with antibiotics (Cravens & Zweig 2000).

Entry of micro-organisms

The body has a range of normal defences against entry of micro-organisms into the urinary tract, including:

- tightly closed folds of urethra
- flushing and scouring action of micturition
- a surface layer of mucus forming a protection against tissue invasion.

In the presence of a urethral catheter the first two defences are compromised since the urethra is held open, effectively providing a 'highway'

for the entry of micro-organisms into the bladder. In addition, urine is usually allowed to drain continuously through the catheter. The risk of catheter-associated infection increases by 5–8% per day (Mulhall et al 1988) and despite modern closed drainage systems, bacteriuria is virtually inevitable in long-term catheterization. Micro-organisms may gain access to the catheterized bladder in three ways (Stamm 1991, Tambyah et al 1999) (Fig. 9.19):

- Extraluminal (early) – during the catheterization procedure
- Intraluminal – by migration within the catheter lumen from the collection bag and/or the catheter–drainage tube junction
- Extraluminal (late) – via the mucus film adherent to the external catheter surface.

The comparative importance of these routes is difficult to determine, although Tambyah et al concluded from their prospective study of 1497 newly catheterized hospital patients that the preponderance of organisms identified gained access extraluminally. However, they also showed that even with excellent adherence to the accepted principles of catheter care, opportunities still exist for organisms to gain access intraluminally and that strategies for prevention of catheter-associated infection, including novel technologies, must address all possible portals of entry. The Department of Health recently published guidelines for preventing infections associated with insertion and maintenance of short-term indwelling urethral catheters in acute care (DoH 2001). Many of these principles are equally relevant to long-term catheterization.

Closed drainage systems

The catheter and drainage bag represent a closed system which is not open to the external environment. It is important that the bag is positioned at a level lower than the bladder, such that there is a free flow of urine into the bag thus preventing collections of stagnant urine within the tubing, which can act as a reservoir for growth of micro-organisms. The bag should also be positioned such that the tap is not resting on the floor. The non-return valve helps to prevent reflux of urine (and bacteria) into the catheter and bladder if the bag is moved, but the drainage tubing should be clamped if the bag needs to be lifted above the level of the bladder (e.g. to assist the patient to get in and out of a bath). A clamp should never be applied to the catheter itself as it may damage the catheter lumen and/or the balloon inflation channel. Clearly it must be released as soon as the procedure is over. Use of a shower may be a preferable alternative.

In order to maintain the effectiveness of the closed system in limiting bacterial access, breaks in the system by disconnecting the bag should be as infrequent as possible. It is generally recommended that bags attached directly to the catheter are changed at weekly intervals unless leakage occurs or the catheter becomes blocked. A high frequency of errors in catheter care including 'breakages' of the closed system have been

documented in some studies (Mulhall et al 1993) and ongoing, frequent monitoring of adherence to procedures and policies remains important.

Meatal cleansing

Catheter-induced urethral secretions commonly produce a discharge at the urethral meatus, which may form hard crusts causing tissue trauma when removed. There is no clear evidence that stringent meatal cleansing with or without the use of antiseptic agents will reduce catheter-associated infection. However, it is recommended that secretions are removed on a daily basis using pure or unperfumed soap and water, with clean wash cloths, to prevent crust formation (Classen et al 1991).

Infecting micro-organisms

A different distribution of micro-organisms, including a significantly higher proportion of Gram-negative bacilli, occurs in the urine from catheterized, compared to non-catheterized patients (Table 9.3). Complex mixed communities of micro-organisms are common (Godfrey & Evans 2001, Kohler-Ockmore & Feneley 1996) and are frequently unresponsive to antibiotic or antiseptic therapy (Stickler et al 1987). The source of these organisms is often the patient's own bowel and micro-organisms identified in the urine have also been isolated from the perineum and urethral meatus (Classen et al 1991, Ehrenkranz & Alfonso 1991).

Whilst bacteriuria presents an undoubted risk of upper urinary tract infection, renal impairment and bacteraemia, the associated risks of morbidity and mortality appear to be related to the underlying health of the patient. Although increased mortality has been associated with

Table 9.3 Common micro-organisms causing catheter-associated urinary tract infections

Gram-negative	Gram-positive
Escherichia coli	*Streptococcus faecalis*
Proteus species	*Staphylococcus aureus*
Pseudomonas species	
Klebsiella species	

urinary catheterization in acutely ill patients (Platt et al 1982, 1983), a similar relationship for long-term catheterized patients in community care is less clear. Systemic symptoms of infection are commonly absent in the latter group. However a further potential complication of long-term catheter-associated urinary tract infection is the increased incidence of neoplastic changes in the bladder (Stickler & Zimakoff 1994), and for spinally injured patients, who form a large proportion of the long-term catheterized population, renal failure is a recognized leading cause of death (see also Chapter 11).

Biofilm mode of bacterial growth

Micro-organisms have a strong tendency to grow on available surfaces in preference to free-living in a surrounding aqueous environment such as urine (Morris et al 1999). A living surface layer, or biofilm, develops as the infecting micro-organisms colonize the surface of the catheter and drainage equipment (Getliffe 1992, Marrie & Costerton 1983, Ramsey et al 1989). Initially only one cell thick, the biofilm gradually becomes thicker and more extensive as its members multiply and spread (Fig. 9.20). Furthermore, the presence of the biofilm becomes effectively irreversible as the

organisms within it 'cement' themselves firmly to the surface by the polysaccharide secretions they produce. It is now well documented that many chronic infections, particularly those involving indwelling devices, such as catheters, implants and prostheses, involve bacterial populations growing as an adherent biofilm enmeshed within a polysaccharide matrix or 'glycocalyx'.

Biofilms can protect the causative organisms from host defences and antimicrobial therapy (Morris et al 1999). Common urinary pathogens such as *Escherichia coli*, although killed in the urine by antimicrobial agents, may persist in the biofilm and restart the cycle of infection (Stickler et al 1989). One possible cause of the apparent resistance of biofilm inhabitants to antimicrobial therapy and host defences is a lack of penetration through the biofilm glycocalyx. A second possible cause is that micro-organisms deep within the biofilm are characterized by a slow and variable growth rate which is influenced by the availability of nutrients. Since growth rate is a primary modulator of antibiotic action (Brown et al 1988) this may be a major determinant of biofilm resistance. The biofilm mode of growth may explain why many patients with heavily colonized urinary catheters experience few overt symptoms of infection. Slow growth rate and nutrient deprivation

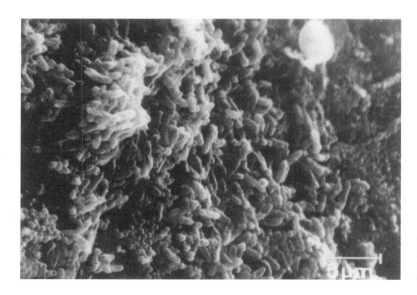

Figure 9.20 Electron micrograph showing a thick layer of adherent bacteria on the catheter surface forming a living biofilm.

are important factors in reducing bacterial pathogenesis (Brown et al 1988), and may also diminish tissue invasion.

One of the aims of catheter material development is to reduce the adherence of microorganisms to the surface. Hydrophobic (water-repelling) surface forces tend to enhance adhesion (Merritt & Chang 1991) and it has been claimed that the hydrophilic (water-attracting) surface of hydrogel-coated catheters may, therefore, resist bacterial colonization more effectively than other catheter materials. This may vary with different micro-organisms as Stickler & Hughes (1999) have shown that *Proteus mirabilis* moves easily across this catheter material. There is evidence of a reduced risk of urinary tract infection in the short term and potential cost saving when silver-alloy-coated catheters are used (Karchmer et al 2000) but the potential for longer term protection and indeed the ability of the silver coating to maintain its integrity are unknown. Whilst short-term benefits may exist, early deposition of proteins or lipid material on catheters in clinical use is likely to rapidly mask specialist surface properties, rendering them less effective in long-term care (Ohkawa et al 1990, Whitfield & Holmes 1991).

Antibiotics and antiseptics

It is generally recognized that antibiotics will not prevent bacteriuria in long-term catheterized patients (Kunin 1987). Whilst systemic antibiotic therapy may be effective in eradicating one episode of infection, bacteriuria soon recurs and resistant strains may emerge (Khardori and Yassien 1995). Similarly, although irrigation of the bladder with antibiotic or antiseptic solutions has been advocated in the past, and continues to be used (Getliffe 1994a), eradication of micro-organisms is rarely achieved and the emergence of resistant strains is again favoured (Gopal Rao & Elliott 1988). The irrigation solutions reviewed by Gopal Rao & Elliott included the antiseptic solutions chlorhexidine, noxythiolin and povidone iodine, a range of antibiotics and other miscellaneous solutions including normal saline and acetic acid, none of which was considered to be effective in limiting the occurrence of bacteriuria.

In particular, the benefits of the widespread use of chlorhexidine in bladder washouts, lubricating gels and antiseptic cleaning solutions have been disputed (Davies et al 1987, Stickler & Chawla 1987). Chlorhexidine is ineffectual against a number of commonly occurring urinary pathogens, but may remove sensitive bacteria in the normal urethral flora, allowing subsequent colonization by more resistant organisms. One study that examined the urogenital flora of female patients following antibiotic therapy showed that the indigenous lactobacillus population had not been restored in the majority of patients. Rather, uropathogenic bacteria were found to dominate (Reid et al 1990). It is therefore difficult to justify continued use of chlorhexidine as an antiseptic agent for catheterized patients.

There is some evidence to suggest that catheter/bladder washouts with mandelic acid (1%) can reduce the numbers of some bacteria commonly found in catheter-associated infections, including *Pseudomonas aeruginosa* and *Proteus mirabilis* (King & Stickler 1991, Robertson & Norton 1990). However, treatment time required may be lengthy and must be weighed against the potential detrimental effects of an acidic solution (pH 2) on the bladder mucosa.

The search for new antimicrobial agents, which are active against biofilm inhabitants, begins under controlled laboratory conditions. King & Stickler (1991) based their conclusions on results from a laboratory model of the catheterized bladder and there have been other promising reports (Seo et al 1990, Stickler & Hewitt 1991). However, the efficacy of such agents in the clinical situation is currently unknown (e.g. tissue reaction engendered; effectiveness of antimicrobial activity in the presence of physiological organic materials in urine). This is particularly important as there is considerable evidence to suggest that many antiseptic and antibiotic agents are inhibited by organic materials such as mucin and cell debris (Thomas 1990).

High fluid intake – myth or magic?

A high fluid intake of more than 2 litres per day has been traditionally recommended for catheterized patients (Wilson 1997). The rationale behind this is twofold:

- diuresis will assist in voiding micro-organisms from the bladder
- a dilute urine will impair bacterial growth and reduce the concentration of encrustation components.

However, catheter drainage not only prevents the normal physiological flushing and scouring action of micturition but, despite continuous drainage, the bladders of catheterized patients are incompletely emptied, since a residual volume of urine remains. Urodynamic mathematical models indicate that incomplete emptying of the bladder reduces the effective voiding of micro-organisms associated with diuresis (Mackintosh et al 1975). Since catheter-associated biofilms adhere strongly to catheter surfaces they are unlikely to be removed by the increased urine flow caused by diuresis, and therefore provide a continuous source of infection.

The major components of catheter encrustations (discussed in more detail below) are all normal constituents of urine and occur in relatively large proportions. It seems likely, therefore, that even dilute urine will contain sufficient quantities of these minerals for them to precipitate under appropriate conditions. However, urine that is very concentrated may cause irritation of the bladder mucosa and potentiate problems of bladder spasm. In addition, concentrated urine commonly has a strong odour, which patients may find upsetting. Deodorizing sprays are available from some manufacturers and some aromatic essential oils such as geranium may be useful in masking smells (but should not be applied directly to the skin).

Although there is no clear evidence that drinking large quantities of fluid will actually prevent catheter-associated infection, it remains sensible to encourage catheterized patients to drink sufficient fluids to avoid constipation or dehydration, especially as many have restricted mobility and may be unable to prepare their own drinks.

Cranberry juice

In American Indian cultures crushed cranberries have been used as a herbal remedy for urinary tract infection for centuries. More recently cranberry juice has become available as a soft drink or in capsule or tablet form from some health shops, and attention has been drawn to its potentially beneficial effects. The mechanism of action against infection may relate to the acidity of the berries and concomitant lowering of the urinary pH, to the bacteriostatic effects of the metabolic byproduct – hippuric acid – which is excreted in the urine (Bodel et al 1959) and/or to an inhibitory effect on the bacterial adherence of some micro-organisms, including *Escherichia coli*, to the bladder mucus (Ofek et al 1991, Schmidt & Sobata 1988, Sobata 1984). The latter property could be particularly advantageous to catheterized patients although effects are likely to vary with differing organisms. For example, *Proteus mirabilis* is a common cause of catheter-associated infection and is characterized by its ability to swarm over catheter and mucosal surfaces but laboratory studies by Stickler & Hughes (1999) were unable to detect any inhibitory effect on its capacity to swarm by oral intake of cranberry juice.

There are relatively few well-controlled studies of the efficacy of cranberry juice and Kahn et al (1967) have indicated that decreases in urinary pH are small and only transient unless large volumes are consumed. A randomized, double blind, placebo-controlled trial to assess the effects of drinking cranberry juice on the incidence of bacteriuria and pyuria in elderly women (who were not catheterized) was conducted by Avorn et al (1994). Within 2 months of drinking 300 ml of a commercially available cranberry beverage daily, only 15% of urine samples from the cranberry juice group showed bacteriuria and pyuria compared to 28% of samples from the placebo group (Fig. 9.21). Rogers (1991) was also able to demonstrate that drinking three glasses of cranberry juice daily reduced the symptoms of urinary tract infection in a small sample of children although this was an uncontrolled study.

Cranberry juice or capsules offers a simple and acceptable form of therapy for most patients and may be beneficial, but much of the evidence is anecdotal and further well-controlled investigations on catheterized patients are necessary to confirm or refute its potential benefits to them. In addition, there are suggestions that drinking in excess of 1 litre a day over prolonged periods may predispose to side-effects including gastritis, increased joint pain in rheumatoid arthritis sufferers and uric acid stone formation (Addison 1997, Rogers 1991).

Summary of key aspects of care in relation to catheter-associated infection

In conclusion, there is no clear evidence that stringent meatal cleansing, addition of antiseptic agents to the drainage bag, bladder washouts with chlorhexidine or similar reagents, drinking large volumes of fluid or regular consumption of cranberry juice will prevent or eradicate catheter-associated infection. Whilst bacteriuria may be almost inevitable in long-term catheterization, it is particularly important to minimize or prevent risks of cross-infection for patients in institutionalized

care and for patients at home, who depend on carers and health professionals coming into the home to provide catheter care. Catheterization is a sterile procedure and modern drainage equipment provides a sealed system that should not be broken more often than absolutely necessary. Effective hand washing techniques and wearing of gloves must be employed whenever catheters and bags are handled, and strict attention paid to infection control protocols.

CATHETER ENCRUSTATION AND BLOCKAGE

Recurrent catheter blockage caused by encrustation affects around 50% of long-term catheterized patients and presents a problem which is both distressing to patients and carers, and costly to health services in terms of time and resources (Fig. 9.22).

Although catheter blockage may result from a number of causes including twisted drainage tubing, bladder spasm or the pressure of a

---

Research study 9.1   Reduction in bacteriuria and pyuria after ingestion of cranberry juice

Avorn and colleagues (1994) carried out a randomized, double-blind, placebo controlled trial on the effects of drinking cranberry juice on the incidence of bacteriuria and pyuria in 153 elderly women (mean age 78.5 years). Subjects were randomly assigned to drink either 300 ml daily of a commercially available cranberry beverage or a specially prepared placebo drink which was indistinguishable in taste, appearance and vitamin C content, during the 6 months of the study. A baseline urine sample and six other, clean voided samples were collected at 1 month intervals and tested for bacteriuria ($>10^5$/ml) and the presence of white blood cells. Both groups were similar in age, number of medications used, and number of medical problems as well as bacteriuria and pyuria and urinary tract symptoms.

Sixty women in the cranberry group, and 61 women in the placebo group, completed the study. Data were analysed by multiple regression. The cranberry group had both bacteriuria and pyuria in 15% of samples compared with 28% of samples from the placebo group. This difference took between 1 and 2 months to develop and then persisted at about the same level (see Fig. 9.21). There was a modest reduction in the rate of antibiotics prescribed for the cranberry group, suggesting that the differences may have manifested themselves as important clinical outcomes. No significant difference was observed in the acidification

of urine in the cranberry group compared to the placebo group (median pH = 6.0 and 5.5, respectively).

The authors suggest that these results provide evidence for the bacteriostatic effects of cranberry juice which may be related to the role of bacterial adhesion in the cause and treatment of urinary tract infection.

NB: The women were not catheterized.

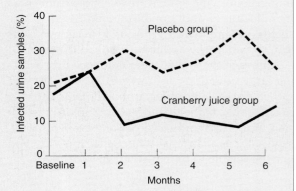

Figure 9.21   The effects of cranberry juice. Reproduced with permission of the American Medical Association from Avorn et al (1994).

constipated bowel on the adjacent urethra (see Box 9.2 on troubleshooting, p. 290), by far the most common cause of recurrent blockage is the deposit of mineral salts or encrustations on the catheter surface. These deposits may occur both within the lumen of the catheter and on outer surfaces of the tip and balloon where they may cause pain and trauma during catheter removal (Fig. 9.23).

Causes of catheter encrustation

The major components of catheter encrustations are struvite (magnesium ammonium phosphate)

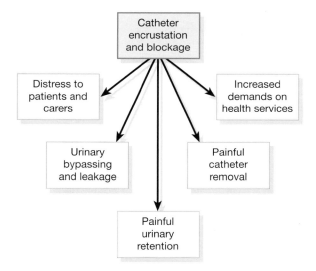

Figure 9.22 Effects of catheter encrustation and blockage.

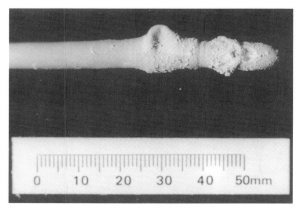

Figure 9.23 An encrusted catheter.

and calcium phosphates (Cox et al 1987, Getliffe 1992, Ohkawa et al 1990) which precipitate from the urine under alkaline conditions. Figure 9.24 is an electron micrograph of the luminal surface of an encrusted catheter showing the large 'coffin-shaped' crystals of struvite surrounded by the 'rubble-like' calcium phosphate.

Urine leaving the kidneys is normally sterile and acidic, with a pH in the region of 6.0 (range 4.5–8.5), depending on diet, medication and acid/base balance within the body. However, in the presence of certain micro-organisms which produce the enzyme urease, an alkaline urine (commonly pH 7.5–9.5) results. Urease catalyses the breakdown of urinary urea to release ammonia. Ammonia in solution is alkaline resulting in an increase in urine pH (Fig. 9.25). A similar association between the presence of urease-producers and the formation of struvite stones in the upper urinary tract (often termed 'infection stones'), has long been recognized (Brown 1901).

The most commonly occurring, potent urease-producer is *Proteus mirabilis*, which is often found in the patient's own bowel flora. Other micro-organisms also produce this enzyme, including *Providencia stuartii*, and some variants of *Staphylococcus aureus, Pseudomonas aeruginosa* and *Klebsiella* species, which may occur as hospital-acquired infections (Table 9.4).

It is interesting to note that the pH of the urine within blocked catheters is usually higher than the pH of urine flowing from a newly inserted catheter (Getliffe 1992, Norberg et al 1980), which suggests a localized production of urease by micro-organisms colonizing the catheter surface as a biofilm. As indicated earlier, biofilms quickly form on catheters and are extremely difficult if not impossible to remove. Laboratory studies have shown that dilute urine can slow swarming (and biofilm development) by *Proteus mirabilis* but there was no evidence that oral consumption of cranberry juice or ascorbic acid contributed to this effect (Stickler & Hughes 1999).

Blockers and non-blockers

There is considerable variation in the tendency of individual patients to develop catheter

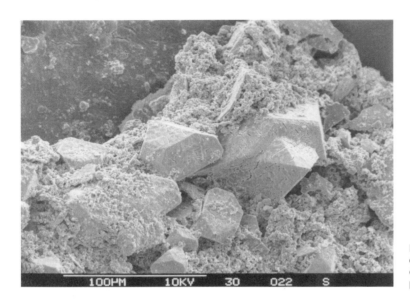

Figure 9.24 Electron micrograph of catheter encrustation showing large crystals of struvite and 'rubble-like' calcium phosphate.

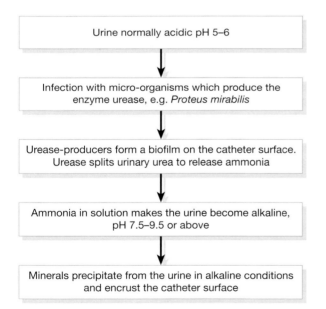

Figure 9.25 Formation of catheter encrustations.

Table 9.4 Micro-organisms which can cause urinary tract infections and which may produce urease

Micro-organism	Usually produce urease (>90% of clinical isolates)	Occasionally produce urease (5–30% of clinical isolates)
Gram-negative	*Proteus mirabilis* *Proteus vulgaris* *Proteus rettgeri* *Providencia stuartii* *Morganella morganii*	*Klebsiella pneumoniae* *Klebsiella oxytoca* *Pseudomonas aeruginosa* *Serratia marcesens*
Gram-positive	*Staphylococcus aureus* *Corynebacterium species*	*Staphylococcus epidermidis*
Mycoplasma	*Ureaplasma urealyticum*	

Adapted from Kunin (1987) and Wickham & Buck (1990).

- *'blockers'* are defined as those patients who consistently and repeatedly develop extensive encrustation on their urinary catheters within a few days to a few weeks, resulting in shorter catheter life because of diminished flow and leakage
- *'non-blockers'* are those patients who do not form encrustations even when the catheter is left in place for weeks to months (Kunin et al 1987b).

encrustation and in the quantity of encrustation produced in a given time period (Getliffe 1994a, Kunin et al 1987a). However, it is generally possible to classify patients into broad categories of 'blockers' or 'non-blockers' (Choong et al 1999, Getliffe 1992, 1994a, Kunin et al 1987b) where:

Research study 9.2 Characteristics and management of patients with recurrent blockage of urinary catheters

In this study by Getliffe (1994a), long-term catheterized patients living in the community were investigated to determine, firstly, whether they could be classified as 'blockers' or 'non-blockers' (or if the occurrence of catheter encrustation was a continuum experienced to some degree by all catheterized patients); and secondly, the factors which contribute to encrustation and blockage.

Forty-seven patients were classified as blockers and non-blockers on the basis of clinical specimens of used catheters. Bladder washouts were witheld during the period of the study and three used catheters replaced at 6-weekly intervals (or earlier if the catheter became blocked) were collected from each patient. The extent of encrustation was observed by cutting the catheter open longitudinally and assigning a score of 0–4 to each 20 mm section. The following definitions were applied:

- A 'blocked catheter' was defined as having at least one score of +3 or +4, where: +4 = catheter lumen completely occluded, and +3 = narrow patent channel
- Patients were defined as 'blockers' if two or more of their catheters became blocked during the study.

Results
Data from 42 patients (18 males and 24 females) who provided a minimum of two catheter samples were analysed. Forty-three per cent of patients were classed as 'blockers'.

Significantly more females (77.8%) than males were 'blockers', but 'blocker status' was not associated with age. 'Blocker' status was significantly associated with high urinary pH and high urinary ammonia, but not with 24 h urinary volume, osmolality or any other urinary component. Therefore, it is unlikely that 'urging patients to drink plenty' will prevent catheter encrustation. Thirty-three per cent of patients who used hydrogel-coated catheters and 52.2% who used silicone–elastomer-coated catheters were 'blockers', but these differences were not statistically significant, nor was there any relationship between 'blocker' status and Charrière size.

Patients were asked if they used bladder washouts during their usual catheter care regimes. Suby G, which is recommended by the manufacturers to reduce encrustation, was the reagent most commonly used (60% of patients using washouts). However, the use of Suby G by 17% of all 'non-blockers' was clearly inappropriate and unnecessary. Furthermore, chlorhexidine was used by 47% of patients using washouts, despite published reports of ineffectiveness against catheter-associated infection (Stickler et al 1987). Although the frequencies with which each reagent was used were too small for statistical analysis, these results suggest that some nurses were unclear about which, if any, bladder washout is appropriate for a particular patient.

Planned catheter changes

The recognition of patients as 'blockers' and 'non-blockers' is useful because it allows proactive care to be planned so as to reduce the likelihood of blockage actually occurring in susceptible patients. Getliffe (1994a) studied 47 long-term catheterized patients in the community. Based on clinical examination of three catheters per subject, removed at 6-weekly intervals (or before, if blocked), it was not only possible to classify patients as 'blockers' or 'non-blockers' but also to identify a characteristic pattern of 'catheter life' for the majority of individual 'blockers'. However, a prevailing tendency towards 'crisis care' appeared to exist, with catheters being replaced only when they had already blocked.

Although there may be some merit in not interfering whilst the catheter is still patent, this practice fails to meet the needs of patients who then require help urgently when their catheter suddenly blocks. If a characteristic pattern of 'catheter life' can be identified for individual patients it becomes possible to plan catheter changes to precede the predicted blockage. Such a policy of planned recatheterization not only reduces the distress caused to patients by blockage but would also reduce the pressures on community and hospital services when urgent unscheduled visits are required, or patients are sent to hospital outpatient/emergency departments for catheter changes.

It is suggested that the 'life' of at least three to five catheters needs to be recorded in order to identify a clear pattern (Norberg et al 1983), since small particles of encrusting material can easily become dislodged and block catheter eyes more quickly than usual on some occasions. Catheters should be examined carefully for signs of encrustation after removal and not simply assumed to be blocked because of failure to drain well (see Box 9.2). It may also be helpful to monitor urinary pH since alkaline urine is a strong indicator of potential encrustation. Urinary pH indicator strips, which change colour in alkaline urine, are available from some manufacturers (e.g. B. Braun Medical Ltd, Aylesbury). An example of a catheter management chart to aid monitoring of 'catheter life' is provided in Figure 9.26.

Whilst planned catheter changes can limit the occurrence of blockage, frequent recatheterization can also be a potential source of trauma. In addition, many patients find catheterization an embarrassing procedure (Getliffe 1994a) and very frequent recatheterizations may be unacceptable to them. Therefore, for patients whose catheters block very frequently (e.g. in less than 7–14 days), alternative approaches to reducing encrustation may be helpful to try to prolong the period the catheter can remain *in situ* before becoming blocked.

Catheter maintenance solutions

The introduction of a catheter maintenance solution into the catheter (commonly termed a 'bladder washout' in earlier literature) has been advocated in the management of both catheter-associated infection and recurrent catheter encrustation and blockage. In the management of recurrent catheter blockage in particular, the main purpose is to reduce the accumulation of minerals encrusting the catheter surface, which will eventually block the catheter. The term 'catheter maintenance solution' is therefore more appropriate as the intention is to 'wash out' the catheter rather than the bladder. Where earlier literature is cited below the term used in the original publication will be retained to avoid confusion.

Since management of these complications by regular use of such solutions may continue for many years there are a number of key questions to be addressed:

- 'Is there a potential risk of damage to the bladder mucosa from regular contact with a catheter maintenance solution in either the short or the long term?'
- 'How effective is the catheter maintenance solution in minimizing catheter-associated complications?'

- 'Is this form of management acceptable to the patient and does it represent effective use of resources?'

The relative lack of either experimental or clinical research-based evidence on the use of catheter maintenance solutions makes it extremely difficult to provide unequivocal answers to these questions. Discussion of the existing research evidence is provided elsewhere (Getliffe 1996, Getliffe et al 2000) but a number of points are considered here.

Research study 9.3 Catheter maintenance solutions and chemical irritations

Various chemical reagents have been used in attempts to dissolve urinary tract calculi but experimental studies usually involve continuous irrigation over several hours (Oosterlink et al 1991, Reckler et al 1986). Tissue damage generally appears greater in the ureters than in the bladder which is protected to a certain extent by a superficial mucous layer. Dilute acid solutions have been shown to cause histological damage to rabbit bladder urothelium (Donmez et al 1990, Parsons et al 1975); however, recovery appeared to occur within 24–48 h. The addition of magnesium to solutions caused less injury and damage was clearly dependent on the period of exposure, which in these experiments was up to 5 h. This is considerably longer than the 15 min normally recommended for bladder washouts used clinically.

Potential risks

Potential risks to the bladder arise from the washout procedure itself, from the reagent used, or from both. Traditional 'bladder washouts' have been performed using a 60 ml bladder syringe fitted to the funnel end of the catheter. This method allows active flushing of the bladder by alternately depressing and withdrawing the plunger causing the washout fluid to disturb any debris so that drainage can occur. However, the physical forces exerted on the bladder mucosa by this procedure may be considerable and there is also a risk that by withdrawing the plunger too forcefully the urothelium can be sucked into the eyes of the catheter causing tissue trauma and catheter blockage.

Indwelling Catheter Management Chart

Name --

G.P. --

Catheter type --

District Nurse --

Catheter size --

Contact Number --

Evaluate the current pattern of 'catheter life' after every three catheters and revise care plan if necessary

Date of catheter change	Previous catheter's 'life' (in days)	Reason for change P – planned B – blocked O – other	Urine pH	Visible encrustation?	Catheter maintenance solution protocol e.g. 50 ml Suby G 2 × weekly	Next catheter change due	Signature
Evaluate							
Evaluate							

Figure 9.26 Catheter management chart.

The bladder mucosa is an important host defence against urinary tract infection and disruption of the urothelium has been associated with increased shedding of urothelial cells. Elliott et al (1989) have demonstrated increased shedding of urothelial cells following bladder washouts with up to 60 ml saline 0.9%, chlorhexidine 0.02% or noxythiolin 2.5%. The response to normal saline and the rapidity of the increase in shedding of cells, which occurred immediately after bladder washouts, is strongly suggestive that the physical force of the washout procedure was largely responsible. Kennedy et al (1992), in a small randomized crossover trial of Suby G, Solution R and saline in 25 female patients with long-term catheters, showed a high percentage of red blood cells in the drainage fluid following use of Suby G, indicating some degree of tissue damage. Increased levels of urothelial cells were also demonstrated following use of all three solutions. Although there were some limitations in the design of this study there is clearly a need for further work on the clinical effects of frequent use of these solutions.

Despite the 'washout' being performed as an aseptic technique, any breakage of the closed drainage system inevitably increases the risk of introducing infection. The availability of prepacked, sterile solutions offers a convenient method for nurses or patients to perform catheter maintenance, and to minimize risks of introducing infection. The most commonly available range of prepacked solutions is shown in Box 9.1.

Saline 0.9%. Saline may be appropriate for use in the removal of small blood clots following surgery but can only remove encrusting material by the physical force of flushing and therefore cannot be recommended as part of a management regime for recurrent catheter blockage.

Chlorhexidine 0.02%. As discussed earlier, neither chlorhexidine nor indeed any antiseptic bladder washout can be recommended as a means of preventing bacteriuria in long-term catheterized patients. This is partly because of reduced susceptibility of biofilm members to antiseptic agents and also because of risks of removal of normal urethral flora and the development of resistant species.

Box 9.1	Catheter maintenance solutions
Suby G	3.23% citric acid solution, pH 4, containing magnesium oxide to minimize tissue irritation, aimed at reducing encrustation
Solution R	6% citric acid solution, pH 2, containing magnesium carbonate, aimed at dissolving encrustations
Mandelic acid 1%	an acidic solution, pH 2, aimed at inhibiting the growth of urease-producers
Saline 0.9%	a neutral solution, pH 7, recommended for flushing of debris and small blood clots
Chlorhexidine 0.02%	an antiseptic solution aimed at preventing or reducing bacterial growth, in particular *E. coli* and *Klebsiella* species

Acidic reagents

Hesse et al (1989), Getliffe (1994b) and Getliffe et al (2000) have reported that in laboratory studies, catheter encrustations were prevented or largely dissolved by irrigation with Suby G and mandelic acid, but that saline was ineffective. Very few clinical studies of the use of catheter maintenance solutions have been conducted, largely because of the difficulty in maintaining adequate controls in the clinical situation.

Application

The catheter maintenance solution is allowed to flow into the bladder under the force of gravity by elevation of the bag above bladder height, or by application of controlled pressure through squeezing a small bellows delivery device (OptiFlo, Bard Ltd, Crawley) (Fig. 9.27). The solution is normally retained in the bladder for 15–20 minutes by clamping the bag tubing or drainage tubing and subsequently allowing it to drain out when the clamp is removed. This method does not involve active flushing and although squeezing the bag device would provide additional force to dislodge debris, this practice is not recommended because the degree of pressure is uncontrolled and potential damage to the bladder mucosa could result

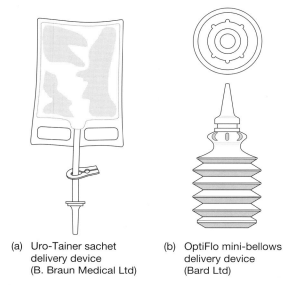

(a) Uro-Tainer sachet delivery device (B. Braun Medical Ltd)

(b) OptiFlo mini-bellows delivery device (Bard Ltd)

Figure 9.27 Catheter maintenance solution delivery devices. Reproduced with permission from Bard Ltd.

from excessive physical force. Squeezing the bellows delivery device allows some controlled agitation of the solution whilst preventing application of excessive force. Although it seems logical that agitation of the maintenance solution may increase the rate of dissolution of mineral deposits in the same way as sugar dissolves more rapidly in tea when it is stirred, further research is required to test both the efficacy and effect on the bladder mucosa.

Catheter maintenance solutions are currently available in 100 ml and 50 ml volumes. Laboratory studies using a model of the catheterized bladder have shown that 100 ml is no more effective than 50 ml at reducing encrustations and also that two sequential washes with 50 ml may be more effective at reducing encrustation than a single washout with either 50 or 100 ml (Getliffe et al 2000). This may be partially due to early saturation of the fluid within the catheter lumen with dissolved minerals limiting further dissolution. Drainage of the first 50 ml followed by the introduction of a further 50 ml fresh solution would then allow further dissolution to take place. Alternatively the application of two 50 ml aliquots may have a cumulative effect in lowering

the pH within the catheter lumen, thus promoting further dissolution.

Since even a large catheter (e.g. 18 Ch) holds little more than 4 ml it is possible that volumes smaller than 50 ml would still completely fill the catheter lumen and bathe the tip without allowing a large excess of solution to be in contact with the bladder mucosa, where it may cause tissue irritation. Smaller volumes could perhaps be used more frequently (e.g. on alternate days) without increasing the risks of tissue damage. On the basis of evidence from animal studies this policy would allow time for re-establishment of the mucous lining of the bladder (Donmez et al 1990, Parsons et al 1975), but clinically based studies are required to establish the efficacy of this approach. The precise frequency with which a catheter maintenance solution should be applied requires an individualized regime for each patient. This should be based on careful recording of catheter life to identify the minimum frequency that will promote patency for an acceptable period. It is not expected that this management approach will necessarily prevent encrustation completely. Pomfret (1995) discusses the instillation of 'mini-bladder washouts' in ten patients experiencing severe problems with catheter encrustation and blockage. Subjective evidence suggested that, for many of them, there appeared to be a reduced frequency of blockage. Clearly further carefully controlled clinical trials are required to provide research-based evidence, but one of the problems of conducting such trials is the difficulty in obtaining adequate numbers of catheterized patients to take part.

Stronger acidic solutions such as Solution R have been used successfully to dissolve fragments of struvite renal calculi following lithotripsy (Holden & Rao 1991). Dissolution of catheter encrustations may be achieved by Solution R also, but the benefits may be outweighed by potential inflammatory tissue reactions to a stronger acid solution, which limit the frequency with which this solution can be used. It is probably of most value used prior to catheter removal if external encrustations on the catheter tip and balloon cause pain and tissue trauma when the catheter is withdrawn. Solution R may also be useful in dissolving encrustations which are blocking the catheter by instilling the solution as far as the blockage and leaving it in place to dissolve the encrustations for up to 15–20 minutes.

Catheter/bladder washouts with mandelic acid 1% have been used with some success to remove Pseudomonas species from the urine of catheterized patients but treatment over several weeks may be necessary (Robertson & Norton 1990). Mandelic acid is also effective in reducing catheter encrustation (Getliffe 1994b) but like Solution R it is a strong acid (pH 2) and does not contain added magnesium oxide to minimize tissue irritation. For this reason long-term use of Solution R or mandelic acid on a regular basis must be questioned.

Fluid intake

Although it seems logical that increased fluid intake should reduce the concentration of the components of catheter encrustations (i.e. magnesium, ammonium, calcium and phosphates) in the urine, Getliffe (1994a) was unable to detect any significant difference in fluid intake or urinary osmolarity between groups of 'blockers' and 'non-blockers'. This is most probably because even in very dilute urine there will still be sufficient quantities of these components to precipitate under alkaline conditions produced by a urease-producing catheter biofilm. However this research was designed to examine differences between groups of patients, i.e. 'blockers' and 'non-blockers'. Consequently it was not possible to identify differences in 'catheter life' between individual patients within the 'blocker' group, which may have been influenced by their fluid intake (see Individualized patient care below).

Oral acidification of urine

Alternative approaches to combat catheter encrustation by decreasing urinary pH through ingestion of acidic liquids such as cranberry juice (Rogers 1991) (discussed above), or acidifying agents such as ascorbic acid (vitamin C) (Nahata et al 1977), have failed to demonstrate clear evidence of effectiveness, although most studies to date have been poorly controlled.

Ascorbic acid has been widely employed as a urinary acidifier, particularly as an adjunct to the treatment of urinary tract infections (Kunin 1987). However, conflicting reports of its efficacy exist (Murphy et al 1965, Travis et al 1965). Interstudy variations in the daily dose of ascorbic acid may have contributed to inconsistent conclusions; however small population size, unclear methodology or lack of rigorous statistical analysis also undermine the validity of some results. The absorption of ascorbic acid is a saturable process (Nahata et al 1977). Large amounts given as a single dose may be only partially absorbed and relatively ineffective at reducing urinary pH. In a well-controlled crossover study of ten subjects taking 4 g or 6 g ascorbic acid daily in divided doses, only the 4 g regimens were associated with a statistically significant decrease in urinary pH (Nahata et al 1977). The maximum drop in overall mean urinary pH for any individual was only 0.24 units and the authors state that such a decrease would be of little clinical consequence. High doses of ascorbic acid (>500 mg/d) are significantly associated with increased intrarenal urinary oxalate concentration and may therefore present an increased risk of calcium oxalate renal stone formation (Urivetzky et al 1992) in susceptible patients.

Attempts to acidify a patient's urine without the elimination of urease-producers is unlikely to prevent catheter encrustation since biofilm urease-producers on the catheter surface will continue to create an alkaline microenvironment within the catheter lumen (Getliffe 1992). Evidence from laboratory-based studies also suggests that attempts to reduce urinary pH in the presence of urease-producers are unlikely to be successful (Bibby et al 1995).

Individualized patient care

In research studies which focus on a population of patients who are all 'blockers' it may be difficult to demonstrate the efficacy of different management approaches because of wide intragroup variations (e.g. in characteristic patterns of catheter

Case study 9.1

Mr P was in his mid-70s and had problems of retention of urine due to benign enlargement of his prostate gland. In view of his age and general health he was considered unfit for surgery and his retention was managed by use of an indwelling urethral catheter. Whilst Mr P was happy with the catheter as an effective alternative to surgery, there were times when the catheter suddenly became blocked and the resulting retention of urine caused him considerable pain and distress. Most often the blockage seemed to occur in the early hours of the morning and Mr P would wake feeling an urgent need to void. He was unwilling to call his GP before surgery hours although the longer he waited the more painful his bladder became. Even when the surgery finally opened at 8.30 am he often had to wait several more hours until the doctor or district nurse was able to visit and change the catheter.

The district nurse was concerned about Mr P's recurrent problem and decided to try to identify the likely cause. She began to keep a chart on which she recorded the characteristics of each 'catheter life' (see Fig. 9.28). Prior to this time Mr P's catheters had been expected to stay *in situ* for approximately 12 weeks, to be changed earlier only if blockage occurred. After monitoring the 'lives' of three catheters a pattern began to emerge. Mr P's catheters appeared to stay patent for about 3 weeks but tended to block soon after that.

Catheter blockage can sometimes be caused by twisted tubing, bladder spasm or by constipation if the loaded rectum presses on the urethra. But the most common cause of recurrent catheter blockage is the build up of mineral deposits, or encrustation, inside the catheter lumen. By observing each catheter carefully when it was removed it was often possible to see evidence of

---

Indwelling Catheter Management Chart — *CASE STUDY*

Name: MR P
Catheter type: BARD BIOCATH (MALE)
Catheter size: 14 CH

G.P.
District Nurse
Contact Number

Evaluate the current pattern of 'catheter life' after every three catheters and revise care if necessary

Date of catheter change	Previous catheter's 'life' (in days)	Reason for change P – planned B – blocked O – other	Urine pH *pH INDICATOR*	Visible encrustation?	Catheter maintenance solution protocol e.g. 50ml Suby G 2 x weekly	Next catheter change due	Signature
22/1/01	23	B	ALKALINE RED	YES AROUND EYES	No	12 WEEKS 16/4/01	RS
19/2/01	28	B	ALKALINE RED	No	No	12 WEEKS 19/5/01	RS
15/3/01	25	B	ALKALINE RED	YES	No	3 WEEKS 5/4/01	RS

Evaluate LAST CATHETER CUT OPEN. ENCRUSTATION BLOCKING LUMEN. URINE CONSISTENTLY ALKALINE — SMELLS OF AMMONIA. SAMPLE TO LAB. SEEMS TO BLOCK AFTER ABOUT THREE WEEKS. PLANNED CHANGES AT 3 WEEKS (BEFORE BLOCKAGE!)

Date of catheter change	Previous catheter's 'life' (in days)	Reason for change	Urine pH	Visible encrustation?	Catheter maintenance solution protocol	Next catheter change due	Signature
5/4/01	21	P	RED	NO	No	3 WEEKS 26/4/01	RS
26/4/01	21	P	RED	YES, ON TIP	No	3 WEEKS 17/5/01	RS
17/5/01	21	P	RED	YES, ON TIP	NO	3 WEEKS 7/6/01	RS

Evaluate 3 WEEK PLAN SEEMS OK. SAMPLE CONTAINS P. MIRABILIS (KNOWN TO CAUSE ALKALINE URINE + CATHETER ENCRUSTATION). LAST CATHETER CUT OPEN. STILL ENCRUSTING BUT STAYS PATENT FOR ABOUT 3 WEEKS. CONTINUE CHANGE AT 3 WEEKS

Figure 9.28 Indwelling catheter management chart.

(continued)

Case study 9.1 *(continued)*

encrustation on the tip or around the eyes. Two catheters were cut open showing encrusting mineral deposits inside filling the lumen. Mineral salts are precipitated if the urine becomes alkaline due to infection with particular bacteria which release ammonia from urinary urea. By monitoring the pH of the urine with indicator paper which turns pink or red in alkaline conditions (B. Braun, Sheffield) it was clear that Mr P's urine was alkaline. The most likely cause was infection with an organism which could release ammonia. This was confirmed when a urine sample was sent for microbiological analysis and the organism *Proteus mirabilis*, which is commonly associated with problems of catheter encrustation, was identified.

Antibiotics are not usually very successful at eradicating this type of catheter-associated infection, partly because bacteria stick firmly to the catheter surface forming a biofilm which is unresponsive to antibiotics and partly because the organism is often present in the patient's

own bowel providing a continued source of reinfection. The catheter could be replaced with a new 'clean' one whilst a course of antibiotics is tried if it is considered that the organism has been introduced by cross-infection, but since Mr P was living at home this seemed unlikely. The district nurse decided to instigate a regime of planned catheter changes at 3-weekly intervals, i.e. just prior to the likely event of a catheter blockage occurring.

Although Mr P's urine remained alkaline and there were signs of encrustation around the tip of some catheters when they were removed, this regime proved effective and further blockage rarely occurred. Mr P was greatly relieved especially as he now felt able to go on holiday with his daughter and family without the uncertainty and fear of his previous catheter problems. A few years later, when it became necessary for Mr P to go into residential care, the fact that his catheter was relatively trouble free was an important factor in his acceptance at the centre of his choice.

---

life). Therefore it is always important for practitioners to look carefully, not only at the research evidence available but also at the way in which it was collected. Strategies which may not appear to be effective for all 'blockers' may nevertheless extend the catheter life of individual patients, since the precise mechanism by which some patients' catheters block very rapidly whilst others may remain patent for several weeks is still unclear. For some individuals therefore, ascorbic acid or cranberry juice therapy may be of some value but the practitioner should monitor and record the characteristic length of catheter life prior to introducing a new regime and then carefully record any consistent increase in 'catheter life'. The chart provided in Figure 9.26 may provide a useful format for monitoring and recording changes.

Catheter material

Although research into new catheter materials continues to focus on materials which will resist biofilm development, encrustation can occur on all currently available catheter materials, both during clinical use or under controlled experimental conditions (Cox et al 1988, 1989, Morris et al 1997). Plain latex and teflon-coated latex show the greatest susceptibility to encrustation but there is

little evidence that any one of three materials recommended for long-term catheter use – silicone, silicone–elastomer-coated latex or hydrogel-coated latex – is significantly more resistant to encrustation than the others (Cox et al 1989). In a clinical study by Bull et al (1991), hydrogel-coated catheters remained *in situ* for significantly longer than silicone–elastomer-coated catheters. Urinary bypassing was cited as the main reason for changes of silicone–elastomer-coated catheters, but a direct relationship with catheter encrustation was not established.

PATIENT EDUCATION AND SUPPORT
Information and practical advice

An explanation of the purpose of the catheter and its care is important for all patients who are not unconscious or cognitively impaired. Such knowledge is essential in helping patients to reach their own potential in terms of self-care and independence, and also in promoting dignity and comfort. As discussed at the outset of this chapter, the initial decision to catheterize should be a joint one between the patient, carer (if at home) and health professionals whenever possible. The potential psychological and social effects must be considered at this stage but ongoing patient education and support should continue to be provided. This should include not only verbal discussion but also provision of written information to which patients and carers can continue to refer. This is particularly important for patients who come home from hospital with a catheter and it is essential that they have adequate supplies of equipment during the first weeks. A range of useful booklets and brochures are available from specialist manufacturers and charities (see Chapter 12).

The main educational issues that should be addressed include the following:

- What a catheter is and why it is needed.
- Simple anatomy and physiology of the urinary tract, illustrating the position of the catheter.
- Personal hygiene, especially hand washing before and after handling the catheter or drainage bag.
- Connecting and disconnecting bags.
- Disposal of urine and cleaning of bags.
- Dietary advice, avoiding constipation, fluid intake.
- Dealing with catheter problems, including when and where to call for help.
- Obtaining supplies.
- Sexual activity.

Sexual activity

Sexual activity is not precluded by the presence of a urethral catheter although catheterization will influence sexuality and may contribute to physical and psychological problems including impaired body image, loss of libido, embarrassment, retrograde ejaculation (in males) and discomfort. In males the catheter can be folded back along the length of the penis and secured in place with a condom. In females it can be helpful to reassure the couple that the catheter is not in the vagina and can be taped across the lower abdomen to keep it out of the way. A 'rear approach' may also be a more comfortable position. KY jelly can be used to aid lubrication. However patients may prefer to consider the possibility of a suprapubic insertion or the temporary removal and subsequent

replacement of the catheter. Healthcare professionals need to be alert to these issues, even in the case of elderly patients. They must be prepared to facilitate discussions, which patients may find difficult to initiate, in a sensitive manner and be able to offer guidance on other sources of advice (see Chapter 12).

Troubleshooting

Some practical hints for dealing with common problems associated with urethral catheterization are offered in Box 9.2.

SUPRAPUBIC CATHETERIZATION

For some patients the insertion of an indwelling catheter suprapubically, into the bladder through the abdominal wall, may offer advantages over the urethral route. This technique may be necessary following urethral or pelvic trauma, and may also be appropriate for urinary retention or voiding problems caused by prostatic obstruction or urethral stricture. The suprapubic route can be particularly useful for women with neuropathy since urethral catheterization forces them to sit on the catheter. A lack of mobility, which prevents changing the seated position, can cause pressure on the catheter, which in turn, could cause erosion of the bladder neck and urethra. Hypercontractility of the neuropathic bladder also increases the risk of the catheter being expelled with concomitant trauma to urethral tissue. Suprapubic insertion can also be the method of choice for patients with restricted hip mobility (e.g. due to arthritis), those with urethral scarring resulting from trauma or tumours, or those who are sexually active. Suprapubic catheterization in patients requiring long-term drainage due to neuropathic bladder dysfunction has been shown to be associated with high levels of satisfaction and an improved quality of life (Sheriff et al 1998).

Some advantages of the suprapubic route

- There is no risk of urethral trauma, necrosis or catheter-induced urethritis.

Box 9.2 Troubleshooting – urethral catheters

Urine does not drain
- Check that the drainage bag is below the level of the bladder.
- Check for kinked tubing.
- Empty the bag – urine will not drain if the bag is very full.
- If it is suspected that the bladder mucosa may be occluding the catheter eyes raise the bag above the level of the bladder briefly to release negative hydrostatic pressure and then position the bag no more than 30 cm below the bladder.
- Check for constipation.
- Change the catheter and inspect for encrustation.

Urinary bypassing
- Check for kinked tubing.
- Check for constipation.
- Change the catheter and inspect for encrustation and blockage.
- If there is a possibility of bladder irritation/spasm:
  —consider increasing fluid intake to dilute urine
  —check for systemic symptoms of infection
  —check for bladder calculi by X-ray or ultrasound
  —replace the catheter with a smaller size
  —consider anticholinergic medication.

Haematuria
- Small amounts of blood may be caused by trauma or infection.
- If severe, seek medical help urgently.

The inflation balloon does not deflate
- Check for kinked tubing.
- Try a different syringe. Leave in place – the water may seep out over a period of time.
- Try to relieve constipation, if present, as this may cause pressure on the inflation channel.
- Try to remove or dislodge debris blocking the deflation channel by gently 'milking' the catheter along its length or inserting a few drops of sterile water into the inflation channel (no more than 1–2 ml).
- Attach a sterile needle to a 10 ml syringe and insert into the catheter arm just above the inflation valve. If the valve is faulty the water may be withdrawn gently via the syringe.
- Never cut the catheter. If it is under traction it may recoil inside the urethra.
- Never cut off the inflation valve. If the balloon does not deflate it will no longer be possible to try alternative simple methods.
- Never attempt to burst the balloon by overinflating it – a cystoscopy will be required to remove fragments! Remaining fragments may result in formation of calculi.
- Consult local nursing policy for further advice.

NB: Always have a spare catheter available!

- There is greater comfort, particularly for patients who are chair-bound.
- Access to the entry site is easier for cleansing and catheter change.
- There is greater freedom for expression of sexuality.
- It facilitates trials of voiding after major/urological surgery. The drainage tubing can be clamped and the ability to void urethrally assessed prior to removal of the suprapubic catheter.

The major contraindication to suprapubic catheterization is in patients with haematuria of unknown origin or with known carcinoma of bladder since there are clear risks associated with inflicting trauma on tumour cells. Suprapubic catheters may also be inappropriate for some very obese patients where the catheter will be trapped between folds of skin and adipose tissue.

Catheter insertion

The catheterization procedure is normally undertaken by a medical practitioner but can be carried out by an appropriately trained and competent nurse, with due adherence to UKCC guidelines (1992). Gujral et al (1999) reported on 164 patients who had their first suprapubic catheter inserted by a continence advisor/urology nurse specialist, with no evidence of serious complications.

The procedure involves insertion of the catheter into the bladder through an incision in the abdominal wall (cystotomy) under local or general anaesthetic, under strict aseptic conditions (Fig. 9.29). After palpating the full bladder, a proposed puncture site is selected one to two finger breadths (approximately 2 cm) above the midline of the symphysis pubis. A trocar and introducer may be used prior to insertion of a standard Foley catheter (usually 12–16 Ch) (Lawrence et al 1989) (Fig. 9.30), or a specifically designed suprapubic catheter which fits over a sharp trocar may be employed (Fig. 9.31). Some suprapubic catheters have coiled tips to reduce the risk of the catheter entering the urethra (Fig. 9.5). Once in place the catheter is anchored by an inflated balloon, a commercially produced seal or by sutures. A small dry

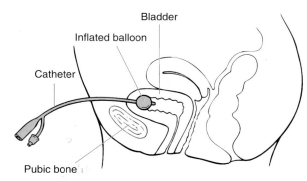

Figure 9.29 Suprapubic catheter in position.

dressing may be placed around the wound for the first 24 hours.

Catheter change

Once the abdominal channel has become established (about 4 weeks) a Foley catheter can be changed routinely by experienced nursing staff on the ward or in the community, usually without the use of local anaesthetic. Patients or carers may also be taught to change the catheter for themselves. A newly inserted catheter is commonly changed after 4–6 weeks and at intervals of between 4–10 weeks after that.

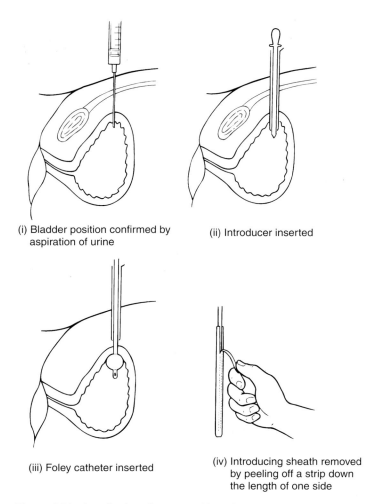

(i) Bladder position confirmed by aspiration of urine

(ii) Introducer inserted

(iii) Foley catheter inserted

(iv) Introducing sheath removed by peeling off a strip down the length of one side

Figure 9.30 Introduction of a suprapubic catheter.

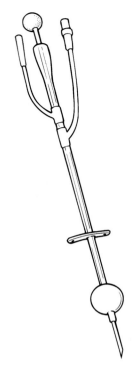

Figure 9.31 Suprapubic catheter with a sharp trocar.

It is important to carefully observe the angle of the catheter as it leaves the abdomen, as this will help insertion of the new catheter along the established pathway. Insertion of a little anaesthetic gel down the side of the old catheter will help to lubricate it and facilitate its removal after deflation of the balloon. If the balloon has not returned to its original flat position or there is some encrustation on the catheter a gentle pull may be necessary to remove it and can result in a little bleeding.

The new catheter should be inserted as quickly as possible whilst the track is still easy to follow. A delay of only a few minutes can result in partial obliteration of the tract as the detrusor fibres contract (Jacovou 1994).

As there may be no immediate flow of urine it is useful to insert the catheter a little further than the previous one, half fill the balloon with water and then withdraw the catheter gently until it feels firm against the bladder wall. The balloon can then be fully inflated. It is possible for the balloon to be inflated outside of the bladder in the abdominal cavity or beyond the bladder in the prostatic bed. It is also possible for the catheter to be inserted so far that the tip appears at the urethra (check by observation of the urethra in females). However, careful comparison of the exposed length of the newly inserted catheter with that of the old one should prevent these occurrences.

It is advisable for patients to have a spare catheter at home so that replacement can take place as quickly as possible should the old catheter fall out. Although this is not a common occurrence it can be very difficult to pass a new catheter following a delay. Sometimes it may be possible to pass a smaller catheter but alternatively, dilatation of the tract may be required under anaesthetic. After permanent removal of the catheter the channel should heal rapidly.

Catheter management

The principles of catheter management are similar to the management of urethral catheters, although there are differences. The suprapubic catheter emerges at right angles to the abdomen and may require support in this position. Its location may also present some difficulties in dressing and carrying out personal hygiene. Secretions around the cystotomy site can be removed while bathing or with soap and water. If staining of clothing by secretions is a problem a simple dressing may be applied but is often unnecessary. One relatively minor complication, which can be a great nuisance to patients, is persistent weeping from small patches of granulation tissue, which develop alongside the catheterization site. Reference should be made to local wound management or catheter care protocols to deal with this problem. If dressings are to be used they should be sterile and applied using an aseptic technique. Evans & Feneley (2000) report on a study of the nursing management of 113 patients with long-term suprapubic catheters in the community. These authors found that 60% of patients required a dressing around their suprapubic site and 42% of patients regularly received either a bladder washout or instillation. Persistent urethral leakage can sometimes be a difficulty, more commonly in females. Similar approaches to management of leakage during urethral catheterization should be initiated (see Box 9.2) but some female patients may require the urethra to be surgically closed.

Despite the greater spatial separation from potential contamination by bowel micro-organisms, suprapubic catheters are nevertheless susceptible to catheter-associated infection, biofilm formation and to catheter encrustation and blockage (Getliffe 1992, Shah & Shah 1998). Other potential risk factors are also similar to those encountered in urethral catheterization and include bladder spasm, loss of bladder tone and pressure necrosis (Addison & Mould 2000, Peate 1997). There is some evidence to suggest that bladder calculi may be more common in suprapubic catheterization and Shah & Shah (1998) recommend annual ultrasound and cystoscopy to check for these.

Common problems with suprapubic catheters

- If no urine drains after changing the catheter, ensure the drainage bag is below the level of the bladder. Also encourage the patient to drink beforehand.
- If there is leakage through the urethra check for kinked tubing. If bladder spasm is a problem, consider anticholinergic medication. Surgical closure of the urethra may be necessary as a last resort.
- Overgranulation of tissue at the insertion site can be ignored if it is not causing concern to the patient. Refer to local wound management or catheter care protocols if further action is required.

INTERMITTENT SELF-CATHETERIZATION

Clean intermittent self-catheterization (ISC), originally introduced by Lapides et al (1972), may be a practical option for many patients who are sufficiently dexterous and motivated, as it provides greater independence and personal control over bladder function. Since the catheter is passed intermittently into the bladder and removed when drainage has ceased, ISC avoids many of the problems associated with the retention of a catheter *in situ*. The importance of regular bladder drainage has been emphasized by Lapides et al (1974) who suggested that as well as providing a reservoir for infection, the increased intravesical pressure caused by build up of residual urine could reduce the vascular supply to the bladder tissue rendering it more susceptible to bacterial invasion. In the absence of regular drainage, dilatation of the upper urinary tract may also occur and carries an associated increased risk of urinary tract infection.

The ISC technique is particularly valuable for patients with neurological disorders that result in bladder emptying problems (see Chapter 11, including Case study 11.1) but it should be considered for drainage of residual urine from any cause, including mechanical outflow obstruction. ISC may sometimes be required following surgery for incontinence (e.g. colposuspension) if outflow obstruction occurs either in the short term or longer term. When a continent urinary diversion such as a 'Mitrofanoff diversion' is performed to create a catheterizable channel into the bladder from the abdominal surface, ISC is required at regular intervals to empty the bladder.

The residual urine should not be less than 100 ml to make the technique worth teaching, and should be measured by catheterization or ultrasound investigation. Provided the importance of regular bladder drainage is understood, ISC can be practised by males or females and can be taught to children as young as 4 years old with parental supervision (Eckstein 1979). An appropriate level of manual dexterity is essential and as a general rule if people can write and feed themselves they have the dexterity to catheterize (Fowler 1998). Disabilities such as blindness, lack of perineal sensation, tremor, mental disability and paraplegia do not necessarily preclude mastery of the technique (Doherty 2001). Location of the urethra may sometimes be more difficult for females but can usually be accomplished easily with practice once they have a better understanding of their own anatomy and often with the use of a mirror in the first instance. If patients are unable to carry out the procedure for themselves the technique can be taught to carers but local protocols on 'consent' must be complied with and health professionals are still responsible for ensuring that the care provided is both effective and safe.

Advantages of ISC

- There is greater opportunity for patients to reach their own potential in terms of self-care and independence.
- The risk of some common catheter-associated problems is reduced:
  —urethral trauma … risk reduced
  —urinary tract infection … risk reduced
  —encrustation … risk removed.
- The upper urinary tract is protected from reflux.
- There is reduced need for equipment and appliances.
- There is greater freedom for expression of sexuality and positive body image.

Frequency of catheterization

Catheterization should follow a regime designed to suit the needs of the individual patient but it is generally accepted that this should be no more than every 2 hours during the day and that sleep should be undisturbed as far as possible. Some patients catheterize far less frequently, and in some cases, where inefficient voiding leads to a gradual collection of a large residual, ISC may be necessary only once a day or even on alternate days. Alternatively, an extra catheterization may be appropriate prior to an activity that may limit access to a toilet for some time or prior to sexual activity. A suitable guideline (Alderman 1988), which is generally accepted, is a frequency of catheterization which maintains:

> Voided urinary volume + residual urine
> = less than 400–500 ml

Assessment of the functional capacity of the bladder either by cystometry or by the use of a frequency chart will help to establish an appropriate regime. Anticholinergic drugs may be helpful for patients experiencing symptoms of frequency, urgency or nocturia (see Chapter 8).

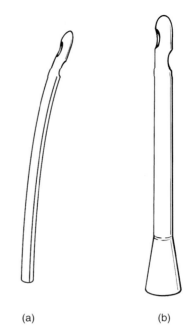

(a) (b)

Figure 9.32 ISC catheters. (a) Scott; (b) Nelaton.

Types of catheter for ISC

Catheters for ISC do not require a retention balloon and are comprised of a plastic tube with two eyes at the tip and a funnel at the other end (Fig. 9.32). The funnel helps patients with poor eyesight to identify the correct end for insertion and also allows patients to observe the colour/concentration of the urine. There are a variety of catheter types, including the standard male length and a shorter length for females. The Scott catheter (for female use only) is made of a slightly more rigid plastic to enable its tip to be inserted into the urethra with one hand. Silver-alloy-coated catheters are preferred for ISC by some female users. A number of manufacturers produce single-use ISC catheters with a hydrophilic coating to aid insertion. Some come as a conveniently packaged 'catheter set' where the catheter is already attached to a urine drainage bag inside the sterile pack. Sizes are in the range 6–20 Ch, most of which are available on prescription. The most common sizes for female use are 10–12, and 12–14 for males. However for males with a history of urethral strictures, larger sizes may be

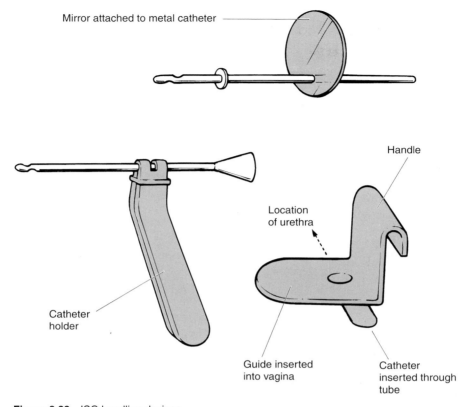

Mirror attached to metal catheter

Handle

Location of urethra

Catheter holder

Guide inserted into vagina

Catheter inserted through tube

Figure 9.33 ISC handling devices.

required (Lawrence & Macdonagh 1988). ISC catheters are usually more rigid than indwelling catheters so as to aid self-insertion; a number of handling devices are also available to assist patients with limited manual dexterity (Fig. 9.33). Patients should have the opportunity to try different catheters and to choose which best suits their needs and lifestyle.

Guidance on the ISC technique for patients, in written form and on videos, is available from a number of manufacturers of ISC catheters (see Chapter 12). Nurses should also ensure that they are competent to teach the technique. A full programme of teaching and follow-up support should be offered after careful assessment and identification of patients who are:

- willing to accept the concept of self-catheterization

- motivated and have sufficient mental ability to understand the technique
- sufficiently agile and manually dexterous to perform ISC.

Patient education

The programme of teaching and support should include:

- discussion with patients about their individual bladder dysfunction and the reasons for self-catheterization
- discussion of personal anatomy and identification of urethral orifice
- performance of ISC, including identification of the most comfortable position, followed by observation of the patient's technique

- discussion of hygiene, including importance of hand washing and cleansing of genitalia
- cleaning, storage and reuse of catheters, and subsequent disposal. Reusable catheters may be washed carefully and stored in an airtight box. They should be disposed of after 3 days. Single-use catheters should not be reused
- possible difficulties and what to do (see Common problems below)
- dietary advice and avoidance of constipation
- obtaining supplies, on prescription
- follow-up visits, usually every 1–2 weeks initially, then as required. Importance of follow-up appointments with consultant as appropriate.

Common problems with ISC

- Relatively high proportions of patients using ISC have chronic bacteriuria although the prevalence is lower than in patients with indwelling urethral catheters (Maes & Wyndaele 1988, Shekelle et al 1999). Prevention of cross-infection is therefore an important issue (Winder 1994). Patients should report any changes in urine, for example blood, sediment and smell. If signs of symptomatic urinary infection occur this should be treated and ISC technique reviewed.
- Sometimes the catheter will not go in at the first attempt. Usually if left for a while the catheter can be inserted at the next try. Dipping the catheter in water may aid lubrication. Lubricants may be used but may be associated with risks of infection (Winder 1994). If the catheter cannot be inserted the GP or clinic should be contacted.
- Sometimes the catheter will not come out. The patient should be advised to leave it for a few minutes, try to relax and 'let go' of the catheter, then cough gently and withdraw it.
- The catheter may be inserted into the vagina by mistake. If this happens it should be withdrawn, washed and reinserted.
- If urethral bleeding occurs it may be helpful to prevent the bladder filling above 450 ml. Atonic bladders can become stretched to hold very large volumes and surface capillaries

---

Box 9.3 Guidelines for intermittent self-catheterization

Helpline number, in case of problems: ....

1. Wash and dry hands immediately before catheterizing, after adjusting clothing.
2. Wash genitals if necessary:
   Females Part labia and cleanse from front to back.
   Males Cleanse tip of penis and pull back foreskin to clean around glans, insert anaesthetic gel if required.
3. Adopt a suitable position such as one of the following, checking that the other end of the catheter is towards the toilet or the container so that you won't spill any urine:
   Females Lying with the knees apart, sitting on a toilet or bidet.
   Standing with one leg raised on the toilet or bath.
   Squatting against a wall.
   Sitting in an empty bath.
   Males Standing over a toilet, sitting on a toilet or chair.
4. Gently insert the catheter, with or without a lubricating agent, or after wetting with water to reduce friction:
   Females Insert inside the urethra sloping slightly down from front to back, until urine begins to come out. If you miss and go into the vagina, remove the catheter, wash it and start again.
   Males Hold the penis at an angle of 60° to horizontal with slight tension applied to straighten urethral curves. Just before the catheter enters the bladder you may notice some resistance as the catheter passes through the external sphincter. If the catheter won't go in, stop and try again later. Don't make yourself sore. Provided you are gentle you won't do any damage; if you push the catheter in too far it will simply curl up in the bladder.
5. When urine flows, stop insertion.
6. Observe colour of urine:
   —pale yellow is desirable
   —dark yellow, strong smelling indicates a concentrated urine. Increase your fluid intake.
7. When urine drainage ceases, slowly withdraw the catheter to ensure that all the urine is drained. It may help to bend forward slightly to aid drainage, or to press on your tummy just above the pubic bone. If the catheter cannot be withdrawn easily, stop, relax by giving a loud sigh and try to imagine letting go, cough slightly and then gently withdraw.
8. Wash the catheter in running water after use, dry and store in its plastic sleeve in a clean, airtight plastic box or bag. Dispose of after 1 week.

NB Self-lubricating catheters are designed for single use only.

become enlarged. This may result in bleeding when the bladder is artificially emptied (Doherty 2001).

ISC requires a high level of patient commitment and may be abandoned, particularly during times of physical or psychological stress, or during pregnancy. With a good, clean technique, ISC may continue to be used during pregnancy although it may be necessary to stop during the later stages (Winder 1994). It is important that patients performing ISC have regular follow-ups with their consultant to ensure there is no evidence of damage to the upper urinary tract.

Children

There is a small though not insignificant number of children who require regular catheterization during the course of the school day per urethra or Mitrofanoff stoma. A care plan should be drawn up by a continence advisor/paediatric community nurse and/or school nurse, together with the child's consultant, the child and the parents. With adequate training and suitable facilities many children are able to carry out ISC themselves either on a toilet or from a wheelchair. Good interagency working between health, education and social services in partnership with the child and parents is essential for effective care. Further detail is beyond the scope of this book but key sources of further information are included in Chapter 12.

EVALUATION OF CATHETER CARE PRACTICE

Documentation

Thorough documentation is important to ensure patient safety, consistency in delivery of high quality care and effective monitoring. It also protects the nurse. If care has not been documented, a court of law may assume that it was not done. This could be used to support accusations of unprofessional conduct. The UKCC guidelines for records and record keeping (1998) should be adhered to. Use of a catheter record card is recommended. This can accompany the patient to hospital if needed. At each catheterization the following data should be recorded in the patient's notes:

- Date of insertion and reason for catheterization
- Catheter type, size including length, balloon size
- Batch number, manufacturer and date of expiry, so that in the event of a fault it can be reported to the manufacturer and/or Department of Health and easily traced
- Any difficulty on insertion or removal of previous catheter

---

Research study 9.4   Clean intermittent self-catheterization: a 12-year follow-up

This study by Wyndaele & Maes (1990) reports a follow up of 75 patients who performed clean intermittent catheterization for a mean of 7 years (maximum 12 years). Most had neuropathic bladders mainly due to spinal cord injury or myelodysplasia, and 92% were continent. In 55 patients other forms of bladder management had failed previously. Chronic or recurrent urinary tract infections were present in 42% of the patients but the fear that regular catheterizations would cause recurrent infections in patients who had sterile urine before clean intermittent self-catheterization proved to be unfounded. Chronic infection may persist if the cause of the chronicity remains, but in patients with recurrent urinary infection and urinary retention prior to commencing clean intermittent self-catheterization, the incidence of infection was found to decrease.

In most acute infections, improper clean intermittent self-catheterization or misuse could often be found. Most acute infections responded well to antibiotic therapy.

Kidney dilatation was relieved or improved in the majority of cases in which it existed prior to catheterization. The upper urinary tract remained normal in most patients who had normal kidneys before they began catheterization. However, the authors point out that hydronephrosis can be a 'silent hazard' of intermittent catheterization and close surveillance is necessary since changes in neuropathic bladder dysfunction may occur, including reduction in bladder compliance.

- Planned care protocol and expected date of review/catheter removal or next change
- Signature of the person inserting the catheter.

Clinical audit

Effective implementation of best practice requires an appropriate tool to monitor quality of care which sets clear definitions of the level of quality to be attained and uses a process that enables practitioners to examine and evaluate their own practice (see also Chapter 1). The clinical audit model described by Redfern & Norman (1996) provides a clear framework that may be usefully adapted to catheter care and comprises the following stages:

- Identification of the issue to be audited
- Setting the standard – based on the best available evidence
- Measuring the quality and checking the results against the standard set
- Identifying whether any change is needed
- Deciding strategies for change
- Implementing necessary changes
- Monitoring the effect of changes against the standard.

FUTURE DIRECTIONS

In this chapter, the use of indwelling and intermittent catheterization techniques in the management of urinary dysfunction have been discussed together with current evidence to support care planning. For all patients careful assessment remains a priority in order to identify the most appropriate form of care, together with evaluation of the efficacy of that care. Future directions in promotion of continence must include further evaluation of non-invasive techniques including behavioural therapies, but it seems likely that there will always be some patients for whom catheterization remains an important aspect of care. Research efforts continue to focus on the development of catheter materials that resist colonization by micro-organisms, thereby reducing the risk of catheter-associated infection and recurrent encrustation. In addition, a design and/or material which would allow the urethra to close while the bladder fills would prevent bladder shrinkage and allow some detrusor muscle tone to be maintained. This would offer patients a more realistic chance of possible removal of the catheter at some future date.

KEY POINTS FOR PRACTICE

- Non-invasive methods for management of urinary dysfunction should be considered as alternatives to long-term catheterization and reviewed on a regular basis.
- Nurses have a responsibility to match careful choice of catheter and drainage equipment with the individual patient, to enhance self-care and independence.

- Good hand washing practice is important before and after handling catheters and drainage equipment to reduce the risks of cross-infection.
- Aim for 'planned care' not 'crisis care'. Monitoring of 'catheter life' can often establish a pattern of recurrent catheter encrustation in susceptible patients and allow recatheterization to be planned prior to problem development.

REFERENCES

Addison R 1997 Cranberry juice; the story so far. Journal of the Association of Chartered Physiotherapists in Women's Health 80: 21–22

Addison R, Mould C 2000 Risk assessment in suprapubic catheterisation. Nursing Standard 14(36): 43–46

Alderman C 1988 DIY catheter freedom. Nursing Standard 2: 25–26

Avorn J, Monane M, Gurwitz J H et al 1994 Reduction in bacteriuria and pyuria after ingestion of cranberry juice. Journal of the American Medical Association 271(10): 751–754

Bell J 1810 Cited in Bloom et al 1994

Bibby J M, Cox A J, Hukins D W L 1995 Feasibility of preventing encrustation of urinary catheters. Cells and Materials 2: 183–195

Blacklock N J 1986 Catheters and urethral strictures. British Journal of Urology 58: 475–478

Blandy J P, Moors J 1989 Urology for nurses. Blackwell Scientific, Oxford, pp 181–195

Bloom D A, McGuire E J, Lapides J 1994 A brief history of urethral catheterisation. Journal of Urology 151: 317–325

Bodel P T, Cotran R, Kass E 1959 Cranberry juice and the anti-bacterial action of hippuric acid. Journal of Clinical Medicine 56: 881–887

British Standards Institution, BS 1695 1990 Urological catheters. Part 1. Specification for sterile single-use urethral catheters of the Nelaton and Foley types. BSI, London

Brown T R 1901 On the relation between the variety of micro-organisms and the composition of the stone in calculous pyelonephritis. Journal of the American Medical Association 36: 1395–1397

Brown M R W, Allison D G, Gilbert P 1988 Resistence of bacterial biofilms to antibiotics: a growth related effect. Journal of Antimicrobial Chemotherapy 22: 777–783

Bruce A W, Sira S S, Clark A F, Awad S A 1974 The problem of catheter encrustation. Journal of the Canadian Medical Association 111: 238–241

Bull E, Chilton C P, Gould C A, Sutton T M 1991 Single-blind, randomised, parallel study of the Bard Biocath catheter and a silicone elastomer-coated catheter. British Journal of Urology 68: 394–399

Choong S K, Hallson P, Whitehead H N, Fry C H 1999 The physicochemical basis of urinary catheter encrustation. British Journal of Urology International 83: 770–775

Classen D C, Larsen R A, Burke J P, Stevens L E 1991 Prevention of catheter-associated bacteriuria: clinical trials of methods to block three known pathways of infection. American Journal of Infection Control 19: 136–142

Cox A J, Harries J E, Hukins D W L, Kennedy A P, Sutton T M 1987 Calcium phosphate in catheter encrustation. British Journal of Urology 59: 159–163

Cox A J, Hukins D W L, Sutton T M 1988 Comparison of in vitro encrustation on silicone and hydrogel-coated latex catheters. British Journal of Urology 61: 156–161

Cox A J, Millington R S, Hukins D W L, Sutton T M 1989 Resistance of catheters coated with a modified hydrogel to encrustation during an in vitro test. Urology Research 17: 353–356

Cravens D D, Zweig S 2000 Urinary catheter management. American Family Physician 61(2): 369–376

Crow R, Mulhall A, Chapman R G 1988 Indwelling catheterisation and related nursing practice. Journal of Advanced Nursing 13: 489–495

Davies A J, Desai H N, Turton S, Dyas A 1987 Does instillation of chlorhexidine into the bladder of catheterised geriatric patients help reduce bacteriuria? Journal of Hospital Infection 9: 72–75

Department of Health 2001 Guidelines for preventing infections associated with the insertion and maintenance of short-term indwelling urethral catheters in acute care. Journal of Hospital Infection 47(Suppl.): S39–S46

Doherty W 2001 Indications for and principles of intermittent self catheterisation. In: Pope Cruikshank J, Woodward S (eds) Management of incontinence and urinary catheter care. British Journal of Nursing Monograph. Mark Allen, Dinton

Donmez T, Erol K, Baycu C, Acikalin E, Cingi M I 1990 Effects of various acidic and alkaline solutions used to dissolve urinary calculi on the rabbit urothelium. Urology International 45: 293–297

Ebner A, Madersbacher H, Schober F, Marbeger H 1985 Hydrodynamic properties of Foley catheters and its clinical relevance. In: Proceedings of the International Continence Society 15th meeting, London

Eckstein H B 1979 Intermittent catheterisation of the bladder in patients with neuropathic incontinence of urine. Zeitschrift fur Kinderchirurgie und Grenzgebiete 28(4): 408–412

Ehrenkranz N J, Alfonso B C 1991 Failure of bland soap handwash to prevent hand transfer of patient bacteria to urethral catheters. Infection Control and Hospital Epidemiology 12: 654–662

Elliott T S J, Reid L, Gopal Rao G, Rigby R C, Woodhouse K 1989 Bladder irrigation or irritation. British Journal of Urology 64: 391–394

Evans A, Feneley R 2000 A study of current nursing management of long-term suprapubic catheters. British Journal of Community Nursing 5(5): 240–245

Fader M, Pettersson L, Brooks R 1997 A multi-centre comparative evaluation of catheter valves. British Journal of Nursing 6(7): 359–367

Fowler C 1998 Bladder problems. In: Multiple sclerosis information for nurses and health professionals. Information pack. MS Research Trust, Letchworth

German K, Rowley P, Stone D et al 1997 A randomised cross-over study comparing the use of a catheter valve and a leg bag in urethrally catheterised male patients. British Journal of Urology 79: 96–98

Getliffe K A 1992 Encrustation of urinary catheters in community patients. PhD thesis, University of Surrey, Guildford

Getliffe K A 1994a The characteristics and management of patients with recurrent blockage of long-term urinary catheters. Journal of Advanced Nursing 20: 140–149

Getliffe K A 1994b The use of bladder washouts to reduce urinary catheter encrustation. British Journal of Urology 73(6): 696–700

Getliffe K A 1995 Long-term catheter use in the community. Nursing Standard 9(31): 25–27

Getliffe K A 1996 Bladder instillations and bladder washouts in the management of catheterised patients. Journal of Advanced Nursing 23: 548–554

Getliffe K A, Hughes S C, Le Claire M 2000 The dissolution of urinary catheter encrustation. British Journal of Urology International 85: 60–64

Godfrey H, Evans A 2001 Catheterisation and urinary tract infections. In: Pope Cruikshank J, Woodward S (eds) Management of continence and urinary catheter care. British Journal of Nursing Monograph, Mark Allen, Dinton

Gopal Rao G, Elliott T S J 1988 Bladder irrigation. Age and Ageing 17: 373–378

Gujral S, Kirkwood L, Hinchcliffe A 1999 Suprapubic catheterisation: suitable procedure for clinical nurse specialists in selected patients. British Journal of Urology 83(9): 954–956

Herman J R 1973 Urology: a view through the retrospectroscope. Harper & Row, Hagerstown, Maryland

Hesse A, Schreyger F, Tuschewitzki G J, Classen A, Bach D 1989 Experimental investigations on dissolution of encrustations on the surface of catheters. Urology International 44: 364–369

Holden D, Rao P N 1991 Management of staghorn stones using a combination of lithotripsy, percutaneous nephrolithotomy, and Solution R irrigation. British Journal of Urology 67: 13–17

Jacovou J W 1994 Supra-pubic catheterisation of the urinary bladder. Hospital Update March: 159–162

Kahn D H, Panariello J S, Simpson J R, Schwartz E 1996 Effect of cranberry juice on urine. Journal of the American Dietetics Association 51: 251–254

Karchmer T B, Giannetta E T, Muto C A, Strain B A, Farr B M 2000 A randomised cross-over study of silver-coated catheters in hospitalised patients. Archives of Internal Medicine 160(21): 3294–3298

Kennedy A P, Brocklehurst J C, Lye M D W 1983 Factors related to the problems of long-term catheterisation. Journal of Advanced Nursing 8: 207–212

Kennedy A P, Brocklehurst J C, Robinson J, Faragher E 1992 Assessment and use of bladder washout/instillations in patients with long-term indwelling catheters. British Journal of Urology 70: 610–615

Khardori N, Yassien M 1995 Biofilms in device related infections. Journal of Industrial Microbiology 15: 41–147

King J, Stickler D J 1991 An assessment of antiseptic bladder washout solutions using a physical model of the catheterised bladder. Journal of Hospital Infection 18: 179–180

Kohler-Ockmore J, Feneley R 1996 Long-term catheterisation of the bladder: prevalence and morbidity. British Journal of Urology 77: 347–351

Kunin C M 1987 Care of the urinary catheter. In: Detection, prevention and management of urinary tract infections, 4th edn. Lea & Febiger, Philadelphia

Kunin C M, Chin Q F, Chambers S 1987a Indwelling catheters in the elderly. Relation of catheter life to formation of encrustations in patients with and without blocked catheters. American Journal of Medicine 82: 405–411

Kunin C M, Chin Q F, Chambers S 1987b Formation of encrustations on indwelling urinary catheters in the elderly: a comparison of different types of catheter materials in 'blockers' and 'non-blockers'. Journal of Urology 138: 899–902

Lapides J, Ananias C D, Silber S J, Lowe B S 1972 Clean intermittent self-catheterisation in the treatment of urinary tract disease. Journal of Urology 107: 458–461

Lapides J, Ananias C D, Lowe B S, Kalis, M D 1974 Follow-up on unsterile intermittent self-catheterisation. Journal of Urology 111: 184–187

Lawrence W, Macdonagh R 1988 The treatment of urethra stricture disease by internal urethrotomy followed by intermittent low friction self catheterisation. Journal of the Royal Society of Medicine 81: 136–139

Lawrence W, McQuilkin P H, Mann D 1989 Suprapubic catheterisation. British Journal of Urology 63(4): 443

Liedberg H, Lundeberg T 1990 Silver alloy-coated catheters reduce catheter-associated bacteriuria. British Journal of Urology 65: 379–381

Mackintosh I P, Watson B W, O'Grady F 1975 Theory of hydrokinetic clearance of bacteria from the urinary bladder. Investigative Urology 12: 473–478

Maes D, Wyndaele J 1988 Long-term experience with intermittent self-catheterisation. Neurourology and Urodynamics 73: 273–274

Marrie T, Costerton J W 1983 A scanning electron microscopic study of urine droppers and urine collecting systems. Archives of Internal Medicine 142: 1135–1141

Merritt K, Chang C C 1991 Factors influencing bacterial adherence to biomaterials. Journal of Biomaterial Applications 5: 185–203

Morris N S, Stickler D J, Winters C 1997 Which catheters resist encrustation by *Proteus mirabilis* biofilms? British Journal of Urology 80: 58–83

Morris N S, Stickler D J, McLean R J 1999 The development of bacterial biofilms on indwelling urethral catheters. World Journal of Urology 17(6): 345–350

Mulhall A B, Chapman R G, Crow R A 1988 Bacteriuria during indwelling urethral catheterisation. Journal of Hospital Infection 11: 253–262

Mulhall A B, King S, Lee K, Wiggington E 1993 Maintenance of closed urinary drainage systems: are practitioners more aware of the dangers? Journal of Clinical Nursing 2: 135–140

Murphy F J, Zelman S, Mau W 1965 Ascorbic acid as a urinary acidifying agent, 2: its adjunctive role in chronic urinary tract infections. Journal of Urology 94: 300–305

Murphy L J T 1972 History of urology. C C Thomas Springfield, Illinois

Nacey J N, Delahunt B 1991 Toxicity of first and second generation hydrogel-coated latex urinary catheters. British Journal of Urology 67: 314–316

Nacey J N, Horsfall D J, Delahunt B, Marshall V R 1986 The assessment of urinary catheter toxicity using cell cultures: validation by comparison with an animal model. Journal of Urology 136: 706–709

Nahata M C, Shrimp L, Lampman L, McLeod D C 1977 Effect of ascorbic acid on urine pH in man. American Journal of Hospital Pharmacology 34: 1234–1237

Norberg A, Norberg B, Lundbeck K, Parkhede U 1980 Urinary pH and the indwelling catheter. Uppsala Journal of Medical Science 85: 143–150

Norberg B, Norberg A, Parkhede U 1983 The spontaneous variation in catheter life in long stay geriatric patients with indwelling catheters. Gerontology 29: 332–335

Ofek I, Coldhar J, Zafriri D et al 1991 Anti-*Escherichia coli* adhesin activity of cranberry and blueberry juices. Letter. New England Journal of Medicine 324(22): 1599

Ohkawa M, Sugata T, Sawaki M et al 1990 Bacterial and crystal adherence to the surfaces of indwelling urethral catheters. Journal of Urology 143: 717–721

Oosterlink W, Verbeek R, Cuvelier C, Vergauwe D, Rappe B 1991 Toxicity to the urothelium of calcium chelating agents for chemolysis. Journal of Urology 146: 1395–1397

Parsons C L, Greenspan C, Mulholland S G 1975 The primary antibacterial defence mechanism of the bladder. Investigative Urology 13: 72–76

Peate I 1997 Patient management following suprapubic catheterisation. British Journal of Nursing 6(10): 555–562

Platt R, Polk B F, Murdock B, Rossner B 1982 Mortality associated with nosocomial urinary-tract infection. New Engand Journal of Medicine 307: 637–642

Platt R, Polk B F, Murdock B, Rosner B 1983 Reduction of mortality associated with nosocomial urinary tract infection. Lancet 1: 893–897

Pomfret I 1995 Bladder irrigation. Journal of Community Nursing December: 24–29

Ramsey J W A, Garnham A J, Mulhall A B et al 1989 Biofilms, bacteria and bladder catheters. A clinical study. British Journal of Urology 64: 395–398

Reckler J, Rodman J S, Jacobs D et al 1986 Urothelial injury to the rabbit bladder from various alkaline and acidic solutions used to dissolve kidney stones. Journal of Urology 136: 181–183

Redfern S, Norman I 1996 Clinical audit, related cycles and types of health care quality: a preliminary model. International Journal of Quality in Health Care 8(4): 331–340

Reid G, Bruce A W, Cooke R L, Llano M 1990 Effect on urogenital flora of antibiotic therapy for urinary tract infection. Scandinavian Journal of Infectious Disease 22: 43–47

Roberts J A, Kaack M B, Fussel E N 1993 Adherence to urethral catheters by bacteria causing nosocomial infections. Urology 41(4): 338–342

Robertson M H, Norton M S 1990 Effect of 1% mandelic acid as a bladder irrigation fluid in patients with indwelling catheters. British Journal of Clinical Practice 44: 142–144

Robinson J 2000 Urethral catheter selection. Nursing Standard 15(25): 39–42

Rogers J 1991 Pass the cranberry juice. Nursing Times 87: 36–37

Scally G, Donaldson L 1998 Clinical governance and the drive for quality improvement in the new NHS in England. British Medical Journal 317(7150): 61–65

Schmidt R D, Sobata A E 1988 An examination of the anti-adherence activity of cranberry juice on urinary and non-urinary bacterial isolates. Microbias 55: 173–181

Seo K, Nakano H, Usui T, Miyake Y, Suginaka H 1990 Removal of adherent bacteria from catheter materials in vitro by N-acylated amino acids. Hiroshima Journal of Medical Science 39: 139–143

Shah J, Shah N 1998 Percutaneous suprapubic catheterisation. Urology News 2(5): 11–12

Shekelle O G, Morton S C, Clark K A, Pathak M, Vickrey B G 1999 Systematic review of risk factors for urinary tract infection in adults with spinal cord dysfunction. Journal of Spinal Cord Medicine 22(4): 258–272

Sheriff M K M, Foley S, McFarlane J, Nauth-Misir R, Craggs M 1998 Long-term supra-pubic catheterisation: clinical outcome and satisfaction survey. Spinal Cord 36(3): 171–176

Sobata A E 1984 Inhibition of bacterial adherence by cranberry juice; potential use for the treatment of urinary tract infections. Journal of Urology 131: 1013–1016

Stamm W E 1991 Catheter-associated urinary tract infections: epidemiology, pathogenesis and prevention. American Journal of Medicine 91(Suppl. 3B): 65–71

Stickler D J, Chawla J 1987 The role of antiseptics in the management of patients with long-term indwelling bladder catheters. Journal of Hospital Infection 10: 219–228

Stickler D J, Hewitt P 1991 Activity of antiseptics against biofilms of mixed bacterial species growing on silicone surfaces. European Journal of Microbiology and Infectious Diseases 10: 416–421

Stickler D J, Hughes G 1999 Ability of *Proteus mirabilis* to swarm over urethral catheters. European Journal of Clinical Microbiology and Infectious Diseases 18(3): 206–208

Stickler D J, Zimakoff J 1994 Complications of urinary tract infections associated with devices used for long term catheter management. Journal of Hospital Infection 20: 177–194

Stickler D J, Clayton C L, Chawla J C 1987 The resistance of urinary tract pathogens to chlorhexidine bladder washouts. Journal of Hospital Infection 10: 28–39

Stickler D J, Dolman J, Rolfe S, Chawla J 1989 Activity of antiseptics against *Escherichia coli* growing as biofilms on silicone surfaces. European Journal of Clinical Microbiology and Infectious Diseases 8: 974–978

Talja M, Andersson L C, Ruutu M, Alfthan O 1985 Toxicity testing of urinary catheters. British Journal of Urology 57: 579–584

Talja M, Korpela A, Jarvi K 1990 Comparison of urethral reaction to full silicone, hydrogel-coated and siliconised latex catheters. British Journal of Urology 66: 652–657

Tambyah P, Halvorson K, Maki D 1999 A prospective study of pathogenesis of catheter-associated urinary tract infections. Mayo Clinic Proceedings 74: 131–136

Thomas S 1990 Wound cleansing agents. In: Wound management and dressings. The Pharmaceutical Press, London

Travis L B, Dodge W F, Mintz A A, Assemi M 1965 Urinary acidification with ascorbic acid. Journal of Paediatrics 67: 1176–1178

UKCC 1992 The scope of professional practice. UKCC, London

UKCC 1998 Records and record keeping. UKCC, London

Urivetzky M, Kessaris D, Smith A D 1992 Ascorbic acid overdosing: a risk factor for calcium oxalate nephrolithiasis. Journal of Urology 147: 1215–1218

Whitfield H N, Holmes S A V 1991 Lipids – a new promoter of encrustation and urinary crystallization? Journal of Urology 145(4) (Suppl. 330A): 471. AUA 86th Annual Meeting, June 2–6

Wickham J E A, Buck A C (eds) 1990 Renal tract stone: metabolic basis and clinical practice. Churchill Livingstone, London

Wilson J 1997 Control and prevention of infection in catheter care. Nurse Prescriber/Community Nurse 3(5): 39–40

Winder A 1994 Intermittent self-catheterisation. In: Roe B H (ed) The promotion and management of continence. Prentice Hall, Hemel Hempstead

Woodward S 1997 Complications of allergies to latex urinary catheters. British Journal of Nursing 6(14): 786–792

Wyndaele J J, Maes D 1990 Clean intermittent self-catheterisation: a 12 year followup. Journal of Urology 143: 906–908

10

Continence training in intellectual disability[1]

Paul Smith
Linda Smith

There is a story about Martin Luther seeing, what we would now regard as, a multiply handicapped child who 'ate, drooled and defaecated.' At a time when such children were regarded as monsters, Luther's remedy was that the child should be taken to the river and drowned.

INTRODUCTION

The prognosis for incontinence in people with learning disabilities has, historically, been rather dismal. Incontinence was formerly a major reason for admission to institutional care (McCoull 1971). Those whose memories of services go back a few decades will remember the pervasive smell of urine and faeces on long-stay wards for people with severe and profound learning disabilities. Incontinence has commonly been regarded as part and parcel of severe intellectual impairment. It is really only since the 1970s that remediation has been considered possible, but as we shall see, incontinence is not intractable.

---

[1] The term 'learning disability', formerly known in the UK as 'mental handicap', refers to people with a global developmental delay in intellectual and social functioning. The term used by the World Health Organization, the USA and the rest of the English-speaking world is 'mental retardation'. In the USA, the term 'learning disability' does not refer to global developmental delay, but is used more specifically to refer to disorders such as hyperactivity and attention deficit disorder, dyslexia and autism. In this chapter, the terms 'learning disability' and 'intellectual disability' are used interchangeably to refer to a global developmental delay.

It is generally accepted that self-help and independence skills-training in people with intellectual disabilities should take a developmental approach. Therefore, before turning to intervention, we shall review the state of knowledge regarding the 'normal' development of continence and the implications of this for the field of learning disability.

NORMAL DEVELOPMENTAL SEQUENCE OF BOWEL AND BLADDER CONTROL

Continence is generally acquired during the second to third year of life, with modesty training occurring after the acquisition of daytime control. Thus, first we teach children to be proud of their toileting prowess then, shortly after, we teach them to keep quiet about it. The feelings of disgust associated with urine and faeces are not, however, universal (Smith & Smith 1987). For example, while adults in all societies regard faeces as offensive, this is not universally true of urine. Furthermore, although in the early years children in Western cultures regard the smell of urine and faeces as pleasant, by school age they have learned to regard these as unpleasant. These are important points, as cultural taboos surrounding toileting affect the attitudes and beliefs of both professional and family carers.

Age of acquisition and sequence of development of bowel and bladder control have been studied in Western children over a number of decades by Largo & Stutzle (1977a,b) and Largo et al (1996). Largo & Stutzle (1977a,b), for example, found that 78% of 3-year-olds had bladder control and 97% had bowel control. A later study (Largo et al 1996) showed a very similar pattern in terms of age of achievement of bladder and bowel control.

The commonly accepted sequence for the acquisition of bowel and bladder control is as follows:

1. bowel control at night
2. bowel control by day
3. bladder control by day
4. bladder control at night.

Some children, however, have a different pattern: Largo & Stutzle (1977a,b), for example, found

that the sequence differed in 8% of the children studied. Brazelton (1962), reporting on over 1000 children, found that 12.3% acquired bowel control first, 8.2% acquired bladder control first, while the majority achieved bowel and bladder control simultaneously. This means that, when considering continence training programmes for those with learning disabilities, there is not one developmental sequence that must be followed rigidly.

Components of bowel and bladder control

A developmental model of acquisition of daytime bladder control, rooted in the views of Gesell & Armatruda (1941) and discussed further by Bettison (1978) and Smith & Smith (1987), may be summarized thus:

- *Infancy:* reflex micturition
- *1–2 years:* some awareness of a full bladder and brief holding of urine
- *3 years:* holding urine for prolonged periods thus increasing bladder capacity
- *3–4 years:* able to initiate urine stream reliably with full bladder when seated on the toilet
- *6 years:* able to commence urine stream without full bladder.

This widely accepted model should not be taken too seriously, however, as there is little hard evidence to support it. By contrast, there is evidence (Blackwell 1991, Duche 1973, Mattson & Lindstrom 1996, Smith & Wong 1981, Yeung et al 1995) to support the following:

- that passing urine in the absence of a full bladder is an early- rather than a late-acquired component
- that complete bladder emptying may be more difficult to acquire than is thought
- that there are wide variations in voiding patterns and in the pattern of acquisition of continence components.

Models such as these need to be more fully developed and researched before models of physiological or biochemical processes can be formulated. If continence training or research is based on false beliefs, training approaches will not be soundly based and basic research on the development of continence may ask the wrong questions.

In the field of learning disability, two issues require consideration. Firstly, how does the acquisition of bowel and bladder control in children with a learning disability differ from that of normal children? In one study, which may be relevant to this question, 140 preterm and 349 full-term children were followed up by Largo et al (1999). Although toilet training started earlier for the preterm children, there was little difference between the two groups in the age at which bladder and bowel control were acquired.

Secondly, does bladder function remain normal for the 'untrained' bladder, which is after all an essentially abnormal condition, given that the bladder did not evolve to function in this uninhibited way over many years? In a study which bears on this question, Vande Walle et al (1995) discuss the issue of 'bladder dysfunction in the commercial television child in a commercial television family in the commercial television society'. Although no data are presented, the authors express the opinion that they have seen an increase in children with bladder dysfunction from the 'TV generation' and that this is because these children are not emptying their bladders completely or regularly. If this is so, this finding may help explain why people with learning disabilities, chronic incontinence and incomplete bladder emptying present such a challenge in terms of continence training.

The implications of developmental sequences for training strategies in learning disabilities are summarized in Box 10.1.

Learning or maturation

A basic question concerns whether the acquisition of continence is learned or whether it is a maturational process. A maturational process would imply that control is innate and unfolds naturally, independent of environmental factors. If this were the case, many incontinent people with a profound learning disability would never mature sufficiently to acquire bladder and bowel control.

> **Box 10.1** Implications of developmental sequences for training strategies in learning disabilities
>
> - If bowel control always preceded bladder control in normal children, continence training should initially focus on this. Given that this is not the case, it is recommended that for practical reasons intervention should focus initially on bladder training where double incontinence is present. This is because emptying the bowel is a less frequent event than emptying the bladder, leading to more training 'opportunities' for bladder than for bowel, even more so if increased fluids are used.
> - Although passing a small amount of urine in the absence of a full bladder is believed to be a late-acquired component, neither the evidence nor the experience of training support this belief.
> - One question often raised concerns whether males with learning disabilities should be taught to pass urine standing or sitting. It is useful to note that Seim (1989), in a study of 266 children aged 24–29 months, records that almost 70% of boys learn to pass urine sitting rather than standing. Although many carers hesitate to train males with learning disabilities to pass urine sitting, this is not only normal, it is also easier.

Training effects

Evidence on training effects includes studies of toilet training practices in different cultures. In some cultures such as hunter–gatherers in arctic climates where there is a survival premium attached to being dry, toilet training starts earlier. Conversely, in hunter–gatherer societies in warmer climates, there may be little or no emphasis on toilet training, yet the children nevertheless achieve control. As well as cultural differences, national and social class differences have been reported in the age at which toilet training begins and is achieved within Western Europe.

The case for toilet 'training' is strengthened by studies discussed later in this chapter which show that behavioural training methods are effective for incontinent children and adults with learning disabilities. Studies of behavioural training approaches have also shown much better outcomes than other methods of continence training in normal children, as well as dramatically accelerated training in infants only a few months of age (Butler 1976, Madsen et al 1969, Smeets et al 1985).

Research study 10.1

Madsen et al's (1969) controlled comparison of different methods of toilet training in normal children was conducted over a 1-week baseline period followed by 4 weeks of training. There were five groups:

1. A maturational control group, where parents were instructed to carry out no training whatsoever.
2. A parents' own control group, where parents were asked to carry out toilet training using whatever procedures they would have used normally.
3. A reinforcement schedule group, where parents were instructed in the use of contingent reinforcement and other behavioural training strategies.
4. A pants alarm group, where parents were provided with miniature urine alarms to signal when a wetting

accident occurred. Parents took their children to the toilet when the alarm sounded, but otherwise used their usual training methods.
5. A pants alarm plus behavioural methods group, where the methods used in groups 3 and 4 were combined.

Analysis of frequency of continent and incontinent passing of urine showed that results for the two behavioural training groups (3 and 5) were significantly better than those of the other three. Also, although outcome was better for older children, behavioural training was more effective than other methods across all age levels. This latter result would not be predicted by maturational theory.

In the study by Smeets et al (1985), three babies aged between 3 and 6½ months, were successfully trained to reach for the potty in response to bladder and bowel sensations, using an intensive, structured behavioural training approach over 4–5 months. Although these babies could not postpone elimination for longer than a few minutes, Smeets et al demonstrated that elimination is not a simple, reflex action at this stage; that babies of only a few months old can be trained to be clean and dry; and that preverbal babies can be taught to communicate bowel and bladder needs.

Maturation effects

So far, a number of studies support the idea that environmental effects are important and that bowel and bladder control can be trained. Evidence to support the role of maturation in the acquisition of continence includes the tendency towards spontaneous improvement with age. In a pioneering, but little known, study of twins (McGraw 1940), one of a pair of identical twins was placed hourly on the potty from the early weeks of life, whereas the second twin was not. Hourly toileting produced a typical learning curve for the first twin which seemed to support a toilet 'training' effect. When a high success rate was achieved around 20 months, the untrained twin was then introduced to the potty. By contrast, no learning curve appeared here, yet the outcome

in terms of continence was indistinguishable (Fig. 10.1).

Largo et al (1996), studying a recent major change in child care, i.e. the introduction of disposable nappies and the consequent more relaxed attitude to training, compared over 300 children born in the 1950s to over 300 born in the 1970s and 1980s. This well-designed study found differences between the two generations in terms of age at onset of toilet training, intensity of prompting and the degree of the child's involvement in 'training'. Despite these, there was no difference in the age at which control was acquired.

Finally, in the case of nocturnal continence, strong evidence has recently emerged on the importance of genetic markers (Eiberg et al 1995) and biological factors such as diurnal variation in vasopressin levels (Rittig 1996) in nocturnal enuresis.

KEY POINT: INNATE OR LEARNED BLADDER CONTROL

Is continence 'trained' or does it mature spontaneously? While bladder control is probably largely innate and would eventually be acquired spontaneously, the considerable variation in the age at which continence is achieved suggests that some aspects of continence are malleable and open to environmental manipulation.

Readiness for training

Just as there is little evidence to support the widely accepted developmental sequence for

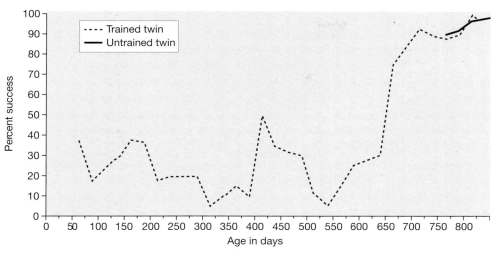

Figure 10.1 Toilet training in infant twins (after McGraw 1940).

continence, so there is no evidence to support popular criteria for determining readiness for training. Michel (1999), for example, has suggested the following guidelines for readiness:

- The ability to ambulate to the potty.
- Stability while sitting on the potty.
- Ability to remain dry for several hours.
- Receptive language skills that allow the child to follow one and two step commands.
- Expressive language skills that allow the child to communicate the need to use the potty with words or reproducible gestures.
- The desire to please based on a positive relationship with caregivers.
- The desire on the child's part for independence and control of bladder and bowel function.

According to these criteria, toilet training would be appropriate for a child or adult with a learning disability who can walk, can understand simple instructions and feed with a spoon or drink from a cup without help.

On the one hand, it is difficult to argue against such plausible guidelines. Certainly, in terms of good practice, an incontinent child or adult with a learning disability who meets the above criteria and has no evidence of bladder or bowel dysfunction should be considered for continence training. On the other hand, no studies have shown that

children who meet these criteria are easier to train than those who do not. People with a profound intellectual disability or additional problems such as autism, cerebral palsy, challenging behaviours or specific language deficits may never meet these criteria, yet many studies have shown that they can be successfully toilet trained.

PREVALENCE OF CONTINENCE PROBLEMS
Children in the general population

There is an impression that the prevalence of continence problems in humans is high compared to other mammals and compared to problems of other basic independence skills. For example, Largo & Stutzle (1977a,b) found that 5% of 5-year-olds and 1% of 10–12-year-olds in the general population were still soiled; Weir (1982), in a study of over 700 3-year-olds in the general population, found that 23% of boys and 12% of girls were still regularly wet by day, of whom the majority were also still wet at night; and in a study of over 2000 children in the general population, Bower et al (1996) found regular nocturnal enuresis in 10% of 5-year-olds and 1.4% of 11-year-olds and regular daytime incontinence in 2.1% of 5-year-olds to 0.6% of 12-year-olds.

Table 10.1 Diurnal urinary incontinence in children and adults

Survey	Sample	Children (%)	Adults[a] (%)
Thomas 1986[b]	General population	18.5	9.5
Smith 1979b	Mild intellectual disability	–	6
Von Wendt et al 1990	Mild intellectual disability	16.7	5.6
DHSS 1972	Mild intellectual disability	25	5

[a] Von Wendt's adults refer to 20-year-olds; Thomas' 15–24-year-olds have been selected as the category closest to that of von Wendt; Smith's figures relate to a 'mainly' adult population – separate figures for children or subdivided adult ages are not provided.
[b] Included for comparison purposes.

Table 10.2 Prevalence of diurnal urinary incontinence by level of intellectual disability (i)

Ability level	% Incontinent by day
Borderline	6
Mild	6
Moderate	11
Severe	18
Profound	58

After Smith (1979b).

Table 10.3 Prevalence of diurnal urinary incontinence by level of intellectual disability (ii)

Ability level	Day wetting at 7 years (%)	Day wetting at 20 years (%)
Mild	16.7	5.6
Moderate	39.4	14.7
Severe	38.1	23.8
Profound	100	64.3

Reproduced with permission of Mac Keith Press from von Wendt et al (1990).

People with learning disability

A number of surveys have looked at the prevalence of incontinence in people with a learning disability (e.g. DHSS 1972, Smith 1979b, Smith et al 1975, von Wendt et al 1990) (Table 10.1).

These surveys support the view that the prevalence of diurnal urinary incontinence in children and adults with a mild learning disability is within the range reported for the general population. Smith (1979b) and von Wendt et al (1990) have provided prevalence of diurnal urinary incontinence by level of intellectual disability (Tables 10.2 and 10.3 respectively).

These studies, whose findings are remarkably consistent, show that diurnal urinary incontinence increases with degree of learning disability and that urinary incontinence is much higher in people with a profound learning disability. Even so, around 40% of those with the most profound intellectual disability will acquire diurnal bladder control by adulthood.

KEY POINTS: DIURNAL URINARY INCONTINENCE IN PEOPLE WITH LEARNING DISABILITIES

- Studies of the prevalence of diurnal urinary incontinence in the field of intellectual disability are few in number.
- The degree to which dependence can be placed on their findings is often unclear and it can be difficult to extract information from some reports.
- Despite these criticisms, the evidence supports the view that: prevalence of diurnal urinary incontinence in mild intellectual disability is within the range reported for the general population; prevalence increases with increasing degree of learning disability; prevalence of diurnal urinary incontinence is considerably greater in people with a profound intellectual disability, although 40% will nevertheless have acquired daytime bladder control by adulthood.

ENCOPRESIS
Prevalence of constipation

Although constipation is believed to be important in around 80% of cases of encopresis in the

Table 10.4 Daytime soiling

	No.	Soiling			
		Daily	Frequently	Sometimes	Never
Smith et al 1975	767	50 (6.5%)	58 (7.5%)	67 (8.7%)	592 (77.3%)
Smith 1979b	1330	142 (10.6%)	115 (8.6%)	189 (14.2%)	884 (66.6%)

Table 10.5 Intellectual disability and soiling

Intellectual disability level	No.	Encopresis at age 7	Encopresis at age 20
Mild	36	1 (2.8%)	0 (0%)
Moderate	34	11 (32.4%)	6 (17.6%)
Severe	21	8 (38.1%)	6 (28.6%)
Profound	14	12 (85.7%)	8 (57.1%)

Table 10.6 Nocturnal enuresis

Ability level	Nocturnal enuresis at age 7		Nocturnal enuresis at age 20	
	No.	%	No.	%
Mild	4	11.1	0	0
Moderate	15	44.1	6	17.6
Severe	7	33.3	4	19.1
Profound	14	100	11	78.6

Reproduced with permission of Mac Keith Press from von Wendt et al (1990).

general population (Doleys et al 1981), little evidence is available on the prevalence of constipation in the field of intellectual disability. There is a widespread belief that chronic constipation and faecal impaction are major problems for high-dependency populations in general (Agnarsson et al 1993, Kobak et al 1962, Thomas et al 1984, von Wendt et al 1990), but the limited available evidence does not support a broad conclusion in people with intellectual disabilities.

Prevalence of encopresis

Smith (1979b) and Smith et al (1975) have provided figures for daytime soiling in a population of institutionalized (mainly) adults with intellectual disabilities (Table 10.4).

Von Wendt et al's (1990) survey of community-living 20 year olds supports the view that: prevalence of encopresis in those with a mild learning disability is within the range reported for the general population; prevalence increases with degree of learning disability; and prevalence is much higher in those with a profound learning disability. Nevertheless, approximately half will have acquired bowel control by adulthood (Table 10.5).

KEY POINTS: PREVALENCE OF ENCOPRESIS

Studies of the prevalence of encopresis in learning disability show that:

- There is less information on the prevalence of faecal incontinence than of urinary incontinence in the field of intellectual disability. Surveys of urinary incontinence often ignore the problem of faecal incontinence or give it less attention.
- The evidence supports the view that the prevalence of faecal incontinence in mild intellectual disability is within the range reported for the general population; prevalence increases with increasing degree of learning disability; the prevalence of encopresis is substantially increased in people with a profound intellectual disability, although 50% will nevertheless have acquired bowel control by adulthood.

NOCTURNAL ENURESIS

Von Wendt et al (1990) report the prevalence of nocturnal enuresis at the ages of 7 and 20 as detailed in Table 10.6.

Again, it is noteworthy that a prevalence of 11.1% at age 7 and 0% at age 20 for nocturnal enuresis in those with mild intellectual disability is within the range reported for the general population.

Finally, although Parker (1984) has expressed the belief that recent years have seen a quiet revolution in the approach taken to incontinence in this field, there is a strong impression that urinary and faecal incontinence continue to present a major problem in the field of intellectual disability. Recent studies of the prevalence of incontinence in community-dwelling samples, though restricted in terms of quantity and quality, offer little evidence of a reduction in incontinence, particularly among those with the most severe degrees of intellectual disability.

AETIOLOGICAL FACTORS

There has been little study of the factors that contribute to the failure to acquire continence, or the breakdown of continence, in the field of learning disability. Why this is so is unclear, but evidence from other high-dependency fields suggests that incontinence in such fields is often perceived as 'normal' and untreatable.

Groves (1982) has expressed the view that, where an incontinent person has an intellectual disability, this is assumed to be *the* causal factor in incontinence. Adults with severe or profound intellectual disabilities are thus assumed to have failed to reach the necessary level of development for bowel and bladder control. People with additional physical disabilities may be assumed to have nervous system lesions incompatible with the acquisition of continence.

Studies of children in the general population have indeed shown that incontinence is often associated with general developmental delay, specific learning and cognitive deficits, speech and language deficits, poor neuromuscular coordination and general neurological immaturity (Gabel 1981, Madge et al 1993, Stern et al 1988). However, most people with neurological abnormalities or immaturity, developmental delay or cognitive deficits are not incontinent and most children with nocturnal enuresis and encopresis do not have general developmental delay or specific cognitive deficits, but are within the average range of intelligence and neurologically intact (Bellman 1966, Fritz & Armbrust 1982).

Intellectual disability as such cannot be the sole cause of incontinence because even where a profound intellectual disability is present, 40–50% of adults acquire bowel and bladder control (DHSS 1972, Smith 1979b, von Wendt et al 1990). On the other hand, increasing degree of intellectual disability must be a factor because prevalence increases with increasing degree of intellectual disability (Dalrymple & Ruble 1992, Lohmann et al 1967, Smith 1979b, von Wendt et al 1990) and intensive continence training takes longer in people with profound intellectual disabilities (Smith & Smith 1977).

As well as the importance of increasing degree of intellectual disability, a number of studies suggest that hyperactivity and challenging behaviours make the acquisition of control harder (Dalrymple & Ruble 1992, Jenkins & Stable 1971, Lohmann et al 1967, Spencer et al 1968). Challenging behaviours include anxiety-related behaviours such as toilet-related fears and poor reactions to environmental change (Dalrymple & Ruble 1992), as well as non-compliance and lack of sociability (Spencer et al 1968). Thus a number of these factors may operate together to reduce the likelihood of continence acquisition.

If it is assumed that intellectual disability causes incontinence, medical causes of incontinence can be overlooked in people with intellectual disabilities. There can be a reluctance to conduct intrusive investigations for diagnostic and treatment purposes in people with severe and profound intellectual disabilities. Reasons for this might include practical, legal and ethical problems associated with conducting invasive examinations of non-consenting adults (Hellstrom et al 1990).

This discourages the study of the acquisition and breakdown of continence processes in people with intellectual disabilities and means that they are less likely to be diagnosed (Groves 1982).

```
KEY POINTS: INTELLECTUAL DISABILITY AND
INCONTINENCE

• Vulnerability to incontinence in the field of intellectual
  disability might be increased by a number of factors,
  of which increasing degree of intellectual disability is
  likely to be one.
• Although it is not yet clear which other factors might
  hinder acquisition of bowel and bladder control in this
  field, other factors might include hyperactivity,
  resulting in failure to sit on the toilet for long enough;
  attention deficit disorder, resulting in failure to respond
  to cues of impending evacuation; lack of social
  responsiveness, resulting in reduced awareness of the
  social consequences of incontinence; and severely
  challenging behaviours, including negativity, non-
  compliance and anxiety-mediated behaviours such as
  toilet-related fears.
• Other barriers to treatment might include lack of toilet
  training opportunities due to negative carer beliefs; the
  availability of free, disposable incontinence pads and
  other aids/appliances for the easier management of
  incontinence; disability benefits disincentives; and
  negative attitudes to investigation and treatment in
  general hospital settings.
```

INTERVENTION
Strategies for different problems

Although there is as yet no consensus on classification or typology, the following distinctions are clinically useful:

- Double or single incontinence due to lack of toileting skills.
- Encopresis due to constipation and retention.
- Toileting problems associated with obsessional behaviours, such as elimination under highly specific conditions, e.g. exclusively into a nappy/pad.
- Repeated accidents in inappropriate locations, such as in corners or against doors, despite the ability to use the toilet.
- Fear or avoidance of toilets other than one specific toilet, such as that at home.
- Wetting accidents shortly after coming off the toilet.

- Messy toileting.
- Faecal smearing.

Baseline assessment of continence skills

The rating scale provided by Smith & Smith (1987) offers a quick and easy way to rate some of the components of continence in a person with learning disabilities (Fig. 10.2). This ad-hoc rating scale is intended to give an initial overall picture of continence skills for the purpose of planning continence training programmes.

Bladder training

By the late 1960s, the key features of behavioural continence training programmes in the field of intellectual disability had emerged (Baumeister & Klosowski 1965, Dayan 1964, Hundziak et al 1965, Kimbrell et al 1967, Miron 1966, Yoder 1966). Although previous programmes had used behavioural techniques, Azrin & Foxx combined a number of these in a package (Box 10.2).

Azrin & Foxx's (1971) study of nine institutionalized adults with profound learning disabilities, whose frequency of wetting was reduced by 90% over an average of 4 days despite being regarded at that time as incapable of learning, is outstanding.

Foxx & Azrin's work stimulated many attempts at replication (Barton 1975, Bettison et al 1976, Butler 1976, Didden et al 2001, Dixon & Smith

```
Box 10.2   Main features of Azrin & Foxx's intensive
daytime continence training

• One-to-one training close to the toilet for a prolonged
  period
• Increased fluid intake to increase the frequency of
  urination
• The use of pants and bowl alarms enabling
  consistent and immediate detection of inappropriate
  and appropriate urination
• Rewards for continent passing urine and
  remaining dry
• Punishment for wetting/soiling accidents
• Prompts to toilet at half-hourly intervals
• Fading of prompts to teach independent toileting
• Shaping of dressing skills
• Emphasizing procedures to maintain progress after
  completion of training
```

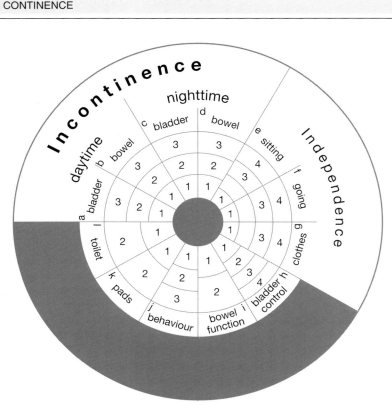

Figure 10.2 Continence skills rating chart. Reproduced from Smith & Smith (1987).

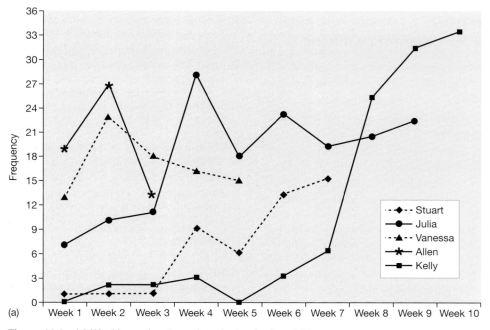

Figure 10.3 (a) Weekly continent passing of urine for five children.

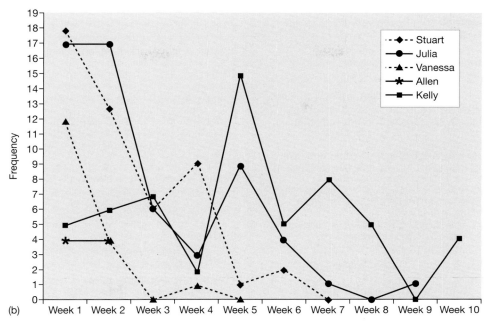

Figure 10.3 (b) Weekly bladder accidents for five children.

1976, Pfadt & Sternlicht 1980, Pfadt & Sullivan 1981, Sadler & Merkert 1977, Singh 1976, Smith 1979b, Smith et al 1975, Trott 1977). For example, Williams & Sloop (1978) reported a similar success rate in six institutional residents between 13 and 23 years old, functioning below a developmental level of 1 year, using Azrin & Foxx's package for only 3 hours per day.

Buchan et al (1989) studied the feasibility of structured behavioural continence training with 53 community-living adults and children with various degrees of learning disabilities, the majority of whom were living at home. Although support to parents was described as intensive, it seems that the parents carried out the training themselves so that Azrin & Foxx's techniques, including urine alarms, were used only 'where possible and appropriate'. Because success was much lower than that reported in any institutional study, the authors concluded that this 'package' was not feasible in the community.

By contrast, Smith & Bainbridge (1991) successfully applied a modified Azrin & Foxx approach to daytime continence training in the case of an 11-year-old boy with a profound learning disability

KEY POINTS: DAYTIME CONTINENCE TRAINING

- Replications of Azrin & Foxx's toilet training approach indicate that the package is an effective one.
- However, training consistently takes longer than that originally reported; there are reports of failure; progress in training is not as smooth as implied; where data are presented for the training period, there is considerable individual variation; ethical issues surrounding the use and role of punishment techniques require serious consideration.

and severe behaviour problems living at home. Punishment techniques were not used and prompts to toilet and dry pants checks were less frequent. Training was conducted in the home by a trainer 5 days per week from 9.00 am to 4.00 pm, the parent carrying out a minimum of pants checks and prompts to toilet during the evenings and at weekends. Results of this and other community toilet training programmes implemented by the present authors demonstrate that intensive continence training is feasible in ordinary family homes. An example is illustrated in Figure 10.3a and 10.3b for five children with severe learning

---

Research study 10.2

The work of Pfadt (Pfadt & Sternlicht 1981, Pfadt & Sullivan 1981), although difficult to access, represents the largest reported continence training programme.

- Sixty three clients with severe learning disabilities progressed through a series of stages comprising intensive training, maintenance and long-term preservation of skills.
- One-to-one intensive training, using Foxx and Azrin procedures for bladder training and independence training, was completed after either nine self-initiated toiletings or 4 weeks' intensive training. Of 63 trainees, 8 failed to reach this criterion and 55 (87%) proceeded to the next stage.
- Maintenance training, which involved one trainer per two trainees, aimed to maintain self-initiated

toileting, reduce accidents further and teach additional skills including washing hands and flushing toilet. This stage was completed after either maintaining independent toileting with fewer than two bladder accidents per week for 2 weeks or 2 months' training. Of the 55 who entered maintenance, 6 were still undergoing maintenance training at the time of the report, 9 had failed to reach criterion and 40 had progressed to the 'preservation' stage.
- Preservation aimed to prepare trainees to maintain their skills in their long-term placements. Staffing ratios at this stage were one to three, preservation being completed after 2 consecutive accident-free weeks or 2 months' training and an accident rate of one per week or less. Of the 40 trainees who entered this stage, 31 reached criterion for full continence.

---

disabilities, living in the community. It can be seen how frequency of passing continent urine increases and frequency of incontinence decreases. However, the intensive nature of these training programmes does raise questions about the feasibility of parents as trainers.

Maintenance of bladder skills

Maintenance of bladder skills is an important issue, as initial success can be reduced in the longer term by unfavourable environmental conditions. Acquisition of bladder control using intensive continence training is well maintained in the short-to-medium term (Bettison et al 1976, Leath & Flournoy 1979, Van Wagenen et al 1969a,b) and the long term (Hyams et al 1992).

A number of factors may influence long-term effectiveness of behavioural continence training approaches. Hyams et al (1992) followed up 15 people with severe learning disabilities, who were by then between 18 and 29 years, 10 years after continence training. Ten had received one-to-one, structured behavioural continence training, while five had received structured continence training as a group. Recording established that continence had been maintained substantially, but independence at toilet less so. A major reason for this seemed to be the fact that current care staff were unaware that these residents had been

independent at toilet and had automatically prompted them to toilet at the same time as other residents. Despite this, intensive training was found to be more cost-effective, the extra investment of resources for intensive training being quickly repaid in terms of carer time. In fact, over a 10-year period, the total savings in carer time for the ten individually trained residents was calculated to be over 50 000 staff hours.

A full discussion of factors which affect long-term maintenance is provided by Pfadt & Sullivan (1981) and Bettison (1982). Some of these factors should present fewer problems in community settings. One factor may be that of less intensive versus more intensive training (Smith 1979a). Less intensive training, though on the face of it cheaper and easier to implement, may in fact be less cost-effective than intensive, one-to-one training (Hyams et al 1992).

Other factors include:

- institutional practices such as shutting or locking doors between day areas and toilets
- ill-fitting clothing or clothing with difficult fasteners
- re-establishing dependency through prompting trainees to toilet (Foxx & Azrin 1973, Hyams et al 1992).

Studies in the USA of problems involved in maintaining continence retraining gains in the elderly with dementia show that staff training is not, by itself, effective in changing institutional attitudes and practices long term. Rather, close monitoring and supervision, regular group and individual feedback and staff motivational systems are necessary (Burgio et al 1990, Engel et al 1990).

Generalization

- The importance of generalizing training across different settings was demonstrated in early studies (Baumeister & Klosowski 1965, Dunlap et al 1985).
- Without generalization training, a sudden return to the regular living situation can erase progress (Baumeister & Klosowski 1965).
- These problems can be avoided by training in the more regular living situation from the outset rather than in special training units (Dayan 1964, Yoder 1966).

Training principles

One type of continence training programme will not suit the needs of every individual. However, although there is a need to consider individual differences and avoid block treatment, certain basic principles should be borne in mind. These include the need for baseline assessment, the use of rewards to motivate learning, the definition of objectives and the type of training procedures used.

Systems of motivation

Some people are concerned about the use of rewards. Carers may worry that rewards may 'spoil' the child or lead to problems later. In fact, the evidence shows that rewards, carefully chosen and used consistently, speed up learning in people with severe intellectual disabilities. Rewards should be given consistently, i.e. on every occasion, and immediately, *not* 5 minutes later. Once goals are achieved, rewards are phased out gradually rather than discontinued abruptly.

Identifying rewards appropriate to the individual and suitable for the needs of the programme can be difficult and calls for a degree of

---

Box 10.3 Systems of motivation

'Social' reinforcement is important for most trainees with a severe learning disability:

- praise
- talking about how pleased other people will be, e.g. family members, teacher and so on
- physical contact – hugs, cuddles, tickle, stroking cheek or head, rubbing back
- play with favourite toys or objects
- favourite tunes or songs
- simple games of anticipation involving peek-a-boo or tickle
- primary reinforcers, i.e. rewards based on biological needs such as food and drink, are often suitable. Edibles, which should be small, easy to administer and easily and quickly consumed, can include small segments or pieces of fruit (fresh or dried), small savoury items such as crisps or savoury biscuits, or small sweets. A variety of drinks may be used.
- a wide range of rewards should be used if possible, in order to avoid satiation.

---

imagination. What is rewarding to one person (e.g. physical contact) may be punishing to another. To identify rewards, it is important not only to ask what a person likes, but also what they choose to spend time doing (Box 10.3).

Defining objectives

Clear and unambiguous definition of goals is not just important for training purposes, but also for purposes of evaluation. For example, the term 'toilet training' is vague: are we talking about bladder or bowel, day or night? Do we expect the trainee to be fully independent at toilet, or be dry and use the toilet while still requiring prompts, help and supervision? Objectives must be stated in a form that can be clearly understood by different care staff, all of whom may have different views on the meaning of 'toilet training'.

Objectives are important at a practical level when formulating a training programme. Once objectives are properly formulated, the outline of the programme should follow and a standard is set by which its effectiveness, or otherwise, can be evaluated (see Box 10.4). Rather than formulate objectives in terms of behaviour(s) to be decreased, turn the formulation round to a behaviour you wish to increase. Focusing on a new skill

---

Box 10.4 Objectives

Example of a badly defined objective:
At the end of training John will stop wetting his pants and be toilet trained.

Example of a well-defined objective:
At the end of training, John will have dry pants during the day, with no more than one accident per week, and will pass urine on the toilet when prompted every 2 hours. He will be able to lower and raise his pants, but will still require to be prompted and will need supervision in the toilet area.

The latter specifies more clearly:

- the aims of the programme
- positive skills or behaviours to be taught
- the degree of success expected
- the support or supervision ultimately expected
- standards by which to evaluate the outcome.

---

immediately emphasizes the positive side. For example, if the problem is daytime incontinence, the objective should be to increase the frequency of dryness and continent passing of urine by day rather than decreasing the frequency of wetting accidents.

Next, consider short-term objectives. Which aspect of continence do you wish to focus on? Is it bladder or bowel training or both? Does it include handling clothes and going to toilet independently, or not? The degree of success expected and how much help, if any, the individual is expected to require when the objective is reached should be included in the statement of objectives.

Training procedures

Having assessed and rated the various components of toileting behaviour, having determined the objectives clearly, and having listed the rewards to be used, the methods of teaching these new skills can now be considered.

Assessment determines the current level of the incontinent individual's bladder and bowel control; objectives specify the goals to be achieved. The task is to break down the distance between these into a series of steps. The structured teaching methods used are the same as those used to teach

other self-help and independence skills. Two of the main methods for teaching new skills are known as 'prompt and fade' and 'backward chaining'.

Prompt and fade

There are three types of prompt: physical prompts, verbal prompts and gestural prompts:

- a *physical prompt* consists of any prompt involving touching. A major physical prompt might consist of walking alongside the trainee, physically guiding to the toilet with an arm round one shoulder, positioning in front of the toilet and physically guiding to sit on the toilet. Physical prompts range from this extreme to holding the trainee's hand lightly or shadowing the back or elbow with your hand.
- a *verbal prompt* consists of any spoken prompt to the child such as 'John, go to the toilet'.
- a *gestural prompt* consists of any other form of prompt in which the trainer prompts the trainee non-verbally and without touching. At one extreme, a gestural prompt can involve an elaborate mime whereby the trainer makes eye contact then looks at the toilet, points to the trainee and then, with a sweeping wave of the arm, points to the toilet, gestures to move to the toilet, then pats the toilet seat and gestures to the trainee to sit on the toilet. At the other extreme, a gestural prompt can consist of a very small point with one finger, or a small head nod. Ultimately, establishing eye contact and following this with a movement of the eyes towards the toilet is the lowest level of gestural prompt.

Prompting. Having established the type and level of prompt required to get the trainee to go to the toilet from a few feet away, the prompts are then broken down into their physical, verbal and gestural components and a series of steps determined to systematically fade these out. Prompts to toilet are always faded in order from physical to verbal to gestural. As physical prompts represent the highest level of prompt related to dependence on others for toileting, they are faded first. Verbal prompts are faded next because, in practice, they are the most difficult to fade: a minimal verbal prompt of just one word spoken softly – 'toilet' – is impossible to fade further. As there is more scope for fading gestural prompts altogether, these are faded last.

Fading. In order to facilitate the correct sequence for fading prompts, the prompts are given in the reverse order: the lowest level of prompt (gestural) is given first, verbal prompts are given next, the highest level of prompt (physical) being given last. These are given with a gap of a second or so in between in order that, when able to respond to a lower category of prompt, the trainee has the full opportunity to do so. Thus, every time a prompt is given, a slightly lower level is first tried than on the previous occasion. As soon as the trainee responds to a lower level of prompt within one category, subsequent prompts never go back up beyond that category or level.

Fading whole categories of prompts is accomplished using the correct sequence of prompts described above, but procedures for facilitating the process further have developed from experience of these programmes. For example, it is possible to fade directly from physical to gestural prompts without the intervening step of verbal prompts. This can be done by first fading the physical prompt to the point where the trainee is held lightly by the hand. The trainer then prompts the trainee from in front, rather than from the side, by reaching out to hold the trainee's hand. The trainer then moves the hand away just as the trainee touches it. If the trainer's hand is moved away, the trainee is likely to step forward to try to hold it. The trainer then points dramatically to the toilet. In this way, fading gestural prompts is achieved more rapidly. Seated close to the toilet and going back and forward to the toilet every half hour or so, with substantial reinforcement for using the toilet and for having dry pants, self-initiated toileting (i.e. going without a prompt) is a relatively easy step to make.

If prompts have been faded to the lowest possible gestural prompt and the trainee has still not self-initiated, the following procedure may be useful. A few minutes before a prompt is due, the trainee should be casually manoeuvred to stand close to the toilet without any overt prompting. Standing next to the toilet, the chances are that after a few minutes the trainee will sit down on the toilet. When this happens, the trainee should be rewarded and training should proceed from there.

Prompts to toilet are reduced as soon as self-initiations appear and discontinued completely when the trainee can self-initiate consistently. After an initial low level prompt in the morning, two or three self-initiations during the day should be sufficient to warrant the complete termination of prompts thereafter. However, because of differences between individuals, it is not possible to set an exact criterion for terminating prompts. It is unwise to stop prompts altogether after the first self-initiated toileting unless self-initiations are very frequent.

When prompts to toilet have been stopped and the trainee has been self-initiating successfully for a few days from close to the toilet, the trainee can be moved gradually away from the toilet and back towards the regular living area, a few feet each day, ensuring consistent self-initiation from each point. The important places to train from are corners, doors or any point where there is a choice of direction on the way to the toilet.

Chaining

Chaining is when a skill is broken down into small steps and taught one step at a time. In *forward chaining*, step 1 is taught first. When this can be executed without assistance, step 2 is added. When step 1 and step 2 can be executed without help, step 3 is added, and so on. *Backward chaining*, by contrast, teaches the last step in the chain first. This step, being closest to the goal to be achieved, is closest to the reward to be earned and is hence, in learning terms, the step most easily and quickly learned. When the last step can be executed without assistance, the second last step is added, and so on. For example, the objective might be to teach lowering pants at toilet without help. Using backward chaining, first the hands are held and guided through the entire procedure, for which the child is rewarded. Once this sequence can be executed with assistance, the trainer guides the trainee through the sequence leaving the last step, the relatively easy one of lowering the pants from below the knees, for the trainee to complete without assistance. When this can be completed without assistance, the trainee is required to lower the pants from above the knees without help, then from the hips and finally the waist. Smaller steps than this may be required, but the concept behind backward chaining involves teaching skills in small steps from the goal backwards.

Fluid intake

In contrast to the long-standing tradition of restricting fluid to incontinent people, increased fluid is common in behavioural continence training programmes. 'Normal' fluid intake is difficult to define because of cultural differences and environmental factors such as ambient temperature and humidity (Vande Walle et al 1995). However, from references to drinking, voiding and defecation habits, Vande Walle et al (1995) assume that an average fluid intake must be 1500 ml/m BSA/day (i.e. 1500 ml per square metre body surface area per day), which results in urine production of 1000 ml/m^2 BSA/day or voiding four to five times with a bladder volume of 200–250 ml/m^2 BSA.

The purpose of increased fluid is to increase training opportunities and speed up training by increasing the frequency of passing urine. Although advice to restrict fluid is still found, a number of studies have established a positive role for increased fluid in bladder function (Hagglund 1965, Spangler et al 1984, Smith & Wong 1981). For example, Smith & Wong studied bladder function data over several weeks in ten children with severe learning disabilities undergoing intensive behavioural continence training utilizing increased fluid intake. When daily frequencies and volumes of continent and incontinent urine were analysed in relation to fluid intake, no association was found between increased fluid intake and incontinence, but a positive association was found with continent passing urine and increased functional bladder capacity.

Box 10.5 Monitoring increased fluids within a behavioural training procedure

Thompson & Hanson (1983) recommend that:

- candidates for behavioural continence training programmes involving augmented hydration should be medically screened
- hydration should not be used with those being treated simultaneously with medication known to increase urinary retention
- hydration should not be used in those with pre-existing epilepsy, a history of spinal injury or impaired cerebrospinal fluid such as hydrocephalus
- fluid intake should be limited to 85–125 ml per hour for children weighing between 27 and 45 kg, and 165 ml per hour for adolescents and adults between 45 and 68 kg, for no more than 12 hours per 24 hours.

Concern has been expressed about the risk of overhydration where fluid intake is increased in association with structured behavioural continence training (Thompson & Hanson 1983) (Box 10.5). Increased fluid in conjunction with intensive behavioural continence training is demonstrably successful (as compared to fluid restriction, which has no merit at all) in people whose incontinence was formerly considered untreatable. There have been no reports of adverse effects of increased fluid intake during structured bladder training programmes (although this could be due to the lack of awareness of symptoms of water intoxication and a tendency to attribute increased agitation to behaviour problems). The success of intensive behavioural continence training programmes does not, however, justify risk to the trainee.

Regular prompting versus timing

A major difference in continence training methods is that of 'regular prompting' versus 'timing', i.e. whether the trainee is prompted to toilet at regular, set intervals of time, or whether toileting occurs at or around the time of an accident. Although 'timing' is popularly recommended, there is little evidence to support its superior effectiveness. In learning disabilities, a small comparison of these methods was undertaken by

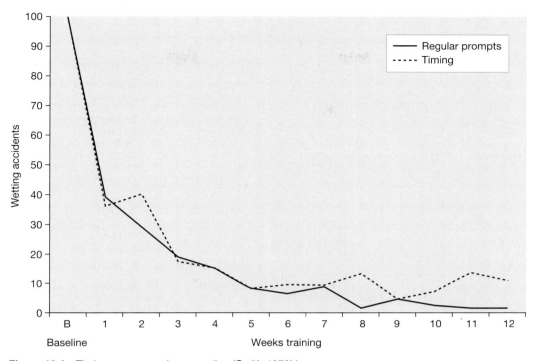

Figure 10.4 Timing versus regular prompting (Smith 1979b).

Smith (1979a). Five children with profound learning disabilities were intensively trained using regular prompts (based on a Foxx & Azrin (1973) approach) and five using a timing approach (based on that outlined by van Wagenen et al 1969b). Both methods were equally effective (Fig. 10.4). In practice, however, timing was more complicated to implement because the untrained bladder does not void reflexively at regular, predictable intervals or volumes. Where two interventions are equally effective but one is simpler, the simpler method should be chosen. There can be exceptions to this rule, however, as is demonstrated by Case study 10.1 and Case study 10.2.

DOUBLE INCONTINENCE

Before considering encopresis separately, it is appropriate to look first at those cases where there has been a failure to acquire control of both bladder and bowel. It might be assumed that the rational approach would be to train bowel control first, as many children acquire bowel control before bladder. This is not always the case, however: some children acquire bladder and bowel control simultaneously and some acquire bladder control first. Where people with severe or profound learning disabilities are doubly incontinent, bladder training carried out first may result in some spontaneous improvement in bowel control, as demonstrated in Figure 10.5.

Bowel training

Treatment approaches to encopresis in children within the general population have included psychoanalytic psychotherapy, family therapy, hypnotherapy, biofeedback and behavioural therapy. With a success rate of 70% or better reported for children within the general population (Bosch 1988, Dawson et al 1990, Kaplan 1985, Young 1973), behavioural approaches, which focus on the appropriate and inappropriate eliminatory behaviours themselves, represent the treatment of choice.

Case study 10.1

Fiona is a young woman with a severe degree of learning disability who lives at home with her mother, a single parent. Fiona has some speech (two-word combinations) and presents with challenging behaviours, including occasional tantrums. She can pass urine on the toilet when taken but still has accidents and her mother complains that Fiona's incontinence has destroyed a new settee. Fiona is described as being wet 'all the time' and her mother thinks she is doing it deliberately to 'get at' her. Two weeks' baseline recording of frequency and times of passing continent and incontinent urine was undertaken (see chart below).

						Time of day							
Time Day	9am	10	11	12	1pm	2	3	4	5	6	7	8	9
Mon	PU	D	D	D	PU	D	D	PU	D	D	PU	D	D
Tues	D	PU	D	D	NPU	PU	D	D	W	D	NPU	PU	D
Weds	NPU	D	PU	D	PU	D	D	PU	D	D	PU	D	D
Thur	PU	D	D	D	D	PU	D	D	D	W	D	PU	D
Fri	D	PU	D	D	PU	D	D	PU	D	D	PU	D	D
Sat	PU	D	D	D	NPU	PU	D	PU	D	D	PU	D	D
Sun	NPU	D	D	D	PU	D	D	PU	D	D	NPU	D	D
Mon	NPU	D	PU	D	D	PU	D	PU	D	D	PU	D	D
Tues	PU	D	D	D	PU	D	D	D	D	W	D	PU	D
Weds	PU	D	D	D	PU	D	PU	D	D	D	PU	D	D
Thur	NPU	D	D	D	D	PU	D	D	W	D	NPU	PU	D
Fri	D	PU	D	D	PU	D	D	PU	D	D	PU	D	D
Sat	D	PU	D	D	PU	D	D	PU	D	D	PU	D	D
Sun	PU	D	D	D	PU	D	D	PU	D	D	NPU	PU	D

Recording key: D = dry; W = wet; PU = prompted to toilet and passed urine;
NPU = prompted to toilet and did not pass urine.

The recording shows that:

- Fiona is not wetting all of the time but only twice a week.
- These accidents occur when Fiona has not been prompted to toilet early in the evenings.

Discussion of baseline records established that missed prompts coincided with mother's favourite TV programmes. The problem was solved by adjusting the times of prompts on those evenings.

Case study 10.2   Developing an intensive daytime bladder training programme

Stewart is a child with a profound learning disability who has reached his teenage years without achieving continence. He has a degree of cerebral palsy but is ambulant. He has single words of speech and can comprehend simple instructions. He can feed with a spoon and drink from a cup. His play tends to involve manipulation of objects rather than imaginative or constructive play. He has no serious behaviour problems but can have temper tantrums when frustrated. He is affectionate and responsive to attention.

Stewart does not communicate the need to eliminate and has frequent bladder and bowel accidents by day, is often wet but never soiled at night, can sit unaided on the toilet, assists with lowering his underpants, passes urine on the toilet occasionally and has regular bowel movements. The priority is daytime

(continued)

Case study 10.2   *(continued)*

bladder control. The objectives are defined as teaching him to remain dry and to pass urine on the toilet every time when toileted on a 2-hourly basis.

Before bringing together the points covered above, we need to consider:

1. fluid intake
2. urine-sensitive alarms
3. clothing
4. the environment in which the training is to be implemented
5. training procedures.

Fluids

Encouraging Stewart to drink additional fluids for the first part of the training day will help increase his bladder capacity as well as increasing the number of training opportunities through increasing the frequency of passing urine. The use of hydration should be discussed with Stewart's general practitioner beforehand in order to confirm it is safe to do so.[1]

Equipment

Two types of continence training are available: toilet bowl alarms and pants alarms. The toilet bowl alarm is a device which attaches to the toilet and signals immediately urine is passed on the toilet.[2] The pants alarm is a small device attached to the underpants which signals the occurrence of a wetting accident. Body-worn nocturnal enuresis alarms are suitable.[3]

Both pants and bowl alarms, used as part of a well-designed training programme, aid immediate detection of urination and hence immediate and consistent reinforcement. Bowl alarms, which emphasize the positive side of training, are more important than pants alarms as well as being more reliable and easier to use in practice. Musical potties are available for smaller or younger children. Do not worry that the use of a musical potty will 'condition' a child to pass urine in response to a particular tune later in life – this does not happen.

---

[1] See earlier discussion of guidelines.
[2] Toilet bowl alarms are available from:
- BIME, Wolfson Centre, RUH, Combe Park, Bath BA1 3NG.
- TFH, 76 Barracks Road, Sandy Lane Industrial Estate, Stockport on Severn, Worcester, DY12 9QB.

[3] A number of companies supply enuresis alarms, including:
- ERIC, 34 Old School House, Britannia Road, Kingswood, Bristol BS15 2DB.
- Ferraris Medical, Ferraris House, Aden Road, Enfield, Middlesex EN3 7SE.
- Malem Medical, 10 Willows Holt, Lowdham, Nottingham NG14 7EJ.

Clothing

Extra clothing should be organized in advance. If a pants alarm is to be used, underpants should be close fitting and made of cotton. Trousers should have elastic waists for easy handling. Dresses or skirts should not be too long. Incontinence pads, tights, dungarees or anything with belts, buttons, clips or zips are to be avoided.

The training environment

As Stewart is beyond the age where spontaneous remission is likely, he is likely to require intensive, structured training. This means that, in the early stages at least, most of the training will be carried out close to the toilet. The toilet area should therefore be as pleasant and comfortable as possible. Although hospital, school and day centre toilets are often more spacious, they are usually less pleasant. If so, the décor, heating, lighting and ventilation should be improved where possible and soft furnishings introduced to deaden echo and noise. A variety of toys and suitable activities should be available while Stewart is being trained. The trainer should have a comfortable chair, radio, access to coffee and a clock. Although intensive toilet training is hard work, it need not be unpleasant. At home, it may be necessary to leave the door open if the bathroom is small, but the space outside the bathroom may be used as the training area provided the toilet is within sight.

Training procedures

Following the work of Foxx & Azrin, the three aspects of training for which we need separate procedures are: bladder training, dry pants training, accident training and independence training.

Bladder training.

- Engage Stewart in play within sight of the toilet.
- Every 30 or 45 minutes, prompt him to sit on the toilet.
- Let him sit on the toilet until he passes urine or for a maximum of 10 minutes.
- Immediately he passes urine and activates the bowl alarm, reward him substantially. A tea trolley with a selection of rewards can be kept out of sight and quickly wheeled in when the bowl alarm is activated. Reward Stewart while he is actually on the toilet and when he starts to pass urine, not when he finishes (this procedure can be reviewed if Stewart begins to stop the urine stream as soon as he is rewarded, or begins to stop and start in the expectation of earning further rewards).

Dry pants training. Teaching Stewart to discriminate between dry and wet pants through feedback and social consequences is an important part of training which is usually insufficiently emphasized. It is important to remember that children who wear disposable incontinence pads with 'stay-dry' liners do not experience feedback for being incontinent.

- Dry pants checks are carried out between prompts to toilet. Every 15 minutes throughout the training day,

(continued)

Case study 10.2 *(continued)*

guide Stewart's hand to check his underpants and praise/reward him for being dry.
- Do this before any activity he enjoys, such as before meals, drinks and activities, or other enjoyable and hence rewarding social interactions.

The purpose of bladder training and dry pants training is to increase Stewart's motivation to pass urine on the toilet and remain dry. Remember that, even if he rarely passes urine on the toilet before training, with increased fluids and prompts to toilet every half hour or so, he will pass urine on the toilet at some point.

Wetting accident procedure.

- When a wetting accident occurs and the pants alarm is triggered, immediately guide Stewart's hand to feel his wet pants. Ensure that you have his attention and say 'No, your pants are wet'. This should be said in a clear but neutral voice. Do not shout – this would be unacceptable and it is important to remember that the purpose of this procedure is not to administer a reprimand but to assist Stewart to discriminate between wet and dry pants.
- Switch the pants alarm off, but do not prompt him to the toilet or change his clothes immediately, as this would afford him one-to-one attention for wetting.
- Quietly withdraw eye contact, praise and attention for a few minutes.
- After 5 minutes, change him into dry clothes in a neutral manner with a minimum of fuss. Then assist Stewart to check his (now) dry pants and praise for being dry. Recommence the bladder training procedure as above.

Training independent toileting. We have trained Stewart to remain dry and pass urine consistently on the toilet. If the aim of training had been to teach him to initiate going to the toilet himself, an additional procedure would have been required which is more complex and requires more intensive training. If Stewart's comprehension is limited, the procedure is as follows:

1. Establish the type and level of prompt required to get Stewart to go to the toilet, then systematically fade (i.e. phase out) prompts. For example, does he require to be physically guided? If so, does he need to be guided with an arm around the shoulders, led by the hand or does he only require the presence of a light touch on his back? Or will he go in response to a verbal prompt only such as 'Stewart, toilet', without the need for any physical prompting?
2. Start training from close to the toilet, then when prompts have been faded and Stewart can self-initiate from close to the toilet, gradually train him backwards from the toilet to all the rooms from which he will be expected to self-initiate.

Relapses in independent toileting. A clear definition of a relapse should be established beforehand, for example, two full days without a self-initiated toileting, or when wetting accidents increase or if Stewart starts to follow others when they are prompted to toilet.

Organizational issues. A well-designed but badly organized or inconsistently implemented programme will have little effect. A little prior planning and organization can pre-empt many of the common problems that affect the integrity of the programme. These include:

- the responsible staff
- maintenance and generalization
- the evaluation of training
- the length of the training programme.

Responsibility for training. Consistent training is easier to achieve if one person has responsibility for coordinating the programme. Whether Stewart lives at home or in residential care, he is likely also to attend school or access day services. It is essential that training is carried out consistently across different situations and that everyone who comes into contact with Stewart is familiar with the programme. Those who will be carrying out the training will need training and practice in the procedures involved. It is useful to enact the training procedures using a simulated training situation and role playing. Morale is also very important, as intensive, structured continence training is tiring. Clear feedback on progress, as well as close supervision and support, should be provided.

Maintenance and generalization (Box 10.6). Maintenance refers to sustaining progress once the objectives have been achieved. As maintenance and generalization can present problems for people with more severe degrees of learning disability, the likelihood that problems will arise should be considered in advance.

Evaluation. Evaluating the effects of training is important. A baseline or pretreatment measure of the behaviour should be obtained. Simple but accurate records of the frequency of passing continent and incontinent urine enable success to be evaluated and decisions to be made about whether to continue the programme unchanged or to modify it.

Length of training. The baseline period must be long enough to establish that the behaviour is stable. There should be evidence that the behaviour is neither increasing nor decreasing in frequency, otherwise it will be difficult to establish conclusively whether change was due to treatment or some other factor. If incontinence is already reducing, introducing a new training programme may not be necessary or desirable. In practical terms, a baseline period of at least 2 weeks, preferably 3, is normal.

A bladder training programme can be expected to last for several weeks, so that there may be little point in starting if Stewart is about to go on holiday. A period should be chosen in which few interruptions are expected. It is important also to specify achievable objectives if there is a time limit on training. If progress is slow and time is limited, objectives may need to be redefined. Progress should be evident in 4 weeks, even though training takes longer to complete.

Box 10.6   Maintenance and generalization

Maintenance

Maintenance of a newly learned skill is achieved as follows:

- Do not terminate the programme suddenly, but phase it out gradually. Reduce the amount of extra attention given during the training period as gradually as possible. Continue to reinforce the desired behaviour with extra rewards for some time after the objective is reached, then phase them out by dropping them intermittently at first. For example, from rewarding the desired behaviour on every occasion, reward on four out of five occasions, then three, two and one out of five occasions, until rewards for passing urine and for dry pants are completely phased out. Social reinforcement, usually praise, should continue indefinitely.
- Ensure that everyone in contact with Stewart knows how to strengthen and support the new behaviour and that no-one reverts to previous toileting procedures. Ensure that occasional occurrences of old behaviours are not inadvertently rewarded, e.g. attention given contingent upon a wetting accident.

- If a relapse occurs, briefly re-implement the original training procedures as quickly as possible.
- Consider carefully the environment(s) where the new skills or abilities are to be maintained indefinitely.

Generalization

- Training should be generalized both to different places and to different people.
- If possible, train initially in one location only, for example at home, and with one trainer. When some progress has been made, extend training to other environments in which the trainee uses the toilet regularly. Finally, extend training to include toilets used less frequently, such as on trips or outings, arranging some trips specifically for the purpose of training in these situations.
- Similarly, start with one trainer conducting most of the training, then introduce others to the programme when progress is underway. The first person should be present until Stewart can perform equally for different people.

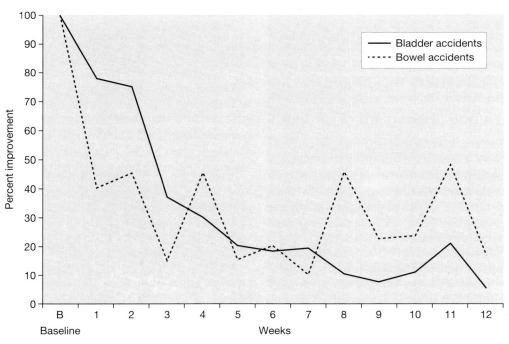

Figure 10.5   Reduction in bowel accidents during intensive bladder training for ten children with profound learning disabilities (Smith 1979b).

In the field of learning disability, because encopresis is often attributed to the presence of a learning disability, treatment for encopresis is rare and there is no consensus on treatment guidelines.

RETENTIVE ENCOPRESIS

Approaches to retentive encopresis in the field of learning disability have included abdominal massage, use of fibre and behavioural training.

Abdominal massage for constipation

Bowel control in people with severe degrees of learning disability and multiple physical handicaps has received little attention. Bowel management can be a major issue in this group of people, many of whom experience chronic constipation. Bowel care may depend heavily on the use of laxatives and enemas. At a clinical level, there has been renewed interest among physiotherapists and nurses in the use of abdominal massage for constipation and retention in this group. The idea

is that the faecal mass is helped to move along the ascending, transverse and descending colon by stimulating peristalsis. The method of massage involves a combination of effleurage (stroking) and petrisage (kneading). Emly (1993) has reported a trial with one young man with a history of constipation and high impacted faeces, in whom thrice-weekly abdominal massage was reported to stimulate regular spontaneous bowel movements. Furthermore, although his communication skills were limited, he was able to indicate when a bowel movement was imminent and could be placed on the toilet. In an unpublished trial with which one of the present authors was associated, several adults with multiple handicaps and severe learning disability received regular abdominal massage for constipation. Although some people showed no improvement, others appeared to benefit, such as a multiply handicapped woman, in the middle years of life, whose results are shown in Figure 10.6.

By contrast, however, in a small trial to investigate the effects of abdominal massage in nine elderly constipated patients and seven healthy young adult volunteers in the general population

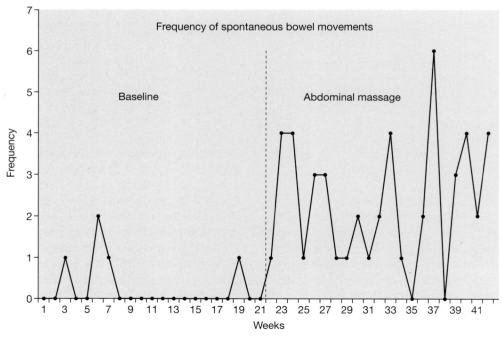

Figure 10.6 Spontaneous bowel movements in one woman with profound and multiple handicaps following abdominal massage.

(Klauser et al 1992), neither stool frequency nor colonic transit time changed significantly in either group. Thus, although two single case studies have found an improvement in people with physical and learning disabilities using abdominal massage, the effectiveness of this technique in the treatment of constipation has not yet been clearly demonstrated. The potential advantages of abdominal massage, if proven effective, are fairly obvious for a client group whose bowel problems can be difficult to treat. In addition, abdominal massage is believed to be a pleasant sensory experience for many people with physical disabilities.

Use of fibre for constipation

Increased fibre and proprietary bulking agents have been demonstrated to increase the urge to defecate in a natural way in the general population (Houts & Peterson 1986) (see also Chapters 7 and 8). Studies where bulk was added to the diets of people with severe intellectual and physical disabilities have shown more variable results (Capra & Hannan-Jones 1992, Fischer et al 1985, Liebl et al 1990, Lupson & Walton 1981, McCallum et al 1978). This may be due to differences in the type of fibre and quantities used.

McCallum et al (1978) found no significant difference in stool frequency in a 9-week randomized trial of bran biscuits, bran or laxatives, each administered for 3 weeks. The authors concluded that bran or bran biscuits could be substituted for laxative use at least in some participants. However, none of the participants with a profound intellectual disability, all of whom had been receiving 'regular' (unspecified) enemas, was enema-free while receiving added fibre.

Prior to the addition of fibre, defecation in six out of seven of Lupson & Walton's (1981) participants occurred only after twice-weekly enemas or two suppositories every 4th day. One participant occasionally self-initiated to the toilet. Four were immobile and unable to self-feed and three were able to feed themselves, of whom two were partially mobile. Within 3 weeks, all were described as passing an average of one soft, normal stool every 2 days without the assistance of artificial elimination aids.

Capra & Hannan-Jones (1992) studied the effects of an added 7 g of fibre for a period of 2 weeks in a random 25% of 37 inpatients, 22 of whom had severe/profound intellectual disabilities together with physical handicaps, while 15 had severe intellectual disabilities but no physical disability. Baseline estimates of daily dietary fibre ranged from 14–23 g with a mean of 18.6 g. None of the 37 was impacted due to the 'regular' (unspecified) use of suppositories and enemas. The authors identified three different outcomes within the experimental 25%: those whose bowel function remained unchanged; those for whom the texture of stools improved, but the frequency of stools and use of elimination aids remained unchanged; those for whom frequency and texture of stools improved and elimination aids reduced.

Fischer et al (1985) found that stool frequency did not increase and elimination aids were only 'very minimally reduced' when fibre was added to the diets of constipated children and young adults with severe physical and intellectual disabilities. There was, however, some improvement in stool size and texture, with the frequency of large-sized stools increasing by 20% (definition of large stools is unclear but 'small' stools were defined as <15 g) and 'a trend towards more soft unformed and soft formed' stools, which was statistically non-significant. The authors state that improvement might be evident with a longer experimental period and higher levels of fibre, as the levels of fibre added here were equivalent to a low-fibre diet.

Liebl et al (1990), studying the effect of a two-stage increase in dietary fibre, found that stool moisture (objectively measured) and consistency (subjectively assessed) improved for some participants during 'Fibre 1', but stool size did not increase during either Fibre 1 or Fibre 2. While 'Fibre 2' did not improve stool consistency or moisture over 'Fibre 1', stool frequency was significantly increased over baseline or 'Fibre 1'.

A number of points are worth making in relation to these studies. Read et al (1986) have concluded that constipation is probably part of a diverse group of disorders with a common presenting symptom. As no reference is made to gastroenterological investigation, participants in these studies may have represented different subgroups, some of whose constipation may represent a relatively simple problem. Problems easily remedied by the simple addition of fibre to the diet would include constipation due to medication such as major tranquillizers and some anticonvulsants commonly used in 'high-dependency' populations, or a low-fibre diet. Constipation in others may represent a range of other, more complex disorders less easily remedied. At present, there has been so little study of constipation in the field of intellectual disability, that the prevalence and aetiology of gastrointestinal disorders is unknown. Constipation in people with severe/profound intellectual disability and/or those with severe physical handicaps should initially address quality of care issues such as fluid intake and dietary fibre.

Some authors, however, have expressed concern about the routine use of increased fibre in high-dependency, immobile or cognitively less able groups (Donald et al 1985, Rosenthal & Marshall 1987). Indeed, the use of increased fibre or bulking agents of any type is not without risk in such populations: phytobezoars (a concretion of undigested, compacted vegetable fibre), though uncommon, have occurred in institutionalized people or those with an acute psychotic mental disorder (Sroujieh 1988). Furthermore, the addition of large amounts of uncooked bran to the diet can compromise the uptake of vitamins and minerals (Agnarsson et al 1993) in those whose diet may already be poor. By contrast, other authors in such fields recommend routine increases in fibre to counteract the constipating effects of certain commonly used tranquillizers (de Silva et al 1992).

KEY POINTS: FIBRE AND CONSTIPATION

- Constipation is symptomatic of a diverse group of disorders, some of which may be improved using the addition of fibre alone and others which may not.
- This may explain the wide variation in response to the use of fibre in people with intellectual disabilities and makes comparison of findings across small sample studies difficult. For some people, increased fibre may improve stool consistency and frequency.
- However, although some of the studies cited have found benefits in the use of added bulk with some severely disabled people, there is a clear need for caution to be exercised through careful monitoring.

Behavioural approaches

Reports of behavioural approaches to encopresis in learning disability are few in number and largely confined to secondary (previously clean) soiling (Carpenter 1989, Chopra 1973, Jansson et al 1992, Matson 1977) and to those with mild rather than severe learning disability (Carpenter 1989, Chopra 1973, Jansson et al 1992, Smith et al 2000). It may be that it is assumed that the chances of success are greater in those with a mild learning disability or those who were previously continent. Behavioural training programmes for both retentive and non-retentive encopresis in the field of learning disability have utilized rewards for clean underwear and for continent elimination, and punishment for soiling, these techniques being used either singly or in combination.

Behavioural approaches to retentive encopresis

Five reports concern behavioural approaches to retentive encopresis (Carpenter 1989, Dalrymple & Angrist 1988, Jansson et al 1992, Piazza et al 1991, Smith et al 1994).

Dalrymple & Angrist (1989) describe the treatment of retentive encopresis in a 15-year-old girl with autism and profound learning disability, whose encopresis had previously been treated unsuccessfully with laxatives, suppositories and enemas. Treatment involved: daily use of mineral oil; scheduled (unspecified) toilet trips; rewards of attention, praise and small edibles for appropriate elimination; and 'positive practice' (unspecified). After 18 months, 86% of stools were passed in the toilet, rising to 100% after 2 years, by which time the majority of stools were self-initiated and a bowel pattern was emerging. Treatment gains were maintained at 1-year follow-up.

Piazza et al (1991) successfully treated primary retentive encopresis over 14 weeks in a 15-year-old boy and a 5-year-old girl with profound learning disabilities. Regular toilet sits, rewards for appropriate elimination, punishment for soiling, increased fibre and the use of elimination aids had all been tried previously but had failed. The programme for both children involved rewarding all stools initially, both continent and incontinent, with praise, snacks and preferred objects, in order to increase the frequency of defecation and thus decrease retention. It was intended to follow this with a discrimination training procedure to teach elimination on the toilet, involving leading the children to the toilet, placing the incontinent stool down the toilet, assisting them to sit on the toilet for 30 seconds then praising them for the stool. However, rewarding all stools resulted in a significant increase in continent bowel evacuation as well as total evacuations.

This multiple-phase study makes an important contribution to the literature. Though limited to two cases, it raises questions about the necessity and effectiveness of punishment procedures, which in these cases had previously exacerbated retention, and the use of artificial elimination aids. The authors suggest that punishment for soiling and elimination aids may reduce the likelihood of continent stools, the latter because the individual's control over bowel function is reduced and the former because punishment may decrease not only incontinent but also continent evacuation in people with severe or profound learning disability.

Smith et al (1994) describe the treatment of chronic faecal impaction and faecal incontinence in four young people aged from 13 to 23 years, three of whom had a severe or profound learning disability. The programme involved supervised, prompted toilet sits after meals for a maximum of 10 minutes, with praise and rewards for appropriate elimination. Neither punishment techniques for soiling nor rewards for clean pants were used lest these should aggravate retention in an effort to keep clean. Artificial elimination aids were stopped or phased out as quickly as possible and replaced with bulk-forming agents such as Normacol or Fybogel. Enemas or suppositories were used only after abdominal examination. Diet was changed to include high-fibre foods or the addition of bran. Stool size and frequency increased, consistency improved, soiling decreased and the use of artificial elimination aids was discontinued in all cases. Improved perception of the need to evacuate was demonstrated by the increased frequency of self-initiated toiletings.

Additionally, retraining of the gastrocolic reflex appeared to occur for three participants. Treatment times were, however, long, ranging from 56 to 132 weeks. Results also indicated a continuing, somewhat erratic pattern of bowel function. Smith et al, like Piazza et al, found little evidence to support a major role for artificial elimination aids in conjunction with a behavioural training approach.

Behavioural approaches to non-retentive encopresis

Six reports concern behavioural treatment of non-retentive encopresis in adults or children with learning disabilities (Chopra 1973, Lyon 1984, Marshall 1966, Matson 1977, Smith 1994, 1996).

Lyon (1984) reduced primary non-retentive encopresis to zero in 5 weeks in an 8-year-old boy with a mild learning disability, using praise and rewards for cleanliness and appropriate evacuation and 'correction' for soiling. Treatment involved four daily underwear checks, with praise and stickers for cleanliness and appropriate toilet use, stickers being exchanged for individual staff time. 'Correction' for soiling involved assuming responsibility for cleaning and changing himself and washing soiled clothing. Results showed that frequency of encopresis reduced from eight episodes in 10 baseline days to zero by the end of 20 days' intervention.

Smith (1994) describes the successful treatment of non-retentive, nocturnal encopresis in a 21-year-old, non-ambulant woman with a hemiplegia and a severe learning disability, who was soiled and smeared between four and seven times a week when her mother entered her bedroom in the morning; she never defecated continently. Soiling appeared to occur around 6.30 am, but when no soiling took place, no stool was passed until the following morning. The programme initially involved waking the client at 6.30 am and attempting to 'catch' and reward a bowel movement on the toilet. However, although this procedure was carried out on two mornings, no stool (either continent or incontinent) was passed. As this could have led to retention, one suppository was administered before breakfast if she failed to defecate of her own accord when toileted at 6.30 am. While this would afford her the opportunity to defecate unaided, should she fail to do so the use of a suppository should serve to increase the urge to defecate, increase the chance of continent evacuation after breakfast and help to condition a gastrocolic reflex in association with eating breakfast. Suppositories were administered for three mornings, after which the client began to defecate continently without their use, sometimes before and sometimes after breakfast. By week 24, she had achieved 4 consecutive clean weeks. After a further 8 weeks, time of waking was gradually shaped back to normal. Punishment techniques for soiling were not used. Rewards included a choice of small edibles from a 'goody' bag.

Smith (1996) used praise and edible rewards for clean pants and appropriate toilet use in the successful treatment of primary non-retentive encopresis in five males between the ages of 18 and 37 years, four of whom had severe learning disabilities. The participants were prompted to the toilet and sat for 10 minutes after each main meal or snack in the hope that an association might develop between the gastrocolic reflex, defecation and the toilet. In addition, underwear was checked at set points throughout the day: on waking, before leaving home, on arrival at school or day centre, mid-morning, before and after lunch, mid-afternoon, before transport home, on arrival home, after tea and before bed. Soiling was briefly drawn to the attention of the participants and minimum assistance given for cleaning and changing. Punishment techniques were not used. Large soilings reduced to zero over periods ranging from 44 to 144 weeks. Underwear checks and rewards were gradually phased out. Stainings or very small bowel accidents continued to occur in some cases.

Long-term maintenance

Huntley & Smith (1999) followed up nine out of ten cases of successful treatment for retentive or non-retentive encopresis reported by Smith (1994, 1996) and Smith et al (1994). Results showed that treatment effects had largely endured over periods ranging from 5 to 17 years. Six of the nine were free of major soiling accidents, although one continued to have minor stainings in connection with imperfect wiping. Of the three still experiencing major soiling accidents, one had relapsed completely a few weeks prior to follow-up after remaining continent for 8 years, in association with a major deterioration in physical health; one experienced one full-sized soiling in 21 consecutive days, but also passed 22 continent stools; and one had experienced a partial relapse which had already responded to retraining, and was currently averaging one soiling per 2 months. Of interest and perhaps surprisingly, those whose encopresis was previously retentive in nature maintained more successfully than those with previously non-retentive encopresis.

OTHER TOILETING PROBLEMS

Not all continence problems are due to 'skills' deficits, that is to say, a simple failure to establish the link between bowel and bladder sensations and the toilet. Functional toileting problems include:

- urinating repeatedly in inappropriate locations such as against doors or in corners
- faecal smearing
- eliminating only under highly specific circumstances such as into an incontinence pad/nappy
- fear or avoidance of toilets other than one specific toilet, usually that at home
- failing to pass urine on the toilet but then passing urine shortly after coming off the toilet
- urinating messily around the toilet.

Some of these behaviours are better explained in terms of anxiety-related or challenging behaviour rather than a lack of continence skills as such. In these cases, the approach should initially involve a functional analysis, as with any challenging behaviour, in order to elucidate the function, purpose or meaning of the behaviour before attempting to change it.

Urinating repeatedly in inappropriate locations

The function or purpose of behaviour is an important issue when considering some of the more unusual toileting behaviours which present in the field of learning disability. It is widely assumed that the main purpose of micturition is simply to discharge urine clear of the skin. This is only part of the story, however, for a major function of passing urine in mammals is scent marking, the function of which is chemical communication. All mammals scent mark and the commonest medium is urine. Dogs, for example, can lift their legs and deposit a small amount of urine on prominent objects in the environment in excess of one hundred times in an hour, a phenomenon which contrasts markedly with a simple waste discharge function of micturition, but is familiar to anyone who takes a dog for a walk. Scent marking using urine is also evident

in primates. None of this is to suggest that we are treating people as animals or with disrespect. The point is, it is important to remember that humans are animals too, that it is important to try to understand the meaning of behaviour in this taboo area, and that our behaviour is rooted in a lengthy evolutionary history.

Scent marking and chemical communication in animals has a large and complex body of literature (Eisenberg & Kleiman 1972, Rolls 1971). The question that arises is whether scent marking occurs in humans. Although there is no definitive evidence, studies bearing on this issue are discussed by Smith & Smith (1987).

Scent marking requires the ability to differentiate the scent of one's own urine. Smith (1988, 1989) describes a young man with a profound learning disability and incontinence, whose habit it was to wet and then sniff his clothing, despite being able to pass urine on the toilet.

As illustrated in Figure 10.7, when presented with samples which included his own urine, an artificial control urine of the type used in standardizing pregnancy tests, water, ammonia solution

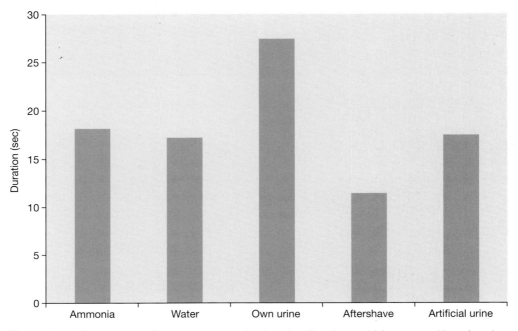

Figure 10.7 Discrimination of own urine: mean duration of sniffing (seconds) for a man with profound learning disabilities.

and aftershave lotion, he showed a marked and statistically significant preference for sniffing his own urine.

KEY POINTS: URINATING IN INAPPROPRIATE LOCATIONS

Where bowel or bladder accidents occur repeatedly in particular locations despite ability to use the toilet:

- reward elimination into the toilet in order to increase motivation for continent elimination
- record accidents and, if these can be predicted from body postures, locations or times of the day, divert to the toilet at these times and reward continent elimination
- consider the possibility of scent marking and introducing an acceptable scent to replace the inappropriate use of urine (Siegel 1977, Smith 1988, 1989).

Faecal smearing

Faecal smearing is found in a small number of people with severe learning disabilities, although its prevalence and aetiology are not well established. A number of factors may be associated with faecal smearing, including sensory play, deprivation, boredom or protest. Faecal smearing can, however, also be seen in favourable living situations. An example is provided here of faecal smearing in a man with a profound learning disability in his early 50s, who had been resettled in a small residential home. Having lived most of his life in a large institution, he had a long history of obsessional and ritualized toileting behaviours including smearing faeces after bowel movements. Functional analysis (e.g. Emmerson 1998) of such behaviours may suggest a relationship to anxiety reduction and the demarcation of personal space. For example, a treatment plan to help an institutionalized middle-aged man with a profound learning disability to feel secure about his new community placement was designed to make toileting a relaxing and pleasant experience, and to reward both continent bowel movements and the absence of smearing after defecation. This resulted in a marked reduction in his faecal smearing over a period of months (Fig. 10.8).

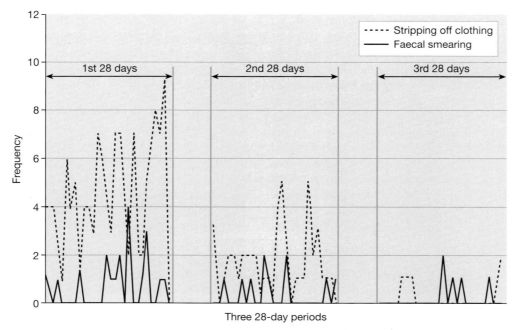

Figure 10.8 Challenging toileting behaviours: reduction in stripping off clothes and in faecal smearing at toilet, over three 28-day periods, in a 52-year-old man with profound learning disabilities.

Transfer of stimulus control

Where a child or adult will urinate/defecate only under specific conditions such as into a nappy or incontinence pad, elimination is said to be under the stimulus control of the pad. Thus, elimination (the response) is stimulated (i.e. is under the control of) by the sensation of the nappy rather than cues associated with the toilet. Quite often such behaviour may be associated with the presence of obsessional behaviours such as are commonly found in autism and fragile X syndrome. In these cases, the solution is to gradually transfer control from the pad to the toilet (Smith et al 2000, Taylor et al 1994). This is done initially by rewarding elimination into the pad, then rewarding elimination into the pad progressively closer to the toilet until the trainee can eliminate into the pad while sitting on the toilet. Finally, either a hole of increasing size is cut in the crotch of the pad, or the pad is more gradually dismantled by progressively removing the wadding and then cutting strips of the outer edges, until elimination takes place without a pad. An example of such change of stimulus control from pad to toilet in six stages is given in Figure 10.9.

Avoidant paruresis

Avoidant paruresis refers to the inability or extreme reluctance to use toilets other than one particular toilet, usually that at home. It is deemed to be anxiety based and associated with body shyness. There are no reports of paruresis in people with autism or learning disability. Paruresis is common in the general population, where techniques of treatment include those commonly used to treat phobic anxiety such as paradoxical intention and *in vivo* desensitization (Jaspers 2001, McCracken & Larkin 1991, Timms 1985, Watson & Freeland 2000).

Wetting shortly after coming off the toilet

This is a common phenomenon. If the client is in the middle years of life or this is a problem of

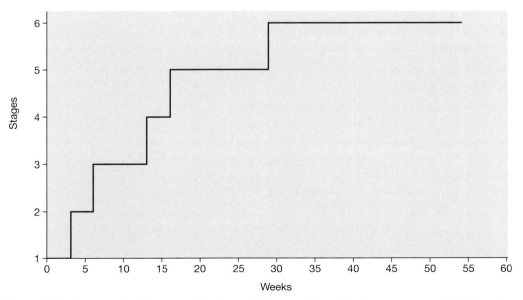

Figure 10.9 An example of change in stimulus control from pad to toilet in six stages in one child. Stage 1 is eliminating in a pad and, following progression through intermediate stages, stage 6 is eliminating into toilet without a pad. (After Smith et al 2000.)

recent onset, refer for consideration of the possibility of stress or urge incontinence.

Assuming that this is a skills deficit or behavioural issue, baseline recording of incontinence should be carried out for 2 weeks.

Where accidents are occurring shortly after unsuccessful prompts to toilet, the client may be trying to perform but in doing so is tensing the wrong muscle groups and inhibiting passing urine.

Take the emphasis off passing urine on the toilet by occupying the client while on, or close to the toilet, in order to encourage relaxation and diversion from the purpose. Do not leave and come back later to check on performance. Play, read, sing or tempt with a favourite activity or even favourite food. When relaxed, the probability is that urine will be successfully passed.

Urinating messily around the toilet

This is a common problem in males in the general population as well as those in the field of learning disability. It concerns standing to pass urine at the toilet but not directing the urine stream accurately. Research has shown that males have a natural tendency to direct the urine stream at objects (see discussion of scent marking in mammals). One solution is to float a target in the toilet. A table tennis ball painted half red, and which spins when hit, is ideal and will not flush away. Whether the problem is due to poor motor control or to poor motivation, this device, which has been empirically validated by Siegel (1977), will greatly improve accuracy.

KEY POINTS FOR PRACTICE

- The origin of many continence problems in learning disability can be complex; there is a need to understand the underlying functions and relationship of these to the evolution of human toileting behaviour.
- Although less attention has been paid to continence problems in people with learning disabilities, a great deal can be done to promote continence in this client group.
- There is much in the broader continence literature that is relevant to the field of learning disability.
- Carers' beliefs about the causes of incontinence in people with severe and profound intellectual disability may determine whether a management or a training approach is taken.

- Despite the fact that continence remains a major area of need in the field of learning disability, it is noteworthy that interest in this problem has declined since the major advances of the 1960s and 1970s. The emerging work of Duker and colleagues is therefore of potentially great interest (Averink et al 2000, Duker et al 2001).
- Treatment studies tend to be small samples and there is a need to progress to larger, controlled trials.
- Ethical issues must always be considered when caring for or supporting clients who are unable to consent to treatment. People with learning disabilities, as with other disabled client groups, have the right to treatment to enable them to achieve as much independence as possible through validated, non-punitive teaching strategies. Continence training should be a positive experience for all concerned.

REFERENCES

Agnarsson U, Warde C, McCarthy G, Clayden G S, Evans N 1993 Anorectal function of children with neurological problems II: cerebral palsy. Developmental Medicine and Child Neurology 35: 903–908

Averink M, Melein L M, Duker P C C 2000 Het gebgruik van response restriction voor zindelijkheidstraining. In: Duker P C C (ed) Handelingsstrategieen bij enuresis und encopresis. Bohn Staflau Van Loghum, Houten

Azrin N H, Foxx R M 1971 A rapid method of toilet training the institutionalised retarded. Journal of Applied Behaviour Analysis 4: 89–99

Barton E S 1975 Behaviour modification in the hospital school for the severely subnormal. In: Kiernan C C,

Woodford F P (eds) Behaviour modification with the severely retarded. Associated Scientific Publishers, Amsterdam

Baumeister A, Klosowski R 1965 An attempt to group toilet train severely retarded patients. Mental Retardation 3: 24–26

Bellman M M 1966 Studies on encopresis. Acta Paediatrica Scandinavica 56(Suppl. 170): 1–151

Bettison S 1978 Toilet training the retarded: analysis of the stages of development and procedures for designing programmes. Australian Journal of Mental Retardation 5: 95–100

Bettison S 1982 Toilet training to independence for the handicapped. C Thomas, Springfield, Illinois

Bettison S, Davison D, Taylor P, Fox B 1976 Long-term effects of a toilet training programme for the retarded. Australian Journal of Mental Retardation 4: 28–35

Blackwell C 1991 Investigation into the acquisition of nocturnal enuresis. Enuresis Resource and Information Centre Annual Conference, Bristol

Bosch J D 1988 Treating children with encopresis and constipation: an evaluation by means of single case studies. In: Emmelkamp P, Everaerd W, Kraimat F R, van Son M J M (eds) Advances in theory and practice in behaviour therapy. Swets & Zeitlinger, Amsterdam

Bower W F, Moore K H, Shepherd R, Adam R 1996 An epidemiological study of enuresis in Australia. In: Norgaard J P, Djurhuus J C, Hjalmas K, Hellstrom A-L, Jorgensen T M (eds) Proceedings of the Third International Children's Continence Symposium. Wells Medical, Tunbridge Wells

Brazelton T B 1962 A child oriented approach to toilet training. Pediatrics 29: 121–128

Buchan L, Chow S, Stoddart A 1989 A one-year continence project for people with mental handicaps. Mental Handicap 17: 162–167

Burgio L D, Engel B T, Hawikins A et al 1990 A staff management system for maintaining improvements in continence with elderly nursing home residents. Journal of Applied Behaviour Analysis 31: 111–118

Butler J F 1976 Toilet training success after reading 'Toilet training in less than a day'. Behaviour Therapy 7: 185–191

Capra S M, Hannan-Jones M 1992 A controlled dietary trial for improving bowel function in a group of training centre residents with severe or profound intellectual disability. Australian and New Zealand Journal of Developmental Disabilities 18: 111–121

Carpenter S 1989 Development of a young man with Prader-Willi syndrome and secondary functional encopresis. Canadian Journal of Psychiatry 34: 123–127

Chopra H D 1973 Treatment of encopresis in a mongol with operant conditioning. Indian Journal of Mental Retardation 6: 43–46

Dalrymple N J, Angrist M H 1988 Toilet training a sixteen year old with autism in a natural setting. British Journal of Mental Subnormality 34: 117–129

Dalrymple N J, Ruble L A 1992 Toilet training. Journal of Autism and Developmental Disabilities 22: 265–270

Dawson P M, Griffith K, Boeke K M 1990 Combined medical and psychological treatment of hospitalised children with encopresis. Child Psychiatry and Human Development 20: 181–190

Dayan M 1964 Toilet training retarded children in a state residential institution. Mental Retardation 2: 116–117

De Silva P, Deb S, Drummond R D, Rankin R 1992 A fatal case of ischemic colitis following long-term use of neuroleptic medication. Journal of Intellectual Disability Research 36: 371–375

DHSS 1972 Census of mentally handicapped people in hospital in England and Wales at the end of 1970. Statistical and Research Report, Series 3. HMSO, London

Didden R, Simone P E, Sikkemam S P E, et al 2001 Use of a modified Azrin–Foxx toilet training procedure with individuals with Angelman syndrome. Journal of Applied Research in Intellectual Disabilities 14: 64–70

Dixon J, Smith P S 1976 The use of a pants alarm in daytime toilet training. British Journal of Mental Subnormality 22(2): 20–25

Doleys D M, Schwartz M S, Ciminero A R 1981 Elimination problems: enuresis and encopresis. In: Mash E J, Terdal L G (eds) Behavioral assessment of childhood disorders. Guilford Press, New York

Donald I, Smith R, Cruikshank J, Elton R, Stoddart M 1985 A study of constipation in the elderly living at home. Gerontology 31: 112–118

Duche D J 1973 Patterns of micturition in infancy: an introduction to the study of enuresis. In: Kolvin I, McKeith R C, Meadows S R (eds) Bladder control and enuresis. Heinemann, London

Duker P C C, Averink M, Melein L M 2001 Response restriction as a method to establish diurnal bladder control. American Journal of Mental Retardation 106: 209–215

Dunlap G, Koegel R L, Koegel L K 1985 Continuity of treatment: toilet training in multiple community settings. Journal of the Association for Persons with Severe Handicaps 9: 134–141

Eiberg H, Berendt I, Mohr J 1995 Assignment of dominant inherited nocturnal enuresis (ENUR1) to chromosome 13q. Nature Genetics 10: 354–356

Eisenberg J F, Kleiman D G 1972 Olfactory communication in mammals. Annual Review of Ecology and Systematics 3: 1–32

Emly M 1983 Abdominal massage. Nursing Times 89(3): 34–37

Emmerson E 1998 Working with people with challenging behaviour. In: Emmerson E, Hatton C, Bromley J, Caine A (eds) Clinical psychology and people with learning disabilities. Wiley, Chichester

Engel B T, Burgio L D, McCormick K A et al 1990 Behavioral treatment of incontinence in the long term setting. Journal of the American Geriatrics Society 38: 361–363

Fischer M, Adkins W, Hall L et al 1985 The effects of dietary fibre in a liquid diet on bowel function of mentally retarded individuals. Journal of Mental Deficiency Research 29: 373–381

Foxx R M, Azrin N H 1973 Toilet training the retarded: a rapid programme for day and night-time independent toileting. Research Press, Champaign, Illinois

Fritz G K, Armbrust J 1982 Enuresis and encopresis. Psychiatric Clinics of North America 5: 283–296

Gabel S 1981 Fecal soiling, chronic constipation and encopresis. In: Gabel S (ed) Behavioral problems in childhood: a primary care approach. Grune & Stratton, New York

Gesell A, Armatruda C S 1941 Developmental diagnosis: normal and abnormal child development. Harper, New York

Groves J A 1982 Encopresis. In: Hollis J H, Meyers C E (eds) Life threatening behaviour: analysis and intervention. American Association of Mental Deficiency Monograph 5, Washington DC

Hagglund R S 1965 Enuretic children treated with fluid restriction or forced drinking. Annales Paediatriae Fenniae 11: 84–90

Hellstrom P A, Jarvelin M R, Konturri M J, Huttunen N P 1990 Bladder function in the mentally retarded. British Journal of Urology 66: 475–478

Houts A C, Peterson J K 1986 Treatment of a retentive encopretic child using contingency management and dietary modification with stimulus control. Journal of Pediatric Psychology 11: 375–383

Hundziak M, Maurer R A, Watson L S 1965 Operant conditioning in toilet training of severely retarded boys. American Journal of Mental Deficiency 70: 120–124

Huntley E, Smith L 1999 Long term follow-up of behavioural treatment for primary encopresis in people with intellectual disability in the community. Journal of Intellectual Disability Research 43(6): 484–488

Hyams G, McCoull K, Smith P S, Tyrer S P 1992 Behavioural continence training in mental handicap: a ten year follow-up study. Journal of Intellectual Disability Research 36: 551–558

Jansson L M, Diamond O, Demb H B 1992 Encopresis in a multihandicapped child: rapid multidisciplinary treatment. Journal of Developmental and Physical Disabilities 4: 83–90

Jaspers J P 2001 Cognitive-behavioral therapy for paruresis: a case report. Psychological Reports 83: 187–196

Jenkins R G, Stable G 1971 Special characteristics of retarded children rated as severely hyperactive. Child Psychiatry and Human Development 2: 26–31

Kaplan B J 1985 A clinical demonstration of a psychobiological application to childhood encopresis. Journal of Child Care 2: 47–54

Kimbrell D L, Luckey R E, Barbuto P, Love J G 1967 Operation dry pants: an intensive habit training programme for severe and profound retardation. Mental Retardation 5: 32–36

Klauser A G, Flaschentraeger J, Gehrke A, Mueller-Lissner S A 1992 Abdominal wall massage: effect on colonic function in healthy volunteers and in patients with chronic constipation. Zeitschrift Fur Gastroenterologie 30: 247–251

Kobak M W, Jacobson M A, Sirca D M 1962 Acquired megacolon in psychiatric patients. Diseases of the Colon and Rectum 5: 373–377

Largo R H, Stutzle W 1977a Longitudinal study of bowel and bladder control in the first six years of life I: epidemiology and the interrelations between bowel and bladder control. Developmental Medicine and Child Neurology 19: 598–606

Largo R H, Stutzle W 1977b Longitudinal study of bowel and bladder control by day and night in the first six years of life II: the role of potty training and child's initiative. Developmental Medicine and Child Neurology 19: 606–613

Largo R H, Molinari L, von Siebenthal K, Wolfensberger U 1996 Development of bladder and bowel control: significance of prematurity, perinatal risk factors, psychomotor development and gender. European Journal of Pediatrics 158: 115–122

Largo R H, Molinari L, von Siebenthal K, Wolfensberger U 1999 Does a profound change in toilet training affect development of bowel and bladder control? Developmental Medicine and Child Neurology 38: 1106–1116

Leath J R, Flournoy R C 1979 Three year follow-up of intensive habit training program. Mental Retardation 8(3): 32–34

Liebl B, Fischer M, Van Calcar S, Marlett J 1990 Dietary fiber and long-term large bowel response in enterally nourished nonambulatory profoundly retarded youth. Journal of Parenteral and Enteral Nutrition 14: 371–375

Lohmann W, Eyman R K, Lask E 1967 Toilet training. American Journal of Mental Deficiency 71: 551–557

Lupson S, Walton D 1981 A trial of bran to relieve constipation in young mentally and physically handicapped patients. Apex 9: 64–66

Lyon M A 1984 Positive reinforcement and logical consequences in the treatment of classroom encopresis. School Psychology Review 13: 238–243

Madge N, Diamond J, Miller D et al 1993 The national encephalopathy study: a ten year follow-up. Developmental Medicine and Child Neurology 68(suppl.): 1–118

Madsen C H, Hoffman M, Thomas D R, Koropsak E, Madsen C K 1969 Comparison of toilet training techniques. In: Gelfand D M (ed) Social learning in childhood. Brookes-Cole, Pacific Grove, California

Marshall G R 1966 Toilet training of an autistic eight-year-old through conditioning therapy: a case report. Behaviour Research and Therapy 4: 242–245

Matson J L 1977 Simple correction for treating an autistic boy's encopresis. Psychological Reports 41: 802

Mattson S, Lindstrom S 1996 How representative are frequency volume charts? In: Norgaard J P, Djurhuus J C, Hjalmas K, Hellstrom A-L, Jorgensen T M (eds) Proceedings of the Third International Children's Continence Symposium. Wells Medical, Tunbridge Wells

McCallum G, Ballinger B R, Presly A S 1978 A trial of bran and bran biscuits for constipation in mentally handicapped and psychogeriatric patients. Journal of Human Nutrition 32: 369–372

McCoull G 1971 Newcastle-upon-Tyne Regional Aetiological Survey (Mental Retardation) 1966–1971. Northern Regional Health Authority, Newcastle

McCracken L M, Larkin K T 1991 Treatment of paruresis with in vivo desensitization: a case report. Journal of Behaviour and Experimental Psychiatry 22: 57–62

McGraw M B 1940 Neural maturation as exemplified in achievement of bladder control. Journal of Pediatrics 17: 580–590

Michel R 1999 Toilet training. Pediatrics in Review 20: 240–245

Miron N 1966 Behaviour shaping and group nursing with severely retarded patients: research monograph 8. Department of Health Hygiene, California

Parker G 1984 Training for continence among children with severe disabilities. British Journal of Mental Subnormality 30: 38–43

Pfadt A, Sternlicht M 1980 Clinical and administrative issues in the large scale implementation of the Azrin–Foxx self initiation training program. Paper presented at the AAMD Annual Meeting, San Francisco

Pfadt A, Sullivan K 1981 Issues in the generalization and long-term maintenance of the treatment gains achieved by the Foxx–Azrin self initiation training procedure. Paper presented at the Eastern Psychological Association Annual Meeting, New York

Piazza C C, Fisher W, Chinn S, Bowman L 1991 Reinforcement of incontinent stools in the treatment of encopresis. Clinical Pediatrics 30: 28–32

Read N W, Timms J M, Barfield L J, Donnelly T C, Bannister J J 1986 Impairment of defecation in young women with severe constipation. Gastroenterology 90: 53–60

Rittig S 1996 Enuresis research: current status and future prospects. In: Norgaard J P, Djurhuus J C, Hjalmas K, Hellstrom A-L, Jorgensen T M (eds) Proceedings of the Third International Children's Continence Symposium. Wells Medical, Tunbridge Wells

Rolls K 1971 Mammalian scent marking. Science 171: 443–449

Rosenthal M J, Marshall C E 1987 Sigmoid volvulus in association with Parkinsonism: report of four cases. Journal of the Geriatric Society 35: 683–684

Sadler O W, Merkert F 1977 Evaluating the Foxx and Azrin toilet training procedure for retarded children in a day training center. Behaviour Therapy 8: 499–500

Seim H 1989 Toilet training in first children. Journal of Family Practice 29: 633–636

Siegel R K 1977 Stimulus selection and tracking during urination. Journal of Applied Behaviour Analysis 10: 255–265

Singh N 1976 Toilet training of a severely retarded non-verbal child. Australian Journal of Mental Retardation 4: 15–18

Smeets P M, Lancioni G E, Ball T S, Oliva D S 1985 Shaping self-initiated toileting in infants. Journal of Applied Behaviour Analysis 18: 303–308

Smith L J 1994 A behavioural approach to the treatment of non-retentive nocturnal encopresis in an adult with a severe learning disability. Journal of Behaviour and Experimental Psychiatry 25: 81–86

Smith L J 1996 A behavioural approach to the treatment of non-retentive encopresis in adults with learning disabilities. Journal of Intellectual Disability Research 40: 130–139

Smith L J, Bainbridge R 1991 An intensive toilet training programme for a boy with a profound mental handicap living in the community. Mental Handicap 19: 146–150

Smith L J, Franchetti B, McCoull K, Pattison D, Pickstock J 1994 A behavioural approach to retraining bowel function after longstanding constipation and faecal impaction in people with learning disabilities. Developmental Medicine and Child Neurology 36: 49–57

Smith L J, Smith P S, Lee S K Y 2000 Behavioural treatment of urinary incontinence and encopresis in children with learning disabilities. Developmental Medicine and Child Neurology 42: 276–279

Smith P S 1979a A comparison of different methods of toilet training the mentally handicapped. Behaviour Research and Therapy 17: 33–43

Smith P S 1979b The development of urinary continence in the mentally handicapped. PhD thesis. University of Newcastle

Smith P S 1988 Can scent marking occur in humans? 18th Annual Meeting of the International Continence Society, Oslo

Smith P S 1989 Education, effets, environmentaux et ethologiques sur l'incontinence associes a un mental handicap. Premier Symposium International Approche Multidisciplinnaire de l'Incontinence de l'Adulte, Paris

Smith P S, Smith L J 1977 Chronological age and social age as factors in daytime toilet training of institutionalised mentally retarded individuals. Journal of Behaviour Therapy and Experimental Psychiatry 8: 269–273

Smith P S, Smith L J 1987 Continence and incontinence: psychological approaches to development and treatment. Croom Helm, London

Smith P S, Wong H 1981 Changes in bladder function during toilet training of mentally handicapped children. Behaviour Research and Severe Developmental Disabilities 2: 137–155

Smith P S, Britton P G, Johnson M, Thomas D A 1975 Problems involved in toilet training profoundly mentally handicapped adults. Behaviour Research and Therapy 15: 301–307

Spangler B F, Risley T R, Bilyew D D 1984 The management of dehydration and incontinence in non-ambulatory geriatric patients. Journal of Applied Behaviour Analysis 17: 109–112

Spencer R L, Temerlin M, Trousdale W W 1968 Some correlates of bowel control in the profoundly retarded. American Journal of Mental Deficiency 72: 879–882

Sroujieh A S 1988 Phytobezoars of the whole gastro-intestinal tract: report of a case and review of the literature. Dirasat 15: 103–109

Stern H P, Prince M T, Stroh S E 1988 Encopresis responsive to non-psychiatric interventions. Clinical Pediatrics 27: 400–402

Taylor S, Cipani E, Clardy A 1994 A stimulus control technique for improving the efficacy of an established toilet training program. Journal of Behaviour Therapy and Experimental Psychiatry 25: 155–160

Thomas T M 1986 The prevalence and health service implications of incontinence – a study in progress. In: Mandlestam D (ed) Incontinence and its management, 2nd edn. Croom Helm, London

Thomas T M, Egan M, Walgrove A, Meade T W 1984 The prevalence of faecal and double incontinence. Community Medicine 6: 216–220

Thompson T, Hanson R 1983 Overhydration: precautions when treating urinary incontinence. Mental Retardation 21: 139–145

Timms M W H 1985 The treatment of urinary frequency by paradoxical intention. Behavioural Psychotherapy 13: 76–82

Trott M C 1977 Application of the Foxx and Azrin toilet training for the retarded in a school programme. Education and Training of the Mentally Retarded 12: 336–338

Van Wagenen R K, Meyerson L, Kerr N J, Mahoney K E 1969a Field trials of a new procedure in toilet training. Journal of Experimental Child Psychology 8: 147–159

Van Wagenen R K, Meyerson L, Kerr N J, Mahoney K E 1969b Rapid toilet training: principles and prosthesis. Proceedings of the 77th Annual Convention of the American Psychological Association, pp 781–782

Vande Walle J, Theunis M, Renson C, Raes A, Hoebeke P 1995 Commercial television bladder dysfunction. Acta Urologica Belgica 63: 105–111

Von Wendt L, Simila S, Niskanen P, Jarvelin M-R 1990 Development of bowel and bladder control in the mentally retarded. Developmental Medicine and Child Neurology 32: 515–518

Watson T S, Freeland J T 2000 Treating paruresis using respondent conditioning. Journal of Behaviour Therapy and Experimental Psychiatry 31: 155–162

Weir K 1982 Night and day wetting among a population. Developmental Medicine and Child Neurology 245: 479–484

Williams F E, Sloop E W 1978 Success with a shortened Foxx–Azrin toilet training programme. Education and Training of the Mentally Retarded December: 399–402

Yeung C K, Godley M L, Ho C K W et al 1995 Some new insights into bladder function in infancy. British Journal of Urology 76: 235–240

Yoder J W 1966 Toilet training the profoundly defective patient at Greene Valley Hospital and School using an S–R reinforcement analysis. Mind Over Matter 11: 28–34

Young G C 1973 The treatment of childhood encopresis by conditioned gastro-ileal reflex training. Behaviour Research and Therapy 11: 499–503

11

Continence problems and neurological disability

Mandy Fader
Michael Craggs

'…from an electrician's point of view rather than a plumbers'

Clare J. Fowler 1999

INTRODUCTION

For people with neurological disorders urinary incontinence is unlikely to be an isolated problem. Difficulties in maintaining continence may be one of the many disabilities that require nursing services. For this reason nurses from a variety of specialties encounter people with neurological disorders, notably in the community, long-stay and respite care, outpatients, elderly care and of course neurological wards. Specialist referral to a continence advisor is often appropriate but there is much that can be done by any nurse with a thorough understanding of the effects that neurological damage can have on continence and the strategies that can be helpful. This chapter aims to provide such a background. It begins with a discussion of the physiological control of bladder and bowel function (see also Chapters 2 and 7) and the changes occurring with neurological disability.

NEURAL CONTROL OF THE BLADDER

Babies are oblivious to their bladders. The baby's bladder fills and then voids as a result of a spinal reflex. Conscious control occurs as the nervous system matures and this reflex can then be inhibited (to 'hold on') or facilitated (to pass urine). Bladder function is therefore partly a conscious activity (normally we can pass urine when we want to) and partly unconscious (the bladder stores urine, whether we like it or not). This requires the interaction of voluntary (somatic) and involuntary (autonomic) aspects of the nervous system.

Bladder and urethral structure

The bladder is made of smooth muscle (detrusor) arranged in spiral, longitudinal and circular bundles. In common with most other visceral organs, this muscle is involuntary and is innervated by the autonomic nervous system.

The urethral sphincter comprises striated (voluntary) muscle and has somatic innervation. The striated muscle of the urethral sphincter is isolated from the pelvic floor and extends along the length of the urethra in women and is distal to the prostate in men (Dixon & Gosling 1987). This muscle is composed of 'slow twitch' fibres and is held in tonic contraction except when micturition occurs.

Detrusor innervation

The detrusor is supplied by both divisions of the autonomic nervous system: the parasympathetic and the sympathetic. The role of the sympathetic nervous supply to the bladder is unclear (Kirby et al 1986); it does not seem to be essential for micturition, but may play a part in maintaining urethral closure (De Groat & Steers 1988). It is the parasympathetic supply that seems to be all-important. The efferent (or motor) parasympathetic neurones arise from the spinal cord between segments S2 and S4 and reach the bladder via the pelvic nerve plexus (Fig. 11.1). The main neurotransmitter released by parasympathetic fibres is acetylcholine, although multiple transmitters have been isolated in the autonomic ganglia (Lincoln & Burnstock 1993).

Afferent (or sensory) parasympathetic supply arises not from sensory receptors but from bare fibre endings in the bladder wall (Gosling et al 1983). This sensory supply is transmitted to the spinal cord along the pelvic nerves (see Table 11.1).

Urethral sphincter innervation

The pudendal nerve conveys motor and sensory impulses to and from the striated muscle of the

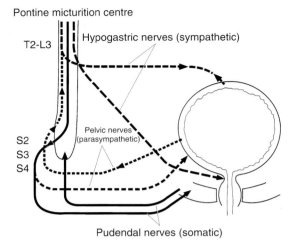

Figure 11.1 Innervation of the detrusor and urethral sphincter. Adapted from 'Objective: Continence' (Teaching Resource) with permission of Coloplast Ltd (1989).

Table 11.1 Comparison of neural control of the detrusor and urethra

	Detrusor	Urethral sphincter
Muscle type	Smooth muscle (involuntary)	Striated muscle (voluntary)
Innervation	Autonomic	Somatic
Nerve supply	Pelvic nerve	Pudendal nerve
Cord segments	S2–S4	S2–S4

urethral and anal sphincters. The anterior horn cells of the motor neurones are grouped together in a nucleus in the ventral horns of the sacral spinal cord at S2, S3 and S4 (Fig. 11.1). This nucleus – called Onuf's nucleus – resembles the sacral parasympathetic nucleus with which it is closely associated. Other characteristics of Onuf's nucleus indicate that the cells are not typically somatic. In motor neurone disease somatic motor cells degenerate, but the cells of Onuf's nucleus are spared.

Central control of bladder function

Three main areas within the central nervous system control micturition: the cortical, the pontine and the sacral centres (Fig. 11.2).

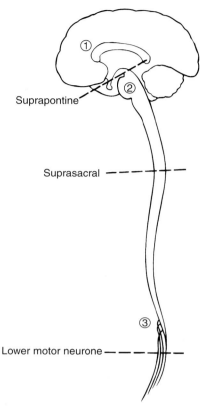

Figure 11.2 Micturition centres: (1) cortical, (2) pontine, (3) sacral. Reproduced with permission from Fowler & Fowler (1993).

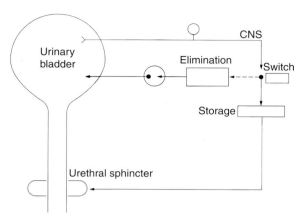

Figure 11.3 Neural 'switch' between storage and voiding proposed by de Groat (1994). Reprinted from de Groat WC (1994) by courtesy of Marcel Dekker. CNS, central nervous system.

De Groat suggests that during urine storage the low level of afferent (sensory) activity activates efferent (motor) input to the urethral sphincter. When the bladder is full and there is a high level of afferent activity the 'switch' is activated, producing firing in the efferent (motor) pathways to the bladder and inhibiting the efferent outflow to the sphincter. Thus, the bladder contracts, the sphincter relaxes and voiding occurs.

Cortical centre

Localized parts within the frontal lobes appear to have a role in inhibiting detrusor contractions; individuals with damage to these frontal areas have been found to develop *detrusor hyperreflexia* (Andrew & Nathan 1964).

Pontine centre

This area within the pons acts as an integration centre. It receives input from the cerebral cortex and coordinates detrusor contraction and urethral relaxation via a spinal–bulbar–spinal reflex. De Groat (1994) proposes that the pontine centre acts as a type of neural 'switch' between the two bladder functions of storage and voiding (Fig. 11.3).

Sacral centre

Spinal reflex mechanisms are not usually evident in adults, but they do mediate voiding in babies and in adults following spinal cord injury above the sacral segments. Voiding via the sacral spinal reflex is often incomplete owing to the failure of detrusor–sphincter coordination (*dyssynergia*), leading to outlet obstruction (the urethral sphincter contracts, rather than relaxes, when the detrusor contracts).

Bladder function: storage and voiding

Continence depends on the bladder being able to store urine without leakage. Three main mechanisms prevent leakage of urine from the urethra:

1. The urethral sphincter is held in tonic contraction so that the urethral pressure is

higher than the pressure within the bladder.

2. The detrusor actively relaxes so that a low pressure is maintained; this is known as *compliance*.
3. Detrusor contractions are inhibited while the bladder fills with urine. Inhibition of detrusor contractions during bladder filling requires unimpaired pathways between the pontine and sacral centres.

The sensation of bladder fullness is transmitted via sensory fibres in the bladder wall; these fibres are sensitive to stretch. In normal adults suppression of voiding is achieved via pathways from the cortical and pontine centres. When voiding is desirable, it begins by relaxation of the voluntary muscles of the pelvic floor and urethral sphincter followed by contraction of the detrusor. Effective voiding is dependent on the synchronization of bladder contraction and urethral relaxation and on sustained detrusor activity to ensure that the bladder is completely emptied (see also Chapter 2).

CONSEQUENCES OF NEUROLOGICAL DAMAGE

The type of continence problem experienced by an individual with neurological damage will depend on which area of the nervous system is affected. Broadly speaking, damage to the central nervous system (the brain and spinal cord, i.e. suprasacral and suprapontine) affects the upper motor neurones; damage to the peripheral nervous system (the pelvic and pudendal nerves) affects the lower motor neurones (Fig. 11.2). The effects on the bladder are similar to upper or lower motor neurone damage anywhere in the body. Upper motor neurone damage causes *spasticity* (too much muscle activity) and lower motor neurone damage causes *flaccidity* (too little muscle activity).

Suprapontine damage

Damage above the pons leaves the spinal–bulbar–spinal reflex intact. The integration of sphincter relaxation and detrusor contraction for voiding is therefore preserved but the inhibitory input

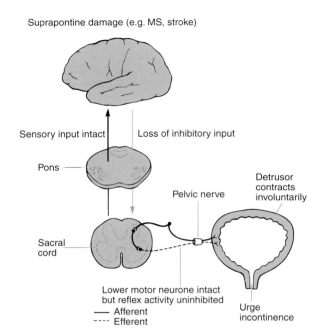

Suprapontine damage (e.g. MS, stroke)

Sensory input intact | Loss of inhibitory input

Pons

Detrusor contracts involuntarily

Pelvic nerve

Sacral cord

Lower motor neurone intact but reflex activity uninhibited
—— Afferent
---- Efferent

Urge incontinence

Figure 11.4 Detrusor hyperreflexia: mediation of the micturition reflex in the sacral cord. Adapted with permission from Popovich & Stewart-Amidei (1991).

to delay micturition may be lost or impaired. The result is an excess of reflex bladder activity, hence *detrusor hyperreflexia*. The person is aware of the need to pass urine but is unable to inhibit the bladder contraction. The consequences are frequency, urgency and possibly urge incontinence (Fig. 11.4).

Suprasacral damage

Lesions that occur above the sacral area and below the pons in the brainstem (suprasacral lesions) cause disruption to the spinal–bulbar–spinal reflex pathways. This results in the loss of the normally coordinated activity of the bladder and sphincter and is termed *detrusor–sphincter dyssynergia*. The urethral sphincter does not relax as the bladder contracts and voiding is obstructed. The bladder may then generate high pressures, which can result in ureteric reflux and renal damage, particularly in patients with traumatic or congenital spinal cord injury. Some urine may be passed if the detrusor contraction persists and the sphincter

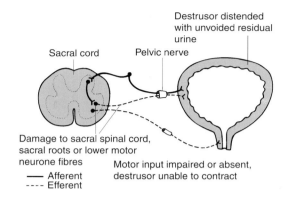

Figure 11.6 Detrusor areflexia. Adapted with permission from Popovich & Stewart-Amidei (1991).

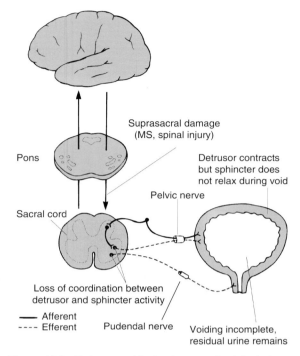

Figure 11.5 Detrusor–sphincter dyssynergia. Adapted with permission from Popovich & Stewart-Amidei (1991). MS, multiple sclerosis.

Box 11.1 Pathophysiological consequences of neurological lesions	
Suprapontine lesions	Detrusor hyperreflexia
Suprasacral lesions	Detrusor hyperreflexia Detrusor–sphincter dyssynergia Unsustained detrusor contractions
Sacral, cauda equina and pelvic nerve lesions	Detrusor areflexia or hyporeflexia (acontractile or hypocontractile detrusor)
Pudendal nerve lesions	Incompetent urethral sphincter

finally relaxes, but the bladder will often not empty completely (Fig. 11.5). In addition the detrusor may not be able to sustain contractions during voiding so that there is incomplete emptying of the bladder. Suprasacral lesions may also result in impairment of inhibitory input to the bladder resulting in detrusor hyperreflexia.

Pelvic nerve, pudendal nerve and infrasacral damage

Damage at and below the sacral spinal cord (i.e. to the cell bodies of the parasympathetic neurones or to the pelvic nerve) causes loss of motor supply to the bladder. The bladder becomes hypocontractile or acontractile (sometimes called *detrusor areflexia*, see Fig. 11.6) and cannot void effectively. When an attempt is made to pass urine the bladder does not empty properly and residual urine remains. Similarly if the pudendal nerve is damaged there may be loss of urethral sphincter muscle tone.

KEY POINTS: NEUROLOGICAL BLADDER PROBLEMS	
Functional problem	**Cause**
Failure to store	Detrusor hyperreflexia
Failure to empty	Detrusor areflexia Detrusor–sphincter dyssynergia Unsustained detrusor contractions
Combined storage/emptying failure	A combination of the above

Figure 11.7 shows the bladder and bowel consequences of damage to the nervous system at different sites; Box 11.1 outlines the pathophysiological consequences of neurological lesions.

Level of lesion	Neurological disease	Bladder dysfunction	Bowel dysfunction
Suprapontine 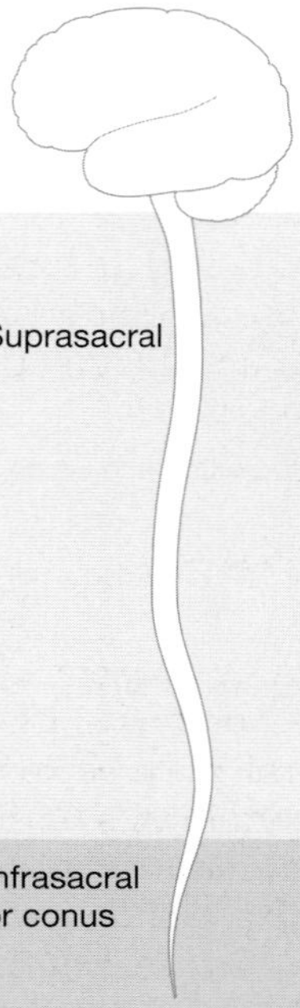	Dementia Parkinson's disease Cerebral vascular accident Cerebral tumour Cerebral palsy Shy-Drager syndrome	Inappropriate toilet behaviour Detrusor hyperreflexia with coordinated external sphincter and bladder neck activity Incontinence	Inappropriate toilet behaviour Incontinence Faecal impaction following immobility
Suprasacral	Multiple sclerosis Traumatic injury Compression (e.g. tumours, cervical spondolysis) Myelitis Spina bifida	Hyperreflexic with uncoordinated external sphincter and uncoordinated bladder neck if above T6 Sensory impairment Incontinence	High cord lesions – colonic mobility reduced and delayed colonic transit Low cord lesions – colonic mobility increased, reduced compliance, instability in rectum Loss of voluntary control over sphincters, pelvic floor and abdominal muscles Rectal prolapse Mixed incontinence
Infrasacral or conus	Sacral agenesis Cauda equina disease Pelvic surgery Childbirth injury Diabetes mellitus	Areflexic/underactive with denervated/underactive external sphincter but coordinated bladder neck Sensory impairment Incontinence	Weakness or loss of pelvic floor and sphincter muscle, voluntary control and spinal reflexes Rectal prolapse Impaired pelvic sensation Areflexic rectum Mixed incontinence

Figure 11.7 Pathophysiology of bladder and bowel function associated with neurological disease at different neuroanatomic sites.

NEURAL CONTROL OF THE BOWEL

As with urinary continence, faecal continence is dependent on the integration of the autonomic and somatic divisions of the nervous system. Peristaltic movements propel food throughout the stomach, small intestine and colon. These movements are controlled by the enteric nervous system of the gastrointestinal wall. Parasympathetic stimulation generally increases the rate of peristalsis whilst sympathetic stimulation has an inhibitory effect (see also Chapter 7).

Defecation

The rectum is usually empty of faeces. The juncture between the sigmoid colon and the rectum is sharply angled (normally 60–105°) to form a flap valve and this prevents faeces from entering the rectum except following mass colonic movements.

The internal sphincter is composed of smooth muscle innervated by motor neurones of the autonomic nervous system which are tonically active. The external sphincter is composed of striated muscle and is under reflex and conscious control. Like the urethral sphincter muscle, the motor neurones that supply these muscles have their cell bodies in Onuf's nucleus and are also tonically active.

Rectal filling and distension result in a transient fall in internal anal sphincter tone. As the rectal volume increases the internal anal sphincter continues to relax until there is a very low resting tone (when the rectum is full). This is known as the *rectoanal inhibitory reflex*. As this reflex is invoked there is an increase in the activity of the external anal sphincter. This increases with rectal filling and is augmented by conscious efforts.

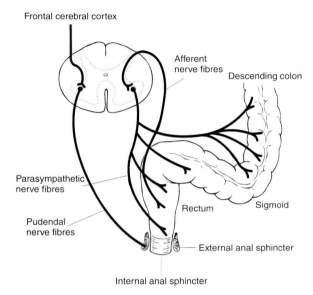

Figure 11.8 Innervation of the lower bowel. Adapted with permission from Popovich & Stewart-Amidei (1991).

Adoption of the squatting position straightens the anorectal angle and voluntary relaxation of the external anal sphincter allows defecation to commence, assisted by raised intra-abdominal pressure caused by straining. Conscious control is not, however, essential for defecation. High rectal volumes ultimately trigger inhibition of the striated sphincter muscle and a sacral reflex results in defecation, even without the assistance of straining (Mathers 1992). Figure 11.8 shows the innervation of the lower bowel and Figure 11.9 shows storage and voiding of faeces.

Consequences of neurological damage

Diseases of the central nervous system are unlikely to have any direct effect on bowel function (although conscious control may be lost), except when the sacral spinal cord (levels S2–S4) is involved. Provided the spinal reflexes remain intact defecation can occur. If the pudendal neurones are damaged then there may be external anal sphincter weakness which can result in faecal incontinence. Waldron et al (1993) found that in women with multiple sclerosis and faecal incontinence, external anal sphincter function was markedly impaired when compared with

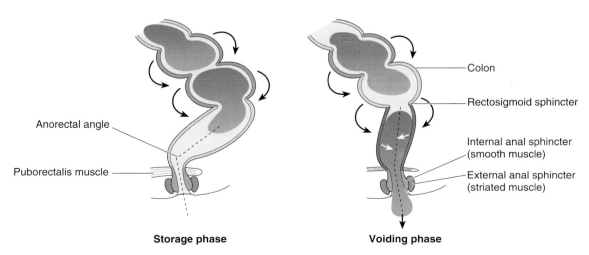

Figure 11.9 Control of the anorectum during continence (storage) and defecation (voiding). Reproduced with permission from Craggs & Vaizey (1999).

controls. If the pelvic nerve is damaged then there may be loss of stool propulsion and difficulty with evacuation.

SPECIFIC NEUROLOGICAL DISORDERS AND BLADDER AND BOWEL DYSFUNCTION

The broad categories of bladder and bowel dysfunction described above outline the basic principles behind neurogenic bladder problems. To a large extent it is more important to consider the site (or sites) of neurological damage rather than what type of disease or disorder the person has. However, the effects that four common neurological disorders have on continence will now be considered in a little more depth.

Multiple sclerosis (MS)

Urinary problems

Urinary problems are a common feature of multiple sclerosis, occurring in up to 90% of people at some time during the course of their disease (McGuire & Savastano 1984). For some people urinary symptoms may occur early on in the disease, or may indeed be the first symptom. More rarely, bladder function is spared despite severe neurological deficits. Overall, bladder dysfunction has been found to correlate well with lower limb deficits (Betts et al 1993); therefore paralysis of the legs is often accompanied by deteriorating bladder function.

Multiple sclerosis is characterized by plaques of demyelinated tissue which can occur anywhere in the central nervous system; pathways to and from the bladder may therefore be disrupted at any level. Detrusor hyperreflexia has been found to be the most common problem: studies reporting urodynamic findings have found a frequency of 52–91% (Betts et al 1993, Schoenburg et al 1979) and this may be complicated by dyssynergia causing bladder emptying problems. Recently Gallien et al (1998) examined a cohort of 149 patients with MS and urinary symptoms and confirmed that detrusor hyperreflexia and detrusor–sphincter dyssynergia were the main

dysfunctions. Hyporeflexia or areflexia seems to occur less frequently and is likely to be the result of demyelination at the sacral (S2–S4) levels of the spinal cord.

Bowel problems

A high prevalence of bowel problems associated with MS has been reported. Constipation has been reported in 36–53% of patients with MS (Chia et al 1995, Hinds et al 1990, Sullivan & Ebers 1983) and faecal incontinence in around 50%. The spinal pathway for defecation is very close to the pathways for micturition, and if spinal cord disease is an important causative factor in bowel disorders the prevalence of bowel problems might be expected to be higher in patients who have bladder dysfunction than in unselected people with MS. However, Chia and colleagues (1992) did not find that bowel symptoms correlated with urinary symptoms; the prevalence of bowel problems in patients with urinary problems was much the same as in unselected patients with MS.

Constipation and difficulty with defecation may be caused by loss of the coordinated activity of the pelvic floor (Chia et al 1992), but may also result from the use of constipating drugs such as anticholinergic medication. Loss of mobility is also very likely to contribute to or cause constipation in this group of patients and alterations in diet and fluid intake due to dysphagia may also play a part.

Faecal incontinence in MS patients may be caused by a variety of factors. There may be impairment of the external anal sphincter (Waldron et al 1993) or of the normal cortical inhibition of colonic motor activity resulting in high intracolonic pressures. Non-neurogenic causes such as obstetric trauma have also been identified in some women with MS (Swash et al 1987).

Associated disabilities

The bladder and bowel symptoms caused by MS are usually compounded by mobility and manual dexterity problems which make toileting access difficult and slow. Other problems such as visual disturbances and dysphagia may also contribute indirectly to continence difficulties.

The pattern and the progress of the disease are variable and problems with continence tend to increase with neurological and functional deterioration. The person with MS is therefore likely to require long-term continence support. Initially management strategies will aim at maintaining independence and will require considerable effort from the individual, such as learning bladder training or intermittent self-catheterization. As disabilities progress carers will often need to be involved and strategies will usually become more supportive – for example, either by carer-performed intermittent catheterization or the use of a long-term suprapubic catheter.

Stroke

Urinary problems

Incontinence has been reported to occur in 44–69% of people admitted to hospital after stroke (Henriksen 1991, Nakayama et al 1997). Incontinence after stroke has been found to be a strong predictor of death and poor outcome regarding general functional status, mobility, cognition and discharge destination (Anderson et al 1994, Brittain et al 1998, Di Carlo et al 1999, Taub et al 1994). Brocklehurst and colleagues (1985) found that about 40% of people regain continence during the first 2 weeks following the stroke. These authors found that 1 year later incontinence is still a problem for about 15% of people, but they point out that this is similar to that of the general elderly population. They suggest that incontinence is commonly a by-product of immobility and dependency rather than of neurological pathway damage.

Barer (1989) suggests that one of the reasons that the association between continence and good recovery is so strong is that continence is important for morale and self-esteem. Barer considers that continence may therefore be a very important goal of therapy. However, it is possible that persistent incontinence is an indicator of more profound neurological damage from which a good recovery is less likely.

Detrusor hyperreflexia seems to be the most common urodynamic finding (Khan et al 1990, Tsuchida et al 1983) in people who have had a stroke, but bladder emptying problems are also frequent. Garrett et al (1989) found that incomplete emptying occurred initially in more than half of 85 stroke patients in a rehabilitation centre and was sustained in about a third.

Whilst urinary incontinence is frequently caused by stroke, incontinence may have been a problem beforehand. Borrie et al (1986) reported that 17% of their patients already had incontinence before their stroke and Jawad & Ward (1999) found that premorbid incontinence was the most significant variable predicting poor functional outcome.

Bowel problems

Bowel function should remain unaffected following stroke although cortical inhibition of defecation may be impaired. Brocklehurst et al (1985) found that faecal incontinence occurred in 30% of stroke patients but this persisted in only two (3%) of the 65 stroke survivors when studied 12 months following stroke.

Constipation is the most likely bowel problem due to functional problems, in particular immobility. But other impairments such as aphasia, dysphagia, cognitive problems or mood changes may also indirectly affect bowel function.

Outcomes

Stroke often results in considerable impairment in the early days or weeks, followed by varying degrees of recovery. Regaining continence would seem to be a significant rehabilitation objective closely linked with regaining mobility and independence in other activities of living. Persistent urinary incontinence (6 weeks after stroke) will need further investigation and intervention and will usually involve strategies to improve detrusor hyperreflexia, sometimes accompanied by bladder emptying problems. Persistent faecal incontinence may be caused by constipation and faecal impaction or may be indirectly caused by other impairments such as severe cognitive or perceptual problems (Barrett 1993).

Parkinson's disease

Urinary problems

Estimates of the prevalence of urinary symptoms associated with Parkinson's disease have been complicated by difficulties in diagnosis. Parkinsonism can be caused not only by idiopathic Parkinson's disease (IPD), but also by multiple system atrophy (MSA). Multiple system atrophy involves the degeneration of certain areas of the nervous system including the motor nucleus of the urethral and anal striated sphincters (Onuf's nucleus). People with MSA generally have more severe incontinence, and in men this is almost always associated with erectile impotence (Beck et al 1994a). Denervation of the urethral sphincter can lead to stress incontinence in women, but in men urinary symptoms are similar to those of prostatic obstruction; surgery may therefore be undertaken but is ineffective (Beck et al 1994b). Sphincter electromyography (EMG) has been found to be valuable in the differential diagnosis of parkinsonism and abnormal sphincter EMG (Box 11.2) is commonly found in people with MSA (Eardley et al 1989). Chandiramani et al (1997) retrospectively studied the clinical features of 52 patients with MSA and determined that the urogenital criteria, which favour a diagnosis of MSA, are:

- urinary symptoms preceding or presenting with parkinsonism
- urinary incontinence
- a significant postvoid residual volume.

In IPD, detrusor hyperreflexia has been found to be the most common urodynamic finding and is probably secondary to degeneration in the basal ganglia. Sphincter EMG in these people is usually normal (Fitzmaurice et al 1985). Myers et al (1999) age matched 14 women with IPD with 28 control women who had urinary symptoms and found that those with IPD had an increased rate of detrusory hyperreflexia (93% vs 50%). Voiding dysfunction also occurs with IPD. Araki &

Box 11.2 Sphincter electromyography

Sphincter electromyography (EMG) is a method of examining the innervation of the striated muscles of the pelvic floor. A concentric needle electrode is inserted into the urethral or anal sphincter and motor unit potentials (electrical activity) are recorded. The duration of each motor unit is measured. The average motor unit duration in normal subjects is about 6 milliseconds (Eardley et al 1989). Motor units of prolonged duration are indicative of denervation (and reinnervation). EMG may also be used as part of a urodynamic investigation to record sphincter activity during filling and voiding. It is particularly useful for the detection of detrusor–sphincter dyssynergia.

Kuno (2000) examined 203 consecutive patients with Parkinson's and found that 27% had symptomatic voiding dysfunction. These authors established that the degree of lower urinary tract symptoms was well correlated with the severity of the disease rather than with disease duration or age.

However, Malone-Lee and colleagues (1993) examined urodynamic data from Parkinson's, stroke and dementia patients together with normal age-matched controls and found that findings were similar. They conclude that urodynamic changes may be age related and not disease specific, and therefore dispute the existence of a disease-specific parkinsonian bladder.

Bowel problems

Constipation is the most frequently recorded problem. A recent study of patients with Parkinson's disease found that three-quarters of patients reported a bowel frequency of less than three evacuations per week and almost all patients (94%) reported hard stool and persistent laxative or enema use (88%) (Stocchi et al 2000). Constipation is likely to be caused by mobility and swallowing problems and gut transit times may be slower in people with Parkinson's disease. Haboubi et al (1988) found prolonged orocaecal transit times in elderly patients with Parkinson's disease compared with elderly patients without the disease and these slow transit times were confirmed by Edwards et al (1993).

Anorectal function using manometry was investigated in patients with MSA and IPD by Stocchi et al (2000). These researchers found that most manometric recordings disclosed an abnormal pattern during straining. However manometric patterns did not differentiate patients with MSA from those with idiopathic Parkinson's disease.

Associated disabilities

The movement disorders that characterize Parkinson's disease (rigidity, bradykinesia, tremor) have profound effects on toileting and the use of aids or devices. Incontinence may therefore be functional or combined with a bladder problem such as detrusor hyperreflexia.

Spinal cord injury

Urinary problems

The management of continence problems for patients with spinal cord injury (SCI) differs somewhat from those with progressive disease. Patients with spinal injury are usually younger and do not face the problem of increasing disability; however they are at higher risk of upper urinary tract damage. Patients with spinal injury will usually require life-long follow-up to monitor renal function and to ensure that continence is managed optimally.

The type of continence problem experienced will depend on the site of injury, with sacral lesions giving rise to detrusor areflexia with a flaccid bladder and sphincters. Suprasacral lesions mainly result in detrusor–sphincter dyssynergia and detrusor hyperreflexia. Thus the bladder is frequently overactive, but voiding is incomplete due to failure of the external sphincter to relax.

Immediately following spinal injury there is a period of 'spinal shock' when spinal reflex activity ceases. During this time (which may last from days to weeks) there is an absence of the usual bladder emptying mechanisms and the bladder must be drained to prevent overdistension. Although this may be achieved by intermittent

catheterization performed by staff, this is labour intensive and an indwelling catheter (either urethral or suprapubic) is commonly used during this time (Arnold 1999). Once reflex activity has reappeared then intermittent catheterization should be instigated to accomplish complete bladder emptying, although anticholinergic medication is likely to be necessary for continence if detrusor hyperreflexia is present. Some patients may benefit from other forms of long-term management and these methods are discussed under treatment options.

A specific problem for some people with SCI is the occurrence of autonomic dysreflexia whereby noxious stimulation (which includes such continence-related factors as catheterization, high bladder pressures or manual evacuation of the bowel) leads to mass sympathetic overactivity below the level of the injury. This causes sudden hypertension, pallor and sweating due to vasoconstriction. Care needs to be taken to check whether the patient has a history of any autonomic dysreflexia before undertaking investigations and procedures that may precipitate such an event and expert advice sought if necessary.

Bowel problems

Spinal injury to the cauda equina area of the sacral spinal cord may affect the lower motor neurones supplying the internal and external anal sphincters and the lower colon. Loss of lower colonic movements causes severe constipation, and faecal incontinence may occur due to lack of sphincteric muscle tone.

Suprasacral lesions will leave the lower motor neurones to the lower colon and anal sphincters intact but there will usually be a loss of voluntary control.

Spinal cord injury usually results in substantial bowel problems, with 11% reporting faecal incontinence weekly or more and only slightly more than a third (39%) declaring reliable continence of bowels (Glickman & Kamm 1996). A further survey of 424 people with paraplegia in Denmark showed that less than a quarter had a normal desire to defecate and more than half used digital stimulation to precipitate defecation

(Krogh et al 1997). A questionnaire sent to 90 spinal cord injury patients in Belgium indicated that 58% suffered from constipation (defined as two or fewer bowel movements per week) (De Looze et al 1998) whereas a study of 221 British patients showed this figure to be 42% (Menter et al 1997).

Associated disabilities

The presence or absence of good hand control is probably the most important determinant of bladder and bowel management. Patients with good hand control will be able to undertake intermittent catheterization for their bladders and digital stimulation for their bowels. The ability to transfer from wheelchair to toilet will also preserve independence in toileting activities. Higher lesions affecting upper limbs will inevitably result in much greater levels of dependence and bladder management is likely to take the form of an indwelling (preferably suprapubic) catheter with the regular use of carer-administered suppositories or enemas to initiate bowel activity.

DISABILITIES AND PROBLEMS THAT AFFECT CONTINENCE

Bladder and bowel problems may occur in isolation in people who have neurological disorders, but often the presence of other disabilities and problems contributes profoundly to the development of incontinence. Indeed continence can be difficult to achieve for some people with neurological disorders, primarily because of their disabilities rather than because of bladder or bowel dysfunction.

Mobility, movement and manual dexterity

Perhaps the most obvious consequence of many neurological disorders is loss of mobility due to paralysis, tremor, rigidity or gait disturbances. Getting to the toilet (or getting the toilet to you) is essential for continence. Loss of mobility may mean that the assistance of carers is essential or that walking aids are needed. The whole business of toileting can be a desperately slow affair and the presence of detrusor hyperreflexia (and therefore urgency) means that urge incontinence is a likely consequence.

Spasticity and contractures make the maintenance of an upright seating position on the toilet difficult or impossible; hip adductor spasticity, resulting in thighs that are 'locked' together, can make the use of a urinal impractical. In addition, contractures to hip adductors may mean that washing the perineum and inner thighs becomes a problem and personal hygiene and skin integrity can be compromised.

Loss of hand control due to tremor or weakness may mean that clothing adjustments for toileting are not possible and even the use of hand-held urinals requires assistance.

Communication, cognition and mental state

Dysarthria and dysphasia accompany many neurological disorders, such as stroke and Parkinson's disease. Loss of the ability to communicate verbally can delay or prevent assistance for toileting.

Mental disabilities may contribute to continence problems as much as physical disabilities. Disinhibition may be a consequence of frontal lobe damage, resulting in urine being passed in inappropriate places such as in a vase, or in public view. Confusion following head injury may affect recognition of the need to pass urine or the place to do so. Loss of motivation and depression may also influence the person's ability to respond to bladder cues and their desire (and ability) to undertake any rehabilitative programme to improve continence.

Constipation

Loss of mobility, alterations in diet and fluid intake, and medications mean that people with neurological problems are likely to become constipated. Constipation is believed to contribute to urinary incontinence in two main ways, either by the faecal mass pressing on the bladder and therefore provoking bladder contractions, or by obstructing voiding. There is, however, a lack of published evidence to support these assertions.

ASSESSMENT AND INVESTIGATIONS

Although many assessment tools have been developed for use by nurses, no specific tool exists for the assessment of neurologically impaired patients (Woodward 1995). However, despite the variety of bladder disorders that are caused by neurological problems, the treatment options available are limited and therefore assessment needs primarily to answer two main questions:

- Is there a failure of bladder emptying?
- Is there a failure of bladder storage?

Fowler & Fowler (1993) suggest that once this information is obtained the results of further urodynamic or other investigations are unlikely to influence management.

Investigations

Urodynamic studies

The problems of performing urodynamic studies on people with multiple disabilities can be considerable (Andrews 1994). It is probably reasonable to minimize the use of this investigation to those with complex problems in whom preliminary treatment is unsuccessful. However, if any invasive treatments such as surgery are contemplated it is particularly important to determine the nature of bladder emptying failure (i.e. whether it is caused by the sphincter not relaxing during voiding or whether the bladder is acontractile) and this is best accomplished using a video cystometrogram.

Investigation of the upper urinary tract (using, for example, intravenous urography or ultrasound) for signs of renal disease should be a priority, given the potentially life-threatening nature of renal damage (Fowler & Fowler 1993). The incidence of renal failure has been reported to be low in people with multiple sclerosis. Betts et al

(1993) found that only two of the 56 subjects in their study had evidence of upper urinary tract disease. But Blaivas & Barbalias (1984) found that dyssynergia in particular is likely to be associated with renal complications.

Measurement of residual volume

The simplest method of identifying if there is a failure of bladder emptying is to measure the postmicturition residual urine volume. This can be done by asking the patient to void and then passing a single-use 10 Ch catheter into the bladder and measuring the volume drained. More than 100 ml on repeated measurements is considered to be clinically significant and interventions to improve bladder emptying are usually required. A catheter specimen of urine should be taken at the same time to screen for urinary tract infection.

Single 'in and out' catheterization is (usually) a simple procedure, but it is nonetheless invasive and there has been a move towards the measurement of postmicturition residual urine with ultrasound. Portable ultrasounds are compact and simple to use and have been used successfully by nurses in various settings (Lewis 1995). For patients with MS, prediction of incomplete bladder emptying can be carried out reasonably accurately by the use of the Kurtzke Functional Systems Scale (Kirchof & Fowler 2000) (see Box 11.3). These authors concluded that unless the pyramidal (corticospinal) or bladder function components of the scale exceeded 1, bladder emptying problems are unlikely.

Decisions about the management of bladder symptoms based on measurement of

---

Box 11.3 The Kurtzke Functional Systems Scale

The Kurtzke Functional Systems Scale involves rating seven different functional systems: (i) pyramidal, (ii) cerebellar, (iii) brainstem, (iv) sensory, (v) bowel and bladder, (vi) visual (or optic) and (vii) cerebral (or mental). Each system is rated on a scale of 0–5 or 0–6. A score of 1 or less for either the pyramidal and/or the bowel and bladder system represents very mild impairment.

postmicturition residual volume have been presented as an algorithm by Holland (1994). Although this algorithm (Fig. 11.10) was designed for bladder management in MS, it can usefully be applied to other neurological patient groups.

History

A detailed history of urinary symptoms, including the presence of frequency, urgency and urge incontinence as well as voiding symptoms such

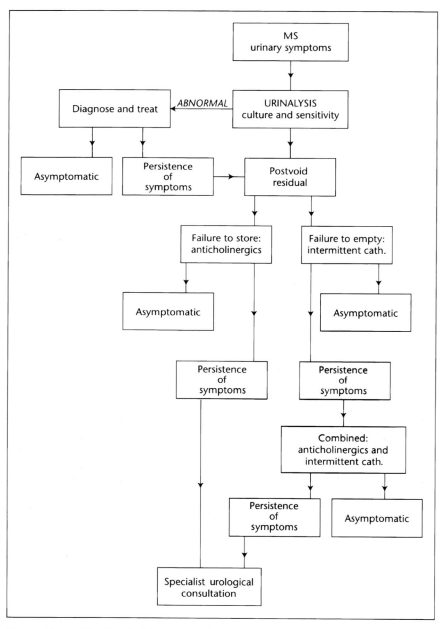

Figure 11.10 Algorithm for bladder assessment and treatment (Holland 1994).

as hesitation, poor stream, difficulty initiating or sustaining voiding, will often elicit the presence of storage and voiding problems. However, the frequency and urgency symptoms of detrusor hyperreflexia may also be caused or exacerbated by voiding problems and treatment of any voiding problem should therefore be initiated before or at the same time as treatment for detrusor hyperreflexia.

It is worth remembering that people with neurological disease may also have non-neurological causes of incontinence, such as prostatism or urethral sphincter incompetence. The history should also aim to help to identify or eliminate these problems as causes of incontinence.

Charting

The use of a continence chart or diary is invaluable to identify objectively the frequency of passing urine and episodes of incontinence. This information also provides a baseline from which to measure improvement once interventions have begun. Where possible, patients should be responsible for keeping their own chart, but cognitively impaired people may be unable to do so. In this case carers may be able to check pads hourly to record this information. If pads with wetness indicators are used it is possible to do this without having to 'feel' that they are wet.

Observations

Disabilities commonly associated with neurological disorders often have a severe effect on toileting (as described above), which may be a crucial factor in losing or gaining continence. Ouslander et al (1987b), having found a strong association between functional disability and incontinence in nursing home settings, suggested that a standard functional assessment of toileting skills is important. The extent and nature of disabilities are also likely to affect the implementation and success of management strategies.

Observation is usually the best method of assessing toileting problems: how the need to pass urine is communicated; how much assistance is needed to get to the toilet; what clothing is worn and how it is removed; how transfer on to the toilet is achieved; and problems with seating position on the toilet. The length of time this whole process takes also needs to be documented.

In the aforementioned study carried out by Ouslander and colleagues, an assessment tool called the 'performance-on-timed-toileting instrument' was used. It comprises a series of five tasks that simulate toileting, including: moving a distance of 5 metres (about 15 feet), transferring to a commode, unfastening a hook, unzipping a zipper on an apron-like garment and then pulling the garment off. The maximum time for all tasks was 195 seconds; maximum times for each task, in the order listed above, were 55, 55, 35, 25 and 25 seconds. Interrater reliability was found to be good. Although nursing home residents took part in this study, similar functional difficulties are found in neurologically impaired people.

INTERVENTIONS FOR URINARY INCONTINENCE

Finding the most acceptable and effective form of continence management for a person with neurological disorders is usually a question of compromise and balance. The best method for preserving renal function may not be the best method for managing continence. For people with static conditions (such as cerebral palsy, spinal injury or spina bifida) preservation of renal function should be a top priority, and emphasis needs to be placed on achieving effective bladder emptying (Fowler & Fowler 1993). For those with progressive disease, more emphasis is placed on reducing incontinence.

However, the importance of achieving continence needs to be balanced against the impact that the strategies used will have on the individual's independence and lifestyle. This will obviously vary from person to person; some people will accept great compromises in their lives if dryness can be achieved, whilst others will prefer to accept good management (without gaining continence) that interferes only minimally with the way they live. Different individuals will have different priorities and negotiation needs to take place in order that both the short-term and long-term needs are met and to achieve a compromise that is acceptable to the patient. The following interventions focus on the medical management of continence problems in neurological disability. Surgical management will be referred to briefly but a detailed discussion of surgical techniques is beyond the scope of this chapter.

Interventions and treatment for detrusor hyperreflexia

Bladder retraining

Bladder retraining is a safe and side-effect-free method for improving frequency, urgency and urge incontinence, although its value in patients with bladder overactivity, resulting from detrusor hyperreflexia rather than idiopathic detrusor instability, has yet to be demonstrated. Following completion of an initial baseline chart the patient is asked to increase the interval between voiding (usually by half an hour); progress is monitored and intervals are then increased gradually until frequency is reduced to 3–4 hourly and incontinence is improved or absent. Although the efficacy of bladder retraining for patients with neurological disease has not been established, this technique may be successful for those patients with mild symptoms. Bladder retraining is particularly valuable when used in conjunction with pharmacological treatments to help the patient monitor and decrease their urinary frequency.

Pharmacological treatment

Oral medications. Until recently oxybutynin was the principal drug in use for the treatment of detrusor hyperreflexia. Oxybutynin has an anticholinergic effect on detrusor muscle and functions by binding with muscarinic receptors, thereby inhibiting the action of acetylcholine and thus reducing the ability of the detrusor to contract. In addition, oxybutynin is a smooth muscle relaxant. In a randomized, multicentre trial of oxybutynin versus propantheline, involving 169 subjects, the efficacy of oxybutynin was found to be superior both on subjective and objective

(urodynamic) measurements (Thuroff et al 1991). Similar results were obtained from a smaller study of 34 patients with MS (Gajewski & Awad 1986). Combining oxybutynin with bladder retraining is likely to be particularly effective, allowing for increased patient participation and behavioural effects.

Unfortunately the side-effects of oxybutynin (and other anticholinergic drugs) can be very troublesome; dry mouth and constipation are common. Constipation can be severe, and for people with neurological disorders who are already likely to have constipation problems this can be intolerable. If treatment with oxybutynin is contemplated then pre-emptive action is essential, either by prescription of laxatives, dietary modification, suppositories or a combination of these. Any current bowel management regime will usually need to become more aggressive if constipation is to be avoided.

More recently other drugs to treat detrusor hyperrflexia have become available, mainly with claims of reduced side-effects. Tolterodine has been found to be as effective as oxybutynin in reducing frequency and symptoms of urgency, but with fewer side-effects (Appell 1997, Drutz et al 1999). Slow-release forms of oxybutynin and tolterodine have also become available. These aim to minimize side-effects and may well come to replace the traditional drugs. However, it is likely to be difficult to completely avoid side-effects in any anticholinergic drug absorbed through the gut given the wide distribution of cholinergic receptors throughout the body.

Intravesical medication. Therapeutic agents applied directly to the detrusor (intravesical medication) are promising alternatives to oral medication and are likely to hold the best hope of side-effect minimization. Oxybutynin chloride delivered directly into the bladder at frequent intervals (once to four times per day) has been found to be effective in studies of spinal cord injured patients (Pannek et al 2000, Vaidyanathan et al 1998) and children with static neurogenic bladder problems (Buyse et al 1998). However intravesical oxybutynin is not currently marketed.

Atropine is a potent anticholinergic and early studies of the intravesical use of this drug in MS patients show increased bladder volumes and decreased frequency (Fader et al 2001a). Atropine is widely available and the likelihood of future availability is therefore more optimistic. The main clinical use for intravesical therapy is for patients who are undertaking intermittent catheterization (usually for dyssynergia) but are experiencing frequency and/or incontinence between catheterizations due to hyperreflexia. Patients with a permanent catheter (see Chapter 9) who experience urinary leakage due to hyperreflexia have also been shown to benefit (Kim et al 1997).

A more long-lasting method of reducing detrusor hyperreflexia is the intravesical use of the neurotoxic agent, capsaicin – the pungent ingredient in chilli peppers. Capsaicin works by damaging sensory nerve endings – they fail to fire as the bladder fills and this moderates (or in some cases eliminates) detrusor activity (Fowler et al 1992a). The advantage is that the effect is relatively long-lived (3 weeks to 6 months has been reported; Fowler et al 1994), but the disadvantage is that it produces an irritative burning sensation in the bladder during installation. De Seze et al (1999) reviewed ten studies of capsaicin treatment and concluded that it was indeed effective for patients with neurogenic detrusor hyperreflexia but less so against detrusor instability. However, the effects of long-term treatment with repeated instillations are unknown. Resiniferatoxin is a capsaicin analogue which does not evoke the acute irritative symptoms during installation (Cruz 1998) and may be a more acceptable treatment for the future. Further developments in the intravesical route may hold the greatest hope in terms of finding an effective, simple and tolerable method of controlling detrusor hyperreflexia.

Other medication. Another approach to the treatment of detrusor hyperreflexia involves the use of desmopressin acetate (DDAVP), a synthetic antidiuretic hormone. Antidiuretic hormone causes less urine to be excreted by the kidneys and consequently the volume of urine in the bladder is reduced. Until fairly recently desmopressin was administered nasally only (it is inactivated in the gut), but this problem has now been overcome and oral tablets are also available. Desmopressin

has been used to control nocturia (passing urine frequently during the night) in particular. Eckford et al (1994b) studied 22 women and 11 men with multiple sclerosis and found that desmopressin caused a significant decrease in nocturnal urinary frequency and volume when compared with placebo. More recently Hoverd & Fowler (1998) showed that desmopressin acetate given during the daytime significantly decreases urinary frequency in patients with MS.

Neuromodulation

Neuromodulation in the form of sacral nerve stimulation has been used successfully for patients with spinal injury as a non-pharmacological method of controlling detrusor hyperreflexia. Neuromodulation describes the physiological process in which the influence of activity in one neural pathway modulates the pre-existing activity in another through synaptic interactions (Craggs & McFarlane 1999). The mechanism of neuromodulation is unclear but there is evidence from animal studies that stimulation of the pudendal afferents results in suppression of the pelvic efferent activity through a central inhibitory effect (Lindström et al 1983).

Sacral nerve stimulation using an implantable device (Fig. 11.11) is an established therapy and has been shown to suppress unstable contractions during urodynamic testing (Koldewijn et al 1994). A recent multicentred randomized controlled trial showed that sacral nerve stimulation markedly improved the quality of life of patients with urge incontinence (Siegal et al 1999). The Medtronic stimulator has been particularly successful in treating urinary retention caused by impaired relaxation of the striated muscle of the urethral sphincter (Fowler et al 1988) but in these cases the mechanism for the treatment is unknown. The disadvantage of this method is that it requires surgery to implant the device.

Magnetic stimulation using brief magnetic pulses to induce electric currents is an alternative and has the very considerable advantage of being able to reach deep into neural structures non-invasively (Fig. 11.12). Direct stimulation of the mixed motor and sensory sacral nerve roots

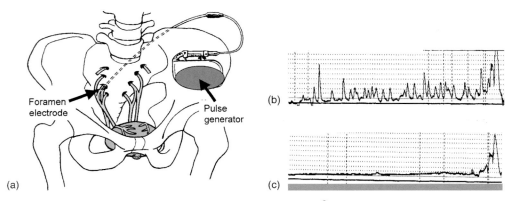

(a)

(b)

(c)

Figure 11.11 (a) Implantable stimulator (using the Medtronic Itrel® stimulator); (b) detrusor instability without stimulation; (c) with stimulation of the S3 sacral nerves.

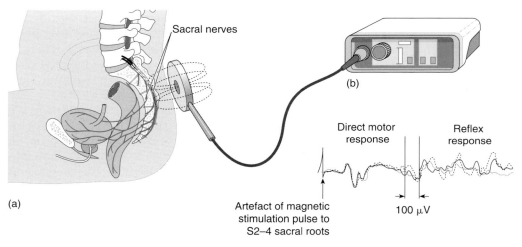

Sacral nerves

(b)

(a)

Direct motor response

Reflex response

Artefact of magnetic stimulation pulse to S2–4 sacral roots

100 μV

Figure 11.12 Functional magnetic stimulator. (a) Powerful magnetic stimulators with a coil over the sacrum can stimulate deep-lying spinal nerves without causing pain. (b) The neurophysiological record shows five superimposed traces of compound muscle action potentials recorded with electrodes near the striated urethral sphincter following five single pulses of stimulation to the S2–S4 nerve roots. (Reproduced with permission from *Urology News.*)

using high frequency magnetic stimulation has been found to inhibit bladder contractions in patients with detrusor hyperreflexia (Craggs et al 1995, Sheriff et al 1996) and detrusor instability (McFarlane et al 1997).

Currently, the size, weight and cumbersome nature of the present generation of magnetic stimulators do not permit easy portable use and their utility is therefore limited. A new generation of smaller, portable devices may make this treatment more practical and widely available.

Behavioural methods

Cognitive impairment may mean that the person does not recognize the need to pass urine and/or is not aware of the appropriate places where urine (or faeces) should be passed. Behaviour modification techniques (see Chapter 10) have been used extensively with people who have congenital neurological disabilities, but also to a lesser extent with people who have acquired neurological disorders in later life. Essentially the problems of learning appropriate toileting behaviour are likely to be similar for both groups. Grinspun (1993) describes a bladder management programme for adults following head injury which involves a behavioural approach based on positive verbal and non-verbal reinforcements. Stokes (1987) details a comprehensive programme based on ABC (antecedents, behaviour, consequences) which is designed for elderly people with dementia. There is, however, little research in this area to demonstrate that these methods are successful with people with other neurological problems and cognitive impairment.

A development that has attracted some attention fairly recently (although the concept is not new) is the 'buzzer': a device that detects urine and produces either a noise, a vibration or a flashing light. This can be used to alert the person (and carers) that urine is being passed. The person is then taken to the toilet to finish emptying their bladder and rewarded with praise. A chart is used to monitor progress and may be used as a further 'reward'. The aim is for the person to recognize the sensation of bladder fullness *before* urine is passed, communicate this need, delay micturition until the toilet is reached, and finally pass urine at the toilet.

Murphy et al (1994) suggest that this type of device has the potential for a number of other uses based on carers being alerted to incontinence episodes. Pads can be changed as soon as they are wet, which may be particularly important for people with skin problems, and individualized toileting can be established (by identification of the patient's usual voiding pattern). Accurate measurement of postmicturition residual volumes can also be made, a measure that can be hard to make accurately because of difficulty in establishing exactly when urine has been voided.

INTERVENTIONS FOR VOIDING PROBLEMS
Intermittent catheterization

Clean intermittent catheterization is the preferred intervention for people with neurogenic voiding problems. Intermittent catheterization has the potential to dramatically improve continence and reduce the likelihood of upper urinary tract problems by overcoming bladder emptying difficulties. Gray et al (1995) interviewed 150 spinal cord injured patients who were intermittently catheterizing after discharge and found that about 50% of the patients experienced no incontinence episodes at all and for those who *did* experience incontinence, this was only episodic in a further 50%.

The aim of intermittent catheterization is to remove the residual urine before the bladder is overdistended (<500 ml) and before incontinence occurs. This can usually be achieved without additional medication for people with detrusor areflexia (i.e. a bladder that does not contract due to lower motor neurone damage). For those with detrusor dyssynergia or combined storage and emptying problems (such as commonly occurs in MS or in SCI), a combination of anticholinergic medication and intermittent catheterization is often required (Fowler et al 1992b) and has been shown to be effective (Kim et al 1997).

Few studies have followed up patients using intermittent catheterization in the long term, but results have generally been encouraging. Kuhn et al (1991) followed up patients on long-term intermittent catheterization for 5 years and found that normal upper tract function was maintained and a low rate of urethral complications occurred. Weld & Dmochowski (2000) reviewed 316 patients with a mean of 18 years since injury (SD 12 years) using upper tract imaging and video urodynamics and categorized them according to method of bladder management (including clean intermittent catheterization and chronic urethral catheterization). The clean intermittent catheterization group had statistically significant lower complication rates compared to the chronic urethral catheterization group and the authors concluded that intermittent catheterization is the safest method of management in terms of urological complications.

Urine infection is not, however, eliminated using this method. Maes & Wyndaele (1988) reviewed 75 patients who carried out intermittent self-catheterization for a mean of 5 years 8 months (range 1–12 years) and found that 59% had chronic bacteriuria. Webb et al (1990) reported the results of 172 adults using intermittent catheterization and found the mean clinical infection rate to be 1 per 14 patient months.

Sterile intermittent catheterization seems to offer no advantage in terms of infection over clean intermittent catheterization, when performed in community settings (Moore et al 1993). Sterile practices for hospital and other residential settings are recommended to prevent cross-infections. Charbonneau-Smith (1993) reported that infection rates were nearly halved when a self-contained, sterile method (the O'Neil catheter) replaced the traditional sterile procedure used in a rehabilitation unit and similar results were reported by Prieto-Fingerhut et al (1997) when comparing sterile and non-sterile procedures.

Catheters with hydrophilic coatings have been introduced for intermittent catheterization to ease insertion and obviate the need for additional lubricant. Although there is some evidence that this type of catheter may reduce urethral trauma (Vaidyanathan et al 1994), substantial differences have been found between coated catheters in terms of their propensity to 'stick' to the urethra on removal (Fader et al 2001b). The long-term benefits of hydrophilic-coated catheters over conventional plastic catheters have yet to be demonstrated and the overall cost of their use is much higher because they cannot be reused.

Other types of catheter, which are short and rigid and made of plastic or metal, are available for women. These may be easier to manipulate and insert than the traditional flexible catheters.

Maintaining intermittent catheterization in the long term does seem to be a problem. Data from the US National Spinal Cord Injury Statistical Center indicate that, although 30% of patients discharged from rehabilitation units were performing intermittent catheterization, fewer than 5% were continuing to use this method 10 years later (Stover & Fine 1986).

The attrition rates for people with progressive disease are also likely to be high: as disabilities increase the procedure becomes more difficult. Devices such as a hip abductor or a catheter handle may help (Norton 1993) and permit independent catheterization for longer, but the procedure may eventually need to be performed by carers, which may be a further burden for some families. Patients and families of people with progressive disease need to be prepared for the possibility that intermittent catheterization may only be practicable for a limited (but often unknown) period of time. Alternative methods of management will possibly need to be considered in order to allow the person and the carer(s) more freedom. The effort and timing considerations of intermittent catheterization may eventually impinge on the patient's (or carers') ability to undertake other activities, and it is important to avoid becoming enslaved to the regime, particularly if other disabilities also compromise quality of life.

Sometimes it may be practicable to instigate a partial intermittent catheterization programme rather than stop catheterizing all together. Catheterizations may, for example, take place only first thing in the morning and last thing at night, when the person is in bed and minimal effort and disruption is required. Incontinence will persist during the day but the total volume will be less than it would be without catheterizations. Problems of urinary tract infection are also likely to be reduced. Reducing the frequency of intermittent catheterization may also be helped by the use of a portable ultrasound. Anton et al (1998) found that the mean frequency of catheterization per day was reduced by more than one catheterization if a portable ultrasound device was used to determine need for catheterization.

All people undertaking intermittent catheterization need the opportunity for long-term support so that help and advice are available when wanted, in order that the benefits of using this method are not lost prematurely owing to potentially solvable problems.

Electrical stimulation and sacral deafferentation

Electrical stimulation of sacral anterior nerve roots, combined with division of posterior sacral nerve roots, was first described by Brindley (Brindley 1994) and is a method that has been used primarily for spinal cord injured patients to control continence (by eliminating hyperreflexia) and to enable complete voiding. Sacral deafferentation

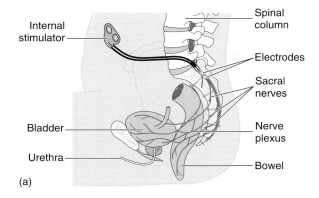

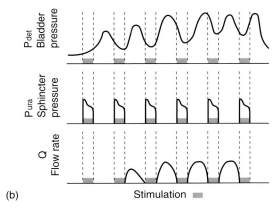

Figure 11.13 (a) Implantable stimulator; (b) bladder/sphincteric pressures and flow rate during stimulation.

produces an areflexic, low pressure bladder and voiding is activated by electrical stimulation of the anterior roots (Fig. 11.13). This produces contraction not only of the detrusor (to enable voiding) but also of the external sphincter and pelvic floor. Applying stimulation in bursts of a few seconds results in the relaxation of these striated muscles between stimulations, whilst the detrusor contraction is maintained. Voiding therefore occurs in bursts. This combination of implant and deafferentation appears to be protective of the upper tracts. A multicentre review of 184 patients with stimulators showed improvement in reflux or upper tract dilatation in 14 out of 17 patients (Van Kerrebroeck et al 1993). A more recent review of 226 patients, by the same research

group (Van Kerrebroeck et al 1997) showed that complete continence during the daytime was achieved in 73% of patients and 86% at night. Van der Aa et al (1999) reviewed 38 patients (from 3 months to 12 years postsurgery) who had had this procedure and found that 31 patients were continent and in 24 patients the residual urine was less than 30 ml. Implant failure occurred in 3 patients.

Voiding triggers, manoeuvres and aids

Simple methods of triggering bladder contractions such as tapping the abdomen can prove effective in precipitating voiding (although voiding may be incomplete) and can enable the patient to gain some control over continence. The Queen Square bladder stimulator is a hand-held vibrating device designed for the same purpose (Dasgupta et al 1997) but is not in widespread use. Methods to aid voiding such as manual expression (the Crede manoeuvre) and the Valsalva manoeuvre have been used for many years but are not now generally recommended. The Crede manoeuvre has been reported to result in dilatation of the upper tracts (Smith et al 1972) and there are concerns that the Valsalva manoeuvre further stretches the pelvic floor (Arnold 1999).

Long-term catheterization

The serious drawbacks of long-term catheterization are well documented and are discussed in Chapter 9. Infection is almost inevitable and there is an increased risk of renal problems, calculi and urethral trauma. For these reasons long-term catheterization should never be considered lightly. However, it is important that long-term catheterization is not perceived as a failure on the part of the patient or a wholly negative management method. The virtues of intermittent catheterizations in particular can be sung so strongly that patients may feel they have failed if they wish to abandon it because their disabilities have made it impractical to continue. For some people a catheter can be a release from all worries of timing, toileting and wet pads, and therefore

---

Case study 11.1

Miss B is a 63-year-old woman with multiple sclerosis living at home with a life-long friend. She was working as a secretary when she noticed her first symptoms at the age of 34. Following episodes of numbness and tingling in her legs she found that she had difficulties going up or down steps because she could not sense the position of her feet. Gradually she started to lose power in her legs and by the age of 48 she needed a wheelchair for all her mobility needs, although she could still stand to transfer with one helper.

Miss B's bladder problems were purely functional to begin with. She could use the toilet only if someone was able to help her and this meant that she sometimes had to 'hold on' for longer than she wanted. Toileting was aided by the use of drop-front pants as these were easier to remove than conventional pants. At night she usually wanted to pass urine once and she used a pan-type urinal.

When she was 55, Miss B started to have problems with frequency and urgency and developed a urinary tract infection. A course of antibiotics improved the symptoms but they persisted and she started to become incontinent of urine at night and in the day if her helper did not get her to the toilet in time. She was very distressed about this and was visited by the district nurse who measured her residual urine by catheterization. This was 200 ml. A trial of daily intermittent catheterization performed by the district nurse was commenced and although this was well accepted by Miss B, and seemed to improve the daytime symptoms, she still had incontinence at night. The intermittent catheterization was increased to include a catheterization at night and this improved the

night problem. Miss B was taught the technique (which she managed with some degree of difficulty owing to hand weakness), and this management continued successfully for about 2 years.

Daytime and nighttime incontinence gradually began again, and Miss B was referred to a continence clinic where urodynamics were performed. This confirmed that she had detrusor hyperreflexia and detrusor–sphincter dyssynergia. After discussions which also involved her friend, it was decided to commence oral oxybutynin and increase catheterizations to four times daily. Miss B was having some problems with catheterizing, because of hand weakness, and it was agreed that her friend would learn the technique. With this regime Miss B was continent. Potential constipation problems were eased by a combination of dietary modification (prunes, moderate fibre) and glycerin or bisacodyl suppositories. Sometimes a micro-enema was necessary. If she went out she would usually be catheterized just before she left and would wear a pad for security.

This management continued for 3 years, but Miss B's general condition deteriorated and she became unable to undertake a stand transfer. Going out became more difficult and catheterizations were difficult to do outside her home, because she needed a hoist and a bed for her friend to catheterize her on. Following review at the continence clinic she decided to try an indwelling catheter. After using a urethral catheter successfully for 1 month, a suprapubic catheter was inserted, to aid reinsertion and to avoid urethral trauma. As Miss B was now dependent on her carer for help with most activities, the suprapubic catheter gave them both greater freedom.

---

provides a considerably better quality of life. In this sense it can be seen as a positive and practical step.

However, whilst a well-managed, patent, long-lasting and leak-free catheter can be a highly successful method of managing incontinence, a constantly blocking, leaking and/or expelling catheter represents the worst of all worlds. These are common catheter-associated problems and the potential for urethral trauma is an additional concern.

Suprapubic catheters are becoming more widely used and offer some substantial advantages over conventional urethral catheters. Recatheterization (particularly for women) is usually easier, particularly if leg abduction is difficult, urethral trauma is avoided and sexual activity can take place much more easily. Eckford et al (1994a) followed up 50 severely disabled

women with multiple sclerosis who had urethral closures and suprapubic catheters following inadequate or problematic conservative measures or urethral catheterization. The mean length of follow-up was 6.5 years and 79% of these women remained completely dry. The main complications related to the presence of the catheter (i.e. recurrent calculi and encrustation/blockage). MacDiarmid et al (1995) reviewed the urological complications in 44 patients with spinal cord injury with a suprapubic catheter. Follow-up (mean 58 weeks) showed no renal impairment or reflux, and the authors concluded that suprapubic catheterization is a safe alternative form of bladder management in selected patients with spinal cord injury.

If long-term catheterization is implemented then thought needs to be given to the drainage containment method. Leg bags are commonly used and may be worn on the thigh, calf or hanging from a belt as a 'sporran'. Generally, for people who use a wheelchair the calf is the most comfortable and convenient location, although for women trousers or a long skirt must then be worn. Consideration needs to be given to the tap on the leg bag because these vary greatly in terms of ease of opening. Larger, bulky taps with a positive 'on/off' action tend to be easier to use for people with manual dexterity problems (MDA 1996), but may also be more obvious under clothing.

Catheter valves (Fig. 11.14) are a positive alternative to leg bags, because the bladder continues to be used as the reservoir for urine rather than an external bag. These valves are very similar to the taps on leg bags and are connected directly to the end of the catheter. The valve needs to be released regularly to drain urine from the bladder. Pettersson & Fader (1997) found that some valves needed two hands for operation and required sustained pressure to enable drainage whilst others could be operated more readily with one hand. It is important that the patient has an opportunity to try out different valves to determine which one they find easiest to use. German et al (1997) found that patients experienced least problems if they used a valve during the day and then attached this to a night drainage bag overnight. To be safe and successful the patient needs to be able to remember to drain the bladder regularly and needs sufficient manual dexterity to operate the valve.

OTHER AIDS AND APPLIANCES

Despite the many advances in the treatment of neurogenic bladder problems, incontinence (or the threat of incontinence) commonly persists and some form of containment using aids or appliances will be necessary. For a man there are two main options, a penile sheath or pads and pants; for women, pads and pants are the main method available. The Continence Product Evaluation (CPE) Network (funded by the Medical Devices Agency, Department of Health) has carried out comparative evaluations of the main product groups and reference to these reports should help make informed product selection by and for patients (www.medical-devices.gov.uk).

Sheaths

Sheath drainage tends to be more popular than absorbent products for men, perhaps to avoid the 'feminine' associations of pads and pants, but also because if they work well they are more convenient. Pads require changing, which can be disruptive for the patient, are more bulky, and hold urine next to the skin. On the other hand sheaths can be difficult to apply successfully and can also cause skin problems; Golji (1981) estimated that 15% of his patients with spinal cord injury who used sheath drainage systems developed some sort of penile or urethral complications. Infection rates have also been found

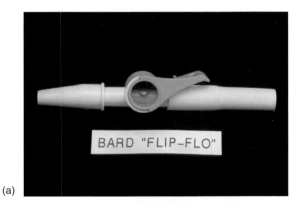

(a)

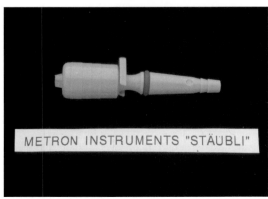

(b)

Figure 11.14 Examples of catheter valves.

to be higher with sheath usage than without. A study by Ouslander et al (1987a) found that nursing home residents who used sheath drainage had significantly higher rates of bacteriuria and urinary tract infection than those who did not.

Self-adhesive sheaths (with adhesive applied to the inner surface of the sheath) have been shown to perform better and are easier to apply than sheaths with a separate adhesive strip (MDA 1995). The use of an applicator does not appear to confer any advantage. Although the majority of self-adhesive sheaths are supplied with an applicator, those without an applicator have been shown to be easier to apply both by carers and by patients (Fader et al 2001b).

Pads

Absorbent pads are available in a variety of forms, both disposable and reusable. Disposable insert pads (to be worn with closely fitting pants) come in a wide range of sizes to accommodate mild incontinence through to heavy nighttime incontinence (Fig. 11.15). For heavier incontinence the all-in-one diaper style pad is more effective at preventing leakage than insert pads (MDA 1999a) but both types can be difficult for the patient to apply. The newer 'pull-up' style pads (Fig. 11.16) are promoted as being much easier for patients to use themselves and may therefore be particularly suitable for those with moderate to

heavy incontinence who are trying to maintain independence.

Reusable pads for heavy incontinence are less commonly used and there are indications that they are much more 'leaky' than their disposable

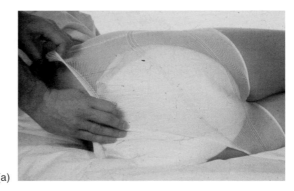
(a)

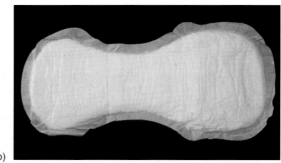
(b)

Figure 11.15 (a) Disposable insert pad with pants; (b) plain insert pad.

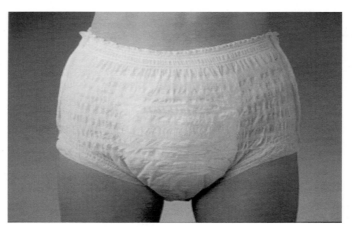

Figure 11.16 'Pull-up' disposable pad.

counterparts (Philp & Cottenden 1993) although they have yet to be systematically evaluated. Reusable pants with an absorbent gusset for light incontinence have advantages over disposable pads because they look like normal underwear, the pad is fixed in position and is very easy to apply (Fig. 11.17) (MDA 2001). Similar pants are available for men and disposable pouches or shields may also be useful for light incontinence.

Whatever type of aid or appliance is used, it is important to remember that people with sensory loss are particularly vulnerable to skin trauma because they cannot feel discomfort or pain. Correct application of aids, skin hygiene and vigilance are essential.

Toileting outside the home

Using the above strategies it should be possible to greatly improve continence for people with neurological disabilities. If the patient continues

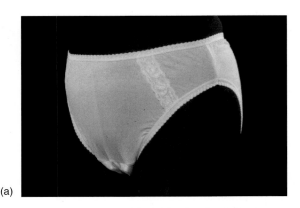

(a)

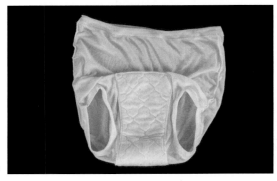

(b)

Figure 11.17 Examples of reusable pants with integral pad.

to use the toilet to remain continent then consideration needs to be given to methods of toileting both in and out of the home environment. At home, toileting is usually (but not always) less of an acute problem. Lifting equipment and carers should be available if needed, and the environment can be modified to enable access to the toilet (such as with grab rails) but people with urgency may still have problems using the toilet quickly enough and frequent toileting is tiring and disruptive.

Outside the home, lack of access to a toilet is a major barrier to participating in social activities. The advent of the 'disabled toilet' in many public places has been of great benefit, but if no lifting equipment is available and the person cannot undertake a stand transfer, then the toilet will remain inaccessible.

A toilet facility that can be used in the wheelchair can be very helpful for use both in and out of the home. For men, a male urinal (or bottle) provides an obvious solution for wheelchair toileting, but close attention to clothing is needed. Clothing can obstruct quick and easy access to the penis, which can be disastrous if there is urgency. Tracksuit bottoms must have waist elastic that is loose enough to pull down below the crotch; trousers with flies often need a longer zip to allow easy bottle access and a large zip-pull can be helpful for men with only one working hand. Alternatively Velcro tabs can be simpler than a zip and dropfront trousers may be useful. If spillage is likely to be a problem, then the addition of a sachet of hydrogel powder such as Verna-Gel (Vernamed) converts urine, after a minute or two, into a solid jelly that is difficult to spill. The jelly can later be washed away with water. Alternatively, a non-spill adaptor (Fig. 11.18) can be used in most male urinals. Male urinals are not discreet, and disposable bottles (Fig. 11.19) are more suitable for outings as they are much smaller and neater.

For women, wheelchair toileting is much more of a problem. Seating adaptations, postural deformities or hip abductor spasticity or contractures may mean that thighs cannot be opened to any useful extent, restricting access to the perineum. A further problem is that many women with severe disabilities need wedged cushions which are built up at the front to maintain a good

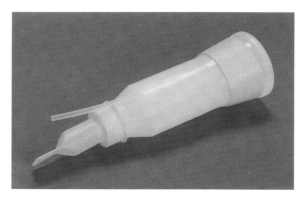

Figure 11.18 Non-spill adaptor.

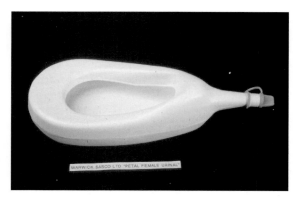

Figure 11.20 Pan-type urinal.

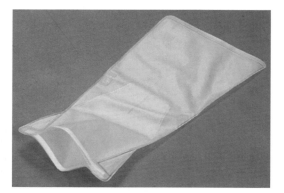

Figure 11.19 Disposable bottle.

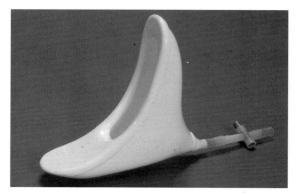

Figure 11.21 Bridge urinal.

seating position. Even with a flat cushion, pressure transmitted through the buttocks means that when in position the mouth of the urinal under the perineal area is lower than the body of the urinal. Urine will therefore tend to run down towards the back of the chair rather than into the urinal.

These design difficulties mean that few female urinals are successful in a wheelchair. Pan-type urinals (Fig. 11.20) can be very useful in the bed for use at night but are less effective in the chair. The Bridge urinal (Fig. 11.21) is designed specifically for toileting in a wheelchair and goes some way to overcoming the problems. Guidance on assessment for appropriate urinals is provided by Macintosh (1998) and an evaluation of a wide range of urinals has been carried out by the CPE Network (MDA 1999b). As with men, appropriate clothing can make a big difference between success and failure. It is not uncommon for disabled people to go

without pants to make toileting easier, but unless this is through personal choice, pants that allow for easy toileting should always be sought. Gussetless pants allow more access to the perineum than French knickers, but attractive front-opening pants are often the most acceptable option (Fig. 11.22).

Whenever a new toileting aid is contemplated it is very helpful to have a practice run at home. Problems can then be identified and skill and confidence increased. Accidents and embarrassment on social occasions can be devastating for self-esteem and self-confidence, and have a lasting impact.

BOWEL INTERVENTIONS AND MANAGEMENT

Before instigating any form of bowel management regimen it is important that any faecal impaction

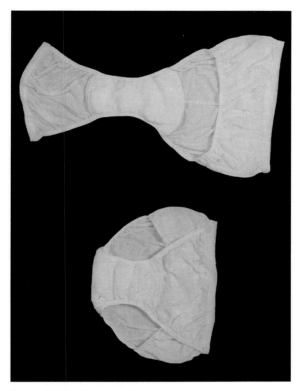

Figure 11.22 Front-opening pants.

be cleared. Regular (daily or alternate day) phosphate enemas seem to be accepted as the most effective form of treatment (Barrett 1993). If faecal loading is with soft stool, stool softeners should be avoided, as this is likely to worsen any faecal incontinence. Micro-enemas may be used as an alternative, particularly if phosphate enemas prove hard to retain (see Chapter 7).

Regular bowel management

Once the bowel is clear then the aim for the majority of neurologically impaired patients is likely to be the planned evacuation of a soft formed stool. Predictable bowel habits mean that constipation can be avoided and social activities can be organized with greater confidence. There is a lack of a research base for much of the recommended bowel management regimens, but most authors agree that the following are key components for a bowel programme.

Timing

The main stimuli for mass colonic movements are physical activity and food (Holdstock et al 1970). Bowel movements are likely to be most effective following a meal (often breakfast), but it is important that the patient's normal routine be followed when possible. Venn et al (1992) studied 46 stroke patients and found that a significantly higher number of subjects were able to establish an effective bowel regime, when their premorbid bowel pattern was used as the scheduled time for their bowel training programme.

Exercise and physical activity

Constipation is an established consequence of immobility. Turning in bed, repositioning in the chair, bathing, and active and passive limb exercises may assist in improving gut motility. If physiotherapy (such as rolling and stretching) are a regular part of the patient's routine, then adjusting the bowel programme so that food is eaten beforehand may help to stimulate bowel activity. However, sometimes physiotherapy can trigger reflex defecation and faecal incontinence can be the unwanted consequence.

Privacy

Defecation is difficult without privacy. Most people are socialized to evacuate their bowels in private and loss of privacy can be embarrassing, stressful and inhibiting. In institutional settings privacy is hard to achieve and efforts need to be made to ensure that toileting is a private affair.

Positioning

An upright position should be adopted whenever possible, to take advantage of gravity and to facilitate abdominal effort. Armrests and back supports are helpful for people with balance problems. It may be difficult to provide effective support for some people with flaccid paralysis or those who have severe postural defects. A toileting sling, used with a hoist, provides considerable

---

Case study 11.2 Spinal cord injury

A young man aged 32 (HM) sustained a complete spinal cord injury (level T6) at the age of 15 after falling out of a tree in his parent's back garden. Luckily he was taken promptly to a nearby specialist unit for spinal cord injuries. There he was stabilized and looked after in an acute trauma ward through the spinal shock phase for about 8 weeks and thereafter for a further 6 months in the rehabilitation unit.

On admission, urological management for an acontractile (areflexic) bladder was introduced immediately with an indwelling catheter per urethra to give continuous drainage. At 2 weeks, bladder emptying was changed to clean intermittent catheterization (CIC) managed initially by the spinal trauma nurses. At about 3 weeks HM himself took over catheterization (CISC – clean intermittent self-catheterization) as by then he had regained good mental and physical faculties whilst remaining bed bound. Complete bladder emptying on a timed basis was possible by this means, giving volumes of about 350 ml with little residual urine. Urine samples were taken routinely for microbiology and any urinary tract infections detected were treated.

At about 8 weeks postinjury HM began to leak urine. A videocystometrogram (VCMG) was performed and demonstrated detrusor hyperreflexia with some small amounts of external urethral sphincter dyssynergia but none at the level of the bladder neck. Detrusor pressures exceeded 40 cmH$_2$O at bladder volumes of 400 ml which led to leakage ('firing-off') of about 100 ml followed by a reduction in bladder pressure but leaving a large residual volume. Management now switched to anticholinergic medication (oxybutynin) to control his detrusor hyperreflexia and CISC for bladder emptying.

He returned home wheelchair bound about 9 months after his injury. HM was an ambitious person and at the age of 18 began training as a journalist and later became a newspaper reporter.

He became intolerant of the side-effects of oxybutynin, which included dry mouth and constipation, so anticholinergics were stopped and new management was introduced using a condom with drainage bag to collect 'fired-off' urine. Unfortunately, leakage of urine from insecure condoms was a frequent problem and this young man also found living with such a containment method not always compatible with his emerging busy social adult life. The consequences of urine leakage aggravated pressure sores on his buttocks which when healed left permanent scarring.

At the age of 25 HM began to suffer from an increasing scoliosis which by the age of 27 was so severe that a spinal correction with fixation rods from about T6 to the sacrum was carried out. He continued to seek better bladder management and it was by referral to a spinal injuries unit closer to his workplace (now in London working as a news editor for a well-know TV company) that he was introduced to the idea of having an implanted Finetech-Brindley sacral anterior root stimulator (SARS) for bladder emptying (see Fig. 11.13). However, there was concern about how the spinal fixation might prevent such a possibility and furthermore he did not want to lose reflex erections. The SARS is often implanted intrathecally through a laminectomy of L3–5 vertebrae and accompanied by posterior rhizotomy (surgical division of sensory nerves) to prevent reflex incontinence and detrusor–sphincter dyssynergia.

In 1999 after much consultation with spinal surgeons and tests using temporary electrodes in the sacral foramen it was decided to implant an extradural SARS on the S2 and S3/4 mixed sacral nerves, made possible by doing a laminectomy of the sacrum between the lower end of the diverging fixation rods. No rhizotomy was performed at this stage. The outcome of this procedure proved to be excellent in terms of bladder emptying (see Fig. 11.11b) and low residual urine (<50 ml). Interestingly good bladder capacity was established with little reflex incontinence despite the preservation of the posterior roots. Bowel evacuation was also greatly facilitated by using a suitably adjusted stimulation programme. Importantly, reflex erections were left intact.

To account for the attenuation of reflex incontinence, it may be that there was some selective nerve damage of the sensory nerves at operation which has persisted, and only time will tell whether a rhizotomy will ultimately become necessary. HM has been delighted with this outcome and, despite other setbacks, it has dramatically improved his overall quality of life since implantation.

---

support if it is left in position while the patient is on the toilet (Fig. 11.23). Elevating the hoist slightly allows the knees to be raised above the hips (whilst keeping the buttocks on the toilet), so that a squatting position can be achieved. Squatting is probably the optimum position for defecation because it increases abdominal pressure and straightens the lower end of the colon (Barrett 1993).

Diet

A high-fibre diet is considered an essential component of an effective bowel programme by some (Gender 1996) but has been found to be associated with an increase in faecal incontinence (Ardron & Main 1990) and colonic faecal loading in immobile elderly patients (Donald et al 1985). The use of dietary fibre in patients with neurological impairments has yet to be studied systematically.

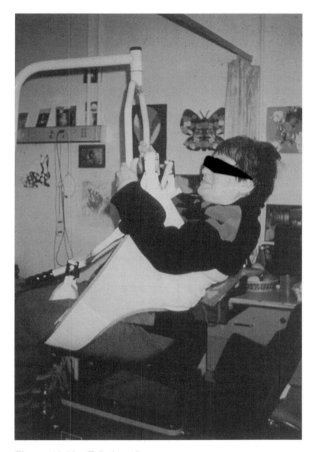

Figure 11.23 Toileting sling.

A judicious approach to the use of fibre is probably wise and the use of a bowel chart (see Chapter 7) can help to establish the efficacy of dietary fibre for an individual.

Digital stimulation, suppositories and enemas

Digital stimulation (inserting a lubricated, gloved finger into the anal canal and rotating it gently in a clockwise motion) is often helpful to initiate reflex defecation. Munchiando & Kendall (1993) used this technique to establish bowel programmes with stroke patients and found a daily programme more effective than an alternate day programme, although interviews with 100 spinal cord injured patients showed that an alternate day programme of bowel intervention was the most commonly used (Kirshblum et al 1998).

Suppositories may be used to stimulate reflex defecation by drawing fluid into the bowel (e.g. glycerin suppositories) or by acting as a bowel irritant (e.g. bisacodyl suppositories). Traditionally bisacodyl suppositories are based on hydrogenated vegetable oil, but a study of 14 spinal cord injured patients showed that polyethylene glycol-based bisacodyl suppositories were faster acting and halved the time taken for total bowel care (Stiens et al 1998). The placement of suppositories involves digital stimulation, which may contribute to the effect. If suppositories alone fail to act, digital stimulation for about 30 seconds may help to trigger defecation. Suppositories have been found to be easier to insert and more effective when inserted blunt end first (Abd-el-Maeboud et al 1991).

Micro-enemas are an alternative to suppositories and are very easy to administer. A comparison between micro-enemas and bisacodyl suppositories in spinal cord injured patients found that patients took 45 minutes more to respond to the suppositories than the enemas (Dunn & Galka 1994) although the suppositories were much cheaper and presumably may have worked faster if they were polyethylene glycol based. Phosphate enemas may be necessary for some patients on a regular basis, but can be messy and difficult to retain. There is also concern that repeated use may stretch the colon wall and cause loss of elasticity (Gender 1996), although this has not been substantiated. Tap water enemas have been suggested as a safer alternative (Harari et al 1993).

Laxatives

Stimulant laxatives (such as senna or bisacodyl) can be taken the night before a planned bowel action, if soft or formed stool is present, but there is concern that regular use may result in damage to the enteric nervous system (Smith 1968) although others do not support this view (Gattuso & Kamm 1993). Faecal softeners such as lactulose are best reserved for those with hard stool. A combination of senna and fibre has been found to be more effective than lactulose in increasing bowel frequency, and facilitating evacuation in frail old people (Passmore et al 1993).

Manual evacuation

For patients with lower motor neurone disorders affecting the lower colon, it may be impossible to evacuate the bowel without manual evacuation. If manual evacuation is necessary then it should be performed gently by trained staff to avoid damaging the anal and rectal mucosa and to avoid stretching the anal sphincter. Guidelines on this procedure have been published by the Royal College of Nursing (Addison 1995).

Antegrade continence enema

The use of the antegrade continence enema requires surgery to open the appendix onto the abdomen to create a continent catheterizable stoma. This stoma may then be irrigated to result in evacuation of the colon. Although this procedure has mostly been used in children with spina bifida there have been more recent reports on adults with neurogenic bowel problems. Teichman and colleagues (1998) reported the results of seven patients with neurogenic bowel disease. Six of the seven patients were continent and reported decreased toileting time and improved quality of life. However complications occurred in four patients. One case report of a single patient with intractable constipation and faecal incontinence indicated a highly successful outcome, with elimination of faecal incontinence and no surgical or medical side-effects. This technique is in need of further evaluation for adults with neurogenic bladder problems.

Electrical stimulation and neuromodulation

Although sacral root stimulators have been used to treat urinary incontinence for many years it is only comparatively recently that attempts have been made to apply the same principle to the bowel. Good outcomes were found by MacDonagh (1990) and colleagues who implanted devices into 12 patients with SCI. Six subjects were able to completely evacuate the rectum without manual removal and most subjects were able to shorten the time taken to complete their regular bowel programme.

Electrical stimulators have also been used in combination with surgical reconstruction of the anal sphincter using the gracilis muscle (Geerdes et al 1996) and recently the use of magnetic stimulation to suppress uninhibited rectal contractions has shown some promise (Shafik 2000).

KEY POINTS FOR PRACTICE

- Continence management in neurological disability represents a substantial challenge for nurses.
- Damage to the nervous system can produce a range of bladder and bowel dysfunctions and careful assessment is needed to ensure that appropriate interventions are used.
- Neurological bladder and bowel problems are frequently associated with other disabilities that can further contribute to incontinence.
- Effective continence management needs to take into account these disabilities, not only to maximize continence but also to ensure that interventions fit into the individual's lifestyle.

REFERENCES

Abd-el-Maeboud K H, El-Nagger T, El-Hawi E M M 1991 Glycerine suppositories – common sense mode of insertion. Lancet 338: 798–800

Addison R 1995 Digital rectal examination and manual removal of faeces. Royal College of Nursing, London

Anderson C S, Jamrozik K D, Broadhurst R J 1994 Predicting survival for 1 year among different subtypes of stroke. Stroke 25: 1935–1944

Andrew J, Nathan P W 1964 Lesions of the anterior frontal lobes and disturbances of micturition and defaecation. Brain 87: 233–262

Andrews K 1994 Bladder disorders in brain damage. In: Rushton D N (ed) Handbook of neuro-urology. Marcel Dekker, New York

Anton H A, Chambers K, Clifton J, Tasaka J 1998 Clinical utility of a portable ultrasound device in intermittent catheterisation. Archives of Physical Medicine and Rehabilitation 79(2): 172–175

Appell R A 1997 Clinical efficacy and safety of tolterodine in the treatment of overactive bladder: a pooled analysis. Urology 50: 90–96

Araki I, Kuno S 2000 Assessment of voiding dysfunction in Parkinson's disease by the international prostate symptom score. Journal of Neurology, Neurosurgery and Psychiatry 68: 429–433

Ardron M E, Main A N H 1990 Management of constipation. British Medical Journal 300: 1400

Arnold E P 1999 Spinal cord injury. In: Fowler C J (ed) Neurology of bladder, bowel and sexual dysfunction. Blue books of practical neurology. Butterworth-Heinemann, Oxford

Barer D H 1989 Continence after stroke: useful predictor or goal of therapy? Age and Ageing 18: 183–191

Barrett J 1993 Faecal incontinence and related problems in the older adult. Edward Arnold, London

Beck R O, Betts C D, Fowler C J 1994a Genitourinary dysfunction in multiple system atrophy: clinical features and treatment in 62 cases. Journal of Urology 151: 1336–1341

Beck R, Fowler C J, Mathias C J 1994b Genitourinary dysfunction in disorders of the autonomic nervous system. In: Rushton D N (ed) Handbook of neuro-urology. Marcel Dekker, New York

Betts C D, D'Mellow M T, Fowler C J 1993 Urinary symptoms and the neurological features of bladder dysfunction in multiple sclerosis. Journal of Neurology, Neurosurgery and Psychiatry 56: 245–250

Blaivas J G, Barbalias G A 1984 Detrusor–external sphincter dyssynergia in men with multiple sclerosis: an ominous urological condition. Journal of Urology 131: 91–94

Borrie M F, Campbell A J, Caradoc-Davies T H 1986 Urinary incontinence after stroke: a prospective study. Age and Ageing 15: 177

Brindley G 1994 The first 500 patients with sacral anterior root stimulation: general description. Paraplegia 32: 795–805

Brittain K R, Peet S M, Castleden C M 1998 Stroke and incontinence. Stroke 29: 524–528

Brocklehurst K C, Andrews K, Richards B, Laycock P J 1985 Incidence and correlates of incontinence in stroke patients. Journal of the American Geriatrics Society 33: 540–542

Buyse G, Waldeck K, Verpooten C et al 1998 Intravesical oxybutynin for neurogenic bladder dysfunction: less systemic side effects due to reduced first pass metabolism. Journal of Urology 160: 892–896

Chandiramani V A, Palace J, Fowler C J 1997 How to recognize patients with parkinsonism who should not have urological surgery. British Journal of Urology 80: 100–104

Charbonneau-Smith R 1993 No-touch catheterization and infection rates in a select spinal cord injured population. Rehabilitation Nursing 18: 296–299

Chia Y W, Gill K P, Forti A D, Henry M M, Shorvon P J 1992 Paradoxical puborectalis contraction is common in multiple sclerosis patients with constipation: a manifestation of multiple sclerosis? Gut 32(Suppl. 2): A204

Chia Y W, Fowler C J, Kamm M A et al 1995 Prevalence of bowel dysfunction in patients with multiple sclerosis

and bladder dysfunction. Journal of Neurology 242: 105–108

Craggs M D, McFarlane J P 1999 Neuromodulation of the lower urinary tract. Experimental Physiology 84: 149–160

Craggs M, Vaizey C 1999 Neurophysiology of the bladder and bowel. In: Fowler C J (ed) Neurology of bladder, bowel and sexual dysfunction. Blue books of practical neurology. Butterworth-Heinemann, Oxford

Craggs M D, Sheriff M K M, Shah P J R, Fowler C, Petersen T 1995 Responses to multi-pulse magnetic stimulation of spinal nerve roots mapped over the sacrum in man. Journal of Physiology 483: 127P

Cruz F 1998 Desensitization of bladder sensory fibers by intravesical capsaicin or capsaicin analogs. A new strategy for treatment of urge incontinence in patients spinal detrusor hyperreflexia or bladder hypersensitivity disorders. International Urogynecology Journal and Pelvic Floor Dysfunction 9(4): 214–220

Dasgupta P, Haslam C, Goodwin R, Fowler C J 1997 The Queen Square bladder stimulator: a device for assisting emptying of the neurogenic bladder. British Journal of Urology 81: 234–237

De Groat W C 1994 Neurophysiology of the pelvic organs. In: Rushton D N (ed) Handbook of neuro-urology. Marcel Dekker Inc, New York

De Groat W C, Steers W D 1988 Neural control of the urinary bladder and sexual organs: experimental studies in animals. In: Bannister R (ed) Autonomic failure: a textbook of clinical disorders of the autonomic nervous system, 2nd edn. Oxford University Press, Oxford

De Looze D, Van Laere M, De Muynck M, Beke R, Elewaut A 1998 Constipation and other chronic gastrointestinal problems in spinal cord injury patients. Spinal Cord 36: 63–66

De Seze M, Wiart L, Ferriere J et al 1999 Intravesical instillation of capsaicin in urology: a review of the literature. European Urology 36: 267–277

Di Carlo A, Lamassa M, Pracucci G et al 1999 Stroke in the very old: clinical presentation and determinants of 3 month functional outcome: a European perspective. European BIOMED Study of Stroke Care Group. Stroke 30: 2313–2319

Dixon J, Gosling J 1987 Structure and innervation in the human. In: Torrens M, Morrison J F B (eds) The physiology of the lower urinary tract. Springer-Verlag, London

Donald I P, Smith R G, Cruikshank J G, Elton R A, Stoddart M E 1985 A study of constipation in the elderly living at home. Gerontology 31: 112–118

Drutz H P, Appell R A, Gleason D, Klimberg I, Radomski S 1999 Clinical efficacy and safety of tolterodine compared to oxybutynin and placebo in patients with overactive bladder. International Urogynecology Journal and Pelvic Floor Dysfunction 10: 283–289

Dunn K L, Galka M L 1994 A comparison of the effectiveness of Therevac SB and bisacodyl suppositories in SCI patients' bowel programs. Rehabilitation Nursing 19: 334–338

Eardley I, Quinn N P, Fowler C J et al 1989 The value of urethral sphincter electromyography in the differential diagnosis of parkinsonism. British Journal of Urology 64: 360–362

Eckford S B, Kohler-Ockmore J, Feneley R C L et al 1994a Long-term follow up of transvaginal urethral closure and suprapubic cystostomy for urinary incontinence in women with multiple sclerosis. British Journal of Urology 74: 319–321

Eckford S D, Swami K S, Jackson S R, Abrams P H 1994b Desmopressin in the treatment of nocturia and enuresis in patients with multiple sclerosis. British Journal of Urology 74: 733–735

Edwards L L, Quigley E M, Pfeiffer R F 1993 Gastrointestinal dysfunction in Parkinson's disease: frequency and pathophysiology. Neurology 42: 726–732

Fader M, Barton R, Malone-Lee J et al 2001a New use for an old drug: results of a dose titration study of intra-vesical atropine. International Continence Society (UK) Proceedings, April, Manchester

Fader M, Pettersson L, Dean G et al 2001b Sheaths for urinary incontinence: a randomized crossover trial. British Journal of Urology International 88(4): 367–372

Fitzmaurice H, Fowler C H, Rickards D et al 1985 Micturition disturbance in Parkinson's disease. British Journal of Urology 57: 652–656

Fowler C, Fowler C 1993 Neurogenic bladder dysfunction and its management. In: Greenwood R, Barnes M P, McMillan T M, Ward C D (eds) Neurological rehabilitation. Churchill Livingstone, Edinburgh

Fowler C, Christmas T J, Chapple C R et al 1988 Abnormal electromyographic activity of the urethral sphincter, voiding dysfunction and polycystic ovaries: a new syndrome? British Medical Journal 297: 1436–1438

Fowler C J, Jewkes D, McDonald W I, Lynn B, de Groat W C 1992a Intravesical capsaicin for neurogenic bladder dysfunction. Lancet 339: 1239

Fowler C J, van Kerrebroeck P E, Nordenbo A, van Poppel H 1992b Treatment of lower urinary tract dysfunction in patients with multiple sclerosis. Committee of the European Study Group of SUDIMS (Sexual and Urological Disorders in Multiple Sclerosis). Journal of Neurology, Neurosurgery and Psychiatry 55: 986–989

Fowler C J, Beck R O, Gerrard S, Betts C D, Fowler C G 1994 Intravesical capsaicin for treatment of detrusor hyperreflexia. Journal of Neurology, Neurosurgery and Psychiatry 57: 169–173

Gajewski J B, Awad S A 1986 Oxybutynin versus propantheline in patients with multiple sclerosis and detrusor hyperreflexia. Journal of Urology 135: 966–968

Gallien P, Robineau S, Nicolas B et al 1998 Vesicourethral dysfunction and urodynamic findings in multiple sclerosis: a study of 149 cases. Archives of Physical Medicine and Rehabilitation 79: 255–257

Garrett V E, Scott J A, Costich J, Aubrey D, Gross J 1989 Bladder emptying assessment in stroke patients. Archives of Physical Medicine and Rehabilitation 70: 41–43

Gattuso J M, Kamm M A 1993 Review article. The management of constipation in adults. Alimentary Pharmacological Therapy 7: 487–500

Geerdes B P, Heineman E, Konsten J et al 1996 Dynamic graciloplasty: complications and management. Diseases of the Colon and Rectum 39: 912–917

Gender A R 1996 Bowel regulation and elimination. In: Hoeman S (ed) Rehabilitation nursing: process and application. Mosby, St Louis

German K, Rowley P, Stone D et al 1997 A randomised cross-over study comparing the use of a catheter valve

and a leg bag in urethrally catheterised male patients. British Journal of Urology 79: 96–99

Glickman S, Kamm M A 1996 Bowel dysfunction in spinal-cord-injury patients. Lancet 347: 1651–1653

Golji H 1981 Complications of external condom drainage. Paraplegia 19: 189–197

Gosling J A, Dixon J S, Himpherson J A 1983 Functional anatomy of the urinary tract: an integrated text and colour atlas. Churchill Livingstone, Edinburgh

Gray M, Rayome R, Anson C 1995 Incontinence and clean intermittent catheterisation following spinal cord injury. Clinical Nursing Research 4(1): 6–18

Grinspun D 1993 Bladder management for adults following head injury. Rehabilitation Nursing 18: 300–305

Haboubi N Y, Hudson P, Rahman Q, Lee G S, Ross A 1988 Small-intestinal transit time in the elderly. Lancet 1: 933

Harari D, Gurwitz J H, Minaker K L 1993 Constipation in the elderly. Journal of the American Geriatrics Society 41: 1113–1140

Henriksen T 1991 Incontinence after stroke. Lancet 338: 1335

Hinds J P, Eidelman B H, Wald A 1990 Prevalence of bowel dysfunction in multiple sclerosis: a population survey. Gastroenterology 98: 1538–1542

Holdstock D J, Misiewicz J J, Smith T, Rowlands E N 1970 Propulsion (mass movements) in the human colon and its relationship to meals and somatic activity. Gut 11: 91–99

Holland N 1994 Bladder management in mutiple sclerosis. MS Management 1(2): 1–11

Hoverd P A, Fowler C J 1998 Desmopressin in the treatment of daytime frequency in patients with multiple sclerosis. Journal of Neurology, Neurosurgery and Psychiatry 65: 778–780

Jawad S H, Ward A B 1999 Study of the relationship between premorbid urinary incontinence and stroke functional outcome. Clinical Rehabilitation 13: 447–452

Khan Z, Starter P, Yan W C, Bhola A 1990 Analysis of voiding disorders in patients with cerebrovascular accident. Urology 21: 315–318

Kim Y H, Bird E T, Priebe M, Boone T B 1997 The role of oxybutynin in spinal cord injured patients with indwelling catheters. Journal of Urology 158: 2083–2086

Kirby R S, Milroy E J G, Mitchell M I 1986 The role of the sympathetic nervous system in the lower urinary tract. Clinical Sciences 70(Suppl. 14): 1–81

Kirchoff K, Fowler C J 2000 The value of the Kurtzke Functional Systems Scales in predicting incomplete bladder emptying. Spinal Cord 38: 409–413

Kirschblum S C, Gulati M, O'Connor K C, Voorman S J 1998 Bowel care practices in chronic spinal cord injury patients. Archives of Physical Medicine and Rehabilitation 79: 20–23

Koldewijn E L, Rosier P F W M, Meuleman E J H et al 1994 Predictors of success with neuromodulation in lower urinary tract dysfunction: results of trial stimulation in 100 patients. Journal of Urology 152: 2017–2025

Krogh K, Nielson J, Dijurhuus J C et al 1997 Colorectal functions in patients with spinal cord lesions. Diseases of the Colon and Rectum 40: 1233–1239

Kuhn W, Rist M, Zaech G 1991 Intermittent urethral self-catheterisation: long-term results. Paraplegia 29: 222–232

Lewis N A 1995 Implementing a bladder ultrasound programme. Rehabilitation Nursing 20: 215–217

Lincoln J, Burnstock G 1993 Autonomic innervation of the urinary bladder and urethra. In: Maggi C A (ed) Nervous control of the urogenital tract. Harwood Academic Publishers, Switzerland, pp 33–68

Lindström S, Fall M, Carlsson C A, Erlandson B E 1983 The neuro-physiological basis of bladder inhibition in response to intravaginal electrical stimulation. Journal of Urology 129: 405–410

MacDiarmid S A, Arnold E P, Palmer N B, Anthony A 1995 Management of spinal cord injured patients by indwelling suprapubic catheterization. Journal of Urology 154: 492–494

MacDonagh R, Sun W M, Smallwood R, Read N W 1990 Control of defaecation in patients with spinal injuries by stimulation of sacral anterior nerve roots. British Medical Journal 300: 1494–1497

McFarlane J P, Foley S J, de Winter P, Shah P J R, Craggs M D 1997 Acute suppression of idiopathic detrusor instability with magnetic stimulation of the sacral nerve roots. British Journal of Urology 80: 734–741

McGuire E J, Savastano J A 1984 Urodynamic findings and longterm outcome management of patients with multiple sclerosis-induced lower urinary tract dysfunction. Journal of Urology 132: 102

Macintosh J 1998 Realising the potential of urinals for women. Journal of Community Nursing 12(44): 1739–1741

Maes D, Wyndaele J 1988 Long-term experience with intermittent catheterisation. Neurourology and Urodynamics 73: 273–274

Malone-Lee J G, Sa'adu A, Lieu P K 1993 Evidence against the existence of a specific parkinsonian bladder. Neurourology and Urodynamics 12: 341–343

Mathers S 1992 Neural control of the pelvic sphincters. In: Henry M M, Swash M (eds) Coloproctology and the pelvic floor. Butterworth-Heinemann, Oxford

Medical Devices Agency 1995 Disability Equipment Assessment Report No. A15. Penile sheaths: a comparative evaluation. Medical Devices Agency, London

Medical Devices Agency 1996 Disability Equipment Assessment Report A20. Sterile 500 ml leg bags for urine drainage: a multi-centre comparative evaluation. Medical Devices Agency, London

Medical Devices Agency 1999a Disability Equipment Assessment Report No. IN4. All-in-one disposable bodyworn pads for heavy incontinence: an evaluation. Medical Devices Agency, London

Medical Devices Agency 1999b Disability Equipment Assessment Report No. IN3. Reusable female urinals: an evaluation. Medical Devices Agency, London

Medical Devices Agency 2001 Disability Equipment Assessment Report No. IN7. Reusable pants with integral pad for light incontinence: an evaluation. Medical Devices Agency, London

Menter R, Weitzenkamp D, Cooper D 1997 Bowel management outcomes in individuals with long-term spinal cord injuries. Spinal Cord 35: 608–612

Moore K N, Kelm M, Sinclair O, Cadrain G 1993 Bacteriuria in intermittent catheterization users: the effect of sterile versus clean reused catheters. Rehabilitation Nursing 18: 306–309

Munchiando J F, Kendall K 1993 Comparison of the effectiveness of two bowel programs for CVA patients. Rehabilitation Nursing 18: 168–172

Murphy K P, Kliever E M, Moore M J 1994 The voiding alert system: a new application in the treatment of incontinence. Archives of Physical Medicine and Rehabilitation 75: 924–927

Myers D L, Arya L A, Friedman J H 1999 Is urinary incontinence different in women with Parkinson's disease. International Urogynecology Journal and Pelvic Floor Dysfunction 10: 188–191

Nakayama H, Jorgensen H S, Pedersen P M 1997 Prevalence and risk factors of incontinence after stroke: the Copenhagen stroke study. Stroke 28: 58–62

Norton C 1993 A helping handle. Nursing Times 89(16): 76–78

Ouslander J G, Greengold M D, Chen S 1987a External catheter use and urinary tract infections among incontinent male nursing home patients. Journal of the American Geriatrics Society 35: 1063–1070

Ouslander J G, Morishita L, Blaustein J et al 1987b Clinical, functional and psychological characteristics of an incontinent nursing home population. Journal of Gerontology 42: 631–637

Pannek J, Sommerfeld H J, Botel U, Senge T 2000 Combined intravesical and oral oxybutynin chloride in adult patients with spinal cord injury. Urology 55: 358–362

Passmore A P, Wilson-Davis K, Stoker C, Scott M E 1993 Chronic constipation in long-stay elderly patients: a comparison of lactulose and a senna-fibre combination. British Medical Journal 307: 769–771

Pettersson L, Fader M 1997 Choosing a catheter valve that suits the patient. Community Nurse 3(4): 9

Philp J, Cottenden A C 1993 Continence consumer test. Elderly Care 5(5): 27–30

Popovich J M, Stewart-Amidei C 1991 Alterations in elimination. In: Bronstein K S (ed) Promoting stroke recovery. Mosby-Year-Book, Missouri

Prieto-Fingerhut T, Banovac K, Lynne C M 1997 A study comparing sterile and non-sterile urethral catheterisation in patients with spinal cord injury. Rehabilitation Nursing 22(6): 299–302

Schoenburg H W, Gutrich J, Banno J 1979 Urodynamic patterns in multiple sclerosis. Journal of Urology 122: 648–650

Shafik A 2000 Suppression of uninhibited rectal detrusor by functional magnetic stimulation of sacral root. Journal of Spinal Cord Medicine 23: 45–50

Sheriff M K M, Shah P J R, Fowler C, Mundy A R, Craggs M D 1996 Neuromodulation of detrusor hyper-reflexia by functional magnetic stimulation of the sacral roots. British Journal of Urology 78: 39–46

Siegal S, Chancellor M, Dijkema H et al 1999 Improvement in quality of life: sacral nerve stimulation for urinary urgency-frequency. Neurourology and Urodynamics 18: 378

Smith B 1968 Effect of irritant purgatives on the myenteric plexus in man and mouse. Gut 9: 139–142

Smith P, Cook J, Rhine J 1972 Manual expression of the bladder following spinal cord injury. Paraplegia 9: 213–218

Stiens S A, Luttrel W, Binard J E 1998 Polyethylene glycol versus vegetable oil based bisacodyl suppositories to initiate side-lying bowel care: a clinical trial in persons with spinal cord injury. Spinal Cord 36: 777–781

Stocchi F, Badiali D, Vacca L et al 2000 Anorectal function in multiple system atrophy and Parkinson's disease. Movement Disorders 15: 71–76

Stokes G 1987 Incontinence and inappropriate urinating. Winslow Press, Bicester

Stover S L, Fine P R (eds) 1986 Spinal cord injury: the facts and figures. University of Alabama at Birmingham, Birmingham, Alabama

Sullivan S N, Ebers G C 1983 Gastrointestinal dysfunction in multiple sclerosis. Gastroenterology 84: 1640

Swash M, Snooks S J, Chalmers D H K 1987 Parity as a factor in incontinence in MS. Archives of Neurology 44: 504–508

Taub N A, Wolfe C D, Richardson E, Burney P G 1994 Predicting the disability of first-time stroke sufferers at 1 year: 12 month follow-up of a population based cohort in southeast England. Stroke 25(2): 352–357

Teichman J M, Harris J M, Currie D M, Barber D B 1998 Malone antegrade continence enema for adults with neurogenic bowel disease. Journal of Urology 160: 1278–1281

Thuroff J W, Bunke B, Ebner A et al 1991 Randomized, double-blind multicentre trial on treatment of frequency, urgency and incontinence related to detrusor hyperactivity: oxybutynin versus propantheline versus placebo. Journal of Urology 145: 813–816

Tsuchida S, Noto H, Yamaguchi O, Itoh M 1983 Urodynamic studies on hemiplegic patients after cerebrovascular accident. Urology 21: 315–319

Vaidyanathan S, Soni B M, Dundas S, Krishnan K R 1994 Urethral cytology in spinal cord injury patients performing intermittent self catheterisation. Paraplegia 32: 493–500

Vaidyanathan S, Soni B M, Brown E et al 1998 Effect of intermittent urethral catheterization and oxybutynin bladder installation on urinary continence status and quality of life in a selected group of spinal cord injury patients with neuropathic bladder dysfunction. Spinal Cord 36: 409–414

Van der Aa H E, Alleman E, Nene A, Snoek G 1999 Sacral anterior root stimulation for bladder control: clinical results. Archives of Physiology and Biochemistry 107: 248–256

Van Kerrebroeck P E, Koldewijn E L, Debruyne F M 1993 Worldwide experience with the Finetech-Brindley sacral anterior root stimulator. Neurourology and Urodynamics 12: 497–503

Van Kerrebroeck P E, van der Aa H E, Bosch J L et al 1997 Sacral rhizotomies and electrical bladder stimulation in spinal cord injury. Part 1: Clinical and urodynamic analysis. European Urology 31: 263–271

Venn M R, Taft L, Carpentier I B, Applebaugh A 1992 The influence of timing and suppository use on efficiency and effectiveness of bowel training after a stroke. Rehabilitation Nursing 17: 116–121

Waldron D J, Horgan P G, Patel F R, Maguire R, Given H F 1993 Multiple sclerosis: assessment of colonic and anorectal function in the presence of faecal incontinence. International Journal of Colorectal Diseases 8: 220–224

Webb R J, Lawson A L, Neal D E 1990 Clean intermittent self-catheterisation in 172 adults. British Journal of Urology 65(1): 20–23

Weld K J, Dmochowski R R 2000 Effect of bladder management on urological complications in spinal cord injured patients. Journal of Urology 163(3): 768–772

Woodward S 1995 Assessment of urinary incontinence in neuroscience patients. British Journal of Nursing 4(5): 254–258

12

Resource information

Mary Dolman
Kathryn Getliffe

This chapter provides information, including addresses, on:

- organizations associated with the promotion of continence
- organizations providing support for people with conditions that may contribute to problems of incontinence
- commercial companies involved in the field of incontinence products, some of which provide educational material and telephone helplines
- useful books and videos for professionals and users
- the Internet for information on incontinence.

Inevitably such material has a dynamic element as changes commonly occur, and therefore it is offered as a source of help rather than an attempt to be fully comprehensive.

This section of the book includes a number of Internet addresses which reflects the exponential increase in sources of information available on the worldwide web. Many people who still find incontinence a social taboo can turn to the Internet for information and get practical advice without face-to-face contact. Many commercial companies involved in continence products also have their own website for information and some offer an advisory service using an email address. Sandvik (1999) evaluated the Internet as a source of information and interactive facilities through 75 sites. There were 25 professional sites, which included hospitals and universities, 25 societies/foundations and 25 commercial sites. Sandvik concluded that the Internet is a source of excellent information and suggests patients can access valuable advice and find comfort from using this service (Sandvik H 1999 Health information and interaction on the internet: a survey of female urinary incontinence. British Medical Journal 319: 29–32).

Wherever possible the websites of organizations and commercial companies have been given but new websites are continually appearing and anyone with access to the Internet should make their own searches.

ORGANIZATIONS ASSOCIATED WITH THE PROMOTION OF CONTINENCE

Association of Chartered Physiotherapists in Women's Health (ACPWH)

Specialist interest group of Chartered Physiotherapists in Obstetrics and Gynaecology. Information from the Physiotherapy Chartered Society, 14 Bedford Row, London WC1R 4ED (Tel: 020 7242 1941)

Association for Continence Advice, 102a Astra House, Arklow Road, New Cross, London SE14 6EB (Tel: 020 8692 4680; Fax: 020 8692 6217). Email: info@aca.uk.com. Website: www.aca.uk.com

The Association for Continence Advice (ACA) is a registered charity. It provides information and advice for professionals working in the field of continence. Membership is multidisciplinary and this provides cross-fertilization of ideas and support. A quarterly newsletter keeps members informed of forthcoming events such as conferences and study days, nationally and internationally, as well as clinical research and new products.

Continence Care Forum (For Nurses), Royal College of Nursing, 20 Cavendish Square, London W1G 0RN (Tel: 020 7409 3333 or RCN Direct 0845 772 6100). RCN Online: www.rcn.org.uk

A specialist group, within the RCN, for nurses interested in continence issues and which supports the specialist Continence Advisor. The activities of the forum include publications for professionals and the public, a newsletter for RCN members and a national annual conference. It produces guidelines for practice, for example Male Catheterization, SupraPubic Catheterization, The Role of the Continence Advisor, Digital Rectal Examination and Manual Removal of Faeces. Videos (commonly sponsored by commercial organizations) are available for instructing nurses in various aspects of care of the incontinent patient.

The current RCN Adviser for the Continence Care Forum is Sue Thomas (Tel: 020 7647 3743 or Email: sue.thomas@rcn.org.uk). The Forum is for members concerned with continence care in any setting to share information and benefit from research.

Continence Foundation, 307 Hatton Square, 16 Baldwins Gardens, London EC1N 7RJ (Tel: 020 7831 9831)

The Continence Foundation provides information and education to professionals and the public. It acts as an umbrella body for the other continence-related organizations in the UK and works closely with relevant groups worldwide. The organization's activities include a national confidential Helpline (*Local call*: 0845 345 0165) which offers counselling and practical advice to incontinent people and their carers; national databases of continence services, continence products and educational resources; publications for public and professionals on prevention and treatment of incontinence; and campaigns on continence issues. The Continence Foundation works closely with the Department of Health and plays a lead role in the planning of Continence Awareness Days. The Helpline is staffed by nurses and is open Monday–Friday 9.30 am to 4.30 pm.

Enuresis Treatment Information Service, 38 Woodstock Road East, Begbrooke, Oxford OX5 1RG (Tel: 01865 841 420)

Provides a helpline and postal information service for children and young adults with bedwetting problems.

ERIC: Enuresis Resource and Information Centre, 34 Old School House, Britannia Road, Kingswood, Bristol BS15 8DB (Tel: 0117 960 3060; Fax: 0117 960 0401). Email: info@eric.org.uk. Website: www.eric.org.uk

ERIC is a national charity that provides information, advice and support on bedwetting, constipation and childhood soiling for children, parents, young adults and professionals. Its activities include a magazine 'ERIC Says', which gives both children and parents an opportunity to share experiences and keep up to date with current treatments; a telephone and postal advice and counselling service; and a pen-pal scheme for children, parents and young people. It has a range of publications for professionals and the public, and sells enuresis alarms and bed protection and literature by mail order. As the first organization worldwide to set up such a resource, ERIC is currently developing its activities in other countries.

Incontact (National Action on Incontinence), Incontact, Freepost Lon 12119, London SE1 1BT (Tel: 020 7717 1225). Website: www.incontact. demon.co.uk

Incontact is a consumer-led organization for people with bladder and bowel problems, and their carers. It offers information and support, puts people in touch with each other and their local continence services, and campaigns for improved services. Its activities include a quarterly newsletter 'Incontact', pen-pals for people wishing to share similar problems, and opportunities for people to test products. It holds a database of members who are willing to share their experiences and views with groups interested in continence issues. Membership is open to all people with an interest in continence issues.

International Continence Society, ICS Office, Southmead Hospital, Bristol BS10 5NB (Tel: 0117 950 3510; Fax: 0117 950 3469). Email: Vicky@ icsoffice.org. Website: www.icsoffice.org

The International Continence Society includes clinicians and other multidisciplinary members representing most countries worldwide. An international research conference is held each autumn. A major achievement of the ICS is the standardization of terminology and techniques in the treatment of incontinence. The International Continence Society, UK, was set up in 1994 to enable professionals in the UK to participate in research and developments in continence.

A 2-day meeting is held annually in the Spring. Abstracts from the international research conference can be accessed on the Internet at www.continent.org/publications.

PromoCon, Disabled Living, 4 St Chad's Street, Cheetham, Manchester M8 8QA (Telephone Helpline 0161 834 2001)

PromoCon is a joint national initiative between the Continence Foundation and the Disabled Living Centres Council which is led by Continence 2001 Disabled Living in Manchester. It provides an information centre and standing exhibition for continence products, situated in Manchester, and nationwide promotes information on continence services and products available for people with disabilities. It provides education to consumer groups and anyone involved in the care of people with incontinence. This group trials new products and makes recommendations. It works closely with some manufacturers to provide a nationwide confidential delivery of products to the door. A choice of products is available which includes washable and disposable pads and a system for disposing of used pads.

ORGANIZATIONS PROVIDING SUPPORT FOR PEOPLE WITH CONDITIONS THAT MAY CONTRIBUTE TO PROBLEMS OF INCONTINENCE

Age Concern England, Astral House, 1268 London Road, London SW16 4ER (Tel: 020 8679 8000)

Alzheimer's Disease Society, Gordon House, 10 Greencoat Place, London SW1P 1PH (Tel: 020 7306 0606)

Association to Aid the Sexual and Personal Relationships of People with a Disability (SPOD), 286 Camden Rd, London N7 0BJ (Tel: 020 7607 8851)

Association for Spina Bifida and Hydrocephalus, ASBAH House, 42 Park Road, Peterborough PE1 2UQ (Tel: 01733 555 988)

British Diabetic Association, 10 Queen Anne Street, London W1M 0BD (Tel: 020 7323 1531)

Digestive Disorders Foundation, 3 St Andrew's Place, London NW1 4LB (Tel: 020 7486 0341; Fax: 020 7224 2012)

This charity exists to fund new research into digestive diseases, help sufferers with practical guidelines on controlling their symptoms, and provides information to the public. The website is http://www/digestivedisorders.org.uk and produces excellent, detailed information led by the medical profession.

Friedreich's Ataxia Group, Copse Edge, Thursley Road, Elstead, Godalming, Surrey GU8 6DJ (Tel: 01252 702 864)

Huntington's Disease Association, 108 Battersea High Street, London SW11 3HP (Tel: 020 7223 7000)

IBS Network (Irritable Bowel Syndrome), Northern General Hospital, Sheffield S5 7AU

The IBS Network is a registered charity set up 10 years ago by S Backhouse and C Dancey to help people with IBS. It is an independent, self-help organization. The homepage website for detailed information is http://homepages.uel.ac.uk/C.P.Dancey/General.html

Interstitial Cystitis support group (icsg), 76 High Street, Stony, Stratford, Bucks MK11 1AH (Tel/Fax: 01908 569169). Website: www.interstitialcystitis.co.uk

An independent group that provides support to people with this debilitating condition. It produces quarterly newsletters and local contact coordinators. The resources include leaflets on diet and various treatments, some of which are self-help remedies as experienced by sufferers.

Multiple Sclerosis Society of Great Britain and Northern Ireland, 25 Effie Road, Fulham, London SW6 1EE (Tel: 020 7736 6267)

National Advisory Service for Parents of Children with a Stoma (and incontinence) (ASPCS), 51 Anderson Drive, Darvel, Ayrshire KA17 0DE (Tel: 01560 22024)

National Association for Colitis and Crohn's Disease (NACC), 4 Beaumont House, Sutton Road, St Albans, Herts AL1 5HH (Tel: 01727 844296 – Information line)

NACC provides support to people with these common disorders. The organization provides information through newsletters and booklets and offers support to both patients and their families through 'Area Groups'. NACC-in-Contact provides trained, supportive listeners available by telephone and raises money for research. A confidential Helpline is offered between 6.30 pm and 9.00 pm Monday, Tuesday and Wednesday evenings (excluding Bank Holidays) (Tel: 0845 130 3344, charged as a local call).

Parkinson's Disease Association, 22 Upper Woburn Place, London WC1H 0RA (Tel: 020 7383 3513)

Royal Association for Disability and Rehabilitation (RADAR), 12 City Forum, 250 City Road, London EC1V 8AF (Tel: 020 7250 3222)

RADAR offers information about keys for disabled toilet facilities and accommodation that caters for people with a disability and continence problems.

Spinal Injuries Association, 76 St James' Lane, London N10 3DF (Tel: 020 8444 2122)

Stroke Association, CHSA House, Whitecross Street, London EC1Y 8JJ (Tel: 020 7490 7999)

COMMERCIAL COMPANIES INVOLVED IN THE FIELD OF INCONTINENCE PRODUCTS

New products are being developed constantly, and it is impossible to include all companies here. The following list is offered as a guide to sources of some commonly used products, but is neither a comprehensive list of all companies nor of all the products they may sell. Many companies provide information on incontinence with their product literature and a Freefone helpline.

3M Health Care Ltd, 3M House, Morley Street, Loughborough LE11 1EP (Tel: 01509 613274; Fax: 01509 623194)

Produces the no-sting skin barrier, Cavilon, that shields skin from body fluids. Available as a spray or in a barrier cream or 1 ml foam stick for easy application.

Astra Tech Ltd, Stroudwater Business Park, Brunel Way, Stonehouse, Gloucester, GL10 3SX (Tel: 01453 791763; Fax: 01453 791001)

Astra Tech was the first company to produce a self-lubricating Nelaton catheter for intermittent catheterization. It has male, female and paediatric length catheters and there is educational support for nurses taking on the skills of male catheterization. Patient booklets for the self-catheterization technique are available, plus videos on male catheterization and children learning the technique, which also includes Mitrofanoff management, for professionals and patients.

Bard Ltd, Forest House, Brighton Road, Crawley, West Sussex RH11 9BP (Tel: 01293 527888; Fax: 01293 552428). Bard Infoline for incontinence information: 0800 591 783

Bard manufactures Foley catheters including the Hydogel and the prefilled range, plus Uriplan leg and night bags for urinary drainage, sheaths, Nelaton catheters, and Contigen (collagen implants). It also supplies a catheter valve and catheter maintenance solution called Opti Flo.

Beambridge Medical, 46 Merrow Lane, Burpham, Guildford, Surrey GU4 7LQ (Tel: 01483 571928 or 07831 692887)

Manufacturers of appliances including urinals contoured for male or female use which are all on the Drug Tariff. The Bridge uricushion has a removable block to allow insertion of a urinal for chairbound people; suppliers of the Bridge catheter valve.

Bional UK Ltd, Unit 2, 149b Histon Road, Cambridge CB4 3JD (Tel: 01223 319 880; Fax: 01223 319 881). Email: afeather@ bional.demon.co.uk

Suppliers of Inurin and Prostanol which are natural products blended from herbs. They aid the bladder and prostate in staying 'healthy'. These are new products in the UK but are used frequently in Europe. Inurin provides nutritional support to the pelvic floor muscles, thus reducing incontinence, whereas Prostanol helps reduce the enlarged benign prostate. They can be purchased from most health food shops but if used in conjunction with other prescribed medication, a physician should give advice as to whether or not the product can be taken.

B Braun (Medical) Ltd, Brookdale Road, Thorncliffe Park Estate, Chapeltown, Sheffield S35 2PW (Tel: 0114 225 9104; Fax: 0114 225 9111). Website: www.bbraun.com

Manufacturers of catheter maintenance solutions and has nurse advisors to provide education in assessment for use of catheter solutions.

Care-Dri International Ltd, 12A Hill Road, Clevedon, North Somerset BS21 7NZ (Tel: 01275 876713; Fax: 01275 349081)

Providers of a good range of washable bed linen and body-worn pants.

CliniMed Ltd, Cavell House, Knaves Beech Way, Loudwater, High Wycombe, Bucks HP10 9QY (Tel: 01628 850 100; Freefone: 0800 585 125). Website: www.clinimed.co.uk. Now part of B Braun (Medical) Ltd

Instillagel local anaesthetic for male and female catheterization and pH paper for testing urine.

Colgate Medical Ltd, Division of Intavent Orthofix, Burney Court, Cordwallis Park, Maidenhead, Berkshire SL6 7BZ (Tel: 01628 594500; Helpline: 0800 526557; Fax: 01628 789400)

Colgate Medical produces the Femina-3 weighted vaginal cones which are only available by mail order. There is an information helpline number for consumers and professionals.

Coloplast Ltd, Peterborough Business Park, Peterborough, PE2 6FX (Tel: 01733 392000; Fax: 01733 233348)

Coloplast manufactures Conveen Products, Stay Dry pads, a dribble pouch for men, sheaths, leg and night drainage bags, and Easicath self-lubricating Nelaton catheters for intermittent self-catheterization. It has a mail order service for most products and produces educational material for consumers and professionals.

de Smit Medical Ltd, 30 Highfields Close, Stoke Gifford, Bristol BS34 8YB (Tel/Fax: 0117 9697865; Mobile: 07970 696246) Email: sersolutions@easynet.co.uk

Distributor for specialist continence products – electrostimulation, biofeedback, enuresis alarms and other related equipment. Product training and support available on request and in conjunction with National Study Days.

EMS Medical Group Ltd, Unit 3, Stroud Industrial Estate, Stonehouse GL10 2DG (Tel: 01453 791791)

Manufacturer of intermittent catheters and catheter valves, and a meatal dilator for stricture therapy. Also the Martex range of washable products for incontinence; bed protection; pants and washable inserts.

Ferraris Medical Ltd, 4 Harforde Court, John Tate Road, Hertford SG13 7NW (Tel: 01992 526300; Fax: 01992 526320). Website: ferrarismedical.com

Ferraris Medical produces enuretic alarms, both for on the bed or worn on the child's nightclothes. It also produces the electrical stimulator Levator CS200 and Biofeedback U-Control unit for home use. All of these products can be purchased direct from the company, but they also offer a rental scheme and have contracts with a number of primary care trusts. Details from the company on the above number. There are two websites giving information for bedwetting and incontinence as follows: www.bedwetting.co.uk and www.treat-incontinence.com, both of which offer an advisory service for patients and professionals, see also Email: info@ferrarismedical.com.

Genesis Medical Ltd, Linton House, 39–51 Highgate Road, London NW5 1RT (Tel: 020 7284 2824; Fax: 020 7284 2675)

Genesis Medical supplies the Unomax and the Duomax electrical stimulator machines with a selection of anal and vaginal probes for purchasing or for leasing by consumers or professionals. Email: mail@genmed.demon.co.uk

Hartmann Ltd, Unit F, Royle Pennine Trading Estate, Royle Road, Rochdale OL11 3EX (Tel: 01706 9393; Fax: 01706 3997)

Hartmann provides a full range of disposable pads called the Moliform range and has stretch pants for the body-worn pads, and all-in-one adult nappies. It also offers a home delivery service where pads are delivered direct to patients' homes.

Hollister Ltd, Rectory Court, 42 Broad Street, Wokingham RG40 1AB (Tel: 0118 989 5009; Fax: 0118 977 5881). Website: www.hollister.com

Hollister Ltd offers a full range of urine drainage bags and sheaths, Nelaton jelled-catheters in all sizes called InstantCath, faecal collectors and the retracted penis pouch, all of which are on the Drug Tariff.

ISIS Medical Ltd, 19 Upper Dicconson Street, Wigan WN1 2AG (Tel: 01942 238359; Fax: 01942 498491)

Distributes the Neuro 4 trophic stimulators for pelvic floor stimulation with the ultra-lightweight vaginal probe, Femelex, which is suitable for both stimulation and biofeedback.

Jade-Euro Med, Unit 14, Old Church Road Industrial Estate, East Hanningfield, Chelmsford CM3 5B9 (Tel: 01245 400413)

Provides body-worn urinals and Drug Tariff continence products. A community nursing service supports NHS nurses working in the community.

Manfred Sauer GmbH, KG/D KG Business Centre, Kingsfield Way, Northampton NN5 7QS (Tel: 01604 588090; Fax: 01604 588091). Website: www.manfred-sauer.co.uk

A company run by people who actually use products and give advice from personal experience. Known for the Bendi Bag, a urinal designed for people in a wheelchair, but a host of good innovations (not all on Drug Tariff) are available from this small company.

Med.I.Pant Ltd, 7 Blundells Road, Bradville, Milton Keynes MK13 7HA (Tel: 01908 220116; Fax: 01908 220566)

Med.I.Pant provides washable products for bed protection and body wear. The shaped insert pads are worn with cotton drop-front pants; this design assists carers in easy changing of pads and for toileting heavy, dependent persons. The inserts vary in size according to absorbency, but there is also a choice of adult nappies for heavy absorbency. Mail order is available and details can be obtained from the above numbers.

Micromedics M.E.D., 135 Harwell Innovation Centre, 173 Curie Avenue H.I.B.C., Didcot, Oxon OX11 0QG (Tel: 01235 838511; Fax: 01235 862838). Email: sales@micromedics-med.com

Distributors of the NeuroTrac4 stimulator and NeuroTrac ETS (Verity Medical Ltd) for stimulation and biofeedback. The periform vaginal and anuform anal probes are also available. The Femsoft urethral insert is available from Micromedics and training is provided for urethral measuring and insertion. Best known for urodynamic equipment and flow meters.

NEEN Health Care, Old Pharmacy Yard, Church Street, Dereham, Norfolk NR19 1DJ (Tel: 01362 698966; Fax: 01362 698967)

Provides the ELPHA 2000C continence stimulator and Peri-Calm stimulator for unstable bladder, plus the biofeedback home unit PFX-2. The periform vaginal and anuform anal probes are available, plus the new Exercisor for exercising the pelvic floor muscles.

Norgine Ltd, Chaplin House, Widewater Place, Moorhall Road, Harefield, Middlesex UB9 6NS (Tel: 01895 826600)

Specializes in Movicol, the laxative for the treatment of faecal impaction and constipation. Supports nurses educationally and provides good educational leaflets for patients.

Pharmacia Ltd, Davy Avenue, Knowlhill, Milton Keynes MK5 8PH (Tel: 01908 661 101; Fax: 01908 603759). Website: www.pharmacia.co.uk

A research-based pharmaceutical company offering Detrusitol and Detrusitol XL for the treatment of detrusor instability. It supports many educational activities for nurses and doctors and has excellent literature.

Portex Ltd, Portex House, 1–3 High Street, Hythe, Kent CT21 5AB (Tel: 01303 260 551; Fax: 01303 265560). Website: www.portex.com

SIMS produces Nelaton catheters, sheaths, leg and night drainage urinary bags, a catheter valve and an enuresis alarm. It has educational literature for professionals and the patient.

Reckitt Benckiser Healthcare (UK) Ltd, Dansom Lane, Hull HU8 7DS (Freephone: 0500 455 456)

A pharmaceutical company well known for Fybogel and Senokot for the relief of constipation. Also Fybogel Mebeverine for bowel dysfunction including IBS. Gives educational support to professionals and patients.

Rusch UK Ltd, PO Box 138, Turnpike Road, Cressex Industrial Estate, High Wycombe HP12 3NB (Tel: 01494 532761)

Well known for manufacturing Foley catheters, this company also supports educational activities for nurses.

SCA Hygiene Health Care Products, Southfields Road, Dunstable LU6 3EJ (Tel: 01582 677400; Fax: 01582 677502). Website: www.tena.co.uk

SCA Hygiene is known for the Tena range of products which caters for very light urinary incontinence through to heavy incontinence. This company offers training for professionals and carers, provides educational material (i.e. videos and literature), and has led the way in the UK for providing a home delivery service whereby products are delivered direct to a patient's home.

Seton Continence Care, Toft Hall, Toft Road, Knutsford, Cheshire WA16 9PD (Tel: 0161 624 5641)

Merged with Thrackraycare and Simpla Plastics and supplies Foley and Nelaton catheters, sheaths and urine drainage bags. Supports NHS nurses in hospital and in the community.

Shiloh Healthcare Ltd, Park Mill, Royton, Oldham OL2 6PZ (Tel: 0161 624 5641; Fax: 0161 627 0902). Website: www.shiloh.co.uk

The largest British-owned UK manufacturer of washable incontinence products. Also produces the Contisure range of disposable pads. Provides educational literature for patients.

Simpla Plastics, a subsidiary of Seton Healthcare Group plc, Tubiton House, Oldham OL1 3HS (Tel: 0161 652 2222; Fax: 0161 620 5795) or Freepost, Cardiff CF4 1ZZ (Tel: 0222 747000)

Manufacturer of urinary catheters and drainage bags, sheaths, catheter valves and the 'G' strap.

TVM Healthcare Ltd, Resolution Road, Flagstaff 42 Business Park, Ashby de la Zouch LE65 1NZ (Customer Services: 0800 521740; Fax: 01530 565120). Website: www.tvm-healthcare.com

TVM has over 30 years' experience sending prescriptions direct to the door and supplying chemists. All the products on the Drug Tariff for continence, ostomy, wound care and laryngectomy care can be dispensed. A sample service of new products is offered to professionals and patients. A quarterly newsletter gives educational information as well as new products on the Drug Tariff. There is literature for professionals and patients in the four specialties they serve. An advice line for continence and stoma care is available through customer services. A resource centre and clinical facilities are available in Reading for patients and professionals (2 Lundy Lane, Reading RG30 2ZZ, Tel: 0800 389 7711). Continence clinics are held regularly by appointment.

Tyco Healthcare Continence Care, 2 Elmwood, Chineham Business Park, Basingstoke RG24 8WG (Tel: 01256 379555; Fax: 01256 379544)

Suppliers of both washable products (Ganmill Range) and disposable products (Cumfie Range). A home delivery service is also available.

For details of other companies and their products, the ACA (*q.v.*) can assist with enquiries, or contact your local specialist nurse.

USEFUL BOOKS FOR PROFESSIONALS

Andrews G 2001 Women's sexual health, 2nd edn. Baillière Tindall, London

Carper J 1988 The food pharmacy. Simon & Schuster, London

Davis P 1992 Aromatherapy: an A–Z, 2nd edn. C W Daniel, Saffron Walden

Low J, Reed A, Dyson M 2000 Electrotherapy explained, 3rd edn. Butterworth-Heinemann, Oxford

Norton C 1996 Nursing for continence, 2nd edn. Beaconsfield Publishers, Beaconsfield Bucks

Schussler B, Laycock J, Norton P, Stanton S (eds) 1994 Pelvic floor re-education: principles and practice. Springer-Verlag, London

---

USEFUL BOOKS FOR PATIENTS

Asbury N, White H 2001 Don't make me laugh. Northumbria Healthcare NHS Trust, available from the Continence Foundation, London

Bladder and bowel problems. Produced by *In*contact, sponsored by Pharmacia & Upjohn. Available from *In*contact, Freepost LON 12119, London SE1 1BT

Fast Facts series. Covers bladder cancer, colorectal cancer, prostate cancer, urinary incontinence, irritable bowel syndrome. Information www.fastfactsbooks.com published by Health Press, Oxford

Norton C, Kamm M A 1999 Bowel control. Beaconsfield Publishers, Beaconsfield, Bucks

Videos for patients are available from most manufacturers but there is also a series from 'Videos for Patients', 18 Denbigh Close, London W11 2QH, introduced by John Cleese. Topics cover cancer of the prostate, constipation, cystitis, enlarged prostate, irritable bowel syndrome, Crohn's disease and ulcerative colitis

USEFUL WEBSITES (there are many, many more)

www.bmj.com – British Medical Journal (many other journals are accessible on-line – consult your library)

www.bowelcontrol.org.uk – information and practical advice for people who have difficulty controlling their bowels. Also very helpful for professionals. Site is provided by St. Mark's Hospital and Academic Institute, written by Christine Norton

www.doh.gov.uk – access to government reports

www.cast.org/bobby – advice on the most beneficial way to present information to people with special needs

www.continenceworldwide.org – global interaction available about any aspect of continence

www.incontinencenet.org – Incontinence Knowledge Centre and has a urology network

www.i-c-c-s.org – International Children's Continence Society

www.incontinencesupport.org – resource centre for products and continence information for carers

www.InContiNet.com – Biofeedback Foundation of Europe

www.medscape.com – abstracts available

www.medscape – includes resource centre/prostate cancer

www.medline.com – access to research publications in health and medical sciences

www.pelvicfloor.com – information on the female pelvic floor, treatment and even a PowerPoint presentation (American)

www.sapien.net/overactivebladder – American information on the overactive bladder

www.surgerydoor.com – health news from Dr Mark Porter often has continence-related subjects

www.wocn.org – the wound, ostomy and continence nursing website

www.31 – provides guidance on accessing information for people with visual impairment

Samples of care pathway forms

Not all information can be provided here, e.g. fluid matrix chart, fibre scoring chart, obstruction checklist, etc. and the reader must use the Reference lists in the relevant chapters to obtain full care pathway forms.

CONTINENCE ASSESSMENT (Stage 1)

FULL NAME:		DATE OF BIRTH:
ADDRESS:		POST CODE:
		TEL:
GP:	PRACTICE:	NHS number:
ASSESSOR:	Line manager:	Date :

Residence		Own home	
Residential	Social services	Private nursing	Supported living

Referral source:

GP   D/N   Consultant   Self   Other

TICK APPROPRIATE BOX:		Other (state)	
Urological	Gynaecological	Neurological	Cardiovascular
Learning disability	Mental health/EMI	Physical disability	Neoplasm

How has your bladder problem affected your life:

How much does your bladder problem bother you? *(circle the choice)*

a lot   ***moderately***   *a little*   ***not at all***

STANDARD STATEMENT	✓	ONLY INITIAL IF VARIANCE FROM STANDARD STATEMENT		
		VARIANCE FROM STANDARD STATEMENT AND REASON	**Initial**	**Date**
Drinks_____cups/mugs of fluid per 24 hours Weighs_____ stones/kgs				
If patient drinks volumes outside parameters of fluid matrix, advise them to drink appropriate amount				
Urinalysis performed:				
GLUCOSE				
KETONE				
S. GRAVITY				
BLOOD				
pH				
PROTEIN				
NITRITE				
LEUCOCYTES				
If leucocytes/nitrite, or symptoms of UTI present, take MSU, refer to GP and discontinue this assessment until treated				
If patient has problems with their bowels, give appropriate advice and literature and arrange onward referral if necessary				

Patient name: _____ **DOB:** _____

STANDARD STATEMENT	✓	VARIANCE FROM STANDARD STATEMENT AND REASON	Initial	Date
Record current medication				
If patient is taking medication on list provided, consider referral to GP for review				
If patient has mobility, dexterity or environmental problems, record any action taken				
If patient has signs of cognitive dysfunction give appropriate literature to patient/carer				
Symptom profile completed by patient				
Is the patient seeing anyone else regarding this problem?				
Patient commenced on appropriate care pathway as indicated from symptom profile				

This patient is unable to commence on a care pathway because:

NB: If no care pathway commenced, return this assessment
with Product Request Form if appropriate to:

CONTINENCE ASSESSMENT (Stage 2)

NAME: _____   DOB: _____   M/F

PAST MEDICAL HISTORY

A) Medical history:

Diabetes	☐	Multiple sclerosis	☐
CVA	☐	Spinal injury	☐
Back pain	☐	Parkinson's	☐

B) Surgical history:

Cystoscopy	☐	Urethral dilatation	☐
Hysterectomy	☐	TUR	☐
Pelvic floor repair	☐	Other	☐

C) Obstetric history:

Number of pregnancies	☐
Forceps	☐
Breech	☐
Other	☐

Large baby: Over 4 kgs (8.5 lbs)   Yes ☐   No ☐

COMPLETE JOURNAL   Yes ☐   No ☐   Reason if not _____

Record current containment if any:

Type of incontinence

Stress	☐	Urge	☐	Stress/urge	☐
Overflow	☐	Reflex	☐	Faecal	☐

Care pathway for stress incontinence

Teach pelvic floor exercises	☐	Give dietary advice	☐	Advise on washable products	☐
Vaginal examination and record result (if appropriate)	☐	Refer to GP re prolapse	☐	Consider oestrogens	☐

Care pathway for urge incontinence

Complete journal	☐	Teach bladder retraining	☐	Check environment	☐
Advise on washable products	☐	Consider anticholinergics	☐		
If neurological dysfunction check for residual urine	☐				

Care pathway for overflow/dribbling incontinence

Check for residual urine	☐	Record flow rate	☐
Check voiding technique	☐	Advise on washable products	☐
Refer to urologist	☐	Consider appliance/sheath	☐
Advise on disposable products	☐	Reassess bowel care	☐

Care pathway for reflex incontinence

Completely wet/dry chart	☐	Consider individual toileting plan	☐
Prompt voiding	☐	Consider urinary catheter	☐
Consider sheath/appliance	☐	Advise on disposable products	☐

Care pathway for faecal incontinence

Complete bowel diary	☐	Complete food diary	☐
Review medication	☐	Teach anal sphincter exercises	☐
Teach 'brace and bulge'	☐	Supply incontinence roll	☐

SUMMARY

Pelvic floor exercises	☐	Refer to Continence Advisor	☐	Biofeedback	☐
Bladder retraining	☐	Medication	☐	Trophic stimulation	☐
Washable products	☐	Catheter	☐	Joint clinic	☐
Disposable products	☐	Appliance	☐	Alarm	☐
Physiotherapist	☐	Intermittent catheter	☐	Training programme	☐
Consultant	☐	Other	☐		

DISCHARGE

Appliance	☐	Improved/cure	☐	Physiotherapist	☐
Primary health care	☐	No further treatment	☐	Surgical intervention	☐
Joint clinic	☐	Intermittent self-catheterization	☐	Trophic stimulation	☐
Deceased	☐	No follow-up/DNA	☐	Other	☐

SUMMARY: **DATE:** _____

_____

_____

_____

_____

PAEDIATRIC DAYTIME WETTING ASSESSMENT CARE PATHWAY (>5 years)

FULL NAME:		DATE OF BIRTH:
ADDRESS:		POST CODE:
		TEL:
GP:	ASSESSOR:	TELEPHONE:
DATE OF REFERRAL:	DATE OF ASSESSMENT:	REFERRED BY:

PAST MEDICAL HISTORY (TICK APPROPRIATE BOX):		Other (state)	
Urological	Urinary tract infections	Neurological	
Learning disability	Physical disability	Congenital	

Has the child had any previous surgery?   Yes   No
If yes indicate nature of surgery

How has the bladder problem affected your child's life (e.g. school)?:

How much does the bladder problem bother your child? *(circle the choice)*

a lot   *moderately*   *a little*   *not at all*

		ONLY INITIAL IF VARIANCE FROM STANDARD STATEMENT		
STANDARD STATEMENT	✓	**VARIANCE FROM STANDARD STATEMENT AND REASON/COMMENTS**	**Initial**	**Date**
Drinks _____ cups/mugs of fluid per 24 hours To have minimum of 6–8				
If patient drinks volumes outside of this amount advise them to drink appropriate amount				
Urinalysis performed:				
GLUCOSE				
KETONE				
S. GRAVITY				
BLOOD				
pH				
PROTEIN				
NITRITE				
LEUCOCYTES				

STANDARD STATEMENT	✓	VARIANCE FROM STANDARD STATEMENT AND REASON/COMMENTS	Initial	Date
If leucocytes/nitrite, or symptoms of UTI present, take MSU, refer to GP and discontinue this assessment until treated				
If child has bowel problems, give family appropriate advice. Refer to constipation guidelines, exclude impaction if indicated				
If child has mobility, dexterity or environmental problems, record any action taken				
If child has signs of cognitive dysfunction (learning disabilities) use 'Continence skills rating chart' to help plan programme				
Symptom profile completed by child and carer				
Child commenced on appropriate numbered care pathway as indicated from symptom profile				
If detrusor instability is suspected, discuss with GP referral of child for pre/postmicturition ultrasound scan of bladder and upper urinary tracts, prior to commencing on pathway				

This child is unable to commence on a care pathway because:

NB: If no care pathway commenced, contact Paediatric Continence Advisor for further advice

TO BE COMPLETED BY ALL STAFF USING THE PATHWAY

SIGN TO CONFIRM THAT YOU HAVE MET ALL STANDARDS OR RECORDED VARIANCES

FULL NAME	DESIGNATION	INITIALS	SIGN	DATE

PAEDIATRIC CONSTIPATION/SOILING ASSESSMENT CARE PATHWAY

FULL NAME:	DATE OF BIRTH:
ADDRESS:	POST CODE:
	TEL:

GP:	ASSESSOR:	TELEPHONE:
DATE OF REFERRAL:	DATE OF ASSESSMENT:	REFERRED BY:

PAST MEDICAL HISTORY (TICK APPROPRIATE BOX):		Other (state)	
Learning disability	Physical disability	Congenital abnormality	Neurological

Primary constipation/soiling problem? (bowel control never really achieved)   Yes   No

Secondary soiling   Y/N   Age child first clean .... Age child began soiling ....
How has the soiling problem affected your child's life (e.g. school)?

STANDARD STATEMENT	✓	ONLY INITIAL IF VARIANCE FROM STANDARD STATEMENT		
		VARIANCE FROM STANDARD STATEMENT AND REASON/COMMENTS	Initial	Date
If child has signs and symptoms of acute obstruction (e.g. vomiting, severe abdominal pain) stop pathway and refer to doctor immediately				
Drinks _____ cups/mugs of fluid per 24 hours To have minimum of 6–8				
If child drinks volumes outside of this amount (including >1 pint/ 568 ml of milk) advice them to drink appropriate amount				
If child has problems with daytime symptoms/wetting, give family appropriate advice. Refer to daytime wetting guidelines				
If child has problems with nighttime wetting, give family appropriate advice. Refer to nighttime wetting guidelines				

STANDARD STATEMENT	✓	VARIANCE FROM STANDARD STATEMENT AND REASON/COMMENTS	Initial	Date
Child has recorded baseline of soiling/bowels opened for 1–2 weeks				
Use fibre scoring chart to establish intake levels. If <5 years give information sheet and advice on increasing fibre in diet				
Establish constipation/soiling using signs and symptom profile and record findings				
If encopresis is suspected liaise with CMHS regarding appropriate interventions				
If child has signs of cognitive dysfunction use 'Continence skills rating chart' to help plan programme				
If child has mobility/physical problems consider discussing abdominal massage with physiotherapist				
Liaise with child's GP regarding appropriate treatment intervention (using drug treatment guidance chart)				
Child commenced on appropriate care pathway, using algorithm – obtaining child/carer's consent to any liaison/treatment/procedures				
Establish follow-up procedure				

TO BE COMPLETED BY ALL STAFF USING THE PATHWAY

SIGN TO CONFIRM THAT YOU HAVE MET ALL STANDARDS OR RECORDED VARIANCES

FULL NAME	DESIGNATION	INITIALS	SIGN	DATE

BOWEL CARE PATHWAY ASSESSMENT

FULL NAME:		DATE OF BIRTH:
ADDRESS:		POST CODE:
		TEL:
GP:	PRACTICE:	CASELOAD HOLDER:
ASSESSOR:	DESIGNATION:	TELEPHONE:

What has been the effect on your life of your bowel problem?

How much does it bother you? *(tick your choice)*

a lot ☐   **moderately** ☐   **a little** ☐   **not at all** ☐

What is your normal bowel habit?

How do you maintain this?

STANDARD STATEMENT	✓	INITIAL ONLY IF VARIANCE FROM STANDARD STATEMENT		
		VARIANCE FROM STANDARD STATEMENT AND REASON/COMMENTS	Initial	Date
If patient has any signs of undiagnosed bleeding, or black tarry stool and is not taking ferrous sulphate, stop pathway and refer to doctor immediately				
Using obstruction checklist observe patient for any signs of obstruction. If present, stop pathway and refer to doctor immediately				
Patient drinks _____ amount of fluid per day				

| STANDARD STATEMENT | ✓ | INITIAL ONLY IF VARIANCE FROM STANDARD STATEMENT | | |
		VARIANCE FROM STANDARD STATEMENT AND REASON/COMMENTS	Initial	Date
If patient drinks volumes outside parameters of fluid matrix, advise them to drink appropriate amount				
If patient is taking medication from the list provided consider review with GP				
Establish constipation using signs and symptoms chart and record findings				
Report any abnormal changes in bowel habit				
If faecal incontinent use algorithm				
Use fibre scoring chart to establish fibre levels. If 12 or less give information sheet and advice on increasing fibre in diet				
If patient unable or unwilling to comply, consider fibre supplements				
If patient is in discomfort consider abdominal massage technique				
Administer and record appropriate treatment. A doctor's opinion may be sought				
Obtain patient's consent to any invasive procedure				
Establish follow-up procedure				

TO BE COMPLETED BY ALL STAFF USING THE PATHWAY

SIGN TO CONFIRM THAT YOU HAVE MET ALL STANDARDS OR RECORDED VARIANCES

FULL NAME	DESIGNATION	INITIALS	SIGN	DATE